Congenital Heart Disease

Congenital Heart Disease

Molecular Genetics, Principles of Diagnosis and Treatment

Editors

Maximilian Muenke Bethesda, Md.
Paul S. Kruszka Bethesda, Md.
Craig A. Sable Washington, D.C.
John W. Belmont Houston, Tex.

93 Figures, 49 in color and 43 tables, 2015

KARGER Basel · Freiburg · Paris · London · New York · Chennai · New Delhi · Bangkok · Beijing · Shanghai · Tokyo · Kuala Lumpur · Singapore · Sydney

Maximilian Muenke
Medical Genetics Branch
National Human Genome Research Institute
National Institutes of Health
Building 35
35 Convent Drive
Bethesda, MD 20892-3717 (USA)

Paul S. Kruszka
Medical Genetics Branch
National Human Genome Research Institute
National Institutes of Health
Building 35
35 Convent Drive
Bethesda, MD 20892-3717 (USA)

Craig A. Sable
Division of Cardiology
Children's National Health System
111 Michigan Avenue, NW
Washington, DC 20010 (USA)

John W. Belmont
Baylor College of Medicine
Department of Molecular and Human Genetics
1100 Bates, Room 8066
Houston, TX 77030 (USA)

Library of Congress Cataloging-in-Publication Data

Congenital heart disease (Muenke)
Congenital heart disease : molecular genetics, principles of diagnosis and treatment / editors, Maximilian Muenke, Paul S. Kruszka, Craig A. Sable, John W. Belmont.
p. ; cm.
Includes bibliographical references and index.
ISBN 978-3-318-03003-7 (hard cover : alk. paper) -- ISBN 978-3-318-03004-4 (eISBN)
I. Muenke, Maximilian, editor. II. Kruszka, Paul S., editor. III. Sable, Craig A., editor. IV. Belmont, John W., editor. V. Title.
[DNLM: 1. Heart Defects, Congenital. WG 220]
RC687
616.1'2043--dc23
2015013896

www.karger.com
Printed in Germany on acid-free and non-aging paper (ISO 9706) by Kraft Druck, Ettlingen
ISBN 978–3–318–03003–7
e-ISBN 978–3–318–03004–4

KARGER 125 YEARS

Contents

6 Evaluation

7 Treatment

Preface

Congenital heart defects are among the most common birth defects affecting millions of families in all populations around the world. Two factors have had a tremendous impact on our understanding of congenital heart diseases: many details of the molecular mechanisms governing normal cardiac and vascular development have been uncovered using model organisms, and, fortuitously, this increased knowledge of molecular embryology has come at a time when the ability to analyze human genetic abnormalities has expanded exponentially. Together these disciplines are providing unprecedented insights into the causes of cardiac malformations.

Cardiology, as discrete discipline in pediatric medicine, has also undergone transformative changes in this same era. New methods for imaging and physiological testing have emerged. These methods help to increase our understanding of cardiac growth in the fetal period and begin to pave the way for earlier and more effective interventions. Less invasive management of septal defects and cardiac valve anomalies have become routine practice. Cardiovascular surgery has become safer and more effective for congenital heart diseases. The dramatic improvements in mortality and long-term morbidity rates in this relatively young field are impressive.

Yet, we have to admit that there is still a huge poorly understood terrain ahead of us. Despite the progress in defining the contributions of chromosomal, genomic and single gene disorders to congenital heart diseases, the causes of these defects in most patients remain unknown. The relative contributions of not yet identified genes, gene variations and teratogens are still poorly understood. The likely interactions of individual genetic variation with nutritional factors, maternal metabolic factors, environmental exposures and commonly used medications are only understood abstractly. Whether and how these factors contribute and how they affect individual patients is still speculative. Much more research will be required to advance our understanding of these apparently complex causal mechanisms.

We felt an international team of authors would best represent the state of the art in this very large and diverse field; these authors chosen encompass all the disciplines necessary to unravel questions of etiology and treatments of congenital heart disease. Hence, this is a book intended for students, trainees and colleagues from a wide variety of disciplines. We hope this volume may prove useful irrespective of whether a researcher is devoted to molecular embryology or skilled at mending a mitral valve.

The editors would like to thank all the authors who graciously contributed to this volume and who took the time to share their expertise and explain their most important discoveries to a wide audience. We also would like to extend our deepest gratitude to all the patients and families whom we have met over the course of our careers for their time, generosity and compassionate spirits.

Maximilian Muenke, Bethesda, Md.
Paul S. Kruszka, Bethesda, Md.
Craig A. Sable, Washington, D.C.
John W. Belmont, Houston, Tex.
April 2015

Foreword

The Editors – Max Muenke, Paul Kruszka, Craig A. Sable, and John W. Belmont – have done a remarkable job assembling international leaders in their respective fields and have created a landmark congenital heart disease volume. After almost 60 years of involvement in pediatric cardiology, I have had the pleasure of watching the field grow into what it is today: an advanced and highly complex discipline. We can make specific genetic diagnoses, identify heritable syndromes, provide genetic counseling, and repair complex heart malformations that would have been previously unimaginable.

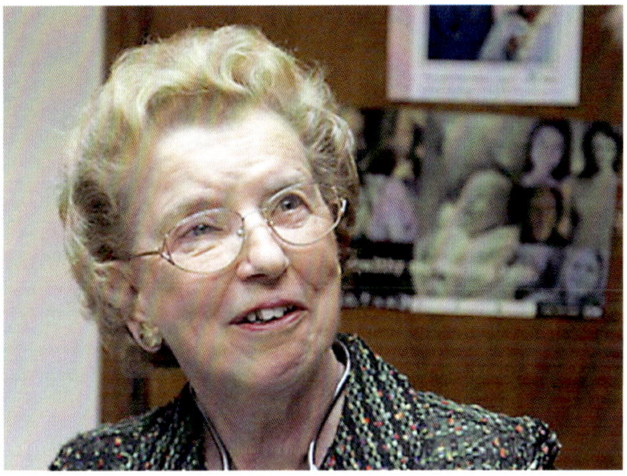

Jacqueline A. Noonan.

Pediatric cardiology began with collections of observations on patients that were made into descriptive studies of congenital heart disease. When I finished my training in the late 1950s, much was known about congenital heart disease associated with Down syndrome, but little was known about other syndromes and noncardiac anomalies associated with congenital heart disease. After starting my first attending physician position at the University of Iowa, I began making 3 × 5 note cards for each patient I saw. After over 800 note cards, I began noticing trends in clinically similar patients. After reporting 9 patients with similar facies and valvular pulmonary stenosis at the Midwest Society for Pediatric Research in 1962 [1], I was able to characterize a syndrome that Dr. Victor McKusick would eventually name 'Noonan syndrome'. This was the beginning of my interest in cardiovascular genetics. I am still in contact with some of these patients that I have diagnosed and taken care of over the last 5 decades and continue to meet new patients as well. Recently, while at a conference in Sweden, I met a 66-year-old gentleman who had self-diagnosed himself by performing an internet search of his physical findings and he was later found to have a mutation in *PTPN11*. I am happy to see that many children with congenital heart disease are becoming productive adults, and I am excited that long-term follow-up studies and research in affected adults are progressing [2].

Now, along with important clinical examination techniques developed in the past, we have a new tool in the form of genomic technology. Over the last 20 years, there has been an explosion in the discovery of genes involved in normal cardiac development as well as the genetic mutations that cause cardiac malformations. Animal models and transgenic experiments have given us a better understanding of human cardiac disease, and the completion of the Human Genome Project, cataloguing our entire genetic code, has allowed for further expansion of our knowledge of cardiac genetics.

This volume begins with a historical overview of congenital cardiovascular anomalies and ends with the potential of stem cells and tissue engineering. In between these chapters are explanations of cardiac embryogenesis, epidemiology of congenital heart diseases, descriptions of syndromes associated with cardiovascular anomalies, single-gene disorders, cardiac imaging, surgical and interventional therapies, and ethical considerations. This thorough account of congenital heart diseases is an invaluable reference and learning tool for pediatric cardiologists, geneticists, and primary care providers.

Even with these new technologies at hand, there is much more to learn. As we are now well into the 21st century, much of the genetic basis of cardiac malformations is still unknown. The editors of this book have assembled the most up-to-date information from many of the leaders in the fields of genetics and both pediatric and adult cardiology. I commend the authors and researchers in this field and look forward to the creative energy that will continue to develop our knowledge of cardiac malformations and benefit both affected children and adults.

Jacqueline A. Noonan, Lexington, Ky.
April 2015

References

1 Noonan JA, Ehmke DA: Associated noncardiac malformation in children with congenital heart disease. Midwest Society for Pediatric Research. Cincinnati, Ohio, Oct. 25 and 26, 1962. J Pediatr 1963;63:468–469.

2 Colquitt JL, Noonan JA: Cardiac findings in Noonan syndrome on long-term follow-up. Congenit Heart Dis 2014;9:144–150.

Dr. Jacqueline A. Noonan
Kentucky Children's Heart Center
Division of Pediatric Cardiology, University of Kentucky
Lexington, KY 40536 (USA)
E-Mail jnoonan@uky.edu

1 Overview

Muenke M, Kruszka PS, Sable CA, Belmont JW (eds): Congenital Heart Disease: Molecular Genetics, Principles of Diagnosis and Treatment. Basel, Karger, 2015, pp 2–10
DOI: 10.1159/000375201

Congenital Cardiovascular Anomalies: A Historical Overview

James H. Moller

Division of Pediatric Cardiology, Department of Pediatrics, University of Minnesota, Minneapolis, Minn., USA

Abstract

Three hundred and fifty years of the history of congenital cardiovascular anomalies are reviewed here. The anatomy of individual anomalies was described in the early years of medical history. By the late 19th century sufficient numbers of patients and specimens had been studied to begin description of the pathophysiology of some conditions. Additionally, during this time, specific murmurs were described, which allowed their clinical identification. Despite these advances, little specific treatment was available for affected children and adults until 1938. In that year, the first cardiac operation was performed when a patent ductus arteriosus was ligated. This was followed 6 years later by two other types of extracardiac operations. The pace quickened in the 1950s as cardiac catheterization was developed for diagnosis and methods to perform open heart operations were elaborated. Since 1954, the variety of operations has grown and become available for a wider range of conditions. Since the 1980s, the various methods to treat particular cardiac anomalies by transcatheter means have expanded and become an important form of therapy. Diagnosis and treatment are now becoming more available throughout the world, improving the outlook for all patients with congenital heart disease.

Since the late 17th century, anatomists reported various malformations of the heart and blood vessels they discovered during dissection. By the mid- to late 19th century, clinicopathologic correlations of malformations were being made. Reports described characteristic murmurs of specific conditions. While patients with congenital heart disease were of interest to physicians, treatment was primarily supportive until 1938, when the first ligation of a patent ductus arteriosus (PDA) was performed. This event opened the era of treatment of cardiac malformations, which affect 1% of children. Treatment methods have dominated the subsequent 75 years. In approaching the history of congenital heart disease, I have chosen to organize the progress in relation to the individuals who made major contri-

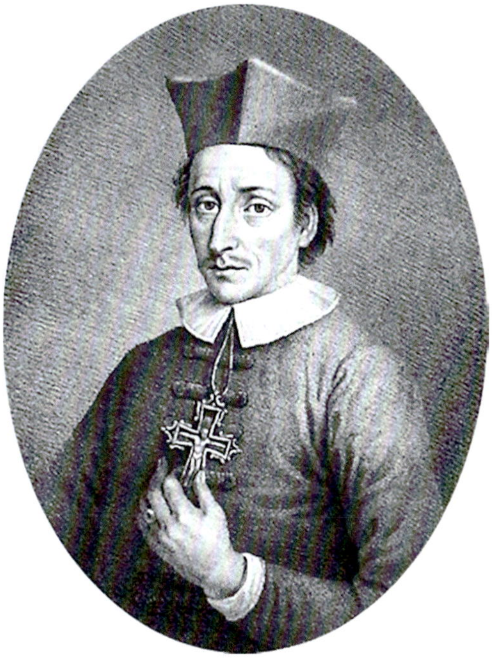

Fig. 1. Nicolas Steno: Danish catholic bishop and scientist. http://upload.wikimedia.org/wikipedia/commons/c/cb/Niels_stensen.png.

butions, realizing that many individuals were involved in developing concepts, performing studies and managing patients. Therefore, the sections which follow will focus on those who made major advancements which have benefitted children in many countries.

Early Descriptions of Anomalies

Nicolas Steno (also known as Niels Stensen; 1636–1686) was a Danish physician and anatomist (fig. 1) who observed and described tetralogy of Fallot for the first time [1]. In a specimen from a fetus he found that the pulmonary artery was much narrower than the aorta. On opening the right ventricle, he passed a probe directly into the aorta and identified a ventricular septal communication. He did not understand why blood did not enter the pulmonary artery but went directly into the aorta. Other instances of tetralogy of Fallot were reported later by Hunter [2], Farre [3] and Baillie [4].

During this early period, Giovanni Battista Morgagani (1682–1771) described coarctation of the aorta in 1760 and James Hope (1801–1841) [5] discussed pulmonary stenosis and its auscultatory findings. In 1866, Wilhelm Ebstein (1836–1912) described for the first time the anomaly which bears his name [6]. Many of these early reports are combined in Maude Abbott's (1869–1940) [7] book, *Atlas of Congenital Heart Disease.*

Correlating Anatomic and Clinical Features

In the late 19th century, the anatomic and clinical features of several important conditions were outlined. One report was by Étienne-Louis Arthur Fallot (1850–1911) [8], for whom little biographic information is available. In a paper, he described his studies with 'maladie bleue' (morbus caeruleus), now called cyanotic congenital heart disease. At the time he wrote, it was virtually impossible to make a correct anatomic diagnosis of cyanotic patients. He indicated that one condition, however, was present in 74% of these patients. This malformation had four components: (1) stenosis of the pulmonary artery, (2) interventricular communication, (3) deviation of the aorta to the right, and (4) right-ventricular hypertrophy. Fallot acknowledged that a number of authors had described various malformations associated with cyanosis. His contribution was that the combination of these four anatomic features accounted for many instances. For his observations, we have called the combination tetralogy of Fallot.

It was a British cardiologist, Paul Wood (1907–1962) [9], who initially gave the name Eisenmenger syndrome to a condition with cyanosis associated with a ventricular septal defect (VSD) but without pulmonary stenosis. Following Victor Eisenmenger's (1864–1932) report, the right-to-left shunt was attributed by many physicians to result from displacement of the aorta to the right so it overrode the VSD [10]. In his paper, however, Eisenmenger expressed that the displacement was the result not the cause of the shunt direction. He described 'endarteric plugs in the pulmonary artery, particularly its branches, without such signs in the aorta, suggesting long-standing stress on the pulmonary artery'. Thus, the cyanosis of such patients was from elevated pulmonary vascular resistance. In his 1957 Connor Lecture of the American Heart Association, Jesse Edwards [11] presented a classification of histologic features of pulmonary vascular disease. In this lecture, he stressed the misconception about the source of cyanosis being the apparent overriding of the aorta rather than the presence of pulmonary vascular disease.

As a pediatrician, Henri Louis Roger (1809–1891) [12] had great interest in auscultation. In his paper presented to the French Academy of Medicine in 1861, he described that while performing an autopsy on a 12-year-old boy, he found a defect in the ventricular septum. Further, he indicated that in listening to thousands of children over 40 years he had identified a prominent murmur associated with a thrill but without symptoms or other physical findings. He reasoned that the murmur was associated with a VSD. When he presented his paper, Roger did not have anatomic evidence of the anomaly in any of his patients. Subsequently, he reported a 26-month-old child who died of a pulmonary 'mishap' who had had the characteristic murmur. The autopsy revealed a VSD [12]. Through the years, the murmur has been called a Roger murmur and a small VSD termed a Roger defect or maladie du Roger.

In his book, George Frederic Still (1868–1941) [13] wrote about a murmur, subsequently called Still's murmur. 'It is usually just below the level of the nipple and half way between the left margin of the sternum and the vertical nipple line; it is not heard in the axilla nor behind, it is systolic and is often so small that only a careful observer would detect it; moreover it is variable in audibility; its characteristic is a twangy sound very like that made by twanging a piece of tense string'. This easily recognized murmur is the most common functional or innocent murmur.

Diagnostic Procedures

More precise identification of cardiac anomalies awaited the development of methods to visualize the heart and to make measurements of pressure and oxygen content within cardiac chambers. Cardiac catheterization and angiography were initially performed in the 1920s and 1930s in several countries. As a surgical intern in Germany, Werner Forssmann (1904–1979) [14] was concerned about the delivery of medications from a peripheral vein to patients in shock. He felt that it would be preferable if the medication could be given directly into the heart. With the aid of a nurse, he assembled the necessary equipment, including a catheter, to perform the first such procedure. Through an incision in his own antecubital fossa, he inserted a catheter into the median basilic vein. He walked to the radiology department and obtained an X-ray which verified that the catheter tip was indeed in the heart. Thus, he had demonstrated that cardiac catheterization of the right side of the heart was possible without ill effects.

In 1956, Forssmann, Cournand and Richards received the Nobel Prize in Medicine for the development of cardiac catheterization. On receiving word of this honor, Forssmann said, 'I felt like the parish priest who has been asked to become the Pope'. In the 1940s, André Frédéric Cournand (1895–1998) and Dickinson Richards (1895–1973), aware of Forssmann's work, used cardiac catheterization to study cardiopulmonary physiology. They were the first to measure the cardiac output by the Fick method (cardiac output equals oxygen consumption divided by arteriovenous oxygen difference) and carried out some of the first hemodynamic studies of children with cardiac malformations [15].

In Cuba, as early as 1931, Agustin Castellanos (1902–2000) et al. [16] were studying peripheral venous angiography and continued this work for a number of years. In 1937, they described the technique and the findings in pulmonary stenosis, PDA with pulmonary hypertension, and transposition of the great arteries. In 1938, they performed the first retrograde aortography to diagnose PDA. These were the initial attempts to visualize cardiac anomalies in children.

Extracardiac Operations

The first operations for cardiac anomalies were performed in 1938 and 1944. The three procedures were extracardiac and did not involve the heart itself.

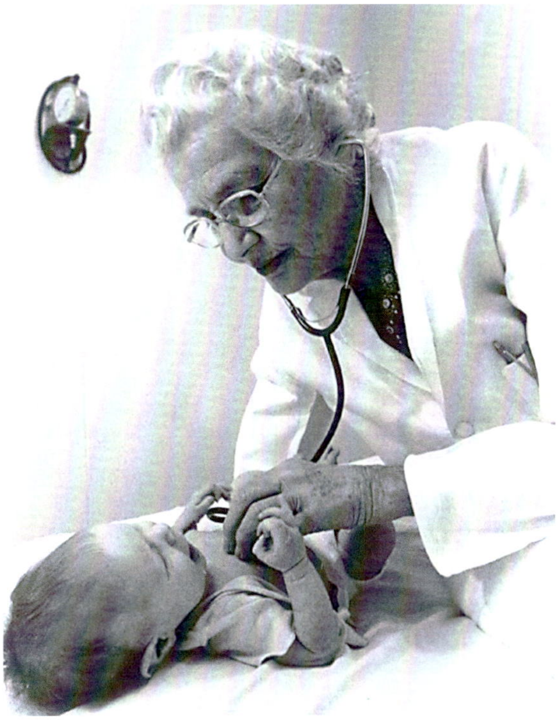

Fig. 2. Helen Taussig with a small patient in 1981. http://www.medicalarchives.jhmi.edu/tausbio.htm.

The first was for a PDA. Robert Gross (1905–1988) commented that a PDA had two major consequences. One was related to the size of the shunt, which could lead to cardiac decompensation, and the other was bacterial endocarditis, which was fatal. At that time, systemic arteriovenous fistulae had been successfully ligated with improvement in cardiac condition, and he reasoned that a PDA was a unique form of fistula. In 1938, he operated upon a 7 year old girl with a large PDA (7–8 mm in diameter) through the left chest [17]. A thrill was palpated over the heart and strongest over the pulmonary artery. When a ligature was placed around the PDA and it occluded the blood pressure, the diastolic pressure rose. Since there were no circulatory changes, it was ligated and the chest closed. She did well postoperatively and she was kept in hospital for 13 days because of the interest in her case.

The second, the Blalock-Taussig (BT) shunt [18], followed in 1944. Helen Taussig (1898–1986; fig. 2) had noted that patients with tetralogy of Fallot and a coexistent PDA were not as cyanotic as most of her patients. She discussed this with Alfred Blalock (1899–1964) who, with the help of his laboratory assistant Vivien Thomas (1910–1985), worked out a technique to create a 'ductus'. This involved dividing a subclavian artery, turning it down and anastomosing it to the ipsilateral pulmonary artery. This provided a new source of pulmonary blood flow. The operation was successful and benefitted many patients with inadequate pulmonary blood flow until corrective operations became available for many patients a decade later. Other 'shunt' operations were developed during this era, including the Pott's [19] procedure (anastomosing the left pulmonary artery to the descending aorta) and the Waterston [20] operation (anastomosing the right pulmonary artery to the ascending aorta). These two procedures did not replace the BT shunt because they often led to pulmonary vascular disease or distortion of the branch pulmonary artery. Now, the concept is continued, but as a modified BT shunt a Gore-Tex tube graft is placed between a subclavian and pulmonary artery.

The third extracardiac operation was performed also in 1944 by Clarence Crafoord (1899–1984) in Sweden. He had performed animal experiments which showed that blood flow could be suspended to all organs for 25 min as long as flow to the brain was preserved. In certain patients with a PDA, he subsequently placed forceps above and below the PDA for 25 min while he repaired the PDA. When the clamps were released, loss of function below the aortic clamping site did not occur. Considering these facts and that in patients with a coarctation a plentiful collateral arterial system develops around the coarctation, he believed that the aorta could be cross-clamped for an even longer period of time. So, in October 1944, Crafoord operated on 2 patients, a 12-year-old boy and a 27-year-old man [21]. Through a left posterior thoracotomy, the coarctation was approached. The coarcted segment was short (4–5 mm) and the distal aorta enlarged. A clamp was placed just below the left subclavian artery and the other proximal to the first intercostal arteries. The coarctation was resected and the aorta repaired with a continuous suture. The patients did well, the upper-extremity blood pressures became normal and the lower-extremity pressures were higher than in the arms.

Three other operations were developed in these early days. One, the Blalock-Hanlon procedure [22], which was designed by Alfred Blalock and C. Rollins Hanlon (1915–2011) with the help of Vivien Thomas [23], created an atrial septal defect (ASD) to mix oxygenated and unoxygenated blood in infants with complete transposition of the great arteries. This palliated these neonates and was often a preliminary step to subsequent operations.

A second operation developed by Russell Brock (1903–1980) [24], the Brock procedure, was described in 3 patients whose pulmonary stenosis was treated through an incision in the right-ventricular wall. This preceded open pulmonary valvotomy.

Finally, William Muller (1920–2012) and J. Francis Dammann (1917–2011) [25] reduced excessive pulmonary blood flow in children with a VSD by placing a polyethylene band around the pulmonary artery. This procedure was widely used to treat associated heart failure and modified until VSD repair with cardiopulmonary bypass became widespread. It is still used as a prophylactic procedure.

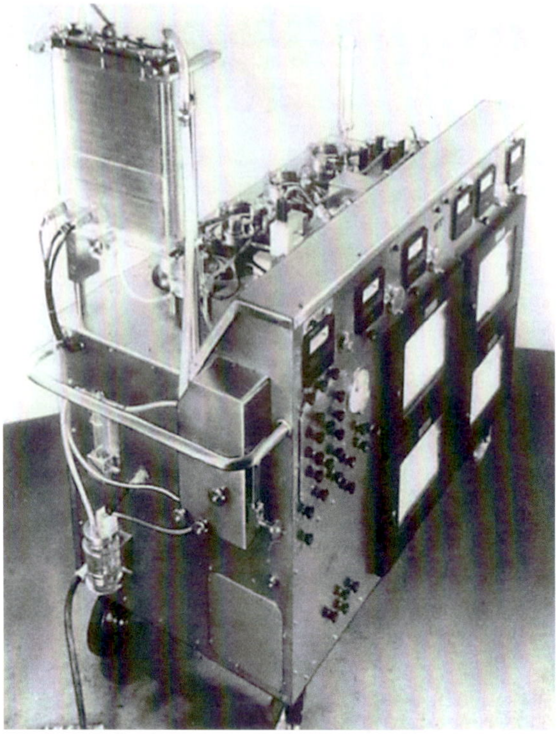

Fig. 3. Gibbon heart-lung machine model II [43].

Intracardiac Operations

The primary challenge to operating inside the heart was the ability to provide oxygenated blood to the patient. Pumps were available to circulate blood, but oxygenating the blood was the problem. The world's first operation within the heart was performed by Clarence Dennis (1909–2005). He had developed a membrane oxygenator which he used twice in 1951 while at the University of Minnesota. The first operation was to close an ASD [26]. At operation, an ostium primum defect with an abnormal tricuspid valve was identified, which was relatively unrecognized at that time. This could not be corrected. His second patient died because of a pump problem. Dr. Dennis left Minnesota to become a Chairman of Surgery at another institution and continued his efforts in bypass methods. John Gibbon (1904–1973) [27] at the Jefferson Medical College had worked for years also developing a membrane oxygenator (fig. 3). Using this oxygenator, he operated upon 6 patients with an ASD and only 1 patient survived. Dennis became discouraged with these results and because of his age retired.

At the University of Minnesota, in September 1952, F. John Lewis (1916–1993) performed the first successful open heart operation with the closure of an ASD in a 5-year-old girl [28]. He subsequently operated upon 59 additional patients with an ASD until June 1956. His technique involved hypothermia (to 80°F) and inflow occlusion of the vena cava and pulmonary veins. The right atrium was opened and the ASD suture closed. The incision in the right atrial wall was closed by a clamp and the wall sutured. In the mean time the right atrium was open was less than 5 min. Fifty-four patients survived including the first one who is now 67 years old. Lewis indicated that this technique was temporary until cardiopulmonary bypass became available.

He had to wait 2 years for that to happen. That first operation was performed on March 26, 1954, at the University of Minnesota by Drs. C. Walton Lillehei (1918–1999), Richard Varco (1912–2004) and colleagues on an 11-month-old boy, who died on the 11th postoperative day of pneumonia [29]. The second and third patients, both under 5 years of age, survived and are still alive 60 years later. A total of 45 patients with VSD, tetralogy of Fallot or atrioventricular septal defect were operated in the next 16 months. The bypass technique was extracorporeal cross circulation. This term describes the procedure in which a donor, usually a parent or relative with the same blood type, served as the oxygenator. Two tables were in the operating room, one for the patient and the other for the donor. Large bore catheters were inserted into the donor's femoral artery and vein. The arterial catheter was passed through one side of a pump into the child's aorta. The blood from the vena cava passed on the other side of the pump and returned to the donor. The pump allowed an equal amount of inflow and outflow from the child. The anomalies were repaired without patch material and by direct suture only, and were performed without cardiac arrest or hypothermia. Thirty patients survived and 20 were still alive over 53 years later.

In their short paper, John W. Kirklin (1917–2004) et al. [30] presented the first group of children with a cardiac anomaly repaired using a pump oxygenator. This further launched intracardiac surgery. Kirklin and the Mayo Clinic had acquired a Gibbon oxygenator. They perfused 8 children, aged 4 months to 11 years, each with severe congenital heart disease, 5 with a VSD, 2 with an atrioventricular septal defect and 1 with an ASD. During the procedure, the circulation was stable and there were no bleeding problems. Postoperatively, 4 of the patients died, 3 within 3 h of the procedure. In none was death attributed to the perfusion. While they had undertaken the operations as a trial, with the results influencing the decision of whether to continue with more operations, they felt encouraged and did continue. Thus, the first two institutions to perform open heart surgery were located 80 miles apart in Minnesota. Soon, more centers around the United States and elsewhere were beginning their own cardiac surgical programs. One important lesson learned from the experience at the Mayo Clinic was the value of a team approach to the patients, an approach involving, in addition to the surgeon, cardiologists, radiologists, physiologists, and pathologists. Each specialty had unique knowledge to address not only the patient but also to develop the field.

Complete transposition of the great arteries is one of the most frequent cardiac anomalies. While an operation to create an ASD had been performed, one to correct the circulation was unavailable. Åke Senning (1915–2000) [31] and William Mustard (1914–1987) [32] developed operations that created a baffle within the atria that allowed blood from the vena cava to pass into the left ventricle and the pulmonary venous return to pass on the opposite of the baffle to the right ventricle. While the operations were successful, the long-term issue remains with the ability of the right ventricle to maintain systemic cardiac output and a systemic blood pressure for a number of years. Many survivors develop cardiac failure and some have undergone cardiac transplantation.

Because of the postoperative issues with a venous switch, a new approach, an arterial switch, was developed. In this operation, the great arteries are moved to the correct ventricle. Performed in neonates, it involved making circumferential incisions above each semilunar valve. The origins of coronary arteries were removed from the root of the aorta arising from the right ventricle and swung posteriorly and anastomosed to the root of the pulmonary artery. The distal part of the aorta was then anastomosed to the proximal part of the pulmonary artery. The pulmonary artery was moved anteriorly and sewn to the root of the previous aorta [33]. As a result, the pattern of the circulation is correct, the great arteries arise from the proper ventricle and the coronary arteries receive fully saturated blood.

Giancarlo Rastelli (1934–1970) was a very creative surgical fellow at the Mayo Clinic. He developed a corrective procedure for truncus arteriosus, which has subsequently been used for coexistent tetralogy of Fallot and pulmonary atresia. He inserted an aortic homograft, complete with aortic valve, into the right ventricle and connected the distal end to the pulmonary artery [34]. The initial report of operations in dogs contained cardiac catheterization studies which showed a small gradient through the graft. In the following years, this procedure has been widely applied.

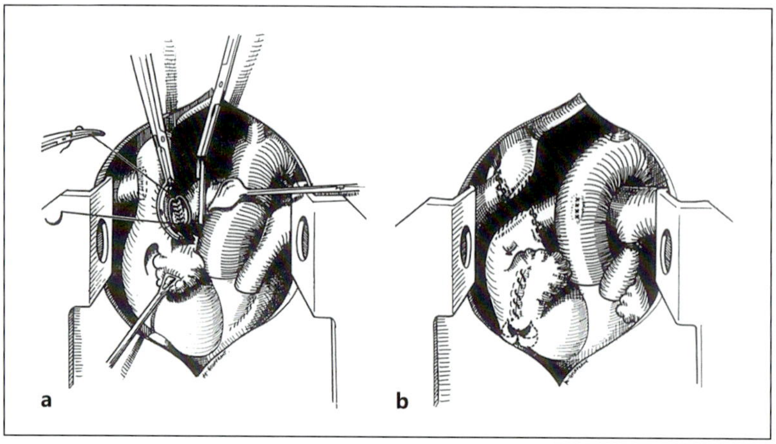

Fig. 4. Fontan procedure. **a** Anastomosis of the proximal end of the right pulmonary artery to the left lateral side of the upper part of the right atrium (left). **b** Appearance at completion of the operation.

Francois Marie Fontan (born 1929) [35] and Guillermo Kreutzer (born 1934) [36] performed their initial operations to create a normal circulatory pattern in children with tricuspid atresia very close in time. Fontan's publication appeared in May 1971 in *Thorax* [35] and Kreutzer's report [36] was presented to the Argentine Congress of Cardiology in November of the same year. These surgeons connected the right atrium to the pulmonary artery. Fontan first created a Glenn connection of the superior vena cava to the right pulmonary artery and then connected the right atrial appendage to the main pulmonary artery with a homograft (fig. 4) [35], while Kreutzer connected the right atrial appendage directly to the main pulmonary artery [36]. Because the right atrium often dilated with time and the pulmonary blood flow decreased, modifications of the procedure have been made subsequently. These initially included an intra-atrial conduit through the right atrium and later an extracardiac conduit from the inferior vena cava to the right pulmonary artery. Despite these improvements, the procedure is palliative, since many patients develop complications, including protein-losing enteropathy or congestive cardiac failure. Both problems remain difficult to treat.

Hypoplastic left-heart syndrome was the last major congenital heart anomaly to be addressed surgically. William Imon Norwood Jr. (born 1941) and his group [37] developed a procedure which created a circulation in which the right ventricle became the systemic ventricle. They divided the main pulmonary artery and tied off the distal end. The proximal end was anastomosed to the hypoplastic ascending aorta. A homograft patch was often used to enlarge the aorta and continue the connection to the proximal descending aorta. A communication was created, either a modified BT shunt or a tube graft, from the right ventricle to pulmonary artery (Sano modification) to maintain pulmonary blood flow. Finally, an atrial septectomy was performed. This was the first of a series of operations which subsequently included a Glenn and then a Fontan procedure. The operative mortality has decreased and many patients survive into early adulthood, but they often develop the complications of a Fontan connection.

Interventional Catheterization Procedures

The first interventional cardiac catheterization was performed by William Rashkind (1922–1986) and William Miller [38] when they created a communication between the right and left atrium in neonates with complete transposition of the great arteries. The intent was to allow mixing venous return from the left and right atria in order to increase arterial oxygen saturation. They passed a balloon-tipped catheter from the right inguinal area through the right atrium and foramen ovale into the left atrium. The balloon was inflated and withdrawn forcefully across the atrial septum with the intent of tearing the septum primum to create a larger atrial communication. This allowed the neonates to grow until they could undergo an atrial or arterial switch operation. It is still used in a variety of neonates where an atrial communication is needed.

In the following years, the ability to treat cardiac anomalies with catheter techniques has grown, perhaps most successfully with conditions on the right side of the heart. Since the early 1980s, balloon pulmonary valvuloplasty has become more popular and nearly supplanted an operative approach to pulmonary stenosis [39]. In patients with pulmonary regurgitation, the valve can be replaced with a Melody valve placed via catheter [40]. Many ASD types are closed using an expandable device, often an Amplatzer occluder, which is self-centering and has disks which are expanded on each side of the septum [41]. Other interventions include occluding a PDA, aortic valvuloplasty, and dilatation of a coarctation.

Other Advances

Two major developments greatly improved the management of critically ill neonates; prostaglandin administration and echocardiographic visualization of the heart. Peter Olley and Flavio Coceani had performed studies in fetal lambs showing that E-type prostaglandins (PGE) were powerful relaxants of the ductus arteriosus and had been used in 2 cyanotic neonates whose parents had refused a cardiac operation for their offspring. In three types of conditions, the ductus is critical for the survival of the neonate: a malformation with severe pulmonary stenosis or atresia, interruption of the aortic arch, and complete transposition. In each of these cases, when the ductus closes, either the pulmonary or systemic blood flow is compromised. If the ductus could be maintained patent with PGE1 or PGE2 treatment, the neonate could survive until an operation could be performed. In their report, Olley et al. [42] described 4 treated neonates who underwent an operation and were doing well postoperatively. PGE1 use in cyanotic neonates has expanded widely and is regularly administered during the transfer of neonates to regional cardiac centers and for stabilizing neonates prior to an operation. Inhibition of prostaglandins by indomethacin has been used successfully in premature neonates to close a symptomatic ductus arteriosus.

Finally, over the past 40 years, echocardiographic techniques have continually improved to image the heart in both adults and children. It has two unique and important roles in pediatrics. Since in many instances cardiac anomalies present soon after birth frequently at a site distant from a referral center, an echocardiogram can reveal the presence of a malformation and prompt the appropriate referral. Secondly, with ultrasound, the structures of a fetal heart can be visualized and if an important anomaly is identified, the baby is delivered at a referral center. Transesophageal echocardiography is used during cardiac surgery to guide the surgeon and assess the adequacy of repair.

Over the past three and a half centuries, tremendous advances have been made in defining cardiac malformations, understanding their effects on the circulation, and treating them. Children around the world are the beneficiaries of this knowledge. Dr. Taussig said, 'The great day will be when we can prevent these conditions rather than merely treating them'. We are slowly uncovering the causes of these anomalies, which is the first step to prevention.

References

1 Stensen N: Embryo monstro affinis Parisiis dissectus. Acta Med Philos Hafneincia 1671/1672;i:202–203.

2 Hunter W: Medical Observations and Inquiries. By a Society of Physicians of London. London, Cadell, 1784, vol 6.

3 Farre JR: Pathological Researches: Essay 1. On Malformations of the Human Heart. London, Longman, Hurst, Rees, Orme & Brown, 1814.

4 Baillie M: The Morbid Anatomy of Some of the Most Important Parts of the Human Body; Rodin AE (ed): The Influence of Matthew Baillie's Morbid Anatomy. Biography, Evaluation and Reprint. Springfield, Thomas, 1973, p 293.

5 Hope J: A Treatise of the Diseases of the Heart and Great Vessels, ed Am 1. Philadelphia, Haswill & Johnson, 1842, pp 376–384.

6 Schiebler GL, Gravenstein JS, Van Mierop LHS: Ebsteins's anomaly of the tricuspid valve: translation of original description with comments. Am J Cardiol 1968;22:867–873.

7 Abbott M: Atlas of Congenital Heart Disease. New York, American Heart Association, 1936, p 62.
8 Fallot A: Contribution a l'anatomie pathologique de la maladie bleue (cyanose cardiaque). Marseille Méd 1888;25:418–420.
9 Wood P: Pulmonary hypertension with special reference to the vasoconstrictive factor. Br Heart J 1958;20:557–570.
10 Eisenmenger V: Die angeborenen Defekte der Kammerscheidewände des Herzens. Zeitschr Klin Med 1897;32(suppl):1–28.
11 Edwards JE: The Lewis A. Connor Memorial Lecture. Functional pathology of the pulmonary vascular tree in congenital heart disease. Circulation 1957;15:164–196.
12 Roger H: Recherches cliniques sur la communication congénitale des coeurs par inocclusion du septum interventriculaire. Bull Acad Méd 1879;8:1074–1094.
13 Still GF: Common Disorders and Diseases of Childhood. London, Frowde, 1909.
14 Forssmann W: Experiments on Myself. New York, Saint Martin's Press, 1974, pp 84–86.
15 Cournand A, Baldwin JS, Himmelstein A: Cardiac Catheterization in Congenital Heart Disease. New York, Commonwealth Fund, 1949.
16 Castellanos A, Pereiras R, Garcia A: La Angio-cardiografia en el nino. Proc 7th Congr Pan Am Med Assoc, Havana, 1939.
17 Gross RE, Hubbard JP: Surgical ligation of a patent ductus arteriosus. Report of first successful case. JAMA 1939;112:729–731.
18 Blalock A, Taussig HB: Surgical treatment of malformations of the heart in which there is pulmonary stenosis or atresia. JAMA 1945;128:189–202.
19 Potts WJ: Anastomosis of the aorta to a pulmonary artery. Certain types in congenital heart disease. JAMA 1946;132:627–631.
20 Waterston DJ: Treatment of Fallot's tetralogy in children under 1 year of age (in Czech). Rozhl Chir 1962;41:181–183.
21 Crafoord C, Nylin G: Congenital coarctation of the aorta and its surgical treatment. J Thorac Surg 1945;14:347–361.
22 Blalock A, Hanlon CR: The surgical treatment of complete transposition of the aorta and the pulmonary artery. Surg Gynecol Obstet 1950;90:1–15.
23 Thomas V: Partners of the Heart: Vivien Thomas and His Work with Alfred Blalock. Philadelphia, University of Pennsylvania Press, 1985.
24 Brock RC: Pulmonary valvulotomy for relief of congenital pulmonary stenosis. Br Med J 1948;i:1121–1126.
25 Muller WH, Dammann JZF Jr: The treatment of certain congenital malformations of the heart by the creation of pulmonic stenosis to reduce pulmonary hypertension and excessive pulmonary blood flow. A preliminary report. Surg Gynecol Obstet 1952; 95:213–229.
26 Dennis C, Spreng DS Jr, Nelson CE, et al: Development of a pump-oxygenator to replace heart and lungs. An apparatus applicable to human patients and application to one case. Ann Surg 1951;134:709–721.
27 Gibbon JH Jr: Application of a mechanical heart and lung apparatus to cardiac surgery. Minn Med 1954;37:171–185.
28 Lewis FJ, Taufic M: Closure of atrial septal defects with the aid of hypothermia; experimental accomplishments and the report of one successful case. Surgery 1953;33:52–59.
29 Lillehei CW, Cohen M, Warden HE, Varco RL: The direct vision intracardiac correction of congenital anomalies by controlled cross-circulation. Results in thirty-two patients with ventricular septal defects, tetralogy of Fallot and atrioventricularis communis defect. Surgery 1955;38:11–29.
30 Kirklin JW, DuShane, JW, Patrick RT, et al: Intracardiac surgery with the aid of a mechanical pump-oxygenator system (Gibbon type): report of eight cases. Proc Staff Meet Mayo Clinic 1955;30:201–206.
31 Senning A: Surgical correction of transposition of the great vessels. Surgery 1959;45: 966–980.
32 Mustard WT: Successful two-stage correction of transposition of the great vessels. Surgery 1964;55:469–472.
33 Lecompte Y, Zannini L, Hazan E, et al: Anatomic correction of transposition of the great arteries: new technique without the use of a prosthetic conduit. J Thorac Cardiovasc Surg 1981;82:629–631.
34 Rastelli GC, Titus JL, McGoon DC: Homograph of ascending aorta and aortic valve as right ventricular outflow. An experimental approach to the repair of truncus arteriosus. Arch Surg 1967;95:698–708.
35 Fontan F, Baudet E: Surgical repair of tricuspid atresia. Thorax 1971;26:240–248.
36 Kreutzer G, Galindez H, Bono H: An operation for the correction of tricuspid atresia. J Thorac Cardiovasc Surg 1973;66: 613–621.
37 Norwood WL, Lang P, Casteneda AR, et al: Experience with operations for hypoplastic left heart syndrome. J Thorac Cardiovasc Surg 1981;82:511–519.
38 Rashkind WJ, Miller WW: Creation of an atrial septal defect without thoracotomy. A palliative approach to complete transposition of the great arteries. JAMA 1966;196: 991–992.
39 Kan JS, White RI, Mitchell SE, et al: Percutaneous transluminal balloon valvuloplasty for pulmonary valve stenosis. Circulation 1984;69:554–560.
40 Bonhoeffer P, Boudjinline Y, Salibu Z, et al: Percutaneous replacement of pulmonary valve in a right-ventricle to pulmonary artery prosthetic conduit with valve dysfunction. Lancet 2000;356:403–405.
41 Du ZD, Hijazi ZM, Kleinman CS, et al; Amplatzer investigators: Comparison between transcatheter and surgical closure of secundum atrial septal defect in children and adults: results of a nonrandomized trial. J Am Coll Cardiol 2002;39:1836–1844.
42 Olley PM, Coceani F, Bodach E: E-type prostaglandins: a new emergency therapy for certain cyanotic congenital heart malformations. Circulation 1976;53:728–731.
43 Romaine-Davis A: John Gibbon and His Heart-Lung Machine. Philadelphia, University of Pennsylvania Press, 1991.

Dr. James H. Moller
Department of Pediatrics, University of Minnesota
MMC 508, 420 Delaware Street SE
Minneapolis, MN 55455 (USA)
E-Mail molle002@umn.edu

Muenke M, Kruszka PS, Sable CA, Belmont JW (eds): Congenital Heart Disease: Molecular Genetics, Principles of Diagnosis and Treatment. Basel, Karger, 2015, pp 11–25
DOI: 10.1159/000375202

Normal Development of the Heart

Marc Sylva · Antoon F.M. Moorman

Department of Anatomy, Embryology and Physiology, Academic Medical Center, Amsterdam, The Netherlands

Abstract

Through the 20th century, the embryonic heart tube was thought to consist of the adult cardiac components in their primordial form. We now know this is not the case and that the early heart contains little more than the precursor cells for the left ventricle or even less, whereas cells are continuously added to the heart tube when it grows and loops. Using new molecular genetic techniques, it is now possible to label cells irreversibly that once expressed a specific gene, thus permitting the composition of fate maps which unveil the origin of the cells building the different components of the heart. This, in turn, provides crucial information when we seek to understand the normal development of the heart and, as a corollary, the causes of cardiac malformations. The question, nonetheless, justifiably arises whether this is of clinical relevance at all, the more because the general building plan of the heart is laid down in the first 2 months of life, a period inaccessible for the pediatric cardiologist. In this chapter, we frame the new molecular and genetic insights into a proper morphological context. These new insights permit us to draw inferences concerning a variety of structural congenital cardiac malformations and potential substrates for arrhythmias, such as atrial fibrillation and outflow tract tachycardias.

Just after birth, two parallel blood flows run through the heart. Oxygen-deprived blood runs from the heart's right atrium though the right ventricle to enter the lungs. The oxygenated blood, in turn, flows through the left side of the heart, entering at the left atrium and is then pumped by the left ventricle into the systemic circulation. The different components of the heart are activated in an organized manner starting at the inflow and ending at the outflow of the heart (fig. 1). At the roof of the right atrium, at the entrance of the right superior caval vein, the sinus node generates an electrical impulse, which travels through the atria and reaches the atrioventricular (AV) node, where its conduction is delayed. From the AV node, the activation front travels through the fast-conducting bundles and bundle branches to the peripheral conduction system of the ventricles, the Purkinje fibers. The rapid propagation of the electrical current in the ventricles ensures simultaneous contraction of the entire ventricular mass, allowing efficient propulsion of blood.

Formation of the Linear Heart Tube

Origin of the Cardiac Mesoderm

Similar to most muscles and vascular structures, the heart is also largely a mesodermal derivative, al-

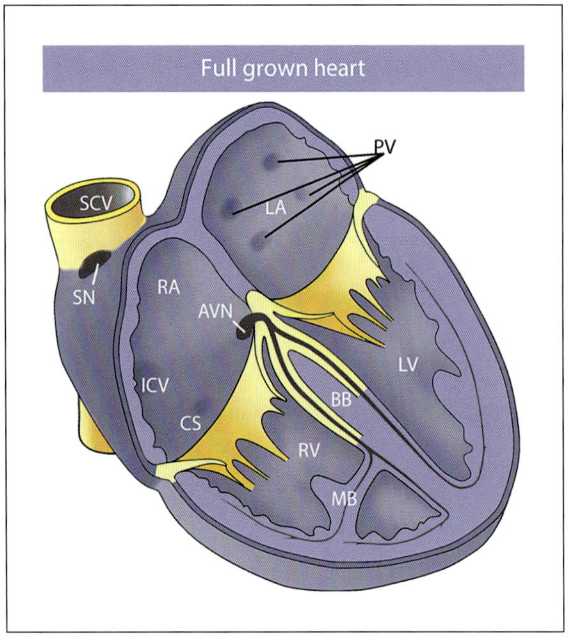

Fig. 1. A schematic representation of the human heart. Different tissue types are depicted in different colors, the nonmyocardial tissues in yellow, the working myocardium in blue, and the myocardium of the conduction system in black. SCV = Superior caval vein; ICV = inferior caval vein; CS = coronary sinus; PV = pulmonary vein; SN = sinus node; AVN = AV node; BB = bundle branches; MB = moderator band; RA = right atrium; LA = left atrium; RV = right ventricle; LV = left ventricle.

beit a contribution from ectoderm-derived cardiac neural crest cells is made to the cushions of the outflow tract. Early in human development, at Carnegie stage (CS) 8 (table 1) [1], when the embryo is a flat disk, the cardiac precursors reside in the mesoderm lateral to the future mouth, i.e. the stomatopharyngeal membrane (fig. 2). The two bilateral precursor pools unite in the midline forming the so-called cardiac crescent [2, 3] (fig. 2).

Folding of the Embryo and Formation of the Heart Tube

As development progresses during CS9, the flat embryo starts to fold. The folding of the embryo brings the heart-forming region in its final position, ventral to the foregut, between the mouth at the cranial side and the future diaphragm (i.e. transverse septum, in which the liver develops) at the caudal side. By the process of folding (fig. 2), the horseshoe-shaped cardiac crescent transforms into a tube with two caudolateral inlets (venous poles) and one craniomedial outlet (arterial pole).

Growth of the Linear Heart Tube

The linear heart tube grows by addition of cardiomyocytes, which differentiate from the surrounding mesoderm. Studies in humans, mice and chicken revealed that the heart tube displays hardly any proliferation, whereas a highly proliferative cardiac precursor pool is present in the dorsal pericardial wall [3–5]. Labeling of these precursor cells with fluorescent dyes in chicken demonstrated that cells from this proliferating pool, while differentiating into cardiomyocytes, are added to the heart tube at all places where the myocardium is attached to the body wall, i.e. at the venous and arterial poles, as well as at the dorsal mesocardium [4] (fig. 2). The stop of cell division of the initially formed cardiomyocytes is reversible, and when the cardiac chambers start to develop a subset of cardiomyocytes reenters the cell cycle and starts to proliferate again [3–5].

Several studies have shown that the identity of a cardiomyocyte is not fixed and that cells can populate different components of the heart depending on the stage of development. For instance, it has been shown that cells that initially reside in the outflow tract eventually end up in the right ventricle, whereas newly added cells form the outflow tract of those hearts in later stages [6, 7]. Cells initially forming the embryonic left ventricle end up as ventricular septum of the formed heart [8].

Based upon molecular genetic studies, the cardiac precursor pool has been divided into two groups of cells, cells that form the initial heart tube (the first heart field) and cells that are added to this linear heart tube at later developmental stages (the second heart field; fig. 2) [9–11]. This concept emphasizes that a distinct population of cells is added to the initial heart tube and has been a major breakthrough in our understanding of cardiac development. Morphological studies never revealed such a distinction, because it is impossible to assess what is the initial heart tube because the

Table 1. Stages of human development with corresponding events in cardiac development

Carnegie stage	Human DPC	Mouse DPC	
CS8	17–19	7	The cardiac crescent forms
CS9	19–21	7.5	The embryo folds, the pericardial cavity is placed in its final position, gully of myocardium forms, the endocardial plexus forms, cardiac jelly forms
CS10	22–23	8	The heart beats, the endocardial tubes fuse, the mesocardium perforates, looping starts, the ventricle starts ballooning
CS11	23–26	8.5	The atria balloon, the proepicardium forms
CS12	26–30	9.5	The septum primum appears, the right venous valve appears, the muscular part of the ventricular septum forms, cells appear in the cardiac jelly, epicardial growth starts
CS13	28–32	10.5	The AV cushions form, the pulmonary vein attaches to the atrium, the left venous valve appears, epicardial mesenchyme appears first in the AV sulcus
CS14	31–35	11.5	The AV cushions approach one another, the outflow ridges become apparent, capillaries form in the epicardial mesenchyme
CS15	35–38	12	The AV cushions oppose one another, the secondary foramen forms, the distal outflow tract septates, the outflow tract ridges reach the primary foramen
CS16	37–42	12.5	The primary atrial septum closes, the outflow tract ridges approach the interventricular septum, the entire heart is covered in epicardium
CS17	42–44	13.5	Secondary atrial septum appears, the sinus node becomes discernable, the left and right AV connection becomes separate, the proximal outflow tract becomes septated, the semilunar valves develop
CS18	44–48	14.5	Papillary muscles appear, the AV valves start to form
CS19	48–51	15	The left venous valve fuses with the secondary septum, the mural leaflets of the mitral and tricuspid valves are released
CS21	53–54	16	The main branches of the coronary artery become apparent
CS22	54–56	16.5	The chordae tendinae form
CS23	56 60	17.5	The septal leaflet of the tricuspid valve delaminates

DPC = Days postconception. A time line of events taking place in human cardiac development is summarized as published previously [1] [data were obtained from ref. 41–43].

Fig. 2. Folding of the embryo and formation of the heart tube. The left column shows from top to bottom the folding of the embryo; the right column depicts the formation of the heart tube. The embryo starts as a flat disk, containing the three germ layers: the ectoderm (Ecto), mesoderm (Meso), and endoderm (Endo). The mesoderm adjacent to the endoderm, between the future transverse septum (TS) and the future pharyngeal mesoderm (PM), will give rise to the heart. The rectangle shows an enlargement of the cardiogenic region and its division into two (sub)fields, the first heart field (1), which will give rise to the linear heart tube, and the second heart field (2), which is gradually added to the initial heart tube. Upon folding of the embryo, the embryonic gut that runs from the stomatopharyngeal membrane (SM) to the cloacal membrane (CM) is formed. The heart (HT) becomes positioned ventrally to the foregut (FG) caudally to the head and cranially to the navel and transverse septum. The pictographs at the right show the formation of the heart tube from a flat horseshoe-shaped cardiac crescent that gradually transforms into a gully and eventually a tube by merging at the back side of the heart. The connection of the heart to the dorsal body wall is termed the dorsal mesocardium (DM). AP = Arterial pole; VP = venous pole.

(For figure 2 see next page.)

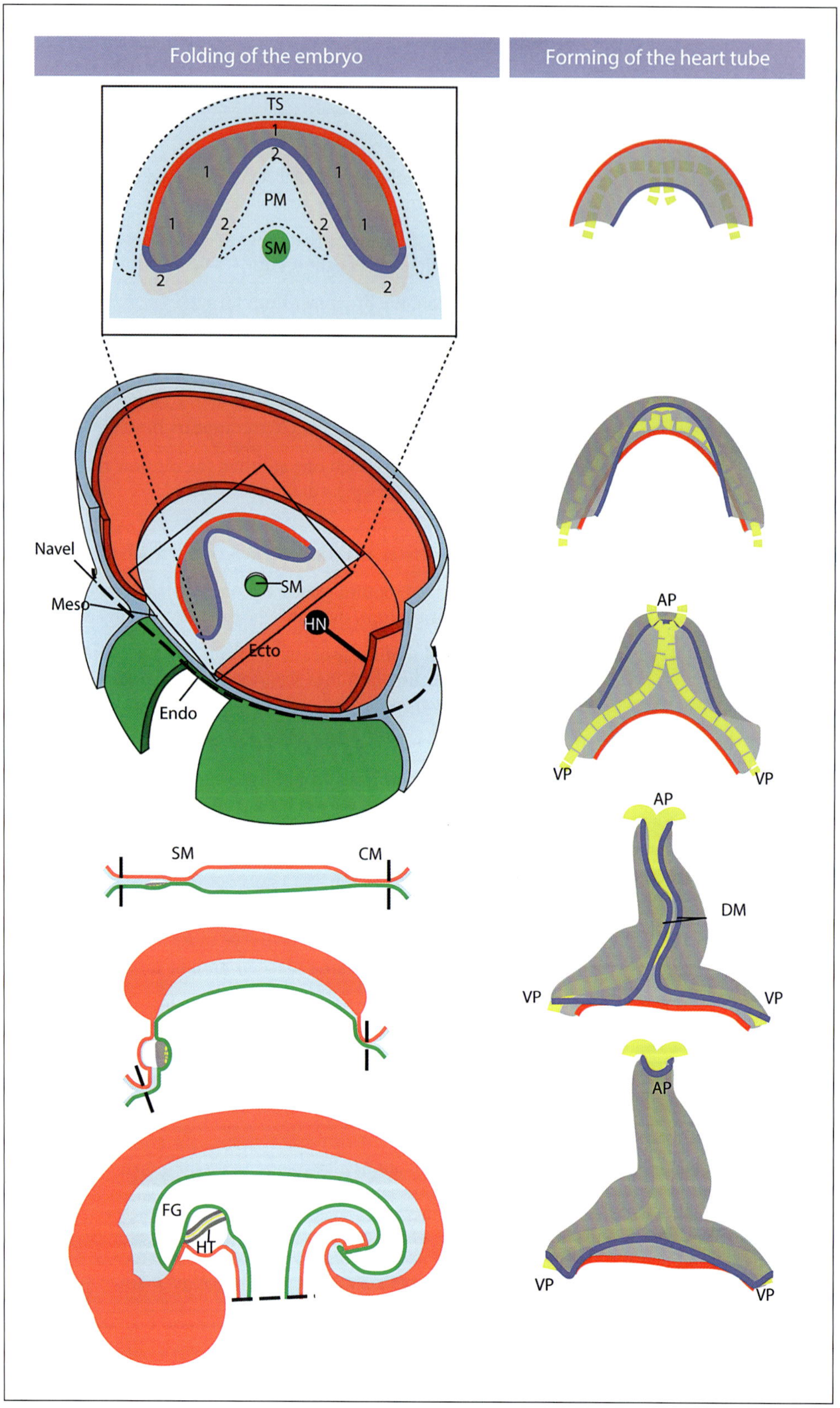
Folding of the embryo
Forming of the heart tube
TS
1
2
1
1
PM
1
2
2
1
SM
2
2
Navel
Meso
SM
HN
Ecto
Endo
SM
CM
FG
HT
AP
VP
VP
AP
DM
VP
VP
AP
VP
VP

2

	Primary	Nodal	His bundle	Purkinje	Compact
Automaticity	High	High	High	Low	Low
Conduction velocity	Low	Low	High	High	High
Contractility	Low	Low	Low	Low	High

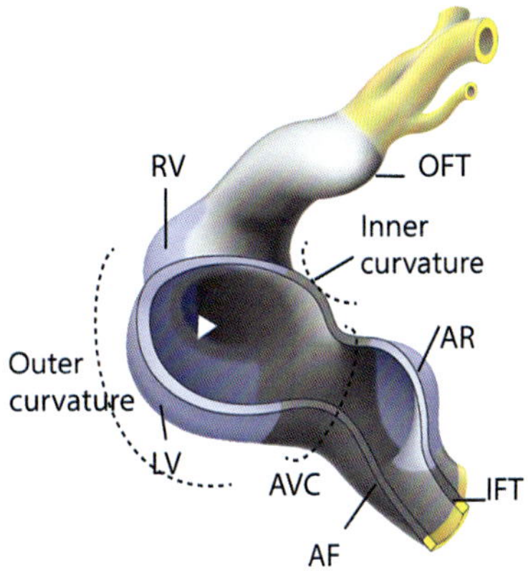

Fig. 3. Different types of myocardium. The table shows the characteristics of different kinds of myocardium in terms of their contraction and electrophysiological behavior. The drawing depicts a lateral view of the chamber-forming, or ballooning, heart viewed with the dorsal side of the embryo on the right side. The primary myocardium is indicated in gray and the secondary, or chamber-forming myocardium, in blue; note the gray area at the top of the ventricular septum (white triangle), which retains characteristics of the primary myocardium. IFT = Inflow tract; AR = atrial roof; AF = atrial floor; AVC = AV canal; LV = left ventricle; RV = right ventricle; OFT = outflow tract.

entire heart grows continuously by the gradual addition of cells from the surrounding visceral mesoderm.

From One Tube to Four Chambers

The Ballooning Model of Chamber Formation

Based on three characteristics being their strength of contractility, firing frequency, and conduction velocity, the cardiomyocytes can be subdivided into different groups (fig. 3) [12].

The myocardium of the tubular heart is called *primary myocardium*, which is composed of 'primitive' or nodal-like cells. These cardiomyocytes have a high frequency of automaticity, have poorly developed sarcomeres, and are poorly electrically coupled to one another resulting in slow conduction, similar to the nodal cardiomyocytes in the adult heart, which, ironically, are called 'specialized' rather than 'primitive'.

At CS9–CS10, the process of looping commences, which transforms the straight heart tube in an S-shaped heart, with inner and outer curvatures. At the outer curvature of the looping heart tube, the primary myocardium differentiates into chamber myocardium and re-initiates cell division, by which the ventricles form (fig. 4). The same process of differentiation and proliferation occurs at the venous pole of the heart tube, by which the atrial appendices form (fig. 4). The differentiating and proliferating myocardium can be termed secondary or chamber myocardium. The myocytes of the atrial and ventricular chambers are fast-conducting cells and have higher contraction forces compared to the primary myocardium of the linear heart tube.

Formation of the Atrial Chambers

The atria are formed bilaterally in a symmetric fashion at the dorsolateral sides of the heart tube. The developing atria receive left-right signals and develop differently according to these signals, mediated by Pitx2c. Upon disruption of Pitx2c-mediated laterality, both atria develop with right atrial appendages, demonstrating the crucial role of Pitx2c in the establishment of atrial sidedness [13; for more details on heterotaxy, see the chapter by Lo et al., Heterotaxy, p. 166].

Initially, the veins draining to the heart are embedded in the mesenchyme at the venous pole of the heart. With ongoing development, the connecting veins are 'excavated' from this mesenchyme, by which they become positioned within the pericardial cavity. The confluence of the left and right superior and inferior cardinal veins, termed the common

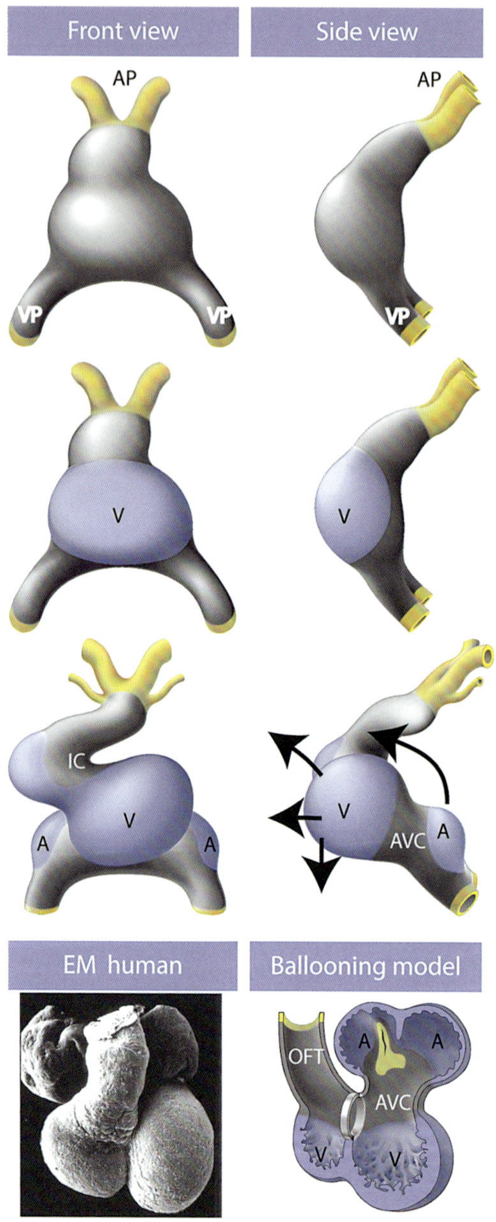

Fig. 4. Ballooning of the heart. Schematic drawings of the chamber-forming heart are shown in frontal and lateral views. Gray = Primary myocardium; blue = chamber-forming myocardium. In the top row, the heart tube consists solely of primary myocardium from the venous (VP) to arterial pole (AP). The first chamber to start ballooning is the embryonic ventricle (V) at the outer curvature of the heart as seen in the panels below. While chamber formation commences, the heart tube starts to loop and acquires an S shape. Apart from the embryonic ventricles, the atria (A) also start to balloon towards the left and right side; the myocardium at the arterial pole, inner curvature (IC), the AV canal (AVC), and venous pole remains primary myocardium. The black arrows in the looping chamber-forming heart indicate the expansion of the chambers eventually leading to the adult configuration, with the ventricles positioned ventrocaudal to the atria and the atria to the left and right of the outflow of the heart. The bottom left panel shows an electron-microscopic photograph of a human heart with a schematic drawing of the same stage next to it. Note that in the schematic drawing the outflow tract is hinged toward the right side, allowing to view the inner curvature.

cardinal veins, which become ensheathed by myocardium, is then called sinus venosus, or left and right sinus horns.

Due to movement of the venous pole to the right of the midline of the body, both sinus horns eventually connect to the right atrium. The right sinus horn becomes incorporated into the dorsal part of the right atrium. In humans, the left sinus horn becomes the coronary sinus, upon which the coronary venous circulation drains.

The formation of the myocardium surrounding the pulmonary venous return differs from the sys-

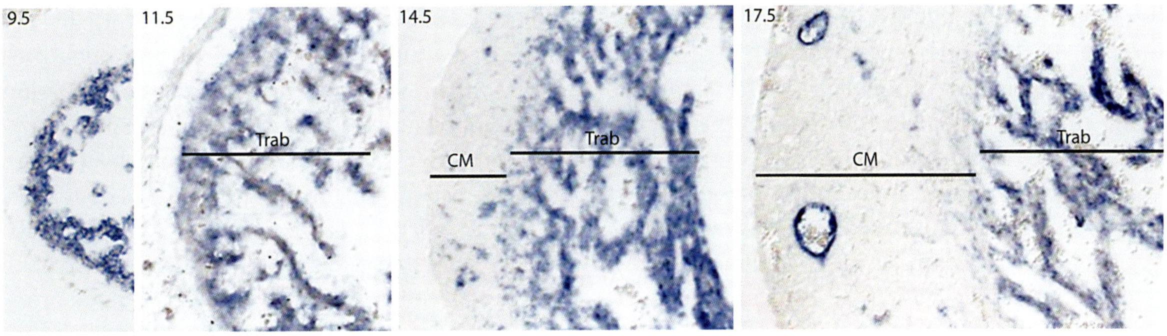

Fig. 5. Development of the compact myocardium. This figure shows a developmental series of mouse hearts (embryonic days of development are in the top left corner). The hearts are stained for the expression of Cx40 mRNA, a trabecular myocardium marker, and photographed at equal magnifications. The growth of the compact myocardium (CM) relative to the inner trabecular (Trab) layer is easily appreciated. Bearing in mind that even after embryonic day 17.5 the compact myocardium will grow, it becomes clear why the trabeculated myocardium becomes inconspicuous at adult stages (modified from Christoffels and Moorman [40]).

temic venous return. Unlike the systemic venous connections, the pulmonary vein develops and connects to the heart after formation of the heart tube. Mesenchyme dorsal to the heart differentiates into a vascular plexus surrounding the embryonic foregut and future lungs. At CS13, this plexus connects as a single pulmonary vein to the heart. Subsequent to its connection to the forming left atrium, the pulmonary vein becomes ensheathed by de novo differentiated myocardium. During further development, the muscularized pulmonary vein is incorporated into the left atrium up to its second bifurcation, resulting into four pulmonary orifices in the left human atrium.

The developing atrial chamber myocardium initially remains flanked by the primary myocardium of the sinus venosus and AV canal [14] (fig. 4). Downstream, with respect to the blood flow, the AV canal myocardium separates the atria from the ventricles. Upstream, the primary myocardium of the sinus venosus separates the systemic veins from the atria.

Formation of the Ventricular Chambers

At the outer curvature of the looped heart tube, at CS10, the ventricles develop with a trabecular phenotype. The trabecules grow by addition of cells at their base, by which the forming ventricles expand, or balloon exteriorly [5].

How the left and right ventricles obtain their different identity and morphology is only partly understood, albeit some differences between the left and the right ventricle in terms of gene expression are known [15–17]. Left-right signaling does not play a major role in the development of the distinct morphology between the left and right ventricles, which is to be expected because the right and the left ventricle develop along the craniocaudal axis of the embryo, which is in contrast to the development of the atrial chambers. Therefore, isomeric atria do occur but isomeric ventricles not. The eventual left-right positioning of the ventricular chambers is determined by the direction of looping, which, in turn, is dependent on left-right signaling. Thus, if the heart loops to the left instead of the normal right side, the morphological right ventricle is positioned on the left side of the morphological left ventricle.

At a later stage, at CS14, the compact layer of the ventricles develops under influence of epicardial-derived fibroblasts. The interaction of these fibroblasts with the ventricular myocytes induces a cascade of proliferation and differentiation of the myocardium resulting in the formation of a compact ventricular layer and expansion of the ventricles [18, 19]. As mentioned above, subsequent to their formation, proliferation of the trabecular myocardium tapers off, whereas proliferation in the forming compact layer continues at high rates. This already starts at a stage that the heart is hardly more than a few millimeters, explaining why in the adult heart the trabeculated myocardium is inconspicuous (fig. 5) [20]. Interestingly, the early markers of chamber formation, atrial natriuretic factor and connexin (Cx40), remain restricted to the original trabeculated myocardium, whereas the compact ventricular layer does not express these markers [3]. Compaction is thus not a process by which trabeculated myocardium becomes compact, but primarily a process by which the myocardium at the epicardial side of the ventricular wall proliferates and differentiates to form the compact layer. The factors that determine the differentiation of the trabecular versus the compact myocardial phenotype have been established only in part. Notch signaling plays an important role in this signaling pathway [21].

Building the ECG

The Earliest ECG Recordings

When chamber formation starts around CS10, or about 3 weeks of human development, the myocardium of the newly formed chambers conducts the depolarizing wave faster than the primary myocardium [22]. The alternating fast and slow conduction in the chamber-forming heart and its surrounding primary myocardium can be registered in an ECG, which resembles that of the formed heart [23]. Thus solely the arrangement of different types of cardiomyocytes results in an adult-like ECG at an embryonic stage where no electrical insulation, differentiated nodes, or conduction system are present.

Sinus Node

From the first beat of the heart tube onward to the last beat of the adult heart, the electrical impulse travels from the venous to the arterial pole. Since the heart grows by addition of cells during development, the most recently differentiated cells added at the venous pole always possess the dominant pacemaker activity.

A gene-regulatory network involving Tbx18-, Shox2-mediated repression of Nkx2.5 expression and Tbx3 inhibition of chamber formation underlies the development of the sinus myocardium, in which eventually the sinus node will develop. Initially, the entire sinus myocardium expresses this gene program, which, among others, results in the expression of the ion channel hyperpolarization-activated cyclic nucleotide-gated potassium channel 4 (Hcn4). Hcn4 is responsible for the spontaneous depolarizing 'funny' current, a major component of pacemaker activity. With subsequent development, this gene program becomes restricted to the sinus node proper via an as yet unknown mechanism, and the remainder of the sinus venosus will differentiate into smooth-walled atria.

Atrioventricular Node

Lineage analyses of the AV node and AV bundles have shown that the AV node is derived from AV canal myocardium, whereas the AV bundle, as well as the bundle branches, is derived from ventricular myocardium [24]. As described above, the myocardium of the AV canal maintains its primary phenotype [25] (fig. 3). In contrast to the sinus node, Nkx2.5 is expressed in the AV canal myocardium. Also, the ion channel Hcn4 is expressed in the AV node, but not the fast-conducting Cx40, explaining its high automaticity but slow conduction.

The AV bundle and bundle branches express the transcriptional repressor Tbx3, but nonetheless express Cx40, allowing the bundles to conduct fast.

Peripheral Ventricular Conduction System

The Purkinje fibers of the formed heart transmit the depolarizing wave from the bundles towards the ventricular working myocardium. The ventricular conduction system is able to conduct fast by virtue of the fast-conducting gap junctions, which are composed of Cx40 and Cx43.

Early in development, when no Purkinje fibers are visible, the trabeculated myocardium expresses these fast-conducting connexins (fig. 5). As described above, the growth of these trabeculations ceases compared to the growth of the compact layer [5], which leaves the initial trabeculations as small structures covering the inner side of the heart and maintaining the expression of fast-conducting connexins. Thus, along with the development of the compact layer, the trabecular layer becomes secondary in force generation and gives rise to the His-Purkinje system.

Septation

Septation of the heart can be subdivided into the septation of four different compartments: (1) the atria, (2) the ventricles, (3) the primary myocardium of the AV canal and primary (or interventricular) foramen, and (4) the outflow tract. Different components contribute to the septation of the heart being the muscular septa that form in the atrial and ventricular chambers, and the nonmuscular endocardial or AV cushions, outflow tract ridges, and the dorsal mesenchymal protrusion, also called vestibular spine (fig. 6). The endocardial cushions are initially acellular structures filled with cardiac jelly produced by the myocardium. Prior to septation, these structures are populated by endocardially derived cells in case of the AV canal and in case of the outflow tract ridges also by neural crest-derived cells.

The dorsal mesenchymal protrusion develops differently at the dorsal side of the heart and is dorsally contiguous with the mesenchyme of the body wall, and ventrally with the dorsal AV cushion and the mesenchymal cap of the primary atrial septum (fig. 6b). The dorsal mesenchymal protrusion has an extracardiac origin, the distinction between endocardium- and dorsal mesenchymal protrusion-derived cells can be observed on the basis of genetic lineage tracings and their anatomical position in the heart [26, 27]. In humans, maldevelopment of the dorsal mesenchymal protrusion would result in AV septal defects as absence of the dorsal mesenchymal protrusion is observed in fetuses with the Down syndrome [28, 29; for more information on Down syndrome, see the chapter by Kruszka, p. 82].

Atrial Septation

During uterine life, the atria are not entirely separated from one another and atrial septation occurs in phases, permitting right-left atrial shunting of blood.

Atrial septation starts with the formation of the primary septum at CS12 (fig. 6). The septum grows towards the AV canal at the right side of the midline. The mesenchymal cap on the edge of the primary septum is contiguous with the ventral AV cushion, and with the dorsal mesenchymal protrusion and the dorsal AV cushion (fig. 6). The primary atrial foramen or ostium primum is lined by this mesenchymal complex and permits shunting. With ongoing growth of the primary septum, the ostium primum closes (fig. 6) at CS16. However, prior to full closure, at CS15, small holes develop in the septum primum, which merge, forming the secondary foramen or ostium secundum (fig. 6), which then permits the right-left shunting of blood.

From CS17 onwards, the dorsal muscular wall of the right atrium folds down to form the secondary atrial septum at the right side of the primary septum, covering the secondary foramen (fig. 6). As fetal blood pressure is higher in the right atrium than in the left, blood flows from the right to the left side. After birth, when the pressure gradient inverts, the secondary foramen closes as the primary and secondary septum are squeezed together. The oval fossa is the part of the primary septum that remains uncovered by the secondary septum (fig. 6).

Ventricular Septation

The interventricular septum in the formed heart has a myocardial and a membranous part. The development of the muscular part is described below; the membranous part will be discussed with the septation of the primary foramen.

When the right and left ventricles form by expansion from the primary heart tube, the cells in between them do not follow the chamber myocardial gene program and form the top of the ventricular septum. The crest of the ventricular septum connects with the caudal, or dorsal, AV cushion. Lineage studies have shown that the cells that make up the ventricular septum are the cells that made up the left embryonic ventricular free wall [8].

Septation of the Atrioventricular Canal and Primary Foramen

Due to the laminar blood in the embryonic cardiovascular system, there is already a separated left- and

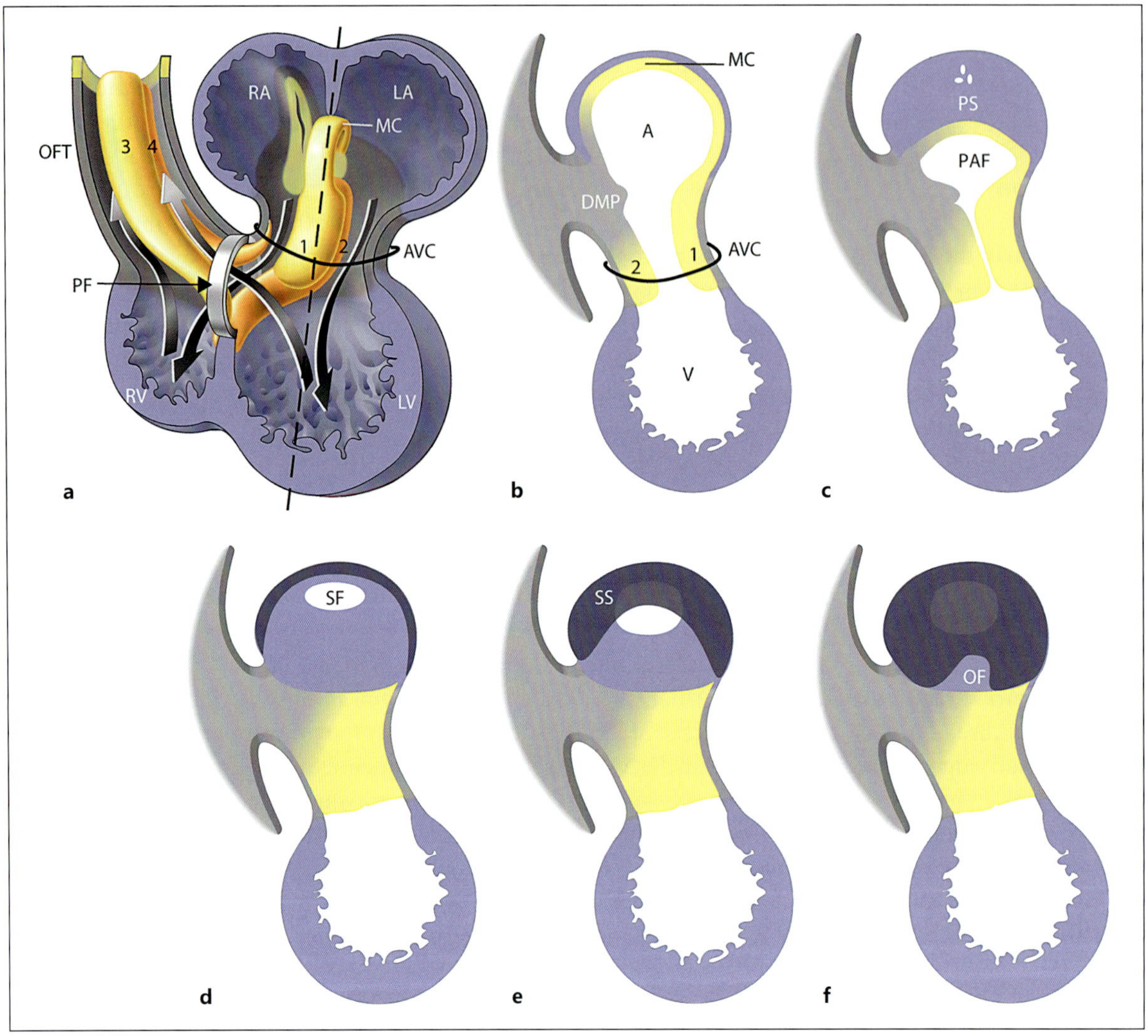

Fig. 6. Septation of the atria and primary foramen. **a** Schematic drawing of the chamber-forming heart with the AV canal (AVC) and outflow tract (OFT) cushions and ridges. The two arrows going down, through the AV canal, in the ventricle, represent the blood flow during diastole. The two arrows pointing toward the direction of the outflow tract represent the blood flow during systole. Note that the primary foramen (PF) is the cross road of the blood running from the right atrium (RA) to the right ventricle (RV), and the blood running from the left ventricle (LV) to the outflow tract. **b–f** Sagittal sections at the level of the dotted line in panel **a**. **b** The ventral and dorsal endocardial cushions (numbered 1 and 2) are growing towards each other. **c** The primary atrial foramen (PAF) is closing due to the ingrowth of the primary atrial septum (PS), with its mesenchymal cap (MC), the dorsal mesenchymal protrusion (DMP), and the endocardial cushions. **c**, **d** Subsequently, holes appear small in the primary septum, which merge forming the secondary foramen (SF). **d–f** The secondary septum (SS) then grows at the right side of the primary septum covering the secondary foramen and the rest of the primary atrial septum, leaving at the right surface of the atrial septum only the oval fossa (OF) uncovered. LA = Left atrium; A = atrium; V = ventricle; 3, 4 = septal and parietal outflow tract ridges.

right-sided circulation before the heart is septated [30]. The primary foramen is the region of the primary heart tube in between the left and right ventricles (fig. 6). This region is often called the interventricular foramen, however, it is never situated between the two ventricles, but on top of them. Through this foramen, the right atrium connects with the right ventricle and the left ventricle connects to the aorta. Obviously, this situation is maintained in adult life, thus the primary foramen becomes divided by the membranous septum into a left and right part at the end of CS18, but never closes.

The AV canal is divided by the ventral and dorsal endocardial cushion into a left and a right half. Also, the outflow tract is divided by two cushions, known as the septal and parietal outflow tract ridges, forming a pulmonary and an aortic channel (fig. 6). Separation of the primary foramen is achieved by the fusion of the AV cushions and outflow tract ridges, resulting into the left-ventricular outlet and the right-ventricular inlet. In the adult heart, the membranous part of the ventricular septum is the remnant of the fused AV and outflow tract cushions.

Separation of the Outflow Tract

At CS12, the outflow tract is a myocardial tube that runs from the developing ventricles to the aortic sac, which is connected to the pharyngeal arch arteries. During development, the ridges separate the outflow tract, resulting into a fully separated pulmonary and aortic channel at CS18 [31].

The separation occurs gradually in a distal to proximal manner, starting at CS14. The ridges lay in a spiral fashion, which gives rise to an 180° twist of the pulmonary and aortic channels, the future pulmonary trunk and ascending aorta. During septation, the outflow tract myocardium becomes incorporated into the right ventricle. The distal myocardial border retracts to the level of the semilunar valves, by which the coronary orifices no longer take origin from cardiac contractile tissue.

The pulmonary trunk is separated from the ascending aorta by protrusion of the pharyngeal mesenchyme, termed the aortopulmonary septum, which grows into the aortic sac and connects distally to the spiraling outflow tract ridges. Along with the separation of the outflow tract, a complex system of three pairs of pharyngeal arch arteries remodels into the aortic arch and pulmonary trunk.

The Cardiac Connective Tissues

Most of the adult heart volume is made up by cardiomyocytes; however, a significant 20% of the cells in the heart is made up by fibroblasts, smooth muscle cells, and endothelial cells [32]. During development, there are four sources of connective tissue cells in the heart: (1) the endocardium, (2) the dorsal mesenchymal protrusion, (3) the cardiac neural crest, and (4) the epicardium. In addition, bone marrow-derived cells also populate the heart in adult life [33]. The first three populations are already discussed; the epicardium develops from the proepicardium as follows.

The proepicardium is a medusa-like structure, which develops at the venous pole of the heart at CS10. At CS11, the villi of the proepicardium make contact with the outer surface of the heart and then grow to cover the entire heart tube with epicardium (CS16). The epicardium then gives rise to a mesenchymal layer between the myocardium and the epicardial outer layer termed the sub/epicardial mesenchyme (CS15). This mesenchyme partly contributes to the fibroblasts populating the heart and the developing coronary arteries.

Development of the Cardiac Vasculature

The coronary veins are formed by sprouting from the sinus venosus and cover the heart by expanding already connected vessels. The coronary arteries develop in the subepicardial mesenchyme between CS16 and CS18. First a plexus forms in the mesenchyme, which later remodels into the coronary artery system. After the coronary tree has developed, the connection with the aorta is established. The signals that promote the coronary arteries to grow toward the aorta and perforate the aortic wall connecting with the systemic circulatory system are as yet unknown.

The Insulating Plane

The insulation separating the myocardium of the atria and ventricles comprises both the annulus fibrosus in the strict sense, the fibrous tissue surrounding the AV junctions, as well as the AV sulcus mesenchyme, which resides at the outer surface of the heart [34].

The annulus fibrosus is contiguous with the fibrous tissues of the valves and is implicated for the support of the valves [35]. Recent lineage studies demonstrated that both endocardially as well as epicardially derived cells contribute to the insulating plane [24, 36–38].

Development of the Valves

Unidirectional Flow in the Primitive Heart

Valves are required for a unidirectional flow of blood preventing regurgitation of blood. However, in the primary heart tube, which is devoid of valves, regurgitation is prevented by the complete closure of the cardiac lumen during the peristaltic waves of contraction. The full closure of the heart tube can be owing to the presence of cardiac jelly, i.e. extracellular matrix depositions in between the endocardium and the myocardium, which functions as a stuffer substance to close the cardiac lumen.

At the site where the chambers are formed, cardiac jelly is no longer produced. The venous pole, AV canal, and outflow tract myocardium retain their primary phenotype. The cardiac jelly in these regions remodels into cushions and ridges, which eventually differentiate into the valves. Before the valves are formed, it is the slow-conducting and long-lasting contractile properties of the primary myocardium and the maintenance of the cushions in these regions that enable these regions to function as sphincters [2].

The Atrioventricular Valves

Within the AV canal, the valves are formed from the dorsal and ventral AV cushions as well as from the lateral AV cushions. To form valves, the cushions need to detach from the underlying myocardium. Different valve leaflets detach from the myocardium via different mechanisms (fig. 7).

The part of the cushions forming the aortic leaflet of the mitral valve protrudes from the outset into the left ventricular lumen and thus is never supported by myocardium (fig. 7). The septal leaflet of the tricuspid valve detaches from the underlying myocardium by apoptosis at CS23 (fig. 7). The anterior and posterior leaflet of the tricuspid valve and the parietal leaflet of the mitral valve are derived from the lateral AV cushions. These valves detach from the ventricle by excavation and not by apoptosis. So the ventricular lumen forms behind the cushions creating a space, liberating the valve leaflets, which starts at CS19 (fig. 7). A small number of cardiomyocytes remain in the forming valves, which are removed by apoptosis during subsequent development.

The Semilunar Valves

In addition to the two outflow tract ridges described in the paragraphs on septation, two intercalated ridges form in the proximal part of the outflow tract. In contrast to the AV valves, the arterial valves are prevented from prolapsing by their semilunar shape and not by chordae tendineae. This shape is achieved by apoptosis of the ridges at the distal side of the leaflet. Subsequently, the initially shaped valves elongate by proliferation of the remaining mesenchyme and eventually thin.

Remodeling of the Embryonic Valves

Finally, the AV and outflow tract valves mature slender valves organized in three layers. (1) The atrialis layer of the AV valve leaflets faces the atrial side and the ventricularis layer of the outflow tract valves faces the ventricular side. These sides, which face the upstream compartment, are primarily composed of elastic fibers, which provide motility to the leaflets. (2) The fibrosa, on the opposite side, is providing stiffness to the valve leaflets. (3) The spongiosa, in between the previous two layers, is composed of proteoglycans for compressibility of the valve leaflets [39].

Future Perspective

Taking together, in the last decades, we have learned a lot about how normal cardiac development takes place. We now know that the linear heart tube contains little more than the precursor cells for the left ventricle. We also learned that the heart grows by addition of cells from the surrounding pericardial wall. Consequently, the linear heart tube does not contain the precursors for all the cardiac chambers. In addition, we now know that the conduction system develops from those regions that are refrained from chamber formation. Despite this enormous leap forward, most congenital cardiac malformations have no identifiable genetic cause. This may find its origin in the robustness of cardiac morphogenesis, as demonstrated by the fact that autosomal dominant mutations in cardiac transcription factors such as Nkx2.5 or Tbx20 lead to a variety of cardiac malformations (see chapter

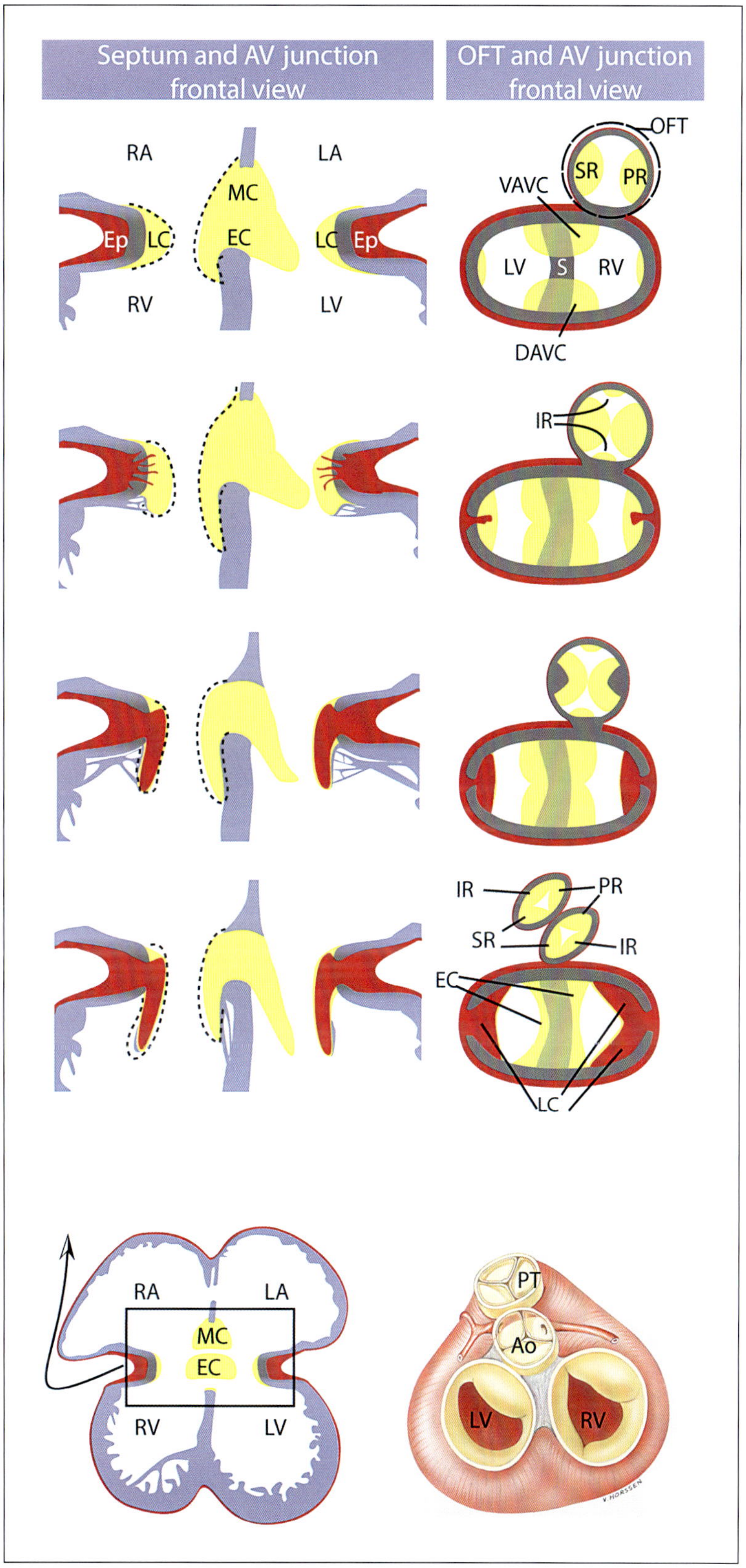

Fig. 7. Development of the AV and outflow tract (OFT) valves and their contributing tissues. The columns show schematic drawings of valve development in the AV canal (left column) and in the developing outflow tract (right column). Red = Epicardium (Ep); gray = primary myocardium; yellow is endocardial cushion tissue (EC) (see online version for colors). Note that in the outflow tract the cells are primarily neural crest derived and in the AV canal endocardial derived. RA = Right atrium; LA = left atrium; RV = right ventricle; LV = left ventricle; MC = mesenchymal cap; LC = lateral cushion; VAVC = ventral AV cushion; DAVC = dorsal AV cushion; SR = septal ridge; PR = parietal ridge; IR = intercalated ridge; S = septum; PT = pulmonary trunk; Ao = aorta.

by Borlak and Ciribilli for discussion on transcription factors on p. 131). On the other hand, it could also indicate that more complex genetic models underlie congenital heart diseases, including copy number variations, coinheritance of common variants with low penetrance, somatic mutations, and mutations in noncoding regions such as enhancers.

References

1 Sylva M, van den Hoff MJ, Moorman AF: Development of the human heart. Am J Med Genet A 2014;164A:1347–1371.

2 Moorman AFM, Christoffels VM, Anderson RH, van den Hoff MJB: The heart-forming fields: one or multiple? Philos Trans R Soc B Biol Sci 2007;362:1257–1265.

3 Sizarov A, Ya J, de Boer BA, et al: Formation of the building plan of the human heart: morphogenesis, growth, and differentiation. Circulation 2011;123:1125–1135.

4 van den Berg G, Abu-Issa R, de Boer BA, et al: A caudal proliferating growth center contributes to both poles of the forming heart tube. Circ Res 2009;104:179–188.

5 de Boer BA, van den Berg G, de Boer PA, Moorman AF, Ruijter JM: Growth of the developing mouse heart: an interactive qualitative and quantitative 3D atlas. Dev Biol 2012;368:203–213.

6 Rana MS, Horsten NC, Tesink-Taekema S, et al: Trabeculated right ventricular free wall in the chicken heart forms by ventricularization of the myocardium initially forming the outflow tract. Circ Res 2007;100:1000–1007.

7 Kelly RG, Brown NA, Buckingham ME: The arterial pole of the mouse heart forms from Fgf10-expressing cells in pharyngeal mesoderm. Dev Cell 2001;1:435–440.

8 Aanhaanen WT, Brons JF, Domínguez JN, et al: The Tbx2+ primary myocardium of the atrioventricular canal forms the atrioventricular node and the base of the left ventricle. Circ Res 2009;104:1267–1274.

9 Buckingham M, Meilhac S, Zaffran S: Building the mammalian heart from two sources of myocardial cells. Nat Rev Genet 2005;6:826–835.

10 Dyer LA, Kirby ML: The role of secondary heart field in cardiac development. Dev Biol 2009;336:137–144.

11 Rochais F, Mesbah K, Kelly RG: Signaling pathways controlling second heart field development. Circ Res 2009;104:933–942.

12 Moorman AFM, Christoffels VM: Cardiac chamber formation: development, genes, and evolution. Physiol Rev 2003;83:1223–1267.

13 Franco D, Campione M: The role of Pitx2 during cardiac development. Linking left-right signaling and congenital heart diseases. Trends Cardiovasc Med 2003;13:157–163.

14 Christoffels VM, Habets PE, Franco D, et al: Chamber formation and morphogenesis in the developing mammalian heart. Dev Biol 2000;223:266–278.

15 Takeuchi JK, Ohgi M, Koshiba-Takeuchi K, et al: Tbx5 specifies the left/right ventricles and ventricular septum position during cardiogenesis. Development 2003;130:5953–5964.

16 Franco D, Meilhac SM, Christoffels VM, et al: Left and right ventricular contributions to the formation of the interventricular septum in the mouse heart. Dev Biol 2006;294:366–375.

17 Vincentz JW, Barnes RM, Firulli AB: Hand factors as regulators of cardiac morphogenesis and implications for congenital heart defects. Birth Defects Res A Clin Mol Teratol 2011;91:485–494.

18 Ieda M, Tsuchihashi T, Ivey KN, et al: Cardiac fibroblasts regulate myocardial proliferation through beta1 integrin signaling. Dev Cell 2009;16:233–244.

19 Lavine KJ, Yu K, White AC, et al: Endocardial and epicardial derived FGF signals regulate myocardial proliferation and differentiation in vivo. Dev Cell 2005;8:85–95.

20 Christoffels VM, Moorman AFM: Development of the cardiac conduction system: why are some regions of the heart more arrhythmogenic than others? Circ Arrhythmia Electrophysiol 2009;2:195–207.

21 Luxan G, Casanova JC, Martínez-Poveda B, et al: Mutations in the NOTCH pathway regulator MIB1 cause left ventricular noncompaction cardiomyopathy. Nat Med 2013;19:193–201.

22 de Jong F, Opthof T, Wilde AA, et al: Persisting zones of slow impulse conduction in developing chicken hearts. Circ Res 1992;71:240–250.

23 Hoff EC, Kramer TC, DuBois D, Patten BM: The development of the electrocardiogram of the embryonic heart. Am Heart J 1939;17:470–488.

24 Aanhaanen WT, Mommersteeg MT, Norden J, et al: Developmental origin, growth, and three-dimensional architecture of the atrioventricular conduction axis of the mouse heart. Circ Res 2010;107:728–736.

25 Christoffels VM, Smits GJ, Kispert A, Moorman AF: Development of the pacemaker tissues of the heart. Circ Res 2010;106:240–254.

26 Snarr BS, Wirrig EE, Phelps AL, Trusk TC, Wessels A: A spatiotemporal evaluation of the contribution of the dorsal mesenchymal protrusion to cardiac development. Dev Dyn 2007;236:1287–1294.

27 Goddeeris MM, Rho S, Petiet A, et al: Intracardiac septation requires hedgehog-dependent cellular contributions from outside the heart. Development 2008;135:1887–1895.

28 Webb S, Anderson RH, Lamers WH, Brown NA: Mechanisms of deficient cardiac septation in the mouse with trisomy 16. Circ Res 1999;84:897–905.

29 Blom NA, Ottenkamp J, Wenink AG, Gittenberger-de Groot AC: Deficiency of the vestibular spine in atrioventricular septal defects in human fetuses with Down syndrome. Am J Cardiol 2003;91:180–184.

30 Hogers B, DeRuiter MC, Baasten AMJ, Gittenberger-de Groot AC, Poelmann RE: Intracardiac blood flow patterns related to the yolk sac circulation of the chick embryo. Circ Res 1995;76:871–877.

31 Sizarov A, Lamers WH, Mohun TJ, et al: Three-dimensional and molecular analysis of the arterial pole of the developing human heart. J Anat 2012;220:336–349.

32 Banerjee I, Fuseler JW, Price RL, Borg TK, Baudino TA: Determination of cell types and numbers during cardiac development in the neonatal and adult rat and mouse. Am J Physiol Heart Circ Physiol 2007;293:H1883–H1891.

33 Zeisberg EM, Kalluri R: Origins of cardiac fibroblasts. Circ Res 2010;107:1304–1312.

34 Becker AE, Anderson RH, Durrer D, Wellens HJJ: The anatomical substrates of Wolff-Parkinson-White syndrome. A clinicopathologic correlation in seven patients. Circulation 1978;57:870–879.

35 Angelini A, Ho SY, Anderson RH, Davies MJ, Becker AE: A histological study of the atrioventricular junction in hearts with normal and prolapsed leaflets of the mitral valve. Br Heart J 1988;59:712–716.

36 de Lange FJ, Moorman AF, Anderson RH, et al: Lineage and morphogenetic analysis of the cardiac valves. Circ Res 2004;95:645–654.
37 Zhou B, von Gise A, Ma Q, Hu YW, Pu WT: Genetic fate mapping demonstrates contribution of epicardium-derived cells to the annulus fibrosis of the mammalian heart. Dev Biol 2010;338:251–261.
38 Wessels A, van den Hoff MJ, Adamo RF, et al: Epicardially derived fibroblasts preferentially contribute to the parietal leaflets of the atrioventricular valves in the murine heart. Dev Biol 2012;366:111–124.
39 Hinton RB, Yutzey KE: Heart valve structure and function in development and disease. Annu Rev Physiol 2011;73:29–46.
40 Christoffels VM, Moorman AF: Development of the cardiac conduction system: why are some regions of the heart more arrhythmogenic than others? Circ Arrhythm Electrophysiol 2009;2:195–207.
41 Arraez-Aybar LA, Turrero-Nogues A, Marantos-Gamarra DG: Embryonic cardiac morphometry in Carnegie stages 15–23, from the Complutense University of Madrid Institute of Embryology Human Embryo Collection. Cells Tissues Organs 2008;187: 211–220.
42 Oostra RJ, Steding G, Lamers WH, Moorman AFM: Steding's and Virágh's Scanning Electron Microsocpy Atlas of the Developing Human Heart Heart. New York, Springer, 2007.
43 O'Rahilly R, Müller F: Developmental Stages in Human Embryos. Washington, Carnegie Institute, 1987.

Dr. Antoon F.M. Moorman
Department of Anatomy, Embryology and Physiology
Academic Medical Center, Meibergdreef 15
NL–1105 AZ Amsterdam (The Netherlands)
E-Mail a.f.moorman@amc.nl

2 Epidemiology

Muenke M, Kruszka PS, Sable CA, Belmont JW (eds): Congenital Heart Disease: Molecular Genetics, Principles of Diagnosis and Treatment. Basel, Karger, 2015, pp 28–45
DOI: 10.1159/000375203

Epidemiology and Prevention of Congenital Heart Defects

Lorenzo D. Botto

Division of Medical Genetics, Department of Pediatrics, University of Utah, Salt Lake City, Utah, USA

Abstract

Congenital heart defects are common, costly, and critical – and they are more so than they ought to be because of the limitations of treatment and the inability to prevent what can be prevented. Major heart defects occur in nearly 1 in 100 births, or 1.2 million babies worldwide every year, and severe heart defects in 1 in 300 births, or approximately 340,000 worldwide. These account for 1 in 3 neonatal deaths and nearly 1 in 10 infant deaths in developed countries. Treatment is costly: heart defects are the most expensive birth defect, and medical costs are only a fraction of the true costs, which accumulate over a lifetime (many complex heart defects are treated, not cured) and affect also the productivity of patients and families. As survival has improved in the last decades, the number of adolescents and adults with heart defects has increased: estimates suggest that, at least in North America, currently more adults are living with heart defects than children, underscoring the need for appropriate services in this population. Potent genetic factors (mostly chromosomal anomalies but also genomic imbalances and rare Mendelian conditions) account for at least 15% (perhaps 30%) of cases. Subtler genetic effects, particularly in the context of gene-environment interactions, have been postulated but to date have not been well characterized. Maternal and environmental factors are also incompletely known, but a few are well characterized and prime targets for primary prevention. These include maternal chronic illnesses, especially diabetes, select medications, and probably smoking and obesity. Multivitamin supplementation is a likely protective factor, though, unlike for neural tube defects, folic acid alone in small amounts may not be. The key for primary prevention is to begin from before conception and target multiple risk factors in an integrated approach aiming at optimal health through the lifespan. This approach will not only reduce the risk for heart defects, but also promote the overall health of the fetus and the woman. Several competing forces and trends will likely modify the epidemiology and prevention of heart defects – prenatal diagnosis and terminations, newborn screening, changing rates of risk factors (e.g. the rise in diabetes in developing countries or new teratogens), etiologic research, approaches to treatment and care, and the increasing focus on preconception care. A concerted effort between researchers, clinicians, and public health professionals will be crucial in improving outcomes and fulfilling the promise of prevention.

Understanding the Problem

Congenital heart defects are common, costly, and critical – epidemiology proves this – and they are more so than they ought to be because even causes that are known are not effectively prevented. This review will briefly summarize the data – the facts but also the gaps – delineating the present but also discussing some trends that will likely shape the future. The review will be necessarily selective. In-depth discussions on the epidemiology and prevention of heart defects are available [1], including recent reviews on modifiable risk factors [1–3]. The statement also underscores an underlying theme of this review – the essential link between epidemiology and prevention. This link is crucial: the epidemiology of heart defects is viewed here not as an obligatory footnote in a textbook but as a key component of an action plan (fig. 1): a self-reinforcing cycle that proceeds from measuring the impact of congenital heart defects *(incentive)* to identifying modifiable causes *(evidence)* and finally implementing global strategies for effective prevention *(strategies)*.

Common, Costly, and Critical: Epidemiology as an Incentive for Action

The 'descriptive epidemiology' of congenital heart defects – frequency, costs, and outcomes – provides crucial measures of impact. When prevention is available but not implemented, these same measures also convey the human cost of inaction – lost lives, unnecessary illness and disability, and wasted money. As springboards for action, these measures must be reliable (valid and possibly precise), relevant to the goals and targets of prevention, and timely. Remarkably, these data can be difficult to come by; when available, they may turn out to be surprisingly fragmentary, imprecise, or old. Yet, with all their limitations, the available data can be used to outline answers to some key questions.

How Common Are Congenital Heart Defects?

Overall, the birth prevalence of major congenital heart defects is approximately 1% [1, 4–7]. Estimating this figure is the subject of many studies, regular reviews, and some debate [4, 7]. The summary estimate is important for one main reason: raising awareness. For most other purposes, however, it is nearly useless. Congenital heart defects are remarkably heterogeneous in their clinical presentation, health impact, and, to a degree, risk factor profile. Examining specific subsets (grouped by anatomy, severity, or embryology, depending on the goal of the analysis), rather than all heart defects combined, is nearly invariably more informative and useful. The following example makes this point with respect to birth prevalence (fig. 2) and will be reinforced when discussing health outcomes and cost.

As a group a few types, the more severe, show limited variability in birth prevalence across studies. Combined, they occur in 2–3/1,000 births. Definitions of what constitutes 'severe' heart defects vary [8, 9], but the overall pattern remains the same. As discussed later, this relatively small group of conditions contributes to a disproportionately high fraction of death, disability, and costs associated with congenital heart defects. The remaining group – mostly septal defects, pulmonic and aortic stenoses – are usually (but not always) milder clinically and are more common (fig. 2), occurring in 4–8/1,000 births. Their birth prevalence is much more variable across studies; in fact, they are the main contributors to the variation in the overall frequency of heart defects across studies (5–15/1,000 in this example) [10–13]. International surveys and meta-analyses reach these same broad conclusions [4, 5]. The variability could be even greater if even the mildest defects are included: for example, small muscular ventricular septal defects, which are nearly always clinically benign and close spontaneously, may be found in 1% or more babies by echocardiography [13–15].

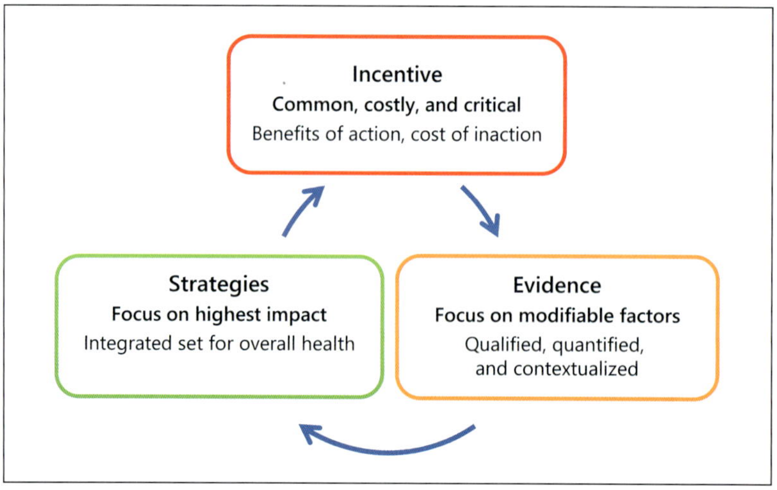

Fig. 1. The cycle from epidemiology to prevention: incentive, evidence, and strategies.

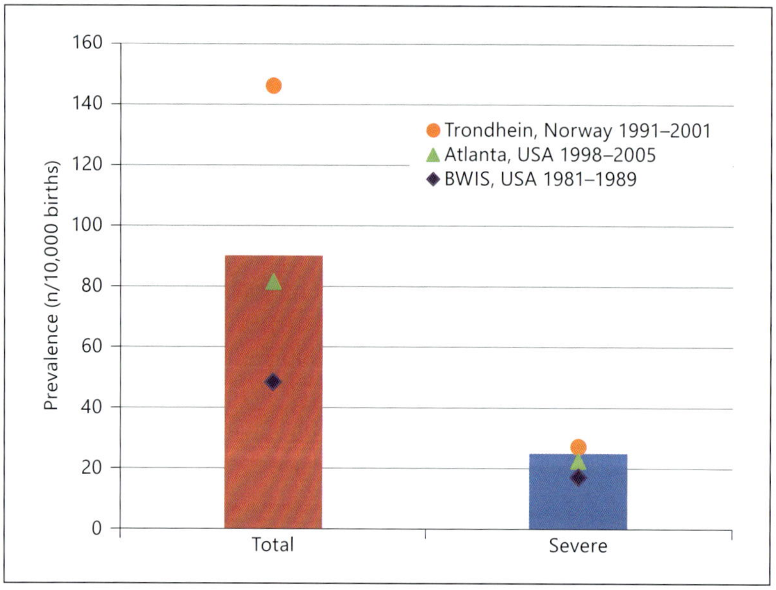

Fig. 2. Birth prevalence of major congenital heart defects (overall and severe) in three studies [11–13] compared to estimated averages from the literature (overall rate, 9/1,000; rate for severe heart defects, 2.5/1,000). Severe heart defects include single ventricle, heterotaxy defects, conotruncal defects, atrioventricular septal defects, total anomalous venous return, hypoplastic left heart, coarctation of the aorta, interrupted aortic arch, and pulmonary atresia. Total major heart defects exclude minor heart defects as well as bicuspid aortic valve and patent ductus arteriosus. BWIS = Baltimore-Washington Infant Study.

These rates can be translated into numbers of babies born in a population in a given time period. Such numbers provide another measure of the frequency of congenital heart defects, one that is more directly helpful for treatment planning and policy development.

Worldwide (fig. 3), 1.2 million affected babies may be born every year (9/1,000 or 135 million births). Of these, at least 300,000 (2–3/1,000) will have severe conditions that require prompt and often complex surgical and medical care to avoid death or disability. Notably, most affected babies will be born in countries with few of the resources needed for treatment and management (fig. 4). In all countries, but particularly these, primary prevention, which costs less, would be particularly beneficial.

What Drives the Variations in Reported Birth Prevalence?

The variation in birth prevalence of the milder defects (which drive the overall rate) has never

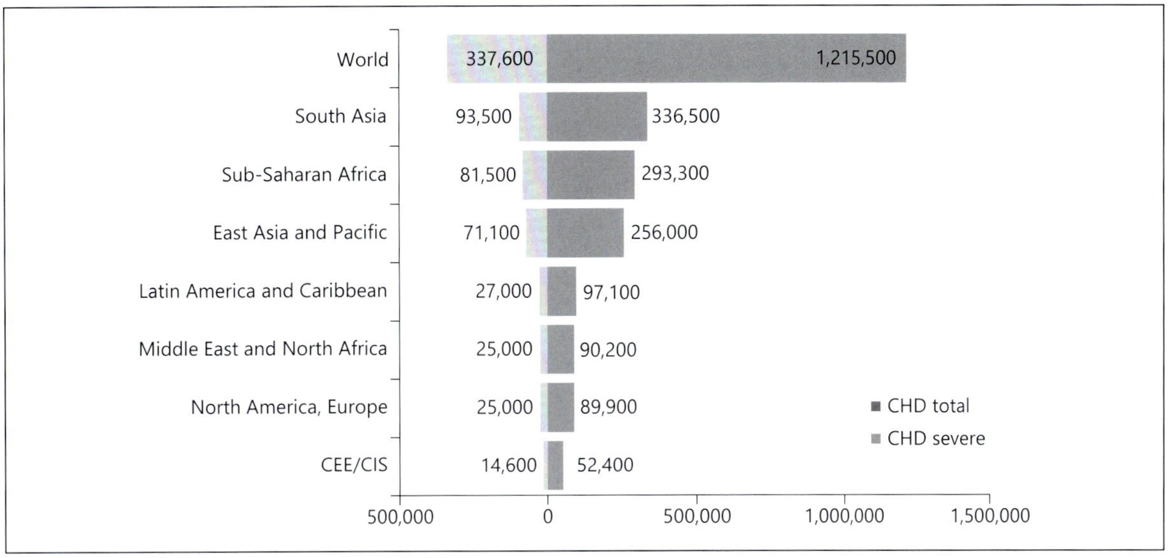

Fig. 3. Estimated number of babies born yearly in different regions of the world with major (birth prevalence, 9/1,000) and severe heart defects (2.5/1,000). CEE/CIS = Central and Eastern Europe/Commonwealth of Independent States; CHD = congenital heart disease.

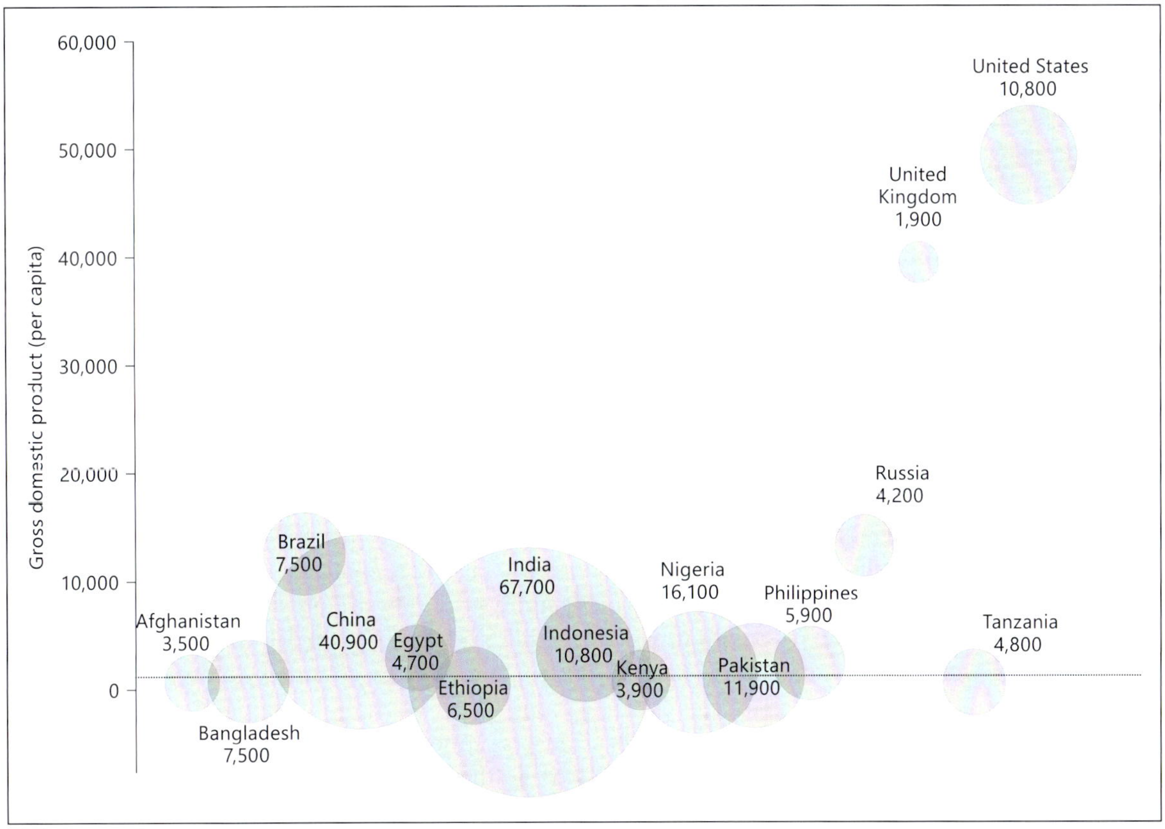

Fig. 4. Estimated number of babies born with severe congenital heart defects (birth prevalence, 2.5/1,000) in selected countries by per capita gross domestic product. The countries represented account for over 60% of all births worldwide. The areas of the circles are proportional to the number of babies affected. Data from UNICEF and World Health Organization, 2011.

been convincingly proven to be real. The severalfold increase in these rates in recent decades [7, 16–18], concomitant with the diffusion of echocardiography, supports the primary role of methodology, rather than biology, in driving these changes. When examining how rates vary by program or over time, even within the same program, it is important to appreciate the many methodological factors that can raise or lower reported rates, and particularly how cases are ascertained, reported, reviewed clinically, classified, and coded [1, 4, 5, 19]. Additional factors include the reporting and inclusion of fetal deaths [20–22], and, particularly in recent years, of pregnancy terminations. The example of hypoplastic left-heart syndrome is telling: the fraction of cases prenatally diagnosed and terminated varies greatly in countries and can exceed 50% [1, 23, 24]. Small changes in how these cases are reported can influence rates considerably; also, not capturing these cases will underestimate, sometimes to a large degree, the burden of congenital heart defects.

Not all variation is necessarily spurious. Small differences in birth prevalence by sex or ethnic origin are probably real. Several studies have indicated slightly higher rates of D-transposition of the great arteries and left-sided obstructive defects in boys than in girls, and in non-Hispanic white than in non-Hispanic black persons [12, 16, 25–27]; these variations have yet to be satisfactorily explained in terms of either biology or methodology.

How Many People Are Living with Congenital Heart Defects – Including Adults?

Simply counting how many people are living with congenital heart defects in the general population has proven remarkably difficult. Surprisingly, few primary data are available. A major challenge is the general lack of accurate, population-based sources of data with validated diagnoses. Instead, available databases are typically dispersed across diverse health delivery systems and service providers, are designed for purposes other than clinical or public health evaluation, and include diagnoses based on administrative coding. In the absence of well-designed national surveillance activities for heart defects in adolescents and adults, it has proven extremely challenging to monitor prevalence and outcome beyond childhood. Unsurprisingly, information on population prevalence is scarce and often relies on statistical modeling [8] or on linkages between administrative databases [28]. Yet, even these preliminary estimates are notable for three main reasons. First, numbers are high: in every 200 persons in the United States, nearly 1 was estimated to be living with a heart defect [8], and 1 in 165 in Quebec [28]. Second, in both studies [8, 28], there were more adults than children living with heart defects. Third, these numbers are expected to increase [8, 28], e.g. by about 5%/year according to one estimate [29]. These findings, despite their limitations, underscore the urgent need to invest in the specialized care of adolescents and adults with congenital heart defects (see Niwa chapter on Adults with Congenital Heart Disease, p. 70). They also highlight the lack of systematic, population-based surveillance programs that can track *over time* the evolution of these trends, which have obvious implications for quality of care, health services planning, and costs.

How Costly Are Congenital Heart Defects?

Congenital heart defects are the most expensive of all birth defects [30, 31]. In the United States, six of the ten birth defects with highest hospital charges were congenital heart defects, and two – hypoplastic left heart and truncus arteriosus – topped the list [30]. In a large survey of children's hospitals, nine types of congenital heart defects were in the top tier of costs [31]. Generating comprehensive estimates of costs has proven difficult – not only do costs vary by institution [32], general cost estimates also depend on the context, perspective, and definitions. The local context is critical: clinical factors (survival or rate of complications) and organizational systems (health delivery systems or payer structure) vary by country and over time in directions which are not always predictable. Cost estimates cannot be simply 'borrowed' from one country to the next. Perspective is also important: depending on whose view is taken – the patient (client), the health delivery system, or society as a whole – estimates can vary considerably. Finally, definitions, and in particular inclusion criteria, are

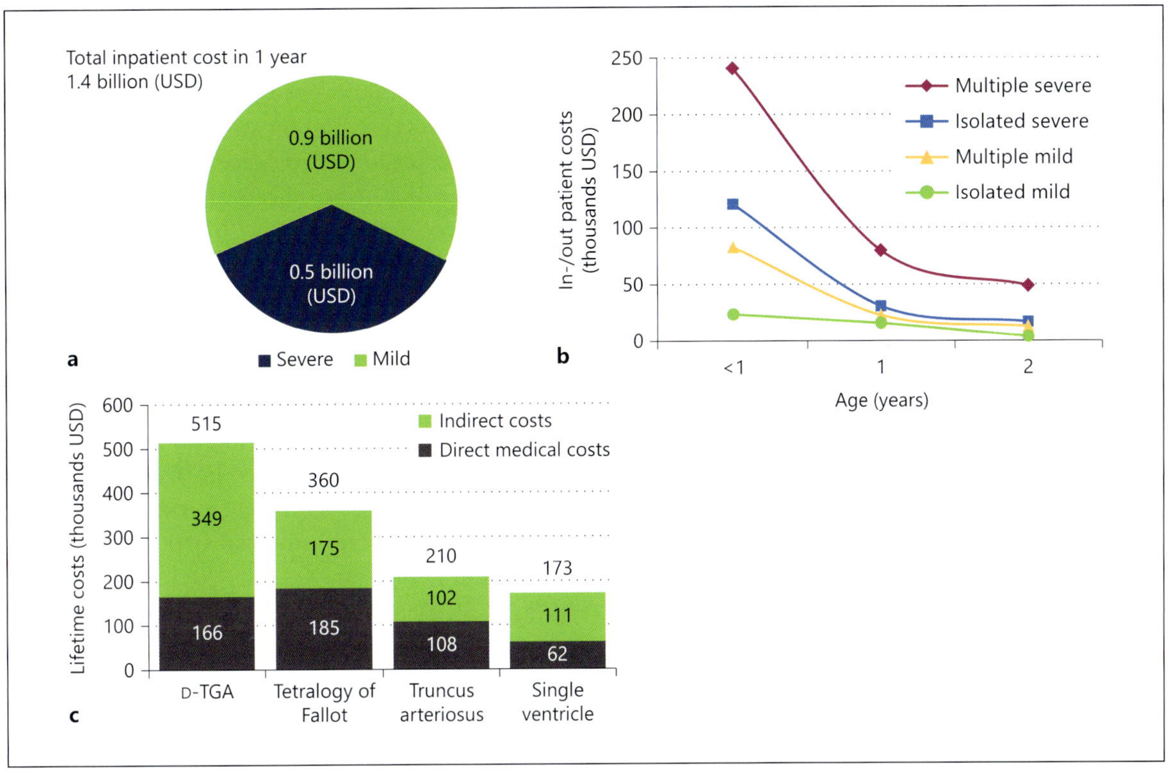

Fig. 5. Estimates of costs for congenital heart defects in the United States: selected data [33, 34]. **a** Estimated inpatient costs for 1 year due to congenital heart defects (overall and for severe types) in 2004. **b** In- and outpatient costs (Mediscan data) for children under 3 years of age by type of congenital heart defect. **c** Estimated lifetime costs (direct and indirect, in 1992) per case. D-TGA = D-Transposition of the great arteries.

crucial: inpatient medical costs are an important component of costs, but not the only one, and other direct and indirect costs, including loss of productivity, can add up quickly. A further challenge is estimating costs over the lifespan, which can provide a realistic assessment of the benefits of prevention. The complexities of cost estimation are many [1, 33–35]. Here only a few summary points are highlighted (fig. 5).

Short-Term Assessment: Cross-Sectional Costs

Cross-sectional costs are useful because they are more easily available than most other estimates and can provide an immediate, if rough, estimate of the potential impact of prevention on cost. For the United States, one study estimated that the nationwide cost in a single year (2004) for *inpatient* admissions of patients with congenital heart defects was 1.4 billion dollars [33, 36]. Over one third of this figure, 511 million dollars, was due to a relatively small subset of severe heart defects – conotruncal defects, single ventricle, hypoplastic left-heart syndrome, Ebstein's anomaly, and endocardial cushion defects. Infants accounted for 95% of these inpatient costs. In an attempt to incorporate also outpatient data, researchers used a different data set limited to a privately insured population and estimated medical costs (of in- and outpatients) associated with major heart defects to be approximately USD 100,000 among children up to 3 years of age [33]. For adults, few data are available, and these are likely underestimates due to the uncertainties of coding in administrative data sets [37].

Long-Term View: Lifetime Costs

Lifetime estimates are particularly important because they provide a more accurate view of the benefits of prevention – for example, preventing a diabetes-associated heart defect saves costs over a lifetime of that baby. Because of the time component, such estimates are understandably challenging, and require modeling, data, and assumptions. Comprehensive lifetime estimates are few. A landmark study in the United States estimated lifetime costs of USD 1.2 billion (in 1992) for a single-year birth cohort for children with one of four congenital heart defects – truncus arteriosus, D-transposition of the great arteries, tetralogy of Fallot, and single ventricle. Of these, direct medical costs, mainly surgical, were approximately USD 0.5 billion [34, 35]; indirect costs, including loss of productivity, were the greater part of the total estimate.

Even from this brief review, it is evident that, for such an important issue, data on costs are remarkably limited; the goal of having comprehensive, recent, nationally representative estimates lies still in the future. With few exceptions, available estimates are far from timely, a major limitation for such a dynamic issue as costs. These gaps reflect in part the limitations and accessibility of current data sources, which are often fragmented and opaque. Greater transparency and integration will be required for reliable cost information.

How Critical Are Heart Defects?

Much like costs, health outcomes – mortality, morbidity, and disability – are best evaluated within one's local setting. Evaluating and tracking outcomes locally can help identify population-specific problems and disparities, and their local determinants. Despite massive variations, some broad qualitative considerations can be made. Nearly everywhere, congenital heart defects are significant contributors to adverse health outcomes [1]. By way of example, mortality will be briefly discussed, though similar arguments can be made for other health outcomes, including morbidity, disability, and quality of life [1].

Internationally, congenital heart defects are the leading cause of *infant* deaths due to congenital anomalies – accounting for approximately 1 in 3 such infant deaths [38, 39]. The contribution to *neonatal* deaths is also significant: in the United States [40] and in several European countries [9], congenital heart defects account for an estimated 1 in 4 neonatal deaths due to birth defects. In developed countries, congenital heart defects are estimated to account for approximately 1 in 10 infant deaths from *any* cause [38, 39].

In infants and young children, a disproportionate fraction of deaths is due to relatively few types of heart defects, particularly hypoplastic left-heart syndrome, conotruncal defects, and atrioventricular septal defects [41]. This finding further underscores the importance of monitoring, preventing, and treating the subset of severe congenital heart defects. Notably, excess mortality does not end in early childhood, but extends for many decades into adult life, as documented in a longitudinal population-based study in Denmark [42] as well as in a study of death certificates in the United States [43].

Prevention: Evidence and Strategies

This brief survey of the epidemiology of occurrence, costs, and outcomes highlights the ongoing and, in fact, growing burden of congenital heart defects on individuals, families, and society. Advances in diagnosis and treatment will improve outcomes among those affected; to this day, however, many complex heart defects are treated, not cured.

The ideal goal is to maximize primary prevention to increase the odds that a baby is born with a normal heart and healthy. Primary prevention is predicated upon identifying and intervening effectively upon modifiable factors. For use in interventions, the evidence of risk factors must be valid and robust, and ideally quite specific – the risk factor must be qualified (what heart defect does it cause?), quantified (how high is the risk?), and contextualized (how many cases does it cause in this population?). Such evidence can provide a measurable basis for intervention. Reviews on many risk factors for congenital heart defects have been published [1–3]. Here, the focus will be on integrating such evidence into a prevention framework.

Integrating Interventions

The scientific evidence characterizing modifiable risk factors is a crucial, but not the only component of effective prevention. Translating such evidence into *maximal* prevention requires strategic thinking, an integrated approach across disciplines, and a combination of personal and population interventions throughout the lifespan [1, 44]. For example, integrating interventions will have benefits beyond a more efficient prevention of congenital heart defects. Many adverse reproductive outcomes, including congenital heart defects, share similar risk factors: diabetes, infections, and smoking are also risk factors for other birth defects, preterm birth, and intrauterine growth restriction, and, beyond pregnancy, they undermine a woman's health, increasing her risk for chronic illness and premature death. For these reasons, when developing recommendations for the primary prevention of heart defects it is reasonable to incorporate information not only on the risk for congenital heart defects, but also the overall benefits to fetal, infant, and maternal health.

When to Start Preventing?

Prevention needs to start before conception. The heart develops early in pregnancy: the primordial cardiac tube starts beating rhythmically at around 21 days after fertilization and continues to develop through complex processes of looping, septation, valve formation, and cell migration (neural crest cells/secondary heart field), all contributing to the final anatomy and function [45]. However, prenatal visits, when screening and pregnancy care typically occur (see chapter by Weinberg and Krishnan on Prenatal Evaluation of Congenital Heart Defects and Fetal Intervention on p. 269), often begin several weeks and even months after the last menstrual period, i.e. too late to prevent heart defects and most other birth defects. Even starting very early in pregnancy may be too late, because for many chronic conditions, such as maternal diabetes or phenylketonuria, metabolic control takes time. In addition, many pregnancies, at least half in the United States and probably most worldwide, are unplanned. Thus, to ensure maximal prevention for the largest population possible, preconception care needs to be promoted and practiced throughout the reproductive lifespan.

What Proportion of Heart Defects Can Be Prevented?

The answer to this crucial question is still unclear, because the cause of most cases that occur is still unknown. Genes, environment, and probably chance, all contribute to the risk for heart defects. As a first step to understanding the potential for prevention, one can reverse the question and examine the proportion that may not be preventable (for now), namely, the proportion of cases due to 'strong' genetic causes – chromosomal anomalies, genomic disorders (deletions or duplications), and single-gene conditions. Chromosomal anomalies alone seem to account for approximately 10–15% of cases of congenital heart defects, as highlighted (fig. 6) in a recent large population-based study [46]. In this study, 1 in 8 cases of major heart defects (12.3%) was associated with chromosomal anomalies. Notably, nearly 85% of these cases were accounted for by four conditions – the three common trisomies (21, 18, and 13, all influenced by maternal age) and deletion 22q11 (independent of maternal age). Also, the contribution of chromosomal anomalies varied greatly by type of heart defect, accounting for about two thirds of cases in some types but many fewer in others. For example, only a small fraction of hypoplastic left-heart syndrome and D-transposition of the great arteries were associated with chromosomal anomalies, leaving open the possibility that many of these cases might be amenable to primary prevention.

As a group, single-gene disorders (e.g. the Noonan, Alagille, and CHARGE syndromes) probably account for a much smaller fraction of cases. However, recent studies using whole exome/genome sequencing suggest that de novo mutations and novel copy number variants play a larger role than previously appreciated. In these initial studies, it has been suggested that de novo mutations might account for 10% of cases [47, 48], and copy number variants for perhaps 5% [49]. If these initial estimates are confirmed, the proportion of cases due to (strong) genetic factors, including chromosomal anomalies,

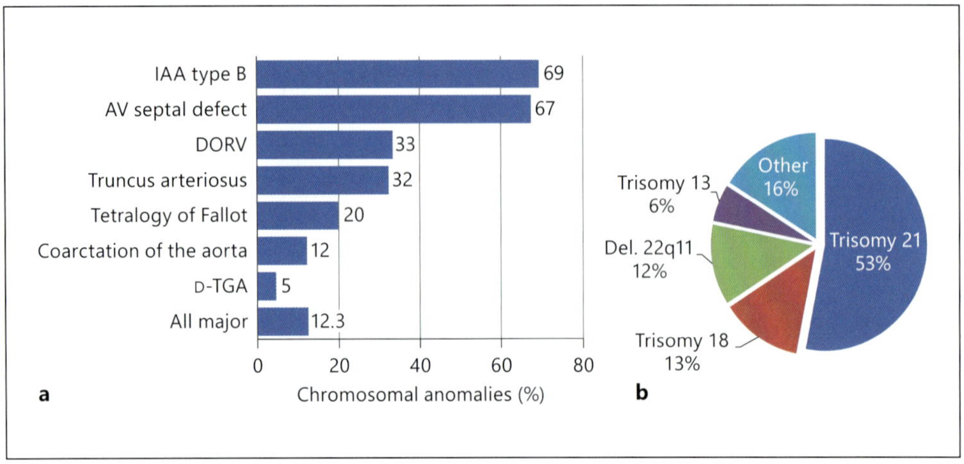

Fig. 6. Contribution of chromosomal anomalies to congenital heart defects overall and by type (**a**), and specific types of chromosomal anomalies identified among all major heart defects (**b**) [data from ref. 46]. AV = Atrioventricular; IAA = interruption of the aortic arch; DORV = double-outlet right ventricle; D-TGA = D-transposition of the great arteries.

could be at least 30%. What remains unclear is to what extent 'weaker' genetic loci can contribute to disease risk and, in particular, to gene-environment interactions that could be modified by preventive interventions.

Estimating How Many Cases Can Be Prevented

Considering now *modifiable* risk factors, it is possible to estimate the fraction of cases *in the population* that are attributable to those factors – in epidemiologic parlance or their etiologic or *population-attributable fraction*. This metric is useful when developing prevention strategies: when computed appropriately [50], the population-attributable fraction can be viewed as an estimate of how many cases might be prevented as the risk factor is progressively reduced. This metric also helps compare the potential impact of different risk factors in the same population. Of course, these estimates are meaningful to the extent that the evidence for causality is strong.

A key concept is that the population-attributable fraction is a function, mathematically determined, not only of the relative risk of disease but also of the *frequency of the risk factor* in the population. A risk factor can vary among countries [51], and several may be quite common in a given country (fig. 7).

As the frequency of risk factors (e.g. smoking rates or obesity) varies in different populations, so will their associated population-attributable fraction: the latter is, therefore, a local metric and can lead to different prevention priorities in different countries. This dependence on exposure rates (not only relative risk) underscores the importance of *surveillance* of risk factors – tracking exposure rates in the population over time: examples of such risk factor surveillance programs include PRAMS (Pregnancy Risk Assessment Monitoring Systems) in the United States [52, 53] and the STEPS program (Stepwise Approach to Surveillance) of the World Health Organization [54]. For similar reasons, even 'weak' risk factors (e.g. with a relative risk of 2 or less) can cause many cases of disease in a population if common enough. For example, smoking or obesity are associated with relatively modest relative risks for heart defects [1–3]; yet, in some areas, they are so common that they could account for a greater fraction of cases than much 'stronger' risk factors (if strength is measured solely on the basis of relative risk) if the latter occur among a tiny fraction of women of childbearing age. Every preventable case is important: however, estimates of the etiologic fraction help to provide a context for the potential benefits in relation to the costs of interventions on specific risk factors.

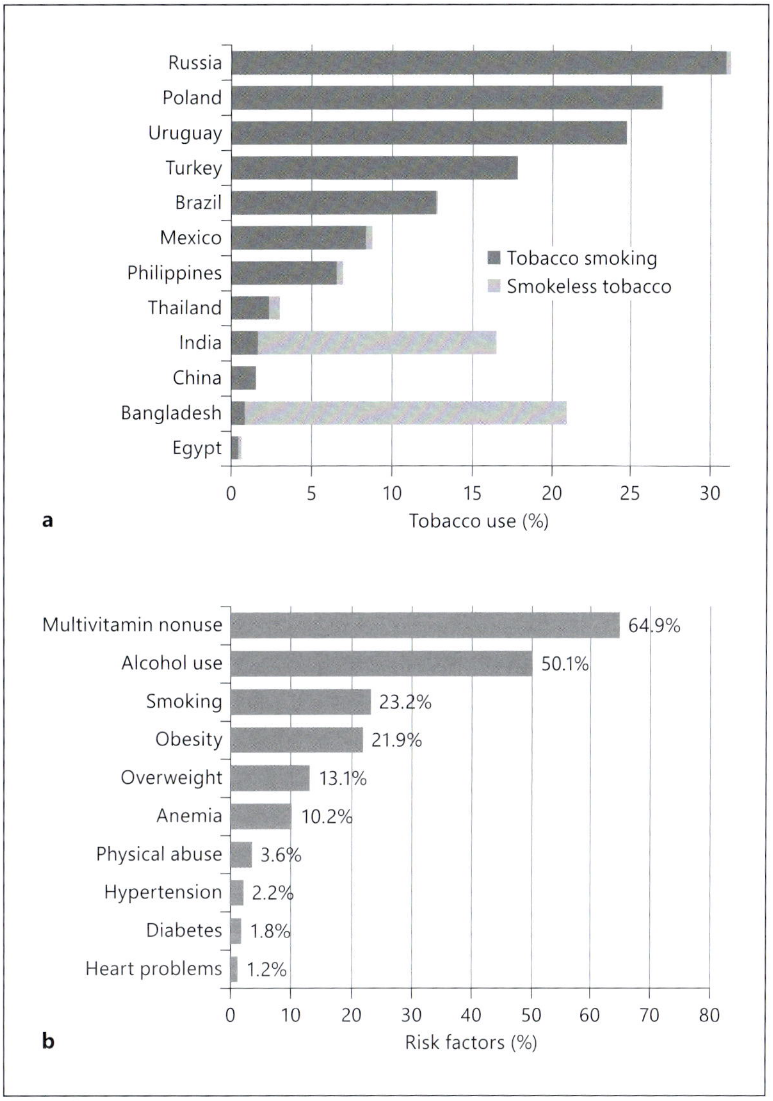

Fig. 7. Examples of risk factor frequencies [51, 53]. **a** Tobacco use in women of reproductive age in different countries from 2008 to 2010. **b** Frequency of different risk factors in women of reproductive age in the United States in 2004.

Maximizing the Impact

Once the evidence for prevention is in place and risk factors are qualified, quantified, and placed in the context of the target population (e.g. with estimates of the population-attributable fraction), one is typically faced with several options for prevention implementation. The Health Impact Pyramid [55] provides a useful framework for the strategic integration of interventions, with the specific goal of maximal penetration in the population at risk (typically women of childbearing age; see chapter by Riehle-Colarruso and Patel p. 57).

This framework emphasizes two key concepts. For maximum impact, tackling even a single risk factor often requires multiple integrated interventions; these interventions are most effective – in terms of population coverage and sustainability – the less individual effort is required. For example, to increase the consumption of folic acid daily in the population, food fortification (where feasible) is typically more efficient, sustainable, and cost-effective than education and counseling about daily use of pills. To illustrate these concepts, two examples (maternal diabetes and multivitamin use) are briefly considered.

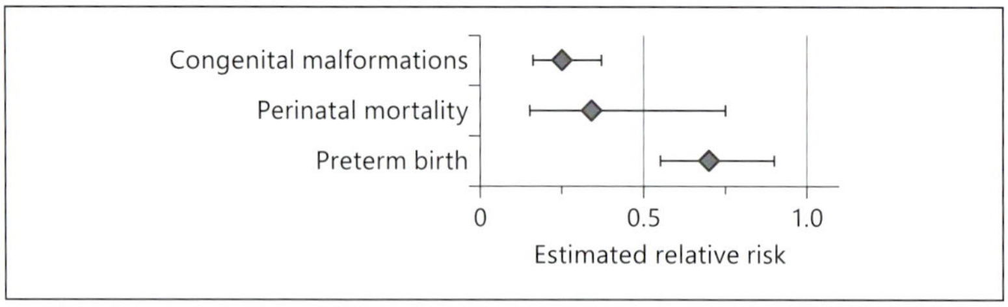

Fig. 8. Risk reduction for diabetes-related pregnancy outcomes with preconception care [meta-analyses from ref. 58, 59].

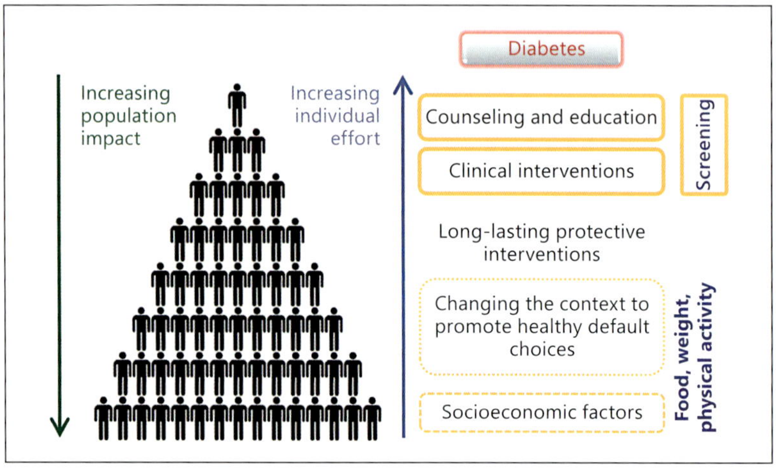

Fig. 9. Health Impact Pyramid: integrating interventions to reduce the diabetes-related risk for congenital heart defects and other adverse fetal and maternal outcomes.

Case Study: Maternal Diabetes

Maternal diabetes is an established and strong risk factor for congenital heart defects [56], as well as for many other fetal and maternal adverse effects [57–59]. The evidence is strong, qualified and quantified, and relative risks have been estimated for several types of heart defects in reviews and meta-analyses [56, 60]. The risk increases as the metabolic control worsens [61], and, conversely, preconception care aimed at reestablishing metabolic control before conception reduces significantly the risk for birth defects as well as for other adverse fetal and infant outcomes (fig. 8) [58, 59].

In terms of 'exposure frequency', maternal pregestational diabetes is fairly common among women of childbearing age in several countries (2% in the United States, higher in some other countries) and is increasing. The population-attributable fraction for major heart defects can be substantial – with a relative risk of 4 for major heart defects combined [56], the population-attributable fraction would increase from 3 to 15% as the frequency of pregestational diabetes increases from 1 to 6% (not an unreasonable disease frequency in some groups of the population). For these reasons, maternal diabetes is a premier target for primary prevention, with potential benefits expanding well beyond congenital heart defects.

Applying the Health Impact Pyramid framework to diabetes (fig. 9) highlights the opportunities and challenges of interventions aimed at reaching the entire population at risk. Clinical interventions, including diabetes screening and counseling, are effective; however, they are also costly, intensive, and require considerable effort on the part of women and health providers. As a consequence, they reach only part of the population at risk, typically the more affluent and educated; coverage is incomplete, with a risk for health disparities. Additional interventions can help increase population coverage by influencing the broader social and economic determinants of health that influence food choices, optimal weight, and physical activity. These interventions require wide-ranging policy and education initia-

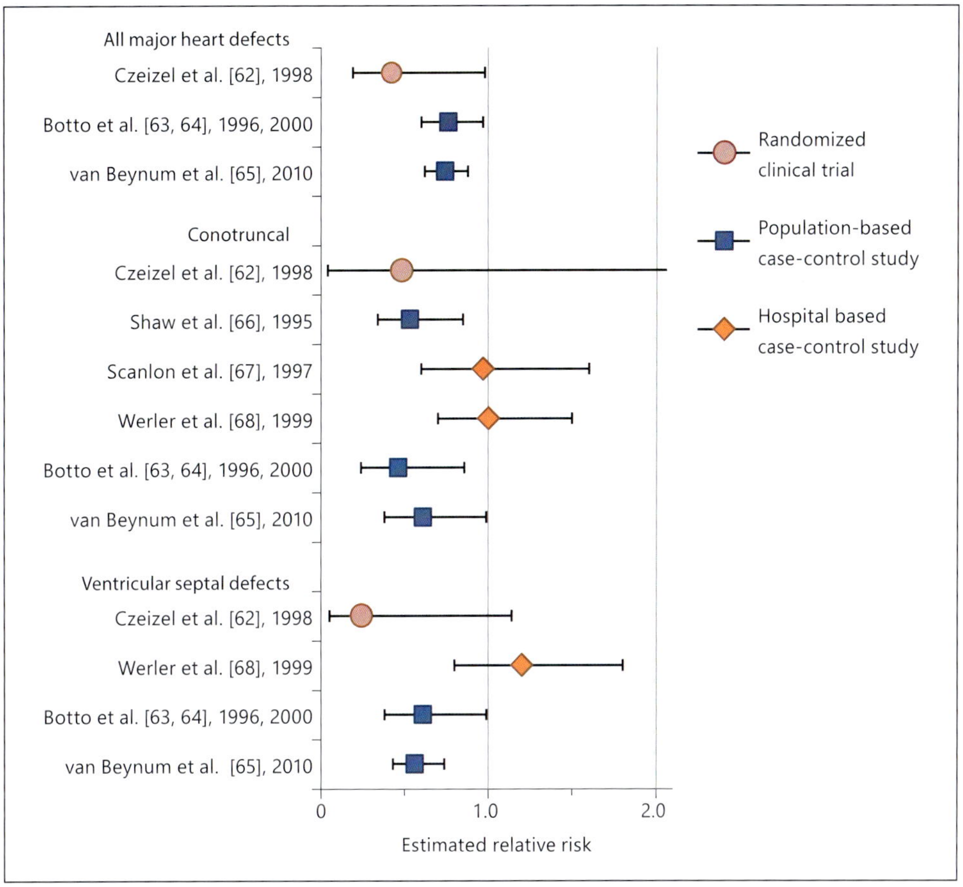

Fig. 10. Estimated relative risk for congenital heart defects associated with the periconceptional use of multivitamin supplements (containing folic acid).

tives, investing for example the school (education, food programs, and exercise) and work (incentives for physical activity, weight control, and screening). Their overall impact over time can be significant and long lasting (as they minimize individual effort), but require a concerted effort that invests policy and law.

Case Study: Folic Acid/Multivitamins

The finding that folic acid, alone or as part of a multivitamin supplement, can prevent most cases of neural tube defects if started before conception has proven to be a significant public health success. The use of folic acid supplements (pills) and, more so, flour fortification with folic acid has led to a population-wide decrease in the rates of neural tube defects in the countries that have fortified effectively. The question of whether folic acid or vitamin supplements can prevent congenital heart defects (and if so, which ones) remains without a definitive answer. One challenge is that randomized controlled trials with a placebo control group are now unethical, given the undisputed benefits of folic acid supplementation. Current data include one randomized clinical trial from the 1990s and a few observational studies [1]. The preponderance of published data (fig. 10) suggests a decreased risk associated with the periconceptional use of a multivitamin supplement [1].

In addition, data from countries that implemented fortification with folic acid show little changes in the rates of congenital heart defects [1], suggesting that either folic acid alone is not effective or that greater amounts are needed (fortification provides a

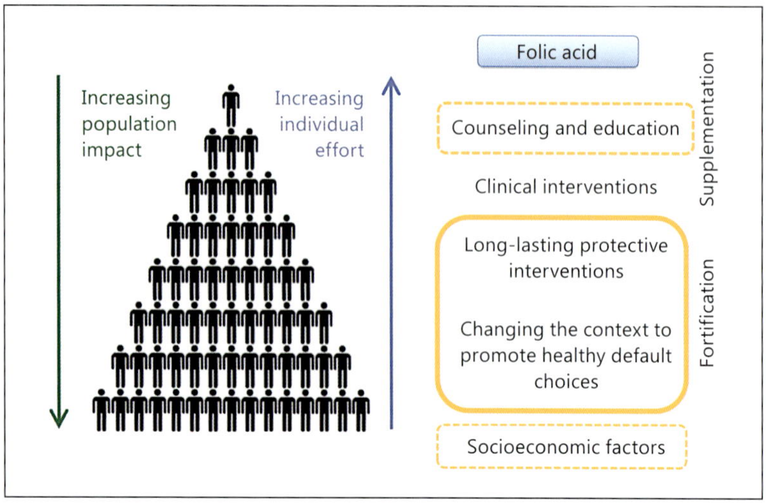

Fig. 11. Health Impact Pyramid: interventions to increase and sustain the periconceptional use of multivitamin/folic acid supplements in the population.

relatively low average dose to most people in the population). Quantifying and qualifying the potential effects of multivitamin supplementation is more challenging than for diabetes, because the data are fewer and the evidence is weaker. Assuming a relative risk of 0.5 associated with multivitamin use (a 50% decrease in risk) for conotruncal and septal heart defects, the relative risk associated with *nonuse* would be 2 (the inverse of 0.5). In many populations (the United States and the Netherlands being two remarkable exceptions), very few women take multivitamin supplements from before conception. The potential effects can be significant: in a population in which half of all women take daily supplements (and half do not), the estimated attributable fraction associated with nonuse is 33% (fig. 11) – about one third of cases of these heart defects in the population are attributable to not using the supplements and are potentially preventable by their use.

The Health Impact Pyramid framework underscores the benefits of integrating supplementation and fortification (fig. 11). Supplementation, promoted by counseling and education, is known to be effective, but requires ongoing efforts, is difficult to sustain, and reaches typically (as many other education efforts) only a segment of the population. Fortification, if it includes commonly eaten foods, requires little or no personal effort on the part of the public or the providers, is long lasting (once fortification is in place, it is easy and inexpensive to maintain), and provides the 'healthy default choice'. Additional interventions may include education on healthy diet (including folate-rich foods), particularly in population groups at greater risk.

Putting Everything Together: Healthy Heart, Healthy Child, and Healthy Parents

Not all causes of heart defects are known. Yet, the available evidence on risks and outcomes is already sufficient to support some recommendations and prevention interventions. Not doing what is known to work contributes to the daily cost of inaction. Primary prevention of congenital heart defects merges in large part with preconception care. Designing sets of intervention that address these risks factors globally promotes efficiency and expands the benefits. Collaboration among the many clinical and public health groups advocating for change and prevention – be it diabetes screening, smoking cessation, adolescent health promotion, or nutrition – is crucial in order to integrate and, importantly, sustain primary prevention over time and in the entire population (table 1). Smoking, for example, may be a relatively minor concern in relation to congenital heart defects if one judges solely in terms of the relative risk of the disease. However, it merits a place in the core set of interventions because of the high rates of smoking in many countries (thus increasing the fraction of attributable cases) and because of its significant impact on many other aspects of maternal and child health.

Table 1. Primary prevention for congenital heart defects: strength of evidence, magnitude of risk, frequency of exposure, and additional benefits for other pregnancy outcomes

Factor	Causes CHD	RR	Common exposure	Additional prevention
Diabetes (pregest.)	Definite	+++	+++ (1–6%)	Definite (birth defects, other)
Medications	Definite	++	+	Definite (NTD, clefts, other)
Obesity	Probable	+	+++ (~15%)	Definite (stillbirth, preterm birth, other)
Nonuse of folic acid/ multivitamins	Probable	++	+++++ (~50%)	Definite (NTD, other)
Smoking	Possible	++	+++ (10–20%)	Definite (clefts, preterm/IUGR)
Fever/influenza	Possible	++	+++ (6–10%)	Probable (NTD)

IUGR = Intrauterine growth restriction; NTD = neural tube defects; RR = relative risk.

2

Likewise, supplementation and fortification may not have yet proven their effectiveness in preventing congenital heart defects: however, they are established protective factors for neural tube defects and, particularly multivitamin supplementation, could have an additional role in decreasing the risk for conotruncal and septal heart defects.

Preconception care has many aspects, which are made explicit in a large set of recommendations [44]. The following set of recommendations for heart defects provides some guidance in harmony with the broader goals of primary prevention and promotion of fetal and maternal health (table 2). These recommendations are simple but not easy. To reach their potential for prevention, these recommendations require not only individual effort (education and counseling), but also adequate policies and laws (e.g. immunizations, fortification, or smoking laws). From a public health perspective, it will be important to have the means to track both process and outcomes – a surveillance system that provides reliable and ongoing information on interventions, risk factor rates, and health outcomes.

Epidemiology and Prevention: Trends and Future

Congenital heart defects are common, costly, and critical. Predicting how this will change is difficult. It may be more helpful to briefly surmise some forces that will likely drive these changes, as these forces will vary in different places and times.

Changes in the total prevalence of congenital heart defects (the sum of live births, stillbirths, and pregnancy terminations) will depend on the balance of risk factor and protective factors in a population. Some trends are not encouraging. Overall, the world is not getting healthier – diabetes, several chronic illnesses, and obesity are affecting more (and sometimes younger) people in many developed and developing countries. Yet, some factors offer hope: there appears to be now greater attention to integrated preconception health and, in the areas of chronic disease, greater action in preventing, screening, or treating diabetes and obesity. Whether these initiatives will reverse the current worrying trends remains to be seen.

Prenatal diagnosis will likely have a significant impact on occurrence and outcomes, though its direction and magnitude are not entirely predictable. Diagnosis is typically easier than treatment; in countries with increasing medical technology, such as large parts of Asia and Africa (see Ekure and Adeyemo chapter Clinical Epidemiology and Clinical Management of Congenital Heart Defects in a Developing Country, p. 46), rates of prenatal diagnosis of severe heart defects will likely increase, at least initially, without corresponding availability of effective and affordable treatment; depending on the social context, pregnancy terminations due to fetal anomalies could increase. Conversely, with better treatment options, family choices may change and birth prevalence of some severe heart defects could even increase if cases previously terminated prenatally are allowed to reach birth. Prenatal diagnosis

Table 2. Increasing the odds for a healthy heart and baby: seven habits of primary prevention and health promotion (based on Botto [1] and Jenkins et al. [2])

(1) Take a multivitamin with folic acid daily Use folic acid (≥0.4 mg) but avoid high retinol intake (>10,000 IU)
(2) Screen/target chronic illnesses Diabetes (may be unrecognized), epilepsy, and phenylketonuria
(3) Screen/stop smoking, no alcohol use Even second-hand smoke is a problem
(4) Screen/assess medication use Seizure medications, retinoic acid, and paroxetine
(5) Avoid immunizations and close contact with ill individuals, especially those with febrile illnesses Hand washing/fever treatment
(6) Avoid exposure to heavy metals, herbicides, pesticides, and organic solvents At work or at home/self or partner
(7) Promote healthy habits Healthy weight, physical activity, nutrition, and early prenatal care

could also decrease morbidity and mortality if it decreases delayed diagnoses and promotes better organization of care.

Newborn screening for critical congenital heart defects using pulse oximetry is being implemented in several areas. Appropriately implemented, newborn screening should increase early diagnoses of some severe heart defects; the rationale is that outcomes should then improve, because treatment would start promptly (before closure of the ductus arteriosus) and in a well-prepared health care setting. As a side benefit, newborn screening could also provide systematic and ongoing data on public health surveillance activities, precisely for those congenital heart defects that have the greatest impact on mortality, disability, and costs.

Trends in costs are difficult to predict. As more babies survive longer, their use of healthcare resources will likely increase. In general, congenital heart defects are likely to remain one of the more costly birth defects; by way of comparison, most children with orofacial clefts can be effectively 'cured' by early surgery and lead an essentially normal and productive life, unlike many children with complex heart defects who will require long-term treatment and repeat surgeries. However, earlier diagnosis, through prenatal or newborn screening, could theoretically decrease costs if it reduces substantially preoperative morbidity and postoperative complications; to date, these benefits remain unproven.

Mortality associated with congenital heart defects is also likely to change. Deaths due to congenital heart defects (as for birth defects in general) will likely increase as a *proportion of infant deaths,* as infant deaths due to other causes (infections or prematurity) decline. In absolute terms, however, mortality should decrease gradually with better treatment and earlier diagnoses. Lower mortality will translate in greater longevity, and prevalence in adults will increase, with greater needs for specialized care. Unless adequate services for older individuals are provided, the peak of mortality for heart defect risks being delayed rather than decreased. Finally, some factors may lead to an *apparent* change in mortality unrelated to true improvements in outcomes. For example, increased pregnancy terminations for fetal cardiac defects can cause an apparent reduction in mortality *as a proportion of the population* (as it is usually tracked using death certificate data), because fewer babies will be born with heart defects and would be at risk for dying. Including pregnancy terminations in birth defect surveillance would help avoid this bias. Conversely, as screening and diagnostic technology is introduced in a country in which it had not been available previously, deaths attributed to heart defects (and attributed to other causes previously) may increase simply because of better ascertainment.

Conclusions

Congenital heart defects remain common, costly and critical, and more so than they ought to be because prevention is lagging. Recent decades have witnessed substantial improvements in diagnosis and care: more babies can now look forward to longer and better lives. Still, large parts of the world are still untouched by these improvements.

Prevention promises to be an additional and powerful tool to improve survival and decrease the personal and societal impact of congenital heart defects. However, making prevention work requires greater investments in research (finding new causes) and implementation (reducing known causes). Known genetic and environmental factors still account for a minority of cases of congenital heart defects. Gene-environment interactions, commonly posited to cause most of the remaining cases, have so far eluded detection. Nevertheless, some environmental and maternal factors have been well characterized. These should be targets of comprehensive prevention interventions. Maternal chronic illness, immunizations, medications, and nutrition appear to be the targets with greatest potential impact in terms of preventing not only congenital heart defects but also many other adverse fetal and maternal outcomes.

Because of how early the embryonic heart develops, the cornerstone of prevention is preconception care, i.e. an integrated set of interventions aimed at lifelong health promotion and addressing multiple risk factors. Implementing these interventions effectively will require not only individual education and clinical interventions, but also long-term, population-based approaches that address the deeper social and economic determinants of health. The challenges are many; however, evidence is available and benefits can be considerable in terms of health, wealth, and lives.

References

1 Botto LD: Epidemiology and prevention of congenital heart defects; in Allen HD, Driscoll DJ, Shaddy RE, Feltes TF (eds): Moss and Adams' Heart Disease in Infants, Children, and Adolescents, Including the Fetus and Young Adult, ed 8. Philadelphia, Lippincott, 2013.

2 Jenkins KJ, Correa A, Feinstein JA, et al: Noninherited risk factors and congenital cardiovascular defects: current knowledge: a scientific statement from the American Heart Association Council on Cardiovascular Disease in the Young: endorsed by the American Academy of Pediatrics. Circulation 2007;115:2995–3014.

3 Riehle-Colarusso T, Patel SS: Maternal nongenetic risk factors for congenital heart defects. Muenke M, Kruszka PS, Sable CA, Belmont JW (eds): Congenital Heart Disease: Molecular Genetics, Principles of Diagnosis and Treatment. Basel, Karger, 2015, pp 57–69.

4 Hoffman JI, Kaplan S: The incidence of congenital heart disease. J Am Coll Cardiol 2002;39:1890–1900.

5 McCrindle BW: The prevalence of congenital cardiac lesions; in Freedom RM, Yoo S-J, Mikailian H, Williams WG (eds): The Natural and Modified History of Congenital Heart Disease. New York, Futura, Blackwell Publishing, 2004.

6 Rosenthal GL: Prevalence of congenital heart disease; in Garson AJ, Bricker JT, Fisher DJ, Neish SR (eds). The Science and Practice of Pediatric Cardiology, ed 2. Baltimore, Williams & Wilkins, 1998, p 1098.

7 van der Linde D, Konings EE, Slager MA, et al: Birth prevalence of congenital heart disease worldwide: a systematic review and meta-analysis. J Am Coll Cardiol 2011;58: 2241–2247.

8 Warnes CA, Liberthson R, Danielson GK, et al: Task force 1: the changing profile of congenital heart disease in adult life. J Am Coll Cardiol 2001;37:1170–1175.

9 Dolk H, Loane M, Garne E: Congenital heart defects in Europe: prevalence and perinatal mortality, 2000 to 2005. Circulation 2011; 123:841–849.

10 Ferencz C, Loffredo CA, Correa-Villasenor A, Wilson PD: Genetic and Environmental Risk Factors of Major Congenital Heart Disease: The Baltimore-Washington Infant Study 1981–1989. Mount Kisco, Futura, 1997.

11 Ferencz C, Loffredo CA, Rubin JD, Magee CA: Epidemiology of Congenital Heart Disease: The Baltimore-Washington Infant Study 1981–1989. Mount Kisco, Futura, 1993.

12 Reller MD, Strickland MJ, Riehle-Colarusso T, Mahle WT, Correa A: Prevalence of congenital heart defects in metropolitan Atlanta, 1998–2005. J Pediatr 2008;153: 807–813.

13 Tegnander E, Williams W, Johansen OJ, Blaas HG, Eik-Nes SH: Prenatal detection of heart defects in a non-selected population of 30,149 fetuses – detection rates and outcome. Ultrasound Obstet Gynecol 2006;27: 252–265.

14 Hiraishi S, Agata Y, Nowatari M, et al: Incidence and natural course of trabecular ventricular septal defect: two-dimensional echocardiography and color Doppler flow imaging study. J Pediatr 1992;120:409–415.

15 Ishikawa T, Iwashima S, Ohishi A, Nakagawa Y, Ohzeki T: Prevalence of congenital heart disease assessed by echocardiography in 2067 consecutive newborns. Acta Paediatr 2011;100:e55–e60.

16 Botto LD, Correa A, Erickson JD: Racial and temporal variations in the prevalence of heart defects. Pediatrics 2001;107:E32.
17 Wren C, Richmond S, Donaldson L: Temporal variability in birth prevalence of cardiovascular malformations. Heart 2000;83:414–419.
18 Oyen N, Poulsen G, Boyd HA, Wohlfahrt J, Jensen PK, Melbye M: National time trends in congenital heart defects, Denmark, 1977–2005. Am Heart J 2009;157:467–473.e1.
19 Bedard T, Lowry RB, Sibbald B, et al: Congenital heart defect case ascertainment by the Alberta Congenital Anomalies Surveillance System. Birth Defects Res A Clin Mol Teratol 2012;94:449–458.
20 Ursell PC, Byrne JM, Strobino BA: Significance of cardiac defects in the developing fetus: a study of spontaneous abortuses. Circulation 1985;72:1232–1236.
21 Chinn A, Fitzsimmons J, Shepard TH, Fantel AG: Congenital heart disease among spontaneous abortuses and stillborn fetuses: prevalence and associations. Teratology 1989;40:475–482.
22 Stoll C, Alembik Y, Roth MP, Dott B, De Geeter B: Risk factors in congenital heart disease. Eur J Epidemiol 1989;5:382–391.
23 International Clearinghouse for Birth Defects Surveillance and Research; in Mastroiacovo P (ed): Annual Report 2009, with Data for 2007. Rome, International Center on Birth Defects, 2009.
24 Garne E, Khoshnood B, Loane M, Boyd P, Dolk H: Termination of pregnancy for fetal anomaly after 23 weeks of gestation: a European register-based study. BJOG 2010;117:660–666.
25 Selected birth defects data from population-based birth defects surveillance programs in the United States, 2003–2007. Birth Defects Res A Clin Mol Teratol 2010;88:1062–1174.
26 Kornosky JL, Salihu HM: Getting to the heart of the matter: epidemiology of cyanotic heart defects. Pediatr Cardiol 2008;29:484–497.
27 Samanek M: Boy:girl ratio in children born with different forms of cardiac malformation: a population-based study. Pediatr Cardiol 1994;15:53–57.
28 Marelli AJ, Mackie AS, Ionescu-Ittu R, Rahme E, Pilote L: Congenital heart disease in the general population: changing prevalence and age distribution. Circulation 2007;115:163–172.
29 Brickner ME, Hillis LD, Lange RA: Congenital heart disease in adults. First of two parts. N Engl J Med 2000;342:256–263.
30 Robbins JM, Bird TM, Tilford JM, et al: Hospital stays, hospital charges, and in-hospital deaths among infants with selected birth defects – United States, 2003. MMWR Morb Mortal Wkly Rep 2007;56:25–29.
31 Keren R, Luan X, Localio R, et al: Prioritization of comparative effectiveness research topics in hospital pediatrics. Arch Pediatr Adolesc Med 2012;166:1155–1164.
32 Pasquali SK, Jacobs ML, He X, et al: Variation in congenital heart surgery costs across hospitals. Pediatrics 2014;133:e553–e560.
33 Boulet S, Grosse SC, Riehle-Colarusso T, Correa-Villasenor A: Health care costs of congenital heart defects; in Wyszynski DF, Correa-Villasenor A, Graham TP (eds): Congenital Heart Defects: From Origin to Treatment. New York, Oxford University Press, 2010, pp 493–501.
34 Waitzman NJ, Romano PS, Scheffler RM: The Cost of Birth Defects. Lanham, University Press of America, 1996.
35 Centers for Disease Control and Prevention, Waitzman NJ, Romano PS, Scheffler RM, Harris JA: Economic costs of birth defects and cerebral palsy – United States, 1992. MMWR Morb Mortal Wkly Rep 1995;44:694–699.
36 Russo CA, Elixhauser A: Hospitalizations for Birth Defects, 2004. HCUP Statistical Briefs. Rockville, US Agency for Healthcare Research & Quality, 2007.
37 Okumura MJ, Campbell AD, Nasr SZ, Davis MM: Inpatient health care use among adult survivors of chronic childhood illnesses in the United States. Arch Pediatr Adolesc Med 2006;160:1054–1060.
38 Lopez AD, Mathers CD: Measuring the global burden of disease and epidemiological transitions: 2002–2030. Ann Trop Med Parasitol 2006;100:481–499.
39 Rosano A, Botto LD, Botting B, Mastroiacovo P: Infant mortality and congenital anomalies from 1950 to 1994: an international perspective. J Epidemiol Community Health 2000;54:660–666.
40 Centers for Disease Control and Prevention (CDC): Racial differences by gestational age in neonatal deaths attributable to congenital heart defects – United States, 2003–2006. MMWR Morb Mortal Wkly Rep 2010;59:1208–1211.
41 Boneva RS, Botto LD, Moore CA, Yang Q, Correa A, Erickson JD: Mortality associated with congenital heart defects in the United States: trends and racial disparities, 1979–1997. Circulation 2001;103:2376–2381.
42 Olsen M, Christensen TD, Pedersen L, Johnsen SP, Hjortdal VE: Late mortality among Danish patients with congenital heart defect. Am J Cardiol 2010;106:1322–1326.
43 Gilboa SM, Salemi JL, Nembhard WN, Fixler DE, Correa A: Mortality resulting from congenital heart disease among children and adults in the United States, 1999 to 2006. Circulation 2010;122:2254–2263.
44 Jack BW, Atrash H, Coonrod DV, Moos MK, O'Donnell J, Johnson K: The clinical content of preconception care: an overview and preparation of this supplement. Am J Obstet Gynecol 2008;199:S266–S279.
45 Gittenberger-de Groot AC, Bartelings MM, Poelmann RE, Haak MC, Jongbloed MR: Embryology of the heart and its impact on understanding fetal and neonatal heart disease. Semin Fetal Neonatal Med 2013;18:237–244.
46 Hartman RJ, Rasmussen SA, Botto LD, et al: The contribution of chromosomal abnormalities to congenital heart defects: a population-based study. Pediatr Cardiol 2011;32:1147–1157.
47 Zaidi S, Choi M, Wakimoto H, et al: De novo mutations in histone-modifying genes in congenital heart disease. Nature 2013;498:220–223.
48 Al Turki S, Manickaraj AK, Mercer CL, et al: Rare variants in NR2F2 cause congenital heart defects in humans. Am J Hum Genet 2014;94:574–585.
49 Warburton D, Ronemus M, Kline J, et al: The contribution of de novo and rare inherited copy number changes to congenital heart disease in an unselected sample of children with conotruncal defects or hypoplastic left heart disease. Hum Genet 2014;133:11–27.
50 Williamson DF: The population attributable fraction and confounding: buyer beware. Int J Clin Pract 2010;64:1019–1023.
51 Centers for Disease Control and Prevention: Current tobacco use and secondhand smoke exposure among women of reproductive age – 14 countries, 2008–2010. MMWR Morb Mortal Wkly Rep 2012;61:877–882.
52 Centers for Disease Control and Prevention. PRAMS: Pregnancy Risk Assessment Monitoring System. http://www.cdc.gov/prams/.
53 D'Angelo D, Willians L, Morrow B, et al: Preconception and interconception health status of women who recently gave birth to a live-born infant – Pregnancy Risk Assessment Monitoring System (PRAMS), United States, 26 reporting areas, 2004. MMWR Surveill Summ 2007;56:1–35.
54 World Health Organization: STEPwise approach to surveillance (STEPS). http://www.who.int/chp/steps/en/.
55 Frieden TR: A framework for public health action: the Health Impact Pyramid. Am J Public Health 2010;100:590–595.
56 Lisowski LA, Verheijen PM, Copel JA, et al: Congenital heart disease in pregnancies complicated by maternal diabetes mellitus. An international clinical collaboration, literature review, and meta-analysis. Herz 2010;35:19–26.

57 Inkster ME, Fahey TP, Donnan PT, Leese GP, Mires GJ, Murphy DJ: Poor glycated haemoglobin control and adverse pregnancy outcomes in type 1 and type 2 diabetes mellitus: systematic review of observational studies. BMC Pregnancy Childbirth 2006;6:30.
58 Wahabi HA, Alzeidan RA, Bawazeer GA, Alansari LA, Esmaeil SA: Preconception care for diabetic women for improving maternal and fetal outcomes: a systematic review and meta-analysis. BMC Pregnancy Childbirth 2010;10:63.
59 Wahabi HA, Alzeidan RA, Esmaeil SA: Prepregnancy care for women with pre-gestational diabetes mellitus: a systematic review and meta-analysis. BMC Public Health 2012;12:792.
60 Correa A, Gilboa SM, Besser LM, et al: Diabetes mellitus and birth defects. Am J Obstet Gynecol 2008;199:237.e1–e9.
61 Guerin A, Nisenbaum R, Ray JG: Use of maternal GHb concentration to estimate the risk of congenital anomalies in the offspring of women with prepregnancy diabetes. Diabetes Care 2007;30:1920–1925.
62 Czeizel AE: Periconceptional folic acid containing multivitamin supplementation. Eur J Obstet Gynecol Reprod Biol 1998;78:151–161.
63 Botto LD, Khoury MJ, Mulinare J, Erickson JD: Periconceptional multivitamin use and the occurrence of conotruncal heart defects: results from a population-based, case-control study. Pediatrics 1996;98:911–917.
64 Botto LD, Mulinare J, Erickson JD: Occurrence of congenital heart defects in relation to maternal mulitivitamin use. Am J Epidemiol 2000;151:878–884.
65 van Beynum IM, Kapusta L, Bakker MK, den Heijer M, Blom HJ, de Walle HE: Protective effect of periconceptional folic acid supplements on the risk of congenital heart defects: a registry-based case-control study in the northern Netherlands. Eur Heart J 2010;31:464–471.
66 Shaw GM, O'Malley CD, Wasserman CR, Tolarova MM, Lammer EJ: Maternal periconceptional use of multivitamins and reduced risk for conotruncal heart defects and limb deficiencies among offspring. Am J Med Genet 1995;59:536–545.
67 Scanlon KS, Ferencz C, Loffredo CA, Wilson PD, Correa-Villasenor A, Khoury MJ, et al: Preconceptional folate intake and malformations of the cardiac outflow tract. Baltimore-Washington Infant Study Group. Epidemiology 1998;9:95–98.
68 Werler MM, Hayes C, Louik C, Shapiro S, Mitchell AA: Multivitamin supplementation and risk of birth defects. Am J Epidemiol 1999;150:675–682.

Dr. Lorenzo Botto
Division of Medical Genetics, Department of Pediatrics, University of Utah
50 North Medical Drive
Salt Lake City, UT 84103 (USA)
E-Mail lorenzo.botto@hsc.utah.edu

Muenke M, Kruszka PS, Sable CA, Belmont JW (eds): Congenital Heart Disease: Molecular Genetics, Principles of Diagnosis and Treatment. Basel, Karger, 2015, pp 46–56
DOI: 10.1159/000375204

Clinical Epidemiology and Management of Congenital Heart Defects in a Developing Country

Ekanem N. Ekure[a] · Adebowale A. Adeyemo[b]

[a]Department of Pediatrics, College of Medicine, University of Lagos, Lagos, Nigeria; [b]Center for Research on Genomics and Global Health, National Human Genome Research Institute, National Institutes of Health, Bethesda, Md., USA

Abstract

Congenital heart defects (CHD) remain one of the most common categories of birth defects worldwide. In many developing countries, high early childhood mortality and limited diagnostic facilities often obscure the true scope of the problem. In this review, we provide an overview of the clinical epidemiology and management of CHD in a developing country: Nigeria, Africa's most populous country. We describe the types of CHD and the clinical presentation, echocardiographic diagnosis, management, and outcome of CHD. Ventricular septal defects are the commonest CHD reported in Nigeria while tetralogy of Fallot is the commonest cyanotic CHD. Their etiology is often unknown, although the congenital rubella syndrome and Down syndrome account for a significant minority of cases. Thus far, there is no modern genetic study of CHD in Nigeria. Diagnosis is often delayed, with only about half of CHD cases getting diagnosed within the 1st year of life and up to 10% diagnosed in adulthood. Echocardiography has played a major role in improving diagnosis. Management remains challenging, but a number of initiatives (especially by nongovernmental organizations) provide access to corrective surgery for a select few. The field of CHD in Nigeria offers opportunities for research into etiology, natural history, clinical management, and outcomes.

In many developing countries (such as Nigeria), congenital malformations are often viewed as less of a priority than communicable diseases, malnutrition, and perinatal conditions, which account for much of the morbidity and mortality observed in such societies. Nonetheless, congenital malformations remain important clinical problems, occurring frequently enough and often posing appreciable burdens on health care systems, which are often ill prepared to manage such complex conditions. Indeed, the first studies of congenital heart defects (CHD) in Nigeria were reported in the 1960s [1] and several other studies [2–16] followed describing various aspects of CHD. The first study of the prevalence of CHD at birth in Nigeria was published in 1966 [17], with an estimate of 3.5 per 1,000 births. In Nigeria, CHD forms an important subset of congenital malformations seen at birth [18–20], in pediatric and/or neonatal admissions [21–24], and at autopsy [18, 25, 26].

Types of Congenital Heart Defects Seen in Nigeria

Ventricular septal defect (VSD) is the commonest CHD reported in Nigeria while tetralogy of Fallot (ToF) is the commonest cyanotic CHD (table 1). Among acyanotic CHD, the three commonest lesions are VSD, patent ductus arteriosus (PDA), and atrial septal defect (ASD), while transposition of the great arteries is the second commonest cyanotic CHD. Other defects make up less than 8% of CHD in most series (fig. 1; table 1).

Detection and accurate diagnosis of CHD is often dependent on the sophistication of the diagnostic methods available. Diagnostic methods used for CHD in Nigeria have evolved over the decades and may have influenced reports on the CHD types seen. In the 1960s–1980s, most cardiovascular evaluations were done by physical examination, ECG, chest X-ray, and selective angiography [1–3]. By the 1990s, echocardiography had become available but, notably, diagnostic cardiac catheterization was used less frequently [4, 5]. In comparing the period before echocardiography became available in Nigeria (pre-echo) with the period thereafter, VSD was the commonest CHD in Nigeria (fig. 1). In the pre-echo era, PDA was the next common type of CHD reported followed by pulmonary stenosis. This is in contrast to most studies in the echocardiography era where ToF or ASD commonly followed VSD, and pulmonary stenosis was absent or occurred not more than 3% in most series. PDA, which made up at least 20% of CHD in all the pre-echo data series, constituted <10% of CHD in more than half of the echocardiography era data series. This trend in PDA may in part be due to a reduction in the prevalence of rubella in the general population.

Complex CHD, including hypoplastic left heart syndrome, was rarely diagnosed in most series, which probably highlights the challenges of non-hospital child delivery coupled with poor health seeking behaviors in developing countries; as a consequence, out-of-hospital deaths are significantly increased. There have been few reports in Nigeria documenting aortic stenosis or coarctation of the aorta, which make up less than 3.5% of the study population even when both are combined. It is, however, pertinent to note that all the studies done in the pre-echo era reported either or both of these lesions, whereas only two studies in the echocardiography era have reported at least one of these lesions. This finding may not be unconnected to an earlier observation by Hoffman et al. [6] stating that coarctation of the aorta is often missed by referring doctors and thus remains undetected until adulthood. In addition, aortic stenosis and coarctation of the aorta are reported to be less common in Black people compared to Caucasians [7]. Frequently, associated extracardiac anomalies are noted in the context of syndromic disorders. Notably, Down syndrome (trisomy 21) is the syndrome most commonly associated with CHD in several series from Nigeria. In the data series by Ekure et al. [8], 64.4% of children with congenital malformations and associated CHD had Down syndrome (see Kruszka chapter on Down syndrome on p. 82). The most frequent defects in these children with Down syndrome in Nigeria are VSD and atrioventricular septal defect (AVSD) [8–11].

In terms of geography, there are no apparent significant differences in the types of CHD encountered between northern and southern regions of Nigeria. In both regions, VSD and ToF are the commonest reported CHD and cyanotic CHD, respectively [1–16].

Although the review above presents a wide profile of CHD in Nigeria, this may still not give a complete picture due to limited accessibility to appropriate diagnosis and early deaths outside the health facilities, especially for critical CHD. In addition, expertise in echocardiography may have improved in recent times with doctors receiving training outside the country. This suggests that in the near future a more complete picture on CHD will emerge.

Table 1. Distribution of CHD reported in studies from Nigeria

Author(s)	City/region of Nigeria	Period of study	Echo era	Age of the study population (all hospital based)	M:F ratio	Pattern of CHD, % of total cases							
						VSD	ASD	PDA	AVSD	PS	AS/CoA	ToF	TGA
Caddell and Morton [1]	Ibadan/South	1963–1965	No	0–12 years most <2 years	–	38.8	0	20.9	9	6	3	3	1.5
Jaiyesimi and Antia [2]	Ibadan/South	1965–1969; 1975–1980	No	Not stated	–	35	7.5	22	0	9	2.6	10	4.3
Fadahunsi [3]	Lagos/South	1974–1981	No	0–15 years	1:1.1	33	4.1	22.6	7.4	8.1	2.6	9.6	3.1
Ibadin et al. [4]	Benin/South	1995–2004	Yes	12 days to 16 years 2.6±3.5*	1:1	55.1	12.2	4.1	0	0	0	28.6	0
Bode-Thomas et al. [5]	Jos/North	1999–2000	Yes	2 months to 16 years 6.5±5.2 years	0.7:1	43.75	6.25	0	12.5	0	0	25	12.5
Wammanda and Danbauchi [15]	Zaria/North	2000–2001	Yes	9 days to 35years 11.5±14.5 years	1:1.3	17	45.7	2.9	2.9	0	0	22.8	0
Sani et al. [10]	Kano/North	2002–2006	Yes	9 days to 35 years 11.5 ±14.5 years	1.5:1	45.9	12.3	2.5	8.2	0	0	26.2	0.8
Okoromah et al. [9]	Lagos/South	2004–2005	Yes	4 weeks to 15 years 3.8±2.5 years	1:1	41.7	20.2	5.7	7.0	3.1	0	11.8	2.2
Kolo et al. [16]	Ilorin/North	2004–2007	Yes	5 days to 79 years 11.5±14.5 years	0.8:1	27.6	21.1	13.1	0	2.6	0	11.8	0
George and Frank-Briggs [13]	Port Harcourt/ South	2007–2008	Yes	<16 years	1:1.3	34.1	22	17.1	7.3	0	0	17.1	0
Chinawa et al. [11]	Enugu/South	2007–2012	Yes	6 months to 12 years 0.82±4.12 years	1:1	19.7	2.8	2.8	7.0	1.4	0	12.7	0
Asani et al. [14]	Kano/North	2009–2011	Yes	5 days to 15 years 3.29±2.56 years	3:2	33.5	13.3	10.9	8.8	0.6	0	16.7	1.7
Sadoh et al. [12]	Benin, Lagos, Abuja/ North and South	2009–2012	Yes	0–17 years 2.06±3.49 years	1:1	46.6	8.7	12.1	8.2	1.7	0.2	7.9	1.5

Means and ranges are shown for age of the study population. AS = Aortic stenosis; CoA = coarctation of the aorta; PS = pulmonary valve stenosis; TGA = transposition of the great arteries.

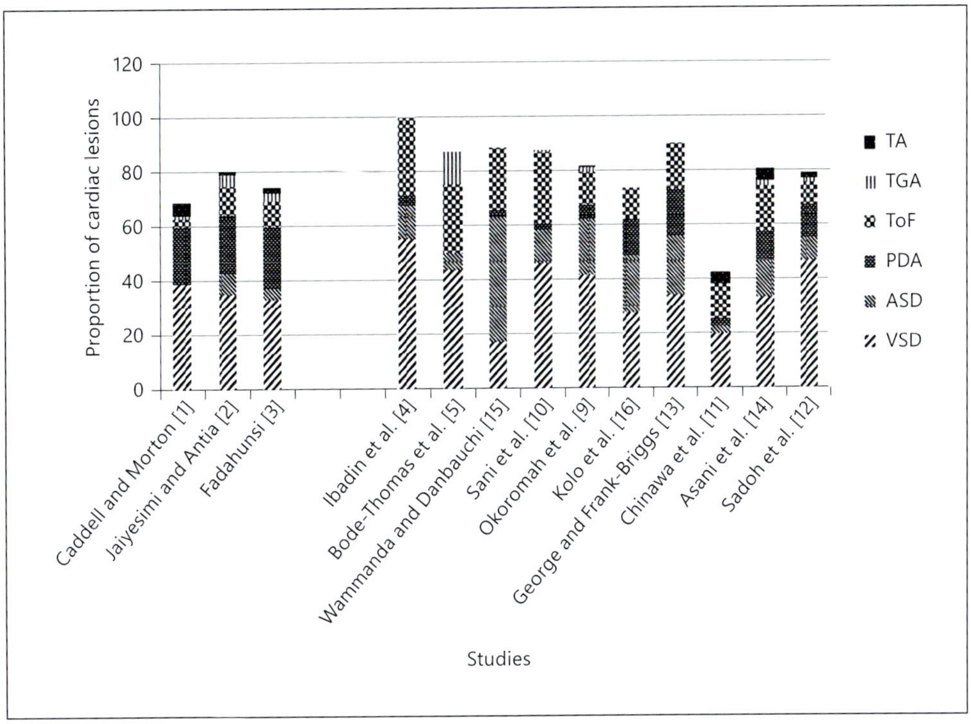

Fig. 1. Pattern of CHD during pre-echo and echo eras (see also table 1 and the reference list). TGA = Transposition of the great arteries. TA = Tricuspid atresia.

Etiology of Congenital Heart Defects in Nigeria

In Nigeria, as it is elsewhere, the etiology of most CHD cases is unknown. Figures from the largest series of CHD in Nigeria [2, 12] suggest that an etiologic or risk factor is identifiable in fewer than 1 in 8 of all CHD cases. The commonest reported environmental risk factors include congenital rubella syndrome [2, 10, 12, 13, 16] and perinatal asphyxia [2]. Genetic risk factors reported have mostly been chromosomal anomalies, of which Down syndrome is the most commonly stated [2, 10–13, 16]. However, it should be noted that a wider range of other genetic or developmental syndromes/associations have been reported in the context of CHD in Nigeria, either in case series or as case reports. These include: the Marfan, Noonan, Holt-Oram, and Ellis-van Creveld syndrome, as well as the VACTERL association (vertebral defects, anal atresia, cardiac defects, tracheoesophageal fistula, and renal and limb abnormalities).

An accurate assessment of the etiology of CHD in Nigeria is hampered by several factors:

(a) Few studies (including those on CHD types) report the etiology or risk factors.

(b) Lack of access to state-of-the art diagnostic facilities limits the risk factors which can be identified; indeed, it is no coincidence that the commonest attributable risk factors (congenital rubella syndrome, Down syndrome, and asphyxia) are those that are most easily diagnosed clinically.

(c) Most studies are retrospective rather than prospective, which implies that patients may not have been evaluated for risk factors using a standard protocol.

(d) Limited sample sizes of most case series (often <100) limit the generalizability of sample estimates (e.g. the proportion of CHD cases with Down syndrome reported from Nigeria range from as low as 2% [2] to as high as 17% [13]).

Table 2. Frequency of reported CHD-associated genetic variants in a Nigerian population in 2013

Study	Ancestry of the study sample	Chromo somal region	Reported gene(s)	SNP	Minor allele frequency	
					CEU	YRI
Cordell et al. [27]	European	4p16.2	STX18; MSX1	rs870142	0.277	0.063
	European	5q11.2	(intergenic)	rs12186641	0.053	0.006
Hu et al. [28]	Han Chinese	1p12	(intergenic – nearTBX15; SPAG17)	rs2474937	0.194	0.352
	Han Chinese	4q31.1	MAML3	rs1531070	0.424	0.006

CEU = Utah residents (CEPH) with Northern and Western European ancestry (source: 1000 Genomes Project); YRI = Yoruba in Ibadan, Nigeria (source: 1000 Genomes Project).

To our knowledge, no genetic studies of CHD using modern high-throughput methods (e.g. genome-wide association studies, structural variant analysis, and sequencing) have been reported from Nigeria. One such study was recently initiated in Lagos, Nigeria, but the findings are not expected for another year or two. We consider such studies essential to the search for genetic risk factors for CHD because of the potential for non-European ancestry populations to confirm and extend reported findings, as well as to find novel loci. In this regard, it should be noted that of the four loci identified in genome-wide association studies for CHD [27, 28], two are sufficiently common (minor allele frequency of at least 5%) in a Nigerian population (the Yoruba in Ibadan, Nigeria) to be directly tested in a replication and/or fine-mapping study (table 2).

Age at Diagnosis

Late diagnosis of illnesses has been the bane of medical diagnosis in developing countries, and diagnosis of CHD is no exception. Advances in cardiac diagnostic technology have enabled CHD diagnosis to be made in utero through fetal echocardiography. Newly introduced pulse oximetry screening for critical CHD complimented by echocardiography has further enhanced early diagnosis of CHD. This is largely nonexistent in most developing countries, including Nigeria.

In Nigeria, only about half of cases of CHD get diagnosed within the 1st year of life, with mean age at diagnosis ranging from 2.06 ± 3.49 to 7.82 ± 4.12 years [4, 9, 11, 12]. Data from five of the six studies that provided detailed age groups at diagnosis show that >10% of the CHD cases are diagnosed after 5 years of age (fig. 2) [2, 4, 9, 12–14]. Documentation of diagnosis in the neonatal period is seen in few reports and makes up <20% of CHD cases [4, 12–14, 16]. The norm is that diagnosis after birth is made from clinical evaluation supported by electrocardiography in most health facilities. A functional echocardiography machine with trained personnel to do the test (often a doctor) is present in just a couple of dozen facilities in Nigeria. This is largely inadequate considering the large population of >160 million people. The echocardiography test costs from USD 10 to 60 and from 150 to 440 in government and private health centers, respectively. This test is largely unaffordable for many average families who do not have medical insurance and have to pay all such expenses out of pocket.

CHD is not infrequently seen or first diagnosed in adults. In Nigeria, most cases of adult CHD are first diagnosed in adulthood with no prior treatment. In northern Nigeria, Sani et al. [10] reported that 10.7% of the 122 CHD cases seen were adults. The commonest defect was ToF. Data from southern Nigeria have also reported cases of VSD, ASD, ToF,

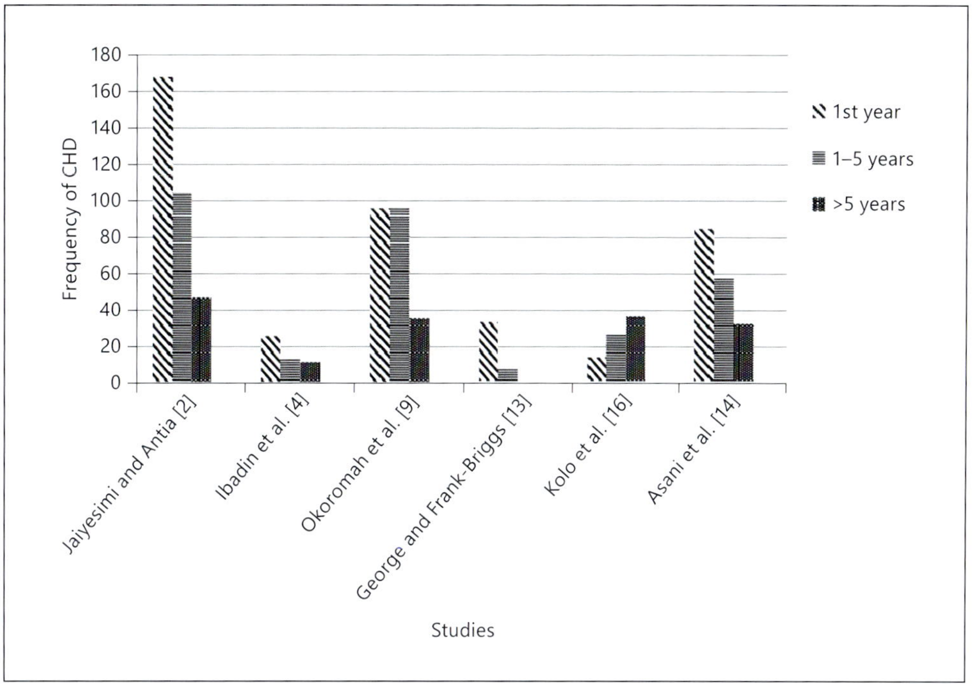

Fig. 2. Age at diagnosis of CHD in Nigeria (see also table 1 and the reference list).

pulmonary stenosis, partial AVSD, and dextrocardia in adults [16, 29–31]. In the series documented by Ejim et al. [31], all 32 ASD cases had initial diagnosis in adulthood, especially in the 3rd decade of life. CHD in adults could be as a result of follow-up of CHD managed from childhood or diagnosed initially in adulthood.

Clinical Presentation

The clinical presentation of CHD varies depending on the type of the defect, severity, and age at presentation. In the newborn period, the child could present with an asymptomatic heart murmur, cyanosis, heart failure, or outright shock. For the infants and young children, the symptoms include heart murmur, poor feeding, failure to thrive, easy fatigability, cough, fast breathing, cyanosis, digital clubbing, squatting, hypoxic spells, and features of heart failure. In adolescence, the symptoms may include murmur, chest pain, arrhythmia, syncope, hypertension, and heart failure.

In Nigeria, institutional delivery occurs in just about 45% of all births [32] while the remaining deliveries occur at home, in traditional birth attendants' facilities or in faith-based centers, frequently without skilled health personnel in attendance. The implication of this is that many critical CHD are missed resulting in early mortality. Adebonojo [33] opined that 40% of these children die in the neonatal period and another 20% within the 1st year of life. The babies born in tertiary hospitals have the benefit of getting early definite diagnosis especially in centers with pediatric cardiologists and functioning diagnostic equipment, such as echocardiography machines. In most cases, the patients are referred to the tertiary institutions when clinical features such as feeding difficulties, poor growth, repeated chest infections, cyanosis, hypoxic spells, or heart murmur are observed.

The most commonly reported clinical presentation seen in children with CHD is difficulty in breathing [4, 13]. Other clinical features include cough, fatigue, heart failure, failure to thrive, or delayed developmental milestones. For children with cyanotic CHD, the commonly reported clinical features are central cyanosis, digital clubbing, easy fatigability, poor weight gain, and hypoxic spells, especially in those with ToF [4, 10, 11, 13]. Most adults with CHD seen in Nigeria are new presentations with no prior treatment and so often have features of heart failure. In a series of adult cases with ASD, Ejim et al. [31] reported findings of dyspnea on exertion, cough, palpitation, leg swelling, chest pain, paroxysmal nocturnal dyspnea, and abdominal distension.

The limited accessibility to definitive management of CHD in Nigeria creates a scenario where those who survive to older age often develop complications. For patients with acyanotic shunt lesions, pulmonary hypertension develops, while those with cyanotic lesions, especially ToF, present with complications such as polycythemia, brain abscess, cerebrovascular accident, and iron deficiency anemia. Reported cases of Eisenmenger's complex have ranged from 0.5 to 9% in available data series, occurring most frequently in patients with VSD, ASD, PDA, and AVSD [10, 12]. Infective endocarditis is currently less reported among children with CHD compared to those with acquired heart diseases in Nigeria [34, 35]. This may not be unrelated to the limited cases of invasive diagnostic or therapeutic cardiac interventions in most centers in the country.

Management of Congenital Heart Defects in Nigeria

Medical and surgical management strategies are important in ensuring survival and better quality of life for CHD patients. For symptomatic CHD patients, definitive treatment often involves cardiac surgery or intervention by cardiac catheterization. As this is often not available in the country, prolonged medical management becomes the mainstay of treatment for most children. For patients with lesions of increased pulmonary blood flow resulting in heart failure, medical management often involves treatment of heart failure, nutritional management, monitoring, and correction of anemia and electrolyte imbalance as well as treatment of recurrent chest infections. Drugs often used to treat heart failure in children include diuretics such as furosemide, hydrochlorothiazide, and spironolactone; angiotensin-converting enzyme inhibitors such as captopril, and positive inotropic agents like digoxin, dopamine, or dobutamine. Since surgery is often delayed and patients develop pulmonary hypertension, drugs such as phosphodiesterase inhibitors are often needed. Dieticians are actively involved in the nutritional management of the patients. The children are seen regularly in outpatient clinics and admitted either to emergency rooms or pediatric wards if necessary.

For patients with ToF, a β-blocker, often oral propranolol, is given routinely to prevent hypoxic spells. Cases of polycythemia with a hematocrit ≥65% are admitted for single exchange plasmapheresis and receive iron supplementation. Where plasma is not available, as is often the case, normal saline is used for the exchange. These treatments are supported with family counseling as parents are often very distraught on being informed of the diagnosis of CHD especially when it becomes clear that a definitive treatment of the illness is beyond their financial capability. Complications, such as a brain abscess, are comanaged with the neurosurgeons.

Currently, there is no center in Nigeria where open heart surgery is performed as a routine procedure. There have, nevertheless, been cardiac surgeries carried out in various centers over the years, usually driven by visiting international medical groups working with local surgeons and physicians. Mitral valvotomy was the first cardiac surgery done in Nigeria (at the University College Hospital, UCH, Ibadan, by Mr. John Weaver) in 1960. Subsequently, palliative cardiac shunts and PDA closure were carried out. It was not until 1974 that the first open heart surgery was done in Enugu, Nigeria, at the University of Nigeria Teaching Hospital by Sir Magdi Yacoub from the UK with the support of the local team led by Prof. Fabian Udekwu [33]. By 2000, 102 surgeries, mostly for mitral valve disease (from rheumatic heart disease), VSD, ToF, and ASD had been done by different visiting teams in that center. In addition to the Hospital in Enugu, open heart surgery subsequently took place at several other centers, including UCH, Ahmadu Bello University Teaching Hospital, Zaria, and Lagos State University Teaching Hospital. After the first case of open heart surgery in Enugu, expectations were high for growth and sustenance of the program, but this was not the case. For various reasons, including financial difficulties, poor training and skills, lack of a national health insurance scheme that covers cardiac care, brain drain, interpersonal conflicts, inter-/intra-institutional conflicts, and poor planning, cardiac surgical activities declined [33, 36, 37]. Currently, there is a renewed zeal to resuscitate and build up open heart surgery programs in Nigeria. In the last decade or so, open heart surgery has been done in five centers, four of which are in the southern part of the country, but the programs are still largely driven by visiting missions and done on carefully selected patients who are not too young and do not have complex heart defects. Open heart surgeries done in these centers included repair of ASD, VSD, ToF, total anomalous pulmonary venous connection, and Glenn shunt. In seven other centers, simple procedures like PDA ligation and Blalock-Taussig shunts are being done, while some of these centers are building up infrastructure to start open heart surgery soon. All these centers are public-funded facilities with only one in the private sector. Some nongovernmental organizations are building dedicated cardiac surgery centers in Nigeria in collaboration with foreign professionals, e.g. the Kanu Heart foundation and the Aruera Reachout Foundation.

With a population of >160 million people, these efforts have been unable to meet the surgical needs of children with CHD in Nigeria. The majority of the patients are referred to health facilities outside the country for their surgery. Although patients obtain surgery in various countries, including both developed and developing countries, India has become very popular because of satisfactory expertise and low costs [38]. The costs of open heart surgery in other African countries and India ranges from USD 5,000 to 12,000, depending on the procedure and the facility; which is much lower than the costs in Europe and North America. In Nigeria, the costs range from USD 6,230 to 11,200 [39]. As expected, funding of these surgeries is a major challenge in a country with a minimum wage of about USD 100 per year.

Funding support for cardiac surgery for Nigerian patients can involve a number of sources, including: not-for-profit or nongovernmental organizations [38], government, employers, and corporate and religious organizations. Nongovernmental organizations that have made significant contributions to cardiac surgery in Nigeria over the years by sponsorship of surgeries or capacity building include: *Save a Child's Heart Foundation, Global Eagle Foundation, Save a Heart Team UK, Kanu Heart Foundation, A. Aruera Reachout Foundation, Murtala Muhammed Foundation, Vama Wave Foundation, Rotary International, MTN Foundation, Down Syndrome Association of Nigeria,* and *Medical Care Corporation.* To access funding from these groups, pediatric cardiologists regularly write medical reports and letters of appeal seeking funds for the cardiac surgery of their patients as part of the management of these patients. Despite all these efforts, few Nigerian children with CHD who require cardiac surgery actually receive it, with reported rates of 5.4 and 6.9% by Ekure et al. [40] and Sadoh et al. [12], respectively.

Follow-up care after cardiac surgery is important in the management of CHD. The patients on return from the trips abroad for surgery or following procedures done locally are investigated and monitored regularly in outpatient clinics. Some parents erroneously believe that the child does not need medical care again after the surgery and so fail to keep clinic appointments. Loss to follow-up is not limited to patients who undergo surgery abroad. Ibadin et al. [4] reported a 73.5% loss to follow-up in patients who did not undergo surgery, while Nwiloh et al. [41] documented a 100% loss to follow-up of all 11 patients with ASD and VSD who underwent open heart surgery locally within 1 year of the surgery.

Medical advances in the area of cardiac catheterization have enabled some CHD to be treated in the cardiac catheterization laboratory without surgery. Cardiac catheterization laboratories were available in two tertiary health facilities in the 1970s but were mostly used for diagnostic purposes, and by the 1990s the equipment had become obsolete. A new catheterization laboratory installed in a private health center facilitated the first intervention procedure in 2010 where a PDA was closed in a 3-year-old child. This was followed by interventions for PDA and ASD in 12 patients over the next 2 years [42]. Recently, a new catheterization laboratory has also been installed in UCH, Ibadan, and it is hoped that in the near future more interventional procedures will be done within the country by cardiac catheterization.

Outcome

Definitive surgical management reduces the risk of morbidity and mortality associated with CHD, but it also exposes the patient to surgery-related morbidity and mortality risks. The cardiac surgical experience in Nigeria is, therefore, not without these associated risks. Cardiac surgical procedures done locally, some of which included acquired heart diseases, have reported inhospital mortality rates ranging from 12.5 to 50% [2, 33, 36, 37, 43]. These are very high rates compared to rates from developed countries. Jaiyesimi and Antia [2] reported a 30-day inhospital mortality rate of 25.7% among 70 patients who underwent cardiac surgery in UCH in the 1970s and 1980s. The majority of the patients were considered to have a poor preoperative state with resulting hemorrhage, respiratory insufficiency, and heart failure postoperatively. Similarly, the report from Enugu on surgeries done a decade ago with a high mortality rate of 50% also cited poor preoperative states as likely underlying causes of death [41]. This may be a reflection of late diagnosis and delay in surgical intervention. Other reasons underlying these high postoperative mortalities included arrhythmia, right ventricular failure, and renal failure [36].

A review of children who had cardiac surgery abroad shows a lower mortality rate. Data on outcome for 68 children referred abroad from a tertiary hospital in Lagos revealed an inhospital mortality rate of 4.4%. The 3 deaths in this report had RACHS-1 risk category 2 surgeries, and a low cardiac output state was common to all 3 cases at the time of death [40]. This lower mortality may be related to selection bias.

As diagnostic, medical, and surgical facilities improve, a rising number of children with CHD are expected to survive into adulthood. For patients who are not opportuned to have definitive treatment, complications such as the Eisenmenger complex, malnutrition, reduced exercise tolerance, developmental delay, behavioral abnormalities, and poor quality of life are common. In many cases, death sadly remains the ultimate outcome.

Challenges and Opportunities

Numerous challenges persist in CHD in Nigeria. Some of these challenges are posed by the health care system and societal factors, such as a high rate of delivery outside the health care system; inadequate numbers of practicing pediatricians, pediatric cardiologists, and pediatric surgeons relative to the size of the population; limited diagnostic facilities; limited access to surgical correction, and few opportunities to conduct genetic and other etiologic research. Nonetheless, several opportunities exist. Firstly, the increasing availability of echocardiography and trained personnel provide an opportunity to carefully characterize the burden and spectrum of CHD seen in Nigeria. Such studies will provide accurate estimates of prevalence of these disorders and the potential burden they pose to the health care system. Secondly, prospective studies of etiology are urgently needed. Such studies provide an opportunity to evaluate the relative roles of environmental (or nongenetic) risk factors that may have an intervention (e.g. rubella) versus other kinds of risk factors (such as genetic and developmental syndromic disorders). A unique puzzle is the potential role of various herbal preparations as teratogens. Such herbal preparations are commonly ingested in pregnancy in Nigeria. Thirdly, genetic studies using high-throughput methods can shed light on the genetic architecture of the various CHD types in this African population. Given that African populations offer opportunities to fine map known genetic loci, discover novel loci, and advance knowledge of the etiopathogenesis of disease [44], such studies could have significant impact. One such study of CHD genetics was recently initiated in Lagos as a collaboration between two NIH Laboratories and the College of Medicine, University of Lagos. The findings should provide an insight into the potential of such studies. Fourthly, studies of natural history, clinical presentation, and outcomes should inform on the ability to better counsel affected families while providing data for use as an evidence base for advocacy and improving health care policies and programs.

References

1 Caddell JL, Morton P: The pattern of congenital heart diseases in Yoruba children of Western Nigeria. Am Heart J 1967;73:431–432.

2 Jaiyesimi F, Antia AU: Congenital heart disease in Nigeria; a ten-year experience at UCH, Ibadan. Ann Trop Paediatr 1981;1:77–85.

3 Fadahunsi HO: Congenital heart disease in Nigerian children: a study from the Lagos University Teaching Hospital. W Afr J Med 1987;6:21–30.

4 Ibadin MO, Sadoh WA, Osarogiagbon W: Congenital heart disease at the University of Benin Teaching Hospital. Nig J Paediatr 2005;32:29–32.

5 Bode-Thomas F, Okolo SN, Ekedigwe JE, Kwache IY, Adewunmi O: Paediatric echocardiography in Jos University Teaching Hospital: problems, prospects and preliminary audit. Nig J Paediatr 2003;30:143–149.

6 Hoffman JIE, Kaplan S: The incidence of congenital heart disease. J Am Coll Cardiol 2002;39:1890–1900.

7 Fixler DE, Pastor P, Chamberlin M, Sigman E, Eifler CW: Trends in congenital heart disease in Dallas county births 1971–1984. Circulation 1990;81:137–142.

8 Ekure EN, Animasahun A, Bastos M, Ezeaka VC: Congenital heart diseases associated with identified syndromes and other extra-cardiac congenital malformations in children in Lagos. West Afr J Med 2009;28:33–37.

9 Okoromah CA, Ekure EN, Ojo OO, Animasahun BA, Bastos MI: Structural heart disease in children in Lagos: profile, problems and prospects. Niger Postgrad Med J 2008;15:82–88.

10 Sani M, Mukhtar-Yola M, Karaye KM: Spectrum of congenital heart disease in a tropical environment: an echocardiography study. J Natl Med Assoc 2007;99:665–669.

11 Chinawa JM, Eze JC, Obi I, Arodiwe I, Ujunwa F, Daberechi AK, Obu HA: Synopsis of congenital cardiac disease among children attending University of Nigeria Teaching Hospital Ituku Ozalla, Enugu. BMC Res Notes 2013;6:475.

12 Sadoh WE, Uzodimma CC, Daniels Q: Congenital heart disease in Nigerian children: a multicenter echocardiographic study. World J Pediatr Congenit Heart Surg 2013;4:172–176.

13 George IO, Frank-Briggs AI: Pattern and clinical presentation of congenital heart diseases in Port-Harcourt. Niger J Med 2009;18:211–214.

14 Asani M, Aliyu I, Kabir H: Profile of congenital heart defects among children at Aminu Kano Teaching Hospital, Kano, Nigeria. J Med Trop 2013;15:131–134.

15 Wammanda RD, Danbauchi SS: An echocardiography analysis of paediatric cardiac diseases. Trop Cardiol 2002;28:29–31.

16 Kolo PM, Adeoye PO, Omotoso AB, Afolabi JK: Pattern of congenital heart disease in Ilorin. Niger Postgrad Med J 2012;19:230–234.

17 Gupta B, Antia AU: Incidence of congenital heart disease in Nigerian children. Br Heart J 1967;29:906–909.

18 Abudu OO, Uguru V, Olude O: Contribution of congenital malformation to perinatal mortality in Lagos, Nigeria. Int J Gynaecol Obstet 1988;27:63–67.

19 Sunday-Adeoye I, Okonta PI, Egwuatu VE: Congenital malformations in singleton and twin births in rural Nigeria. Niger Postgrad Med J 2007;14:277–280.

20 Ekanem TB, Okon DE, Akpantah AO, Mesembe OE, Eluwa MA, Ekong MB: Prevalence of congenital malformations in Cross River and Akwa Ibom states of Nigeria from 1980–2003. Congenit Anom (Kyoto) 2008;48:167–170.

21 Adeyemo AA, Okolo CM, Omotade OO: Major congenital malformations among paediatric admissions at University College Hospital, Ibadan, Nigeria. Ann Trop Paediatr 1994;14:75–79.

22 Adeyemo AA, Gbadegesin RA, Omotade OO: Major congenital malformations among neonatal referrals to a Nigerian university hospital. East Afr Med J 1997;74:699–701.

23 Ambe JP, Madziga AG, Akpede GO, Mava Y: Pattern and outcome of congenital malformations in newborn babies in a Nigerian teaching hospital. West Afr J Med 2010;29:24–29.

24 Chinawa JM, Eze JC, Obi I, Arodiwe I, Ujunwa F, Daberechi AK, Obu HA: Synopsis of congenital cardiac disease among children attending University of Nigeria Teaching Hospital Ituku Ozalla, Enugu. BMC Res Notes 2013;6:475.

25 Akang EE, Osinusi KO, Pindiga HU, Okpala JU, Aghadiuno PU: Congenital malformations: a review of 672 autopsies in Ibadan, Nigeria. Pediatr Pathol 1993;13:659–670.

26 Ekure EN, Abdulkareem FB: A review of 10 years autopsy of children with cardiovascular disorders. Clin J Med Sci 2005;5:35–39.

27 Cordell HJ, Bentham J, Topf A, Zelenika D, Heath S, Mamasoula C, Cosgrove C, Blue G, Granados-Riveron J, Setchfield K, Thornborough C, Breckpot J, Soemedi R, Martin R, Rahman TJ, Hall D, van Engelen K, Moorman AF, Zwinderman AH, Barnett P, Koopmann TT, Adriaens ME, Varro A, George AL Jr, dos Remedios C, Bishopric NH, Bezzina CR, O'Sullivan J, Gewillig M, Bu'Lock FA, Winlaw D, Bhattacharya S, Devriendt K, Brook JD, Mulder BJ, Mital S, Postma AV, Lathrop GM, Farrall M, Goodship JA, Keavney BD: Genome-wide association study of multiple congenital heart disease phenotypes identifies a susceptibility locus for atrial septal defect at chromosome 4p16. Nat Genet 2013;45:822–824.

28 Hu Z, Shi Y, Mo X, Xu J, Zhao B, Lin Y, Yang S, Xu Z, Dai J, Pan S, Da M, Wang X, Qian B, Wen Y, Wen J, Xing J, Guo X, Xia Y, Ma H, Jin G, Yu S, Liu J, Zhou Z, Wang X, Chen Y, Sha J, Shen H: A genome-wide association study identifies two risk loci for congenital heart malformations in Han Chinese populations. Nat Genet 2013;45:818–821.

29 Ejim EC, Ike SO, Anisiuba BC, Onwubere BJ, Ikeh VO: Ventricular septal defects at the University of Nigeria Teaching Hospital, Enugu: a review of echocardiogram records. Trans R Soc Trop Med Hyg 2009;103:159–161.

30 Ogah OS, Adegbite GD, Akinyemi RO, Adesina JO, Alabi AA, Udofia OI, Ogundipe RF, Osinfade JKL: Spectrum of heart diseases in a new cardiac service in Nigeria: an echocardiographic study of 1441 subjects in Abeokuta. BMC Res Notes 2008;1:98.

31 Ejim EC, Anisiuba BC, Ike SO, Essien IO: Atrial septal defects presenting initially in adulthood: patterns of clinical presentation in Enugu, South-East Nigeria. J Trop Med 2011;2011:251913.

32 UN Children's Fund (UNICEF), The State of the World's Children 2014 in numbers: Every child counts. Revealing disparities, advancing child rights, January 2014;75. eISBN: 978-92-806-4731-0, available at: http://www.unicef.org/sowc2014/numbers [accessed June 4, 2014].

33 Adebonojo SA: Open heart surgery in Nigeria; in Adebonojo SA (ed): Development of Open Heart Surgery in West Africa: A Historical Perspective. Eruwa, Acecool Medical, 2008, pp 21–36.

34 Ifere OA, Masokano KA: Infective endocarditis in children in the Guinea savannah of Nigeria. Ann Trop Paediatr 1991;11:233–240.

35 Bode-Thomas F, Ige OO, Yilgwan C: Childhood acquired heart diseases in Jos, north central Nigeria. Niger Med J 2013;54:51–58.

36 Falase B, Sanusi M, Majekodunmi A, Animasahun B, Ajose I, Idowu A, Oke A: Open heart surgery in Nigeria; a work in progress. J Cardiothorac Surg 203;8: 1–9.
37 Nwiloh J, Edaigbini S, Danbauchi S, Babaniyi I, Aminu M, Adamu Y, Oyati A: Cardiac surgical experience in northern Nigeria. Cardiovasc J Afr 2012;23:432–434.
38 Maheshwari S, Animasahun BA, Njokanma OF: International patients with congenital heart disease: what brings them to India? Indian Heart J 2012;64:50–53.
39 Falase B, Sanusi M, Majekodunmi A, Ajose I, Idowu A, Oke D: The cost of open heart surgery in Nigeria. Pan Afr Med J 2013;14:61.
40 Ekure EN, Okoromah CAN: In-hospital outcome of children referred for cardiac surgery abroad from a developing country. Nig J Paediatr 2009;36:80–86.
41 Nwiloh JO, Oludara MA, Adebola PA: Heart surgery practice in Sub Saharan Africa: single Nigerian institutional midterm results and challenges. World J Cardiovasc Surg 2014;4:35–41.
42 Animasahun BA, Johnson A, Ogunkunle OO, Idowu OA, Bode-Thomas F, Maheshwari S, Omokhodion SI, Njokanma OF: Transcatheter closure of patent ductus arteriosus and atrial septal defect without on-site surgical backup: a two-year experience in an African community. Pediatr Cardiol 2014;35:149–154.
43 Ugochukwu O, Jerome A: An audit of intensive care unit admission in a pediatric cardio-thoracic population in Enugu, Nigeria. Pan Afr Med J 2010;6:10.
44 Adeyemo A, Rotimi C: What does genomic medicine mean for diverse populations? Mol Genet Genomic Med 2014; 2:3–6.

Dr. Adebowale A. Adeyemo
Center for Research on Genomics and Global Health
National Human Genome Research Institute, NIH
12 South Drive, Bethesda, MD 20892-5635 (USA)
E-Mail adeyemoa@mail.nih.gov

Muenke M, Kruszka PS, Sable CA, Belmont JW (eds): Congenital Heart Disease: Molecular Genetics, Principles of Diagnosis and Treatment. Basel, Karger, 2015, pp 57–69
DOI: 10.1159/000375220

Maternal Nongenetic Risk Factors for Congenital Heart Defects

Tiffany J. Riehle-Colarusso[a] · Sonali S. Patel[b]

[a]National Center on Birth Defects and Developmental Disabilities, Centers for Disease Control and Prevention, Atlanta, Ga., and [b]Department of Pediatrics, Section of Pediatric Cardiology, University of Colorado School of Medicine, Aurora, Colo., USA

Abstract

The development of congenital heart defects (CHDs) is likely a combination of genetic and nongenetic influences. Unfortunately, CHD prevention has been hindered by a lack of conclusive information on modifiable risk factors. This chapter discusses general concepts about risk assessment and synthesizes current knowledge about nongenetic maternal risk factors, which have at least one significant finding showing evidence of a positive association with CHDs overall. Risk factors for individual CHD phenotypes are not discussed. Maternal nongenetic risk factors reviewed include sociodemographic characteristics, health conditions, therapeutic medication use, and nontherapeutic drug use. Some risk factors are clear prevention targets based on current evidence, such as diabetes and obesity. Others, such as febrile illness and antidepressant use, have inconsistent risk estimates in the literature, warranting further investigation. Prepregnancy planning, which includes a discussion with a health care provider of the various risk factors for CHDs, may improve a woman's chances of having a healthy pregnancy and delivery. Additional information regarding these and other risk factors for CHDs can be found in the primary citations, published reviews, and through the Teratogen Information Services.

The causes of most congenital heart defects (CHDs) are largely unknown. Some CHDs have been linked to genetic disorders, maternal conditions, or environmental exposures, but the development of CHDs is likely a combination of genetic and nongenetic influences (see chapter by Botto p. 28). For the purpose of this chapter, nongenetic risk factors are defined as specific maternal characteristics, conditions, or exposures for which published studies have found a positive association with CHD occurrence. Understanding these fac-

The findings and conclusions in this report are those of the authors and do not necessarily represent the official position of the Centers for Disease Control and Prevention.

tors is important for the development and implementation of targeted primary prevention strategies.

CHD prevention has been hindered by a lack of conclusive information about many potentially modifiable risk factors. Teratogens are environmental factors that affect fetal development, leading to permanent abnormalities or death. They cause approximately 10–15% of all birth defects as a result of exposure early during critical organogenesis [1]. To be a teratogen, the agent must have a well-characterized link to the adverse outcome, including exposure dose, route, and pregnancy timing [1]. One important cardiac teratogen is maternal rubella infection early in gestation, causing congenital rubella syndrome in the offspring [2].

Besides teratogens, other risk factors have been less well characterized for their association with CHDs. Studies on CHD risk factors are frequently published with updated or new information, often conflicting with earlier publications. Two well-designed, comprehensive literature reviews of nongenetic, noninherited CHD risk factors have been published synthesizing the literature. The first was a scientific statement from the American Heart Association published in 2007 [3] and the second was an updated review by Patel and Burns [4] published in 2013. This chapter provides a framework for interpreting the analyses of risk factors and summarizes the current knowledge about maternal nongenetic risk factors which have evidence of a positive association with CHDs. This information may help providers and families take actions which could decrease the likelihood of having a child with a CHD.

Understanding Risk Factors for Congenital Heart Defects

Measurements of Associations for Risk Factors with Congenital Heart Defects

Observational epidemiologic studies assess risk factors by investigating relationships between exposures and outcomes within a population. Study findings are influenced by factors such as study type and design, inclusion criteria, sample size, and analytic methods. Studies referenced in this chapter include population-based case-control and cohort studies, and meta-analyses. In a case-control study, persons with CHD in a source population are compared to a sample of the source population who do not have CHDs to provide measures of association for one or more potential risk factors. A cohort study compares persons with similar exposures to unexposed persons to evaluate the occurrence of one or more outcomes relative to the exposure. Meta-analyses combine and compare previous study results to find similarities and differences across studies. While it is beyond the scope of this chapter to describe individual studies, complete information can be found in the original papers or in the two published reviews [3, 4].

This chapter reports study results of how maternal risk differs between persons with and without CHD. The measures of associations of a study are quantified relationships between the exposure and the health problem. Depending on the study design, these could be the odds ratio (OR), relative risk (RR), or prevalence ratio (PR). An OR estimates the *odds* that CHDs will occur in an exposed group compared to the odds that CHDs will occur in an unexposed group. The RR estimates the *risk* of CHDs occurring in an exposed group compared to the risk of CHDs occurring in an unexposed group (fig. 1) [5]. The RR is more intuitive than the OR because it directly measures and compares the risks. Case-control studies are frequently used to assess risk factors associated with CHDs, and the case-control study design precludes direct estimation of RRs. Thus, ORs are more common in the CHD literature than RRs [5]. However, when a disease is rare (e.g. CHD), the OR is approximately equal to the RR. When a study calculates CHD prevalence at a point in time, then the prevalence of characteristics can be compared between groups. The PR indicates the *prevalence* of CHDs in individuals with a particular characteristic (e.g. maternal age ≥35 years) relative to those without the characteristic (e.g. maternal age 18–24 years) [5]. Confidence intervals (CIs) are usually reported with measures of association. We interpret CIs that

	Disease Yes	Disease No	Total with and without disease
Exposure yes	A	B	A+B
Exposure no	C	D	C+D

$$OR = \frac{\text{odds of disease in exposed}}{\text{odds of disease in unexposed}} = \frac{\frac{A/(A+B)}{B/(A+B)}}{\frac{C/(C+D)}{D/(C+D)}} = \frac{\frac{A}{B}}{\frac{C}{D}} = \frac{A*D}{B*C}$$

$$RR = \frac{\text{probability of disease in exposed}}{\text{probability of disease in unexposed}} = \frac{A/(A+B)}{C/(C+D)} = \frac{A*(C+D)}{C*(A+B)}$$

Fig. 1. Disease and exposure table for understanding OR and RR [5]. When a disease is rare (e.g. CHDs), the OR is approximately equal to the RR.

contain the value 1.0 as indicating that the risk estimate does not differ statistically from the null value, suggesting no association [5].

Challenges of Studying Risk Factors for Congenital Heart Defects

There are several challenges to investigating risk factors for CHDs, some of which are discussed here. How a study addresses these issues influences findings and comparisons among studies. Case definitions and case detection may vary between studies due to lack of a standard CHD nomenclature and imprecise diagnostic codes. Secondly, since CHDs are rare birth outcomes and some exposures are rare in the population, a large sample size may be necessary to detect significant associations. For example, given the prevalence of CHDs is approximately 1 in 100 births, it would take 10,000 births to find 100 infants with CHDs. Then, if 20% of mothers smoked, there might only be 20 infants with CHD and mothers who smoked in a birth cohort of 10,000.

Another challenge to studying CHD risk factors is that CHDs are a heterogeneous group of phenotypes, and an exposure may not affect the occurrence of all phenotypes uniformly. While phenotype-specific assessments of associations are more informative, this specificity is difficult to obtain in small study populations. Thus, investigations often study CHDs combined as one group of birth defects.

Additionally, estimates of measures of associations may be confounded by factors which distort the true association and need to be controlled for in the analysis. For example, the association between alcohol and CHDs could be confounded by smoking if smoking is associated with both alcohol consumption and the occurrence of CHDs. If confounding by smoking is not controlled for in the analysis, the effect estimate suggesting an association between alcohol and CHDs might be erroneous. Another potential threat to validity is recall bias, which occurs when there is a difference between study participants in the accuracy or completeness of exposure reporting. For example, mothers of infants with CHDs may be more likely to remember and report exposures than mothers of infants without CHDs. Lastly, there could be misclassification of either case status or exposure status, which could result in under- or overestimation of associations.

Measurements of associations do not necessarily establish a causal relationship between a risk factor and CHDs. The likelihood of causality is strengthened by consistent findings from multiple well-designed studies which control for confounding variables, minimize bias, account for chance findings, and have biologic plausibility [6].

Select Risk Factors

This chapter reviews maternal nongenetic risk factors for which at least one study identified a statistically significant positive association (i.e. the CI of the measure of association did not include 1.0) with CHDs. This is not an exhaustive review as exhaustive reviews have been published previously [3, 4]. However, previous review methodology [4] was utilized to identify studies published between January 1990 and April 2014 which evaluated risk factors for CHDs overall. This chapter excludes potential risk factors for individual CHD phenotypes and investigations which only evaluated specific CHD phenotypes or subgroups. Furthermore, it excludes the discussion of potential mediating factors, such as the intake of folic acid-containing multivitamins, on associations with risk factors. Risk factors meeting these criteria are further discussed in four categories: maternal sociodemographic characteristics, maternal health conditions, maternal therapeutic medications, and maternal nontherapeutic drugs. Table 1 summarizes published investigations regarding each risk factor described in this review. All investigations published during the review period with a positive measure of association, regardless of statistical significance, are included in table 1 for completeness as well as to demonstrate the range of findings. For many risk factors, findings have not been consistently significant, suggesting further investigations are warranted to inform prevention strategies. Additional information regarding these risk factors and others can be found in the primary citations, published reviews, and through the Teratogen Information Services (TIS).

Maternal Sociodemographic Characteristics

Age. Given the frequency of women delivering babies after the age 35 years as well as before the age 20 years, defining the risk of maternal age on the development of CHDs has been the focus of numerous investigations [7–9]. Advanced maternal age, defined as mothers over the age of 35 years, has been consistently associated with CHDs [8–10]. Although the risk of chromosomal aberrations increases with maternal age, it has also been hypothesized that in children without identified chromosomal abnormalities, the structural abnormalities observed are related to unknown or undetectable genetic defects. Younger maternal age, defined as mothers younger than 20 years, has had less consistent findings with CHDs [8, 9]. In contrast to chromosomal etiologies as seen with older mothers, it is hypothesized that other factors, such as less prenatal care, nutritional status, and gynecological immaturity, may play a role in CHD development in infants of younger mothers, although studies evaluating these factors have not been performed.

Maternal Reproductive History. Other maternal sociodemographic factors have been investigated for their potential association with CHDs, including maternal reproductive history and maternal stress. It is difficult to directly quantify reproductive history, but common proxies include the number of prior pregnancies, number of prior live births, and use of assisted reproductive technologies. A maternal history of greater than three pregnancies and/or live births has been identified as a risk factor for CHD development [9–13]. It has been hypothesized that this may be due to nutrient depletion. In addition, use of assisted reproductive techniques, such as in vitro fertilization, has been associated with CHDs [14].

Maternal Stress. Maternal stress has also been investigated for its role in CHD development. Maternal stressors may lead to birth defects through increased production of corticosteroids. Increased glucocorticoid levels are associated with hyperinsulinemia and insulin resistance, which may be associated with an increased risk of CHDs. Additionally, stress increases catecholamine production, which in turn decreases uterine blood flow and increases the risk for fetal hypoxia. An investigation performed in China identified an association between CHD development and maternal self-reported mental stress levels during pregnancy [12]. While maternal stress may impact CHD development, accurate measurement of stress is challenging and warrants further study.

Maternal Health Conditions

Diabetes. Diabetes is a major health concern worldwide, with increasing rates in developed and developing countries [15]. Multiple studies demonstrate consistent associations between maternal pregestational diabetes and multiple birth defects, including CHDs [16–19]. Although the mechanisms are not well understood, it appears there is a positive

Table 1. Estimates of select maternal risk factors associated with CHDs

Risk factor	Data source (study years)	Study design	OR, PR, and RR (95% CI)
Age			
Advanced (35–39 years)	Canadian Institute for Health Information (2002–2010) [9]	Cohort	**1.1 (1.1–1.2)**^{OR}
	Metropolitan Atlanta Congenital Defects Program (1968–2005) [8]	Cohort	**1.2 (1.1–1.3)**^{PR}
	Polish Registry of Congenital Malformations (1998–2002) [7]	Cohort	1.1 (1.0–1.1)^{OR}
	Baltimore-Washington Infant Study (1981–1989) [10]	Case-control	**1.3 (1.1–1.5)**^{OR}
Advanced (≥40 years)	Canadian Institute for Health Information (2002–2010) [9]	Cohort	**1.6 (1.5–1.7)**^{OR}
Young (≤20 years)	Canadian Institute for Health Information (2002–2010) [9]	Cohort	**1.2 (1.1–1.2)**^{OR}
	Metropolitan Atlanta Congenital Defects Program (1968–2005) [8]	Cohort	0.9 (0.8–1.1)^{PR}
Reproductive history			
Multigravidity (≥3 pregnancies)	Polish Registry of Congenital Malformations (2005–2006)[13]	Cohort	**1.2 (1.1–1.4)**^{OR}
	Shandong Peninsula, China (2004–2005) [12]	Case-control	**2.5 (1.5–4.0)**^{OR}
Multiparity (≥3 live births)	Canadian Institute for Health Information (2002–2010) [9]	Cohort	**1.3 (1.3–1.4)**^{OR}
	National Birth Defects Prevention Study (1997–2007) [11]	Case-control	1.0 (0.9–1.1)^{OR}
	Baltimore-Washington Infant Study (1981–1989) [10]	Case-control	**1.3 (1.1–1.5)**^{OR}
Use of assisted reproductive techniques	Paris Registry of Congenital Malformations (1987–2006) [14]	Case-control	**1.4 (1.1–1.7)**^{OR}
Stress	Shandong Peninsula, China (2004–2005) [12]	Case-control	**2.7 (1.5–4.8)**^{OR}
Diabetes mellitus (pregestational)	EUROCAT (1990–2005) [16]	Cohort	**2.2 (1.9–2.6)**^{OR}
	HCCSCA (1980–1996) [17]	Case-control	**2.5 (1.6–3.9)**^{OR}
	National Birth Defects Prevention Study (1997–2003) [18]	Case-control	**4.6 (2.9–7.5)**^{OR}
	Baltimore-Washington Infant Study (1981–1989) [19]	Case-control	**3.0 (1.9–4.8)**^{OR}
Prepregnancy weight			
BMI 25–29 kg/m^2	National Birth Defects Prevention Study (1997–2004) [22]	Case-control	**1.2 (1.1–1.3)**^{OR}
	Swedish Medical Birth Registry (1995–2007) [23]	Cohort	1.1 (1.0–1.1)^{OR}
	Atlanta Birth Defects Risk Factor Surveillance Study (1993–1997) [24]	Case-control	**2.0 (1.2–3.1)**^{OR}
BMI ≥25 kg/m^2	National Birth Defects Prevention Study (1997–2004) [22]	Case-control	**1.2 (1.1–1.3)**^{OR}
BMI 30–35	National Birth Defects Prevention Study (1997–2004) [22]	Case-control	**1.2 (1.1–1.4)**^{OR}
	Swedish Medical Birth Registry (1995–2007) [23]	Cohort	1.1(1.0–1.2)^{OR}
BMI ≥30 kg/m^2	Canadian Institute for Health Information (2002–2010) [9]	Cohort	**1.9 (1.7–2.2)**^{OR}
	Atlanta Birth Defects Risk Factor Surveillance Study (1993–1997) [24]	Case-control	**2.0 (1.2–3.4)**^{OR}
BMI ≥35 kg/m^2	National Birth Defects Prevention Study (1997–2004) [22]	Case-control	**1.4 (1.2–1.7)**^{OR}
	Swedish Medical Birth Registry (1995–2007) [23]	Cohort	**1.3 (1.1–1.4)**^{OR}
Epilepsy	Canadian Institute for Health Information (2002–2010) [9]	Cohort	**2.7 (2.2–3.2)**^{OR}
Febrile illness	National Birth Defects Prevention Study (1997–2005) [25]	Case-control	1.1 (1.0–1.3)^{OR}
	Baltimore-Washington Infant Study (1981–1989) [26]	Case-control	1.1 (0.9–1.5)^{OR}
	Atlanta Birth Defects Case-Control Study (1968–1980) [27]	Case-control	**1.8 (1.4–2.4)**^{OR}
Influenza	Baltimore-Washington Infant Study (1981–1989) [26]	Case-control	1.1 (0.9–1.4)^{OR}
	HCCSCA (1980–1996) [29]	Case-control	**1.7 (1.3–2.3)**^{OR}

Table 1. Continued

Risk factor	Data source (study years)	Study design	OR, PR, and RR (95% CI)
	Atlanta Birth Defects Case-Control Study (1968–1980) [27]	Case-control	2.1 (0.8–5.5)^{OR}
Genitourinary infections	National Birth Defects Prevention Study (1997–2005) [30]	Case-control	1.7 (1.0–2.9)^{OR}
	HCCSCA (1980–1996) [28]	Case-control	**2.6 (1.2–5.4)**^{OR}
Upper respiratory infection	National Birth Defects Prevention Study (1997–2005) [25]	Case-control	1.1 (0.9–1.3)^{OR}
	Shandong Peninsula, China (2004–2005) [12]	Case-control	**5.9 (2.7–13.1)**^{OR}
	Finnish Register of Congenital Malformations (1982–1983) [31]	Case-control	**1.5 (1.1–2.1)**^{OR}
Hypercholesterolemia/atherosclerotic heart disease	HAVEN (2003–2010) [32]	Case-control	**1.5 (1.1–2.1)**^{OR}
	Canadian Institute for Health Information (2002–2010) [9]	Cohort	**2.2 (1.9–2.6)**^{OR}
Hyperhomocysteinemia	Arkansas Reproductive Health Monitoring System (1998–2008) [33]	Case-control	**1.5 (1.2–1.8)**^{OR}
	HAVEN (2003–2005) [34]	Case-control	**2.9 (1.4–6.0)**^{OR}
	Alabama Prenatal Genetics Clinics (1988–1998) [35]	Case-control	**3.5 (1.2–10.2)**^{OR}
Hypertension	Canadian Institute for Health Information (2002–2010) [9]	Cohort	**1.8 (1.6–2.0)**^{OR}
	Kaiser Permanente Northern California (1995–2008) [38]	Cohort	**1.4 (1.3–1.5)**^{OR}
	National Birth Defects Prevention Study (1997–2003) [37]	Case-control	**1.8 (1.1–2.7)**^{OR}
	Finnish Register of Congenital Malformations (1982–1983) [31]	Case-control	**2.6 (1.1–5.2)**^{OR}
Phenylketonuria (PKU)	Maternal PKU Collaborative Study (1984–1995) [39]	Cohort	–*
Rubella	Review of 11 studies (1965–1996) [2]	Meta-analysis	–*
Antiasthmatics	NY State Congenital Malformations Registry (1988–1991) [43]	Case-control	**2.4 (1.2–4.8)**^{OR}
	Swedish Medical Birth Registry (1995–2004) [42]	Cohort	1.1 (1.0–1.3)^{OR}
Bronchodilators	NY State Congenital Malformations Registry (1988–1991) [43]	Case-control	**2.2 (1.1–4.6)**^{OR}
	Swedish Medical Birth Registry (1995–2004) [42]	Cohort	**1.4 (1.1–1.7)**^{OR}
Antibiotics			
Penicillins	National Birth Defects Prevention Study (1997–2003) [44]	Case-control	1.0 (0.8–1.1)^{OR}
	Swedish Medical Birth Registry (1995–2001) [48]	Case-control	1.0 (0.8–1.2)^{OR}
	Baltimore-Washington Infant Study (1981–1989) [10]	Case-control	**1.3 (1.1–1.6)**^{OR}
Dihydrofolate reductase inhibitors	Clalit Health Maintenance Organization (1998–2007) [47]	Cohort	**2.3 (1.3–3.9)**^{OR}
	Slone Epidemiology Unit Birth Defects Study (1976–1988) [46]	Case-control	**3.4 (1.8–6.4)**^{RR}
Combination (dihydrofolate reductase inhibitors and sulfonamides)	Clalit Health Maintenance Organization (1998–2007) [47]	Cohort	**2.3 (1.3–3.9)**^{OR}
	National Birth Defects Prevention Study (1997–2003) [44]	Case-control	1.5 (1.0–2.2)^{OR}
	Swedish Medical Birth Registry (1995–2001) [48]	Case-control	**1.6 (1.1–2.3)**^{OR}
	HCCSCA (1980–1996) [45]	Case-control	**2.1 (1.4–3.3)**^{OR}
Antidepressants	Baltimore-Washington Infant Study (1981–1989) [10]	Case-control	**3.0 (1.2–7.6)**^{OR}
Selective serotonin reuptake inhibitors	Finnish Register of Congenital Malformations (1996–2003) [49]	Cohort	**1.3 (1.1–1.6)**^{OR}
	Swedish Medical Birth Registry (1995–2007) [51]	Cohort	1.0 (0.8–1.2)^{PR}

Table 1. Continued

Risk factor	Data source (study years)	Study design	OR, PR, and RR (95% CI)
Serotonin-norepinephrine reuptake inhibitors	National Birth Defects Prevention Study (1997–2007) [50]	Case-control	**2.7 (1.5–5.0)**^{OR}
	Swedish Medical Birth Registry (1995–2007) [51]	Cohort	1.3 (0.8–2.1)^{PR}
Tricyclic antidepressants	Swedish Medical Birth Registry (1995–2007) [51]	Cohort	**1.6 (1.1–2.4)**^{PR}
Antiepileptics	National Birth Defects Prevention Study (1997–2005) [52]	Case-control	1.4 (1.0–2.1)^{OR}
	Slone Epidemiology Unit Birth Defects Study (1976–1988) [46]	Case-control	**2.2 (1.4–3.5)**^{RR}
Phenobarbital	Malformation and Drug Exposure Collaborative (1990–1996) [53]	Case-control	**2.2 (1.2–4.0)**^{OR}
Antifungals (metronidazole)	Baltimore-Washington Infant Study (1981–1989) [10]	Case-control	**2.5 (1.1–5.8)**^{OR}
Antihypertensives	HCCSCA (1980–1996) [36]	Case-control	1.3 (1.0–1.5)^{OR}
	Kaiser Permanente Northern California (1995–2008) [38]	Cohort	1.5 (1.0–2.2)^{OR}
	National Birth Defects Prevention Study (1997–2003) [37]	Case-control	**1.8 (1.1–2.7)**^{OR}
	Swedish Medical Birth Registry (1982–2006) [54]	Cohort	**2.6 (1.9–3.5)**^{OR}
β-Blockers	National Birth Defects Prevention Study (1997–2003) [37]	Case-control	**2.6 (1.2–5.3)**^{OR}
	Swedish Medical Birth Registry (1982–2001) [48]	Cohort	**1.9 (1.2–2.8)**^{OR}
Angiotensin-converting enzyme inhibitors	Kaiser Permanente Northern California (1995–2008) [38]	Cohort	1.5 (0.9–2.6)^{OR}
	National Birth Defects Prevention Study (1997–2003) [37]	Case-control	1.9 (0.5–7.2)^{OR}
	Swedish Medical Birth Registry (1982–2006) [54]	Cohort	2.9 (0.9–6.8)^{OR}
	Tennessee Medicaid (1985–2000) [55]	Cohort	**3.7 (1.9–7.3)**^{RR}
Anti-inflammatory agents			
Ibuprofen	Norwegian Mother and Child Cohort Study (1999–2007) [56]	Cohort	0.9 (0.5–1.5)^{OR}
	Baltimore-Washington Infant Study (1981–1989) [10]	Case-control	**1.4 (1.1–1.8)**^{OR}
Naproxen	Swedish Medical Birth Registry (1995–2001) [48]	Case-control	**1.7 (1.1–2.5)**^{OR}
Alcohol (≥5 drinks/sitting)	Pregnancy Risk Assessment Monitoring System (1996–2005) [57]	Case-control	**3.0 (1.2–7.5)**^{OR}
	Baltimore-Washington Infant Study (1981–1989) [10]	Case-control	1.1 (0.9–1.4)^{OR}
Cigarette smoking	Canadian Institute for Health Information (2002–2010) [9]	Cohort	**1.3 (1.1–1.5)**^{OR}
	Analysis of 33 studies (1971–2011) [58]	Meta-analysis	1.1 (1.0–1.2)^{OR}
	Baltimore-Washington Infant Study (1981–1989) [59]	Case-control	1.1 (1.0–1.2)^{OR}
	National Birth Defects Prevention Study (1997–2002) [60]	Case-control	**1.2 (1.1–1.4)**^{OR}
Cocaine	Boston City Hospital (1988–1990) [62]	Cohort	**3.7 (1.4–9.4)**^{RR}
	Baltimore-Washington Infant Study (1981–1989) [10]	Case-control	**1.6 (1.1–2.3)**^{OR}

Data source: studies are listed in descending order of publication date. Significant values are in bold. –* = Measure of association not provided; HAVEN = Heart Defects, Vascular Status, Genetic Factors and Nutrition Study; HCCSCA = Hungarian Case-Control Surveillance of Congenital Abnormalities; NY = New York.

association between hyperglycemia during embryogenesis and the risk for congenital malformations among infants of diabetic mothers [18]. While the prevalence of birth defects among diabetic women with optimal glycemic control is similar to that of the general population, achieving and maintaining euglycemia early in pregnancy remains a challenge, especially since many pregnancies are unplanned [20]. Glycemic control has been proposed as a prevention strategy for birth defects; however, as the prevalence of diabetes continues to rise, this may not be solely effective [15].

Prepregnancy Weight. The prevalence of overweight and obesity is also increasing in the United States at an alarming rate [8]. Adult weight is categorized by use of the body mass index (BMI), a measure of weight for height: overweight is a BMI between 25 and 30 kg/m^2, obesity is a BMI between 30 and 40 kg/m^2, and morbid or severe obesity is a BMI greater than 40 kg/m^2 [21]. Given the rise in excess weight among potential mothers, multiple studies have investigated the role of prepregnancy weight on the development of CHDs. Each category of excess weight has been significantly associated with the development of CHDs [9, 22–24]. However, interpretation of these studies is challenging as it remains unclear whether associations are due to causality or confounding. For example, obesity may co-occur with pregestational diabetes, making it difficult to separate contributory from interactive effects. Given the increasing prevalence of overweight and obesity, preventive and management strategies for prepregnancy weight are important for reducing the occurrence of CHDs.

Epilepsy. Epilepsy is a chronic condition which has been investigated for its association with CHD. A cohort study conducted in Canada identified an increased risk of CHDs among infants born to mothers with a history of epilepsy [9]. It is unclear whether this association is solely from the condition or from the medications used to treat it, suggesting the need for further investigations.

Febrile Illness. Evidence for the role of maternal febrile illness during the first trimester of pregnancy in the development of CHDs has been mixed [25–27]. Fever can have multiple infectious etiologies (e.g., influenza, genitourinary infections, or upper respiratory infections), and can be difficult to define or establish retrospectively. Additionally, reporting a history of fever is subject to recall bias. Studies of individual infectious etiologies of fever have demonstrated inconsistent findings related to CHDs [12, 25–31], suggesting further investigations examining the role of maternal fever and its etiologies are needed to inform prevention strategies.

Hypercholesterolemia and Atherosclerotic Heart Disease. Lipids act as ligands for receptors and transcription factors involved in intracellular signaling processes and gene expression during cardiac embryogenesis. As the majority of embryonic cholesterol is derived from the mother, it is hypothesized that excess maternal lipids may have differential effects on fetal genes and tissues of the fetus. A case-control study performed in Holland identified an increased risk of CHDs in infants born to mothers with abnormal lipid profiles, including elevated total and low-density lipoprotein cholesterol levels [32]. In addition, a population-based cohort study identified an association between atherosclerotic heart disease and the formation of congenital heart defects, again suggesting a role of excess lipids in CHD development [9].

Hyperhomocysteinemia. Folate is a key factor in cardiovascular development. Folate and vitamin B_{12} are involved in the remethylation of homocysteine into methionine. A compromised folate and/or vitamin B_{12} status results in hyperhomocysteinemia. In animal models, high levels of homocysteine have resulted in cardiac defects. Three studies have demonstrated an increased risk of CHD in infants born to mothers with high homocysteine levels [33–35]; however, these studies were conducted with small sample sizes, suggesting further work is warranted.

Hypertension. Hypertension is a common condition during pregnancy, occurring in up to 5% of women [36]. Multiple studies have identified nearly a twofold increase in the risk of CHDs among infants born to mothers with hypertension during pregnancy [9, 31, 37, 38]. As was discussed in the epilepsy section, it is unclear whether the excess risk lies with the condition or the medication, and needs further investigation.

Phenylketonuria. Two other conditions, maternal phenylketonuria (PKU) and maternal rubella infections, have well-established teratogenic associations with CHDs in recently published studies. Uncontrolled maternal PKU can be teratogenic on the fetal brain and heart. In one study, CHDs occurred in 14% of pregnancies exposed to high maternal phenylalanine levels compared to only 1% among nonexposed pregnancies [39]. This risk for CHDs can be reduced with controlled phenylalanine levels through diet regulation prior to and during pregnancy; however, implementation of these preventive strategies is challenging and complex [40].

Maternal Rubella Infection. The teratogenicity of maternal rubella infection during pregnancy has also been demonstrated. A review suggests approximately 45% of infants with congenital rubella syndrome have some form of CHD [2]. The risk of rubella embryopathy can be virtually eliminated by ensuring women of child-bearing age are immunized against rubella, highlighting the effectiveness of primary prevention [41].

Maternal Therapeutic Medications

Management of chronic conditions frequently necessitates the use of medications during pregnancy. Studies examining the relationship of medication use during pregnancy and CHDs are challenging to interpret as findings may be a consequence of the condition or the medication. Although there are elevated risks identified for some classes of medications, there are valid reasons for pregnant women to continue to take the medication for the management of their chronic conditions, which should be discussed with their health care provider.

Antiasthmatics. Asthma medications are utilized by women during pregnancy. Some results have shown a significant relationship between antiasthmatic medication use during pregnancy and CHDs, but other results were not significant [42, 43]. When separated by class of medication, however, an increased risk of CHDs has been identified with maternal bronchodilator use during pregnancy [42, 43].

Antibiotics. Antibiotics are commonly prescribed during the periconceptional period of pregnancy. An increased risk of CHDs has been observed among mothers who reported use of a dihydrofolate reductase inhibitor (e.g. sulfasalazine), penicillin, or dihydrofolate reductase inhibitor combined with sulfonamide (e.g. trimethoprim-sulfamethoxazole) [10, 44–48].

Antidepressants. Given that depressive symptoms can affect up to 20% of women during pregnancy [49], studies have examined the association of maternal antidepressant use during pregnancy with the development of CHDs [10, 49–51]. Any maternal antidepressant use, as well as medications within the three classes of antidepressants (i.e. selective serotonin reuptake inhibitors, serotonin-norepinephrine reuptake inhibitors, and tricyclic antidepressants), have been associated with CHDs [49–51].

Antiepileptics. There have been conflicting results regarding the risk of any antiepileptic medication use during pregnancy and CHD development [46, 52]. In addition, a large collaborative surveillance system study identified the increased risk of CHDs associated with phenobarbital, a type of antiepileptic [53]. However, study variability, multiple medication use, and the small number of exposed cases make it difficult to establish the true cardiac risk [52, 53]. Mechanisms for the formation of CHDs may include a direct teratogenic effect or an indirect effect by interfering with folate metabolism [46].

Antifungals. Antifungal medications are another class of medications prescribed during the periconceptional period. A significant association between metronidazole use and the development of CHDs has been observed [10]; however, this association has not been replicated or evaluated in other studies.

Antihypertensives. Antihypertensive medications may be prescribed during the periconceptional period. Investigation of maternal use of these medications associated with CHD development has yielded conflicting results. Analyses of the Swedish Medical Birth Register and the National Birth Defects Prevention Study databases identified a two- to threefold increased risk of CHDs [37, 54], but more recent studies have not reported significant associations [36, 38]. Given the reported increased risk, investigations into specific classes of medications have been performed. β-Blocker medications have been consistently identified to have an increased risk of CHD development [37, 48], while investigation results of angiotensin-converting enzyme inhibitors have been mixed [37, 38, 54, 55]. As with other medications, it has been postulated that the apparent increased risk may be due to the underlying condition (i.e. hypertension), highlighting the need for further investigations.

Nonsteroidal Anti-Inflammatory Drugs. Nonsteroidal anti-inflammatory drugs are commonly used over-the-counter medications. Studies on these drugs as a group have not found a significant association with CHDs. However, two particular medications have been observed to have a slightly significantly increased risk of CHD development: ibuprofen and naproxen [10, 48, 56].

Maternal Nontherapeutic Drugs

Alcohol. There is a wide range of teratogenic effects of alcohol consumption during pregnancy on birth outcomes. Alcohol may impact cardiac development through its contribution to impaired conversion of retinol to retinoic acid, antagonism of the N-methyl-D-aspartate receptor, compromised nutritional status, or vascular disruptive events [4]. Conflicting results have been reported for maternal alcohol consumption during the periconceptional period and CHD development, likely due to the challenge of documenting exposure and potential interaction with other risk factors such as cigarette smoking [10, 57]. However, given the multiple adverse birth outcomes, prevention of this exposure is of public health importance.

Smoking. Although maternal cigarette smoking has been established as a risk factor for preterm birth and low birth weight, it may only be a modest risk for CHD development. Studies, including a recent meta-analysis [58], have yielded inconsistent results for CHDs [9, 58–60]. The mechanisms by which cigarette smoke and/or the chemical compounds contained within it might result in CHDs remain to be elucidated; however, fetal hypoxia, alterations in essential nutrients, direct teratogenic effects, and DNA damage have been hypothesized as potential pathways of harm [61]. Given the prevalence of exposure to cigarette smoke (both active and passive) and potential infant morbidity burden, as well as suggestive evidence associating it with CHDs, efforts to reduce smoking prior to conception and during pregnancy should be employed [61].

Cocaine. An increased risk of CHD development has been observed among mothers who reported prenatal cocaine use [10, 62]. Cocaine may exert direct toxic effects on fetal myocytes. Exposure of myocardial cells from near-term fetal rats to cocaine resulted in apoptotic cell death, which may play a role in the development of structural malformations [63].

Conclusion

In summary, this chapter reviews maternal nongenetic risk factors which have evidence in the last 25 years for being significantly associated with CHD development. Only risk factors for CHDs as a group were discussed. Since CHDs are a heterogeneous group of defects, the associations reviewed in this chapter may not be uniform across all CHD phenotypes. Furthermore, it excludes risk factors that may be associated with individual CHDs, but have not shown evidence for CHDs as a group. Table 1 shows the range of results for maternal sociodemographic characteristics, maternal health conditions, maternal therapeutic medication use, and maternal nontherapeutic drug use. While all risk factors discussed have at least one study showing a statistically significant association, many of the risk factors have conflicting results. Given the inconsistent results and challenges with studying risk factors, additional investigations are warranted for many risk factors. Well-designed, population-based epidemiologic studies are important to guide prevention policies and interventions.

Improved awareness of maternal nongenetic risk factors for CHDs among women and healthcare providers may provide opportunities for preventive actions to decrease the occurrence of CHDs. For example, there is evidence for prevention strategies such as maintenance of a healthy weight, good glycemic control of diabetes, and avoidance of alcohol and cigarette smoking. Other factors, such as advanced maternal age, maternal stress, reproductive history, febrile illness early in pregnancy, chronic health conditions, such as epilepsy and cardiovascular disease, and use of certain medications, such as some antibiotics, antiasthmatics, antidepressants, antihypertensives, and antiepileptics, may also increase the risk of having a baby with CHD. It may also help women who take medications for chronic health conditions to discuss the therapeutic options during pregnancy with a health care provider. Additionally, all pregnant women or women planning to become pregnant should be encouraged to discuss all medications and herbal or dietary supplements they are taking or planning to take with their health care provider. Prepregnancy planning which includes a discussion with a healthcare provider of various risk factors for CHD may improve a woman's chances of having a healthy pregnancy and delivery.

References

1 Brent RL: The causes and prevention of human birth defects: what have we learned in the past 50 years? Congenit Anom (Kyoto) 2001;41:3–21.
2 Reef SE, Plotkin S, Cordero JF, Katz M, Cooper L, Schwartz B, Zimmerman-Swain L, Danovaro-Holliday MC, Wharton M: Preparing for elimination of congenital rubella syndrome (CRS): summary of a workshop on CRS elimination in the United States. Clin Infect Dis 2000;31:85–95.
3 Jenkins KJ, Correa A, Feinstein JA, Botto L, Britt AE, Daniels SR, Elixson M, Warnes CA, Webb CL; American Heart Association Council on Cardiovascular Disease in the Young: Noninherited risk factors and congenital cardiovascular defects: current knowledge: a scientific statement from the American Heart Association Council on Cardiovascular Disease in the Young: endorsed by the American Academy of Pediatrics. Circulation 2007;115:2995–3014.
4 Patel SS, Burns TL: Nongenetic risk factors and congenital heart defects. Pediatr Cardiol 2013;34:1535–1555.
5 Blair RC, Taylor RA: Biostatistics for the Health Sciences. Upper Saddle River, Pearson Prentice Hall, 2008.
6 Botto LD: Epidemiology and Prevention of Congenital Heart Defects; in Allen HD, Driscoll DJ, Shaddy RE, Feltes TF (eds): Moss and Adams' Heart Disease in Infants, Children, and Adolescents: Including the Fetus and Young Adult. Philadelphia, Lippincott, Williams & Wilkins, 2013, chapt 25.
7 Materna-Kiryluk A, Wisniewska K, Badura-Stronka M, Mejnartowicz J, Wieckowska B, Balcar-Boron A, Czerwionka-Szaflarska M, Gajewska E, Godula-Stuglik U, Krawczynski M, Limon J, Rusin J, Sawulicka-Oleszczuk H, Szwalkiewicz-Warowicka E, Walczak M, Latos-Bielenska A: Parental age as a risk factor for isolated congenital malformations in a Polish population. Paediatr Perinat Epidemiol 2009; 23:29–40.
8 Miller A, Riehle-Colarusso T, Siffel C, Frias JL, Correa A: Maternal age and prevalence of isolated congenital heart defects in an urban area of the United States. Am J Med Genet A 2011;155A:2137–2145.
9 Liu S, Joseph KS, Lisonkova S, Rouleau J, Van den Hof M, Sauve R, Kramer MS; Canadian Perinatal Surveillance System (Public Health Agency of Canada): Association between maternal chronic conditions and congenital heart defects: a population-based cohort study. Circulation 2013;128: 583–589.
10 Ferencz C, Rubin JD, Loffredo C, Magee CA: Epidemiology of Congenital Heart Disease: The Baltimore-Washington Infant Study: 1981–1989. Mount Kisco, Futura, 1993.
11 Duong HT, Hoyt AT, Carmichael SL, Gilboa SM, Canfield MA, Case A, McNeese ML, Waller DK; National Birth Defects Prevention Study: Is maternal parity an independent risk factor for birth defects? Birth Defects Res A Clin Mol Teratol 2012;94:230–236.
12 Liu S, Liu J, Tang J, Ji J, Chen J, Liu C: Environmental risk factors for congenital heart disease in the Shandong Peninsula, China: a hospital-based case-control study. J Epidemiol 2009;19:122–130.
13 Materna-Kiryluk A, Wieckowska B, Wisniewska K, Borszewska-Kornacka MK, Godula-Stuglik U, Limon J, Rusin J, Sawulicka-Oleszczuk H, Szwalkiewicz-Warowicka E, Walczak M; Members of PRCM Working Group: Maternal reproductive history and the risk of isolated congenital malformations. Paediatr Perinat Epidemiol 2011; 25:135–143.
14 Tararbit K, Houyel L, Bonnet D, De Vigan C, Lelong N, Goffinet F, Khoshnood B: Risk of congenital heart defects associated with assisted reproductive technologies: a population-based evaluation. Eur Heart J 2011; 32:500–508.
15 Mokdad AH, Bowman BA, Ford ES, Vinicor F, Marks JS, Koplan JP: The continuing epidemics of obesity and diabetes in the United States. JAMA 2001;286:1195–1200.
16 Garne E, Loane M, Dolk H, Barisic I, Addor MC, Arriola L, Bakker M, Calzolari E, Matias Dias C, Doray B, Gatt M, Melve KK, Nelen V, O'Mahony M, Pierini A, Randrianaivo-Ranjatoelina H, Rankin J, Rissmann A, Tucker D, Verellun-Dumoulin C, Wiesel A: Spectrum of congenital anomalies in pregnancies with pregestational diabetes. Birth Defects Res A Clin Mol Teratol 2012;94:134–140.
17 Banhidy F, Acs N, Puho EH, Czeizel AE: Congenital abnormalities in the offspring of pregnant women with type 1, type 2 and gestational diabetes mellitus: a population-based case-control study. Congenit Anom (Kyoto) 2010;50:115–121.
18 Correa A, Gilboa SM, Besser LM, Botto LD, Moore CA, Hobbs CA, Cleves MA, Riehle-Colarusso TJ, Waller DK, Reece EA: Diabetes mellitus and birth defects. Am J Obstet Gynecol 2008;199:237.e1–e9.
19 Loffredo CA, Wilson PD, Ferencz C: Maternal diabetes: an independent risk factor for major cardiovascular malformations with increased mortality of affected infants. Teratology 2001;64:98–106.
20 Dunne F, Brydon P, Smith K, Gee H: Pregnancy in women with type 2 diabetes: 12 years outcome data 1990–2002. Diabet Med 2003;20:734–738.
21 National Institutes of Health: Clinical guidelines on the identification, evaluation, and treatment of overweight and obesity in adults – the evidence report. Obes Res 1998; 6(suppl 2):51S–209S.
22 Gilboa SM, Correa A, Botto LD, Rasmussen SA, Waller DK, Hobbs CA, Cleves MA, Riehle-Colarusso TJ; National Birth Defects Prevention Study: Association between prepregnancy body mass index and congenital heart defects. Am J Obstet Gynecol 2010; 202:51.e1–e10.

23 Blomberg MI, Kallen B: Maternal obesity and morbid obesity: the risk for birth defects in the offspring. Birth Defects Res A Clin Mol Teratol 2010;88:35–40.
24 Watkins ML, Rasmussen SA, Honein MA, Botto LD, Moore CA: Maternal obesity and risk for birth defects. Pediatrics 2003;111(5 pt 2):1152–1158.
25 Botto LD, Panichello JD, Browne ML, Krikov S, Feldkamp ML, Lammer E, Shaw GM; National Birth Defects Prevention Study: Congenital heart defects after maternal fever. Am J Obstet Gynecol 2014;210: 359.e1–e11.
26 Oster ME, Riehle-Colarusso T, Alverson CJ, Correa A: Associations between maternal fever and influenza and congenital heart defects. J Pediatr 2011;158:990–995.
27 Botto LD, Lynberg MC, Erickson JD: Congenital heart defects, maternal febrile illness, and multivitamin use: a population-based study. Epidemiology 2001;12:485–490.
28 Acs N, Banhidy F, Puho EH, Czeizel AE: Possible association between acute pelvic inflammatory disease in pregnant women and congenital abnormalities in their offspring: a population-based case-control study. Birth Defects Res A Clin Mol Teratol 2008;82:563–570.
29 Acs N, Banhidy F, Puho E, Czeizel AE: Maternal influenza during pregnancy and risk of congenital abnormalities in offspring. Birth Defects Res A Clin Mol Teratol 2005; 73:989–996.
30 Cleves MA, Malik S, Yang S, Carter TC, Hobbs CA: Maternal urinary tract infections and selected cardiovascular malformations. Birth Defects Res A Clin Mol Teratol 2008;82:464–473.
31 Tikkanen J, Heinonen OP: Risk factors for cardiovascular malformations in Finland. Eur J Epidemiol 1990;6:348–356.
32 Smedts HP, van Uitert EM, Valkenburg O, Laven JS, Eijkemans MJ, Lindemans J, Steegers EA, Steegers-Theunissen RP: A derangement of the maternal lipid profile is associated with an elevated risk of congenital heart disease in the offspring. Nutr Metab Cardiovasc Dis 2012;22:477–485.
33 Hobbs CA, MacLeod SL, Jill James S, Cleves MA: Congenital heart defects and maternal genetic, metabolic, and lifestyle factors. Birth Defects Res A Clin Mol Teratol 2011; 91:195–203.
34 Verkleij-Hagoort AC, Verlinde M, Ursem NT, Lindemans J, Helbing WA, Ottenkamp J, Siebel FM, Gittenberger-de Groot AC, de Jonge R, Bartelings MM, Steegers EA, Steegers-Theunissen RP: Maternal hyperhomocysteinaemia is a risk factor for congenital heart disease. BJOG 2006;113:1412–1418.
35 Wenstrom KD, Johanning GL, Johnston KE, DuBard M: Association of the C677T methylenetetrahydrofolate reductase mutation and elevated homocysteine levels with congenital cardiac malformations. Am J Obstet Gynecol 2001;184:806–812; discussion 812–817.
36 Czeizel AE, Banhidy F: Chronic hypertension in pregnancy. Curr Opin Obstet Gynecol 2011;23:76–81.
37 Caton AR, Bell EM, Druschel CM, Werler MM, Lin AE, Browne ML, McNutt LA, Romitti PA, Mitchell AA, Olney RS, Correa A; National Birth Defects Prevention Study: Antihypertensive medication use during pregnancy and the risk of cardiovascular malformations. Hypertension 2009;54:63–70.
38 Li DK, Yang C, Andrade S, Tavares V, Ferber JR: Maternal exposure to angiotensin converting enzyme inhibitors in the first trimester and risk of malformations in offspring: a retrospective cohort study. BMJ 2011;343:d5931.
39 Levy HL, Guldberg P, Guttler F, Hanley WB, Matalon R, Rouse BM, Trefz F, Azen C, Allred EN, de la Cruz F, Koch R: Congenital heart disease in maternal phenylketonuria: report from the Maternal PKU Collaborative Study. Pediatr Res 2001;49: 636–642.
40 Yano S, Moseley K, Bottiglieri T, Arning E, Azen C: Maternal Phenylketonuria International Collaborative Study revisited: evaluation of maternal nutritional risk factors besides phenylalanine for fetal congenital heart defects. J Inherit Metab Dis 2014;37: 39–42.
41 Ergenoglu AM, Yeniel AO, Yildirim N, Kazandi M, Akercan F, Sagol S: Rubella vaccination during the preconception period or in pregnancy and perinatal and fetal outcomes. Turk J Pediatr 2012;54:230–233.
42 Kallen B, Otterblad Olausson P: Use of anti-asthmatic drugs during pregnancy. 3. Congenital malformations in the infants. Eur J Clin Pharmacol 2007;63:383–388.
43 Lin S, Herdt-Losavio M, Gensburg L, Marshall E, Druschel C: Maternal asthma, asthma medication use, and the risk of congenital heart defects. Birth Defects Res A Clin Mol Teratol 2009;85:161–168.
44 Crider KS, Cleves MA, Reefhuis J, Berry RJ, Hobbs CA, Hu DJ: Antibacterial medication use during pregnancy and risk of birth defects: National Birth Defects Prevention Study. Arch Pediatr Adolesc Med 2009;163: 978–985.
45 Czeizel AE, Rockenbauer M, Sorensen HT, Olsen J: The teratogenic risk of trimethoprim-sulfonamides: a population based case-control study. Reprod Toxicol 2001; 15:637–646.
46 Hernandez-Diaz S, Werler MM, Walker AM, Mitchell AA: Folic acid antagonists during pregnancy and the risk of birth defects. N Engl J Med 2000;343:1608–1614.
47 Matok I, Gorodischer R, Koren G, Landau D, Wiznitzer A, Levy A: Exposure to folic acid antagonists during the first trimester of pregnancy and the risk of major malformations. Br J Clin Pharmacol 2009;68:956–962.
48 Källén BA, Otterblad Olausson P: Maternal drug use in early pregnancy and infant cardiovascular defect. Reprod Toxicol 2003;17: 255–261.
49 Malm H, Artama M, Gissler M, Ritvanen A: Selective serotonin reuptake inhibitors and risk for major congenital anomalies. Obstet Gynecol 2011;118:111–120.
50 Polen KN, Rasmussen SA, Riehle-Colarusso T, Reefhuis J; National Birth Defects Prevention Study: Association between reported venlafaxine use in early pregnancy and birth defects, National Birth Defects Prevention Study, 1997–2007. Birth Defects Res A Clin Mol Teratol 2013;97:28–35.
51 Reis M, Kallen B: Delivery outcome after maternal use of antidepressant drugs in pregnancy: an update using Swedish data. Psychol Med 2010;40:1723–1733.
52 Werler MM, Ahrens KA, Bosco JL, Mitchell AA, Anderka MT, Gilboa SM, Holmes LB; National Birth Defects Prevention Study: Use of antiepileptic medications in pregnancy in relation to risks of birth defects. Ann Epidemiol 2011;21:842–850.
53 Arpino C, Brescianini S, Robert E, Castilla EE, Cocchi G, Cornel MC, de Vigan C, Lancaster PA, Merlob P, Sumiyoshi Y, Zampino G, Renzi C, Rosano A, Mastroiacovo P: Teratogenic effects of antiepileptic drugs: use of an International Database on Malformations and Drug Exposure (MADRE). Epilepsia 2000;41:1436–1443.
54 Lennestal R, Otterblad Olausson P, Kallen B: Maternal use of antihypertensive drugs in early pregnancy and delivery outcome, notably the presence of congenital heart defects in the infants. Eur J Clin Pharmacol 2009;65:615–625.
55 Cooper WO, Hernandez-Diaz S, Arbogast PG, Dudley JA, Dyer S, Gideon PS, Hall K, Ray WA: Major congenital malformations after first-trimester exposure to ACE inhibitors. N Engl J Med 2006;354:2443–2451.
56 van Gelder MM, Roeleveld N, Nordeng H: Exposure to non-steroidal anti-inflammatory drugs during pregnancy and the risk of selected birth defects: a prospective cohort study. PLoS One 2011; 6:e22174.

57 Mateja WA, Nelson DB, Kroelinger CD, Ruzek S, Segal J: The association between maternal alcohol use and smoking in early pregnancy and congenital cardiac defects. J Womens Health (Larchmt) 2012;21:26–34.
58 Lee LJ, Lupo PJ: Maternal smoking during pregnancy and the risk of congenital heart defects in offspring: a systematic review and metaanalysis. Pediatr Cardiol 2013;34:398–407.
59 Alverson CJ, Strickland MJ, Gilboa SM, Correa A: Maternal smoking and congenital heart defects in the Baltimore-Washington Infant Study. Pediatrics 2011;127:e647–e653.
60 Malik S, Cleves MA, Honein MA, Romitti PA, Botto LD, Yang S, Hobbs CA; National Birth Defects Prevention Study: Maternal smoking and congenital heart defects. Pediatrics 2008;121:e810–e816.
61 US Department of Health and Human Services: The Health Consequences of Smoking: 50 Years of Progress. A Report of the Surgeon General. Atlanta, US Department of Health and Human Services, Centers for Disease Control and Prevention, National Center for Chronic Disease Prevention and Health Promotion, Office on Smoking and Health, 2014.
62 Lipshultz SE, Frassica JJ, Orav EJ: Cardiovascular abnormalities in infants prenatally exposed to cocaine. J Pediatr 1991;118:44–51.
63 Xiao Y, Xiao D, He J, Zhang L: Maternal cocaine administration during pregnancy induces apoptosis in fetal rat heart. J Cardiovasc Pharmacol 2001;37:639–648.

Dr. Tiffany J. Riehle-Colarusso
National Center on Birth Defects and Developmental Disabilities
Centers for Disease Control and Prevention
1600 Clifton Road NE, Atlanta, GA 30333 (USA)
E-Mail tcolarusso@cdc.gov

Muenke M, Kruszka PS, Sable CA, Belmont JW (eds): Congenital Heart Disease: Molecular Genetics, Principles of Diagnosis and Treatment. Basel, Karger, 2015, pp 70–79
DOI: 10.1159/000375205

Adults with Congenital Heart Disease

Koichiro Niwa

Department of Cardiology, Cardiovascular Center, St. Luke's International Hospital, Tokyo, Japan

Abstract

Improvements in the surgical care of pediatric patients with congenital heart disease (CHD) have resulted in a growing population of adult CHD (aCHD) patients. These adults are developing a host of new issues and complications that many adult cardiologists have not been trained to recognize and treat. Additionally, some of this cohort are facing stressors, such as pregnancy, that are new to pediatric cardiologists. Fortunately, research in the natural history of adults with CHD, their psychosocial issues, and treatment of aCHD is taking place. This chapter explores the unique issues associated with this special CHD population, which the next generation of adult cardiologists will need to understand.

Improvements in the quality and level of care in the fields of pediatric cardiology and cardiovascular surgery have resulted in the survival and increased life expectancy of patients with congenital heart disease (CHD) (see chapters by Costello et al. p. 280 and by Morgan and Qureshi p. 289). Today, 85–90% of those born with CHD grow up to become adults. Even though surgical treatment has made survival to adulthood possible for CHD patients, it is seldom curative. Unoperated and postoperative patients with moderate to complex lesions require lifelong surveillance. Postoperative residua, sequelae and long-term surgical complications (see table 1 for definitions) vary in severity and require regular medical attention by experienced cardiologists (tables 1, 2). Because of this, a number of specialized centers have been established in the last 3–4 decades, first in Europe and North America, and then in East Asia, to respond to this need. This evolving field of adult congenital heart disease will now include board-certified specialists as one of the internal medicine subspecialties in North America, and, possibly, the trend will spread into other international regions.

Frequency of Adult Congenital Heart Disease

Data from large referral centers in Europe and North America revealed that the number of adult CHD (aCHD) patients continues to increase due to

Table 1. Residua, sequelae, and late complications

Residua	Lesions which existed before surgery and left over after surgery or getting worse with age (i.e. left-axis deviation or mitral regurgitation)
Sequelae	Lesions which inevitably happen as a results of surgery (pulmonary regurgitation after ToF repair or surgical scar)
Complications	Lesions that happen unexpectedly due to surgery (nerve palsy)
Late complications	Complications that occur (un)expectedly in (un)operated lesions with age (heart failure, sudden death, arrhythmias, thrombosis, or cyanotic organ damage)

Table 2. Exacerbating factors in adults with CHD

Residua, sequelae, complications after initial cardiac surgery, reoperation
Catheter intervention, ablation
Noncardiac surgery
Reproductive issues, inheritance
Arrhythmia, cardiac failure, sudden death
Multisystem systemic disorders in cyanotic CHD
Infective endocarditis
Influence of aging and metabolic syndrome
Smoking, alcohol abuse
Exercise, recreational sports
Travel by aircraft, driving license
Psychosocial considerations
Health and life insurance, disability benefits
Liver disease (hepatitis, liver cirrhosis, hepatic cancer)

the success of medical and surgical care of pediatric patients [1, 2]. As a consequence of advanced treatment, the proportion of aCHD patients surviving outnumbers children with CHD in many countries of the Western World. In the Asia-Pacific region, however, available data are limited to only a few countries and the proportion of adults with CHD varies from country to country: from 75% in Singapore, 51% in Japan, 32% in Thailand, 22–26% in Korea to 20% in Taiwan [3, 4].

Treatment Facilities and Human Resources

With few exceptions, however, reparative surgery is followed by residua and sequelae that require long-term if not life-long surveillance [5]. Because of the complexities inherent in the comprehensive care of these patients, specialized tertiary-care facilities emerged in the late 1970s in North America and Europe [6, 7]. The comprehensive care by multidisciplinary teams, including adult and pediatric cardiologists, cardiac surgeons, specialized nurses, and other cardiac and noncardiac consultants, has made the care of aCHD patients with moderate-to-severe CHD unique. Centers have emerged within teaching hospitals having preexisting pediatric cardiology units with capabilities in multi-imaging modalities and surgical treatment to care for aCHD. Availability of other cardiovascular specialists (vascular medicine, electrophysiology, and imaging), obstetricians-gynecologists, psychiatrists, infectious disease specialists, hematologists, nephrologists, rheumatologists, clinical geneticists, pulmonologists, and specialized nurses is also important to address other issues associated with CHD. However, there appears to be a significant shortfall in tertiary-care provisions for aCHD, which will require further planning and resource allocation [8]. As aCHD has high rates of health care utilization, particularly aCHD with moderate-severe lesions, appropriate resource allocation is required to serve this growing population. Patients with severe CHD had higher adjusted rates of outpatient cardiologist care, emergency department utilization, hospital ization, and days in critical care compared to patients with other CHD types [8].

Regarding cardiac providers for aCHD, proper transition from pediatric cardiologists and cardiovascular surgeons to aCHD specialists and/or cardiologists that are well trained in the field of aCHD is necessary [9]. Other than some areas in North America and Europe, this system has not been developed. In many parts of the world, such as the Asia-Pacific area, pediatric cardiologists are still principal caregivers for aCHD.

Table 3. Cardiac failure, especially right-ventricular (RV) failure in aCHD: background morphology and physiology

RV failure – subpulmonary and systemic
Systemic RV failure with/without atrioventricular valve regurgitation
Complete transposition of the great arteries after atrial switch
Congenital corrected transposition of the great arteries
Single RV
Subpulmonary RV failure
Left-right shunt (atrial septal defect)
Tricuspid regurgitation (Ebstein disease, ToF after repair)
Pulmonary stenosis, pulmonary hypertension, Eisenmenger syndrome
Pulmonary regurgitation (ToF after repair)
Left-ventricular (LV) failure
Pressure overload
Coarctation of the aorta, aortic stenosis
Volume overload
Aortic regurgitation (bicuspid aortic valve, ToF or cyanotic CHD with pulmonary atresia or stenosis)
Left-to-right shunting (ventricular septal defect, patent ductus arteriosus)
Mitral regurgitation

Current Status and Future Prospects of Adult Congenital Heart Disease

In postoperative patients with CHD, even if the procedure is performed at the proper time and without complication, disease-specific and/or operative procedure-specific anatomical and functional abnormalities can progress. These abnormalities are classified as residua, sequelae, and complications (table 1) [5]. Residua are observed before surgery and continue postoperatively, such as right-ventricular (RV) outflow stenosis in repaired tetralogy of Fallot (ToF). Sequelae occur after surgery, such as pulmonary regurgitation in repaired ToF. An example of a complication is unexpected nerve palsy secondary to a surgical procedure. In moderate and severe CHD, there are residua and sequelae specific to the type of CHD. With few exceptions, reparative surgery is not curative and requires long-term surveillance. Residua and sequelae may progress in severity with age and induce late complications, such as arrhythmias, cardiac failure, thromboembolism due to RV failure, sudden death, reoperation, cardiac intervention, and ablation. There are many other obstacles that further complicate aCHD (table 2), including pregnancy and delivery, noncardiac surgery, hepatitis, psychosocial problems such as depression, cognitive abnormalities, health insurance coverage problems, and extra-cardiac complications inherent in the comprehensive care of these patients, making close follow-up and proper management mandatory. The most common cause of death is postoperative arrhythmia [10].

Common Problems and Specific Pathophysiological Issues in Adult Congenital Heart Disease

Cardiac Failure

Chronic heart failure is widespread in aCHD, with RV failure being most common. Table 3 outlines the morphology and physiology of heart failure in aCHD. Potential pathogenetic factors for cardiac failure in aCHD are shown in table 4. Chronotropic incompetence and exercise intolerance are present even in asymptomatic patients. Volume/pressure overload, neurohormonal activation, impaired autonomic nervous function, and operative scar formation in aCHD may all play a contributory role in congestive heart failure (CHF) and may be followed by arrhythmias and sudden cardiac death (SCD). Additionally, atrial/ventricular chamber dilatation,

Table 4. Possible pathogenetic factors for heart failure in aCHD

Cyanosis
Pressure/volume overload
Residua and sequelae after repair
Poor intraoperative myocardial preservation
Artificial material (large ventricular patch)
Ventricular incisions/scar
Arrhythmias (brady- and tachyarrhythmias)
Abnormal ventriculoarterial coupling (decreased aortic stiffness)
Abnormal ventricular-ventricular interaction
Myocardial ischemia (LV hypertrophy, abnormal coronary supply)

fibrosis, and dysfunction may also be risk factors for cardiac failure. In considering therapy for cardiac failure or coexisting arrhythmias, care must be taken for the underlying hemodynamic substrate in each CHD, particularly repairable ones that might favor a surgical or catheter-based approach to treatment. Typical aCHD substrates for CHF, arrhythmias, and SCD are: severe aortic stenosis and/or aortic regurgitation (superimposed coarctation of the aorta), Ebstein's disease, congenital corrected transposition of the great arteries, ToF after repair, extracardiac conduit repair (Rastelli procedure), complete transposition of the great arteries after Mustard or Senning operation, single-ventricle physiology, Fontan surgery, and unrepaired or palliated cyanotic CHD.

Management of CHF in aCHD includes medication, cardiac resynchronization therapy (CRT), reoperation and cardiac/cardiopulmonary transplantation with or without intracardiac repair. Reoperation combined with arrhythmia surgery, such as in reoperation of repaired ToF with subsequent extracardiac conduit repair, is popular in the aCHD field, and this concept is generally different from patients with acquired heart disease in that reoperation can be rare other than patients with valve surgery. In patients with repaired ToF with sustained ventricular tachycardia (VT) and a history of syncope, reoperation with cryoablation of VT is recommended in order to stabilize hemodynamics and reduce the incidence of recurrent VT. Cardioverter defibrillator implantation is indicated if the patients have no severe residual lesions that can be repaired [11].

As the pathophysiology and symptoms of cardiac failure, such as exercise intolerance, cardiac dysfunction, and neurohormonal abnormalities, are very similar between patients with CHD and acquired heart disease, management strategies for CHF in acquired heart disease, such as treatment with angiotensin-converting enzyme inhibitors, angiotensin II receptor blockers, and β-blockers, can be applied to aCHD patients. These medications have been shown to work in patients with left-ventricular (LV) failure; however, no evidence for efficacy in RV failure exists [11–15]. Regarding CRT, there are several reports on its usefulness for aCHD. CRT can work in CHD and cardiac failure, but experience is still limited and specific conditions such as RV failure, complete right bundle branch block (not left bundle branch block) and coronary vein abnormalities could possibly make CRT difficult [16]. Other future possibilities include cardiac transplantation and artificial heart. Further experience for managing cardiac failure in aCHD is necessary.

Arrhythmias

Arrhythmia and SCD in aCHD is a big issue (see chapter on Genetic Arrythymias by Mazzanti and Priori on p. 198). Repaired ToF patients with severe pulmonary valve regurgitation associated with RV dysfunction are prone to SCD following VT. Measurement of QRS duration, RV size by MRI, and inducible VT by electrophysiological study are advocated and have been proven to be useful for the prediction of SCD in repaired ToF patients [17]. Reoperation with cryoablation for VT is effective for the prevention of these crucial events. Cardioverter defibrillators are also used for primary and secondary prevention of sudden death, but inappropriate firing and a high frequency of complications are still observed in some cases [18]. Supraventricular tachyarrhythmias such as atrial flutter or atrial fibrillation are common in aCHD patients long after repair. Antiarrhythmic medication and catheter ablation including the catheter maze procedure (creating atrial scar tissue that interrupts abnormal electrical impulses) have been successful, but there is no consensus regarding the management of atrial

Table 5. Defect type and treatment options in PAH patients

Type of defect	Treatment
Small restrictive defects (ASD <2 cm, VSD <1 cm) with normal PVR (<3 WU) and net left-right shunting	No contraindication for closure
Large nonrestrictive defects (ASD >2 cm, VSD >1 cm) in cyanotic patients with elevated PVR and shunt reversal (right to left)	Closure contraindicated Treat with advanced therapies for PAH
Moderately restrictive defect in patients who have not undergone closure and have mild/moderately elevated PVR (3–6 WU) but no cyanosis	Treat with advanced therapies Rule out desaturation with exercise Serial right-heart catheterizations with vasodilator and exercise testing Consider closure or partial closure (with fenestration) if on treatment: PVR <3 WU No desaturation with exercise Q_p:Q_s between 1.6:1 and 2:1 PAH reversible with vasodilator therapy PAP <2/3 systemic BP, PVR <2/3 SVR Tolerates temporary occlusion in catheterization laboratory
Defects previously closed in childhood, now with elevated PVR and evidence of irreversible PAH	Treat with advanced therapies for PAH

ASD = Atrial septal defect; BP = blood pressure; PAP = pulmonary artery pressure; Q_p:Q_s = pulmonary:systemic blood flow; SVR = systemic vascular resistance; VSD = ventricular septal defect; WU = Wood's units.

fibrillation in aCHD. In addition to warfarin, there are new oral anticoagulants available for atrial fibrillation in Fontan patients and patients with other disorders, but their efficacy is still under review. New guidelines are needed for these latest anticoagulants, and for the role of catheter and surgical cryoablation in aCHD.

Pulmonary Hypertension

Pulmonary arterial hypertension (PAH) in CHD develops as a result of vascular remodeling secondary to increased pulmonary blood flow, increased pulmonary vasculature pressure due to left-to-right shunting, and increased sheer stress. Despite significant advances in pediatric cardiology and surgery, about 3–10% of adults with CHD will develop PAH [19, 20].

There are no clear guidelines for the treatment of PAH-CHD. However, the data available seem to demonstrate that with the advancement of PAH-targeted therapies, the quality of life, exercise capacity, and outcomes in these patients are improving [21–24]. Targeted therapies for PAH may be useful in select patients with a combined medical-surgical approach (table 5).

Correcting a defect on the wrong patient could lead to progression of pulmonary hypertension, RV failure, and a worse prognosis than prior to repair [22]. An adult with cyanosis at rest or with exertion should probably not undergo closure of a septal defect, as this is a sign of advanced PAH-CHD and reversal of shunting, and patients being considered for surgery should get a right-heart catheterization to measure hemodynamics. In aCHD, pulmonary vascular resistance (PVR) and the pulmonary to systemic blood flow ratio (Qp/Qs) are important indicators of severity of disease and reversibility with surgery. High pulmonary pressures due to high Qp/Qs, with a normal or low PVR, are potentially reversible. On the other hand, high pulmo-

Table 6. Physiological changes during pregnancy and delivery

Hemodynamic changes (similar reaction during exercise)
Pregnancy
Increased blood volume: 140–150% of normal
Increased cardiac output: 140–150% of normal
Dilatation of peripheral arteries
Labor
Increase in blood volume: 500 ml/contraction
Blood loss during delivery: 500–900 ml
Venous return after delivery: 500 ml
Return to normal hemodynamics within 1 month
Hypercoagulability, anemia (relative)
Tachypnea
Increased cortisol and estrogen levels
Autonomic nerve dysfunction (increased heart rate)
Histologic changes in aortic media (elastic fiber fragmentation, aortic dilatation)

Table 7. Risk factors (high) for pregnancies in women with CHD

Pulmonary hypertension (Eisenmenger syndrome)
LV out- and/or inflow stenosis
Severe aortic stenosis (pressure gradient >80 mm Hg)
Severe mitral stenosis
Cardiac failure (NYHA class III or IV, ejection fraction <35%)
Marfan syndrome (aortic root >40 mm), CHD with dilated aortic root (>45 mm)
Mechanical valve
Cyanotic CHD with or without pulmonary hypertension (SaO_2 <85%)
Fontan-type circulation
Systemic RV with decreased function
Complete transposition of the great arteries after atrial switch
Congenital corrected transposition of the great arteries

nary pressures secondary to a high PVR could be a contraindication to surgery. A recent extensive review suggested that PVR values <6 Wood's units can be considered operable, although these numbers should be used as a guide and not an absolute [22]. In patients that are borderline operable, the best strategy is to treat with targeted therapy and then reevaluate. Patients with the Eisenmenger syndrome (PVR and remodeling secondary to chronic elevation in pulmonary pressures) could possibly be treated with targeted medical therapy, especially pulmonary vasodilators [24]. Residual defects can be present years after the initial operation and can be the cause of PAH-CHD decades later [20].

Pregnancy and Delivery

Half of the aCHD patients are female and many will face pregnancy in their lifetime, which results in hemodynamic and other physiologic changes (table 6). Cardiac disease is the leading cause of maternal death in some countries, and most pregnant women with cardiac disease have CHD. The number of such patients at risk for child bearing is expected to grow [25]. Women with PAH, severe LV outflow tract stenosis, cyanotic CHD, aortic root dilatation, cardiac dysfunction, and mechanical valves carry a high risk for pregnancy-related morbidity (table 7). The most frequent complications in these patients during pregnancy and delivery are CHF or arrhythmia followed by thrombosis. Risk stratification for pregnant patients with CHD is related to the functional status of the patient and lesion specificity [26]. Timely prepregnancy counseling should be offered to all women with CHD to prevent avoidable pregnancy-related risks [27]. Adequate care during pregnancy, delivery, and the postpartum period requires a multidisciplinary team approach with cardiologists, obstetricians, and anesthesiologists, especially in women with moderate or severe risks. Successful pregnancy is feasible for most women with CHD with mild-to-moderate severity when appropriate counseling and optimal care are provided. Registration systems on pregnancy and delivery in cardiac disease, including aCHD, have been initiated in Europe and Japan. In Asian and developing countries, rheumatic heart disease is still common, so proper management planning during pregnancy for women with this disorder is also important.

Psychosocial Issues

Most aCHD patients with proper therapy will have a longer life span and may experience psychological stressors associated with chronic disease. Consequently, many studies are now focusing not only on medical support, but also on their psychosocial features and their quality of life. These studies are conducted by means of questionnaires or interview surveys, such as semistructured interviews or structured clinical interviews. The results regarding the psychosocial state of patients compared to controls are inconsistent in emotional and social functioning, depression, anxiety, and mood disorders [29–32]. However, adult patients with cyanosis after the Fontan procedure are at higher risk for depressive symptoms [33]. Additionally, there have been inconsistent results when evaluating self-esteem in patients with aCHD [34, 35].

The reasons for these inconsistent findings could be explained by differences in sample size (including low response rates), recruiting sources (e.g. the sample is not from a homogeneous group), study methods, and sociocultural background (e.g. the health care system and mental health treatment [35]) in different countries. In a Japanese study [34], aCHD patients often have psychosocial difficulties, which influence the patients' mental health, social problem solving, independence, and self-esteem.

Table 8. Factors for low incidence of atherosclerosis in cyanotic aCHD

Cyanotic aCHD patients have low levels of low-/high-density lipoprotein and total cholesterol, which persist after surgical elimination of cyanosis
Increased nitric oxide levels
Increased serum bilirubin levels
Low platelet counts

Possibility of Acquired Cardiovascular Disease

In spite of the theoretical risk of atherosclerosis in patients with aCHD due to various risk factors, cyanotic CHD is noted to have a minimal incidence of coronary artery disease (CAD) [28, 36–39]. Perloff [36] found that atherosclerosis was absent on coronary angiography of 49 cyanotic patients with CHD in their early 40s. A more recent series, describing 250 patients with CHD who underwent selective coronary angiography for reasons other than suspected CAD in the United Kingdom, revealed that the prevalence of significant CAD (9.2%) was similar to the general population: no patient younger than 40 years had significant CAD, and none of the cyanotic patients had significant CAD [40]. In general, cyanotic CHD is a preventive factor for cardiovascular disease [36] (table 8).

Cardiovascular risk may also vary by type of CHD (table 9) [41]. Specific conditions in which the coronary arteries are directly affected or altered surgically may confer a greater risk for premature atherosclerotic CAD. Coronary artery re-implantation at the time of arterial switch repair in transposition of the great arteries has been shown to result in abnormal coronary flow, and intracoronary ultrasound reveals that some patients develop intimal proliferation, a precursor to atherosclerosis [42]. Left-sided obstructive lesions may also be associated with CAD. Coarctation of the aorta, even after repair, is commonly associated with systemic hyper-

Table 9. Clinical manifestations of cardiovascular disease (CVD) in aCHD

aCHD patients have a similar prevalence of risk factors for CVD as the general population
Cyanotic aCHD patients have a lower incidence of CVD
Acyanotic aCHD patients have a similar prevalence of CVD as the general population
Increased risk of coronary atherosclerosis is observed in congenital coronary artery anomalies, complete transposition of the great arteries after arterial switch, and coarctation of the aorta
Aortopathy may be an additional risk factor for CVD
Prevention of CVD is even more important in young adults with CHD

tension; aortic stenosis can be associated with LV hypertrophy and diastolic dysfunction, known risk factors for adult-onset cardiovascular morbidity and mortality [43].

According to a recently published paper, 141/12,124 (1%) of aCHD patients had CAD, which is lower than the prevalence of CAD in the general population, most likely due to the young age of adults in this study; however, 109 of these 141 (77%) experienced coronary artery interventions [44]. The most frequent background CHD in this study were atrial septal defects, bicuspid aortic valve, ToF and coarctation of the aorta, and 82% of these patients had traditional risk factors for CAD, such as hypertension, hyperlipidemia, diabetes mellitus, or obesity [44]. Surprisingly, 7 of the patients had the Eisenmenger syndrome, and all of these patients had at least one of the traditional risk factors for CAD [44].

aCHD patients have a similar prevalence of traditional risk factors for CAD as the general population, and noncyanotic aCHD patients have a similar prevalence of CAD as the general population. However, patients with cyanotic aCHD, even after repair, have a lower incidence of CAD. In cyanotic patients with risks such hypertension, dyslipidemia, diabetes mellitus, and the metabolic syndrome, atherosclerosis is still possible [40, 44–47].

Aortopathy

Bicuspid aortic valve and/or coarctation of the aorta are consistently associated with medial wall abnormalities in the ascending aorta, which are prevalent in a variety of CHD types, such as single ventricle, persistent truncus arteriosus, transposition of the great arteries, hypoplastic left-heart syndrome and ToF, and may predispose to dilatation, aneurysm, rupture, and aortic regurgitation [48, 49]. This dilatation can develop in CHD patients even without a stenotic region of the aorta. CHD patients who exhibit ongoing dilatation of the aortic root and reduced aortic elasticity may have wall abnormalities intrinsic to the aortic root [50]. The paradigm in aortic dilatation has shifted from the idea of so-called poststenotic dilatation to primary intrinsic aortopathy. The effects of aortic dilatation and increased stiffness can induce aortic regurgitation, LV hypertrophy, reduced coronary artery flow, and LV failure. This aortic pathophysiological abnormality has been labeled as a new clinical entity: 'aortopathy'. These patients should be followed for progression of aortic root dilatation. Also, we should evaluate therapies that prevent this dilatation and stiffness, such as β-blockers/angiotensin-converting-enzyme inhibitors or angiotensin II receptor antagonists.

Conclusion

Formal education and training systems for CHD practitioners are still lacking in developing countries such as Asia. Collaborative work and support of addressing the shortage of adult cardiologists knowledgeable in CHD is necessary. Further expansion of this population and the need for the evolution of specialized care facilities for pediatric cardiology and aCHD can be anticipated throughout the world. Training and education focused on the trainees who represent the next generation of pediatric and adult cardiologists will allow them to assume responsibility for this patient population.

References

1 Marelli AJ, Mackie AS, Ionescu-Ittu R, et al: Congenital heart disease in the general population: changing prevalence and age distribution. Circulation 2007;115:163–172.

2 van der Bom T, Bouma BJ, Meijboom FJ, et al: The prevalence of adult congenital heart disease, results from a systematic review and evidence based calculation. Am Heart J 2012;164:568–575.

3 Shiina Y, Toyoda T, Kawasoe Y, et al: Prevalence of adult patients with congenital heart disease in Japan. Int J Cardiol 2011;146:13–16.

4 Niwa K: ACHD achievements in the Asia-Pacific region. Prog Pediatr Cardiol 2012; 34:57–60.

5 Perloff JK: Adults with surgically treated congenital heart disease: sequelae and residua. JAMA 1983;250:2033–2036.

6 Niwa K, Perloff JK, Webb GD, et al: Survey of specialized tertiary care facilities for adults with congenital heart disease. Int J Cardiol 2004;96:211–216.

7 Marelli AJ, Therrien J, Mackie AS, et al: Planning the specialized care of adult congenital heart disease patients: from numbers to guidelines; an epidemiologic approach. Am Heart J 2009;157:1–8.

8 Mackie AS, Pilote L, Ionescu-Ittu R, et al: Health care resource utilization in adults with congenital heart disease. Am J Cardiol 2007;99:839–843.

9 Sable C, Foster E, Uzark K, et al: Best practices in managing transition to adulthood for adolescents with congenital heart disease: the transition process and medical and psychosocial issues: a scientific statement from the American Heart Association. Circulation 2011;123:1454–1485.

10 Oechslin EN, Harrison DA, Connelly MS, et al: Mode of death in adults with congenital heart disease. Am J Cardiol 2000;86:1111–1116.

11 Hechter SJ, Fredriksen PM, Liu P, et al: Angiotensin-converting enzyme inhibitors in adults after the Mustard procedure. Am J Cardiol 2001;87:660–663.

12 Lester SJ, McElhinney DB, Viloria E, et al: Effects of losartan in patients with a systemically functioning morphologic right ventricle after atrial repair of transposition of the great arteries. Am J Cardiol 2001;88: 1314–1316.

13 Dore A, Houde C, Chan KL, et al: Angiotensin receptor blockade and exercise capacity in adults with systemic right ventricles: a multicenter, randomized, placebo-controlled clinical trial. Circulation 2005;112: 2411–2416.

14 Therrien J, Provost Y, Harrison J, et al: Effect of angiotensin receptor blockade on systemic right ventricular function and size: a small, randomized, placebo-controlled study. Int J Cardiol 2008;129:187–192.

15 Shaddy RE, Boucek MM, Hsu DT, et al: Carvedilol for children and adolescents with heart failure: a randomized controlled trial. JAMA 2007;298:1171–1179.

16 Dubin AM, Janousek J, Rhee E, et al: Resynchronization therapy in pediatric and congenital heart disease patients: an international multicenter study. J Am Coll Cardiol 2005;46:2277–2283.

17 Gatzoulis MA, Balaji S, Webber SA, et al: Risk factors for arrhythmia and sudden cardiac death late after repair of tetralogy of Fallot: a multicenter study. Lancet 2000; 356:975–981.

18 Khairy P, Harris L, Landzberg MJ, et al: Implantable cardioverter-defibrillators in tetralogy of Fallot. Circulation 2008;117:363–370.

19 Mulder BJ: Changing demographics of pulmonary arterial hypertension in congenital heart disease. Eur Respir Rev 2010;19:308–313.

20 Kaemmerer H, Mebus S, Schulze-Neick I, et al: The adult patient with Eisenmenger syndrome: a medical update after dana point part I: epidemiology, clinical aspects and diagnostic options. Curr Cardiol Rev 2010;6: 343–355.

21 Rosenzweig EB, Kerstein D, Barst RJ: Long-term prostacyclin for pulmonary hypertension with associated congenital heart defects. Circulation 1999;99:1858–1865.

22 Giglia TM, Humpl T: Preoperative pulmonary hemodynamics and assessment of operability: is there a pulmonary vascular resistance that precludes cardiac operation? Pediatr Crit Care Med 2010;11(2 suppl): S57–S69.

23 Sakazaki H, Niwa K, Nakazawa M, et al: Clinical features of adult patients with Eisenmenger's syndrome in Japan and Korea. Int J Cardiol 2013;167:205–209.

24 Dimopoulos K, Inuzuka R, Goletto S, et al: Improved survival among patients with Eisenmenger syndrome receiving advanced therapy for pulmonary arterial hypertension. Circulation 2010;121:20–25.

25 Siu SC, Sermer M, Colman JM, et al; Cardiac Disease in Pregnancy (CARPREG) Investigators: Prospective multicenter study of pregnancy outcomes in women with heart disease. Circulation 2001;104:515–521.

26 Tateno S, Niwa K, Nakazawa M, et al: Arrhythmia and conduction disturbances in patients with congenital heart disease during pregnancy: multicenter study. Circ J 2003;67:992–997.

27 Drenthen W, Pieper PG, Roos-Hesselink JW, et al: Outcome of pregnancy in women with congenital heart disease. A literature review. J Am Coll Cardiol 2007;49:2303–2311.

28 Roos-Hesselink JW, Ruys TP, Stein JI, et al: Outcome of pregnancy in patients with structural or ischemic heart disease: results of a registry of the European Society of Cardiology. Eur Heart J 2013;34:657–665.

29 van Rijen EHM, Utens EM, Roos-Hesselink JW, et al: Psychosocial functioning of the adult with congenital heart disease: a 20–33 years follow-up. Eur Heart J 2003;24:673–683.

30 Kovacs AH, Saidi AS, Kuhl EA, et al: Depression and anxiety in adults with congenital heart disease: prevalence and predictors. Int J Cardiol 2009;37:158–164.

31 Müller J, Hess J, Hager A: General anxiety of adolescents and adults with congenital heart disease is comparable with that in healthy controls. Int J Cardiol 2013;165: 142–145.

32 Müller J, Hess J, Hager A: Minor symptoms of depression in patients with congenital heart disease have a larger impact on quality of life than limited exercise capacity. Int J Cardiol 2012;154:265–269.

33 Popelová J, Slavík Z, Skovránek J: Are cyanosed adults with congenital cardiac malformations depressed? Cardiol Young 2001; 11:379–384.

34 Enomoto J, Nakazawa J, Mizuno Y, Shirai T, Ogawa J, Niwa K: Psychosocial factors influencing mental health in adults with congenital heart disease. Circ J 2013;77: 749–755.

35 Kovacs AH, Sears SF, Saidi A: Biopsychosocial experiences of adults with congenital heart disease: review of the literature. Am Heart J 2005;150:193–201.

36 Perloff JK: The coronary circulation in cyanotic congenital heart disease. Int J Cardiol 2004;97:79–86.

37 Duffels M, Mulder KM, Trip MD, et al: Atherosclerosis in patients with cyanotic congenital heart disease. Circ J 2010;74:1436–1441.

38 Perloff JK: Cyanotic congenital heart disease the coronary arterial circulation. Curr Cardiol Rev 2012;8:1–5.

39 European Association for Cardiovascular Prevention & Rehabilitation, Reiner Z, Catapano AL, De Backer G, et al: ESC/EAS Guidelines for the management of dyslipidaemias: the Task Force for the management of dyslipidaemias of the European Society of Cardiology (ESC) and the European Atherosclerosis Society (EAS). Eur Heart J 2011;32:1769–1818.

40 Giannakoulas G, Dimopoulos K, Engel R, et al: Burden of coronary artery disease in adults with congenital heart disease and its relation to congenital and traditional heart risk factors. Am J Cardiol 2009;103:1445–1450.
41 Sahara M, Takahashi T, Morita T, et al: Three-vessel coronary artery disease complicated with congestive heart failure in a highly aged patient with tetralogy of Fallot having undergone palliative surgeries. Intern Med 2006;45:1147–1151.
42 Pasquali SK, Marino BS, Powell DJ, et al: Following the arterial switch operation, obese children have risk factors for early cardiovascular disease. Cong Heart Dis 2010;5:16–24.
43 Pemberton VL, McCrindle BW, Barkin S, et al: Report of the National Heart, Lung, and Blood Institute's Working Group on obesity and other cardiovascular risk factors in congenital heart disease. Circulation 2010;121:1153–1159.
44 Yalonetsky S, Horlick EM, Osten MD, et al: Clinical characteristics of coronary artery disease in adults with congenital heart defects. Int J Cardiol 2011;164:217–220.
45 Javier DA, Niwa K: Cardiovascular risk factors among adults with congenital heart disease. Nihon Shoni Junkanki Gakkai Zasshi 2013;29(suppl):S137.
46 Zaidi AN, Bauer JA, Michalsky MP, et al: The impact of obesity on early postoperative outcomes in adults with congenital heart disease. Cong Heart Dis 2011;6:241–246.
47 Kavey RE, Allada V, Daniels SR, et al: Cardiovascular risk reduction in high-risk pediatric patients: a scientific statement from the American Heart Association Expert Panel on Population and Prevention Science; the Councils on Cardiovascular Disease in the Young, Epidemiology and Prevention, Nutrition, Physical Activity and Metabolism, High Blood Pressure Research, Cardiovascular Nursing, and the Kidney in Heart Disease; and the Interdisciplinary Working Group on Quality of Care and Outcomes Research: endorsed by the American Academy of Pediatrics. Circulation 2006;114:2710–2738.
48 Niwa K, Perloff JK, Bhuta SM, et al: Structural abnormalities of great arterial walls in congenital heart disease: light and electron microscopic analyses. Circulation 2001;103:393–400.
49 Niwa K, Siu S, Webb G, et al: Progressive aortic root dilatation in adults late after repair of tetralogy of Fallot. Circulation 2002;106:1374–1378.
50 Senzaki H, Iwamoto Y, Ishido H, et al: Arterial haemodynamics in patients after repair of tetralogy of Fallot: influence on left ventricular after load and aortic dilatation. Heart 2008;94:70–74.

Dr. Koichiro Niwa
Department of Cardiology, Cardiovascular Center
St. Luke's International Hospital
9-1 Akashi-cho, Chuo-ku
Tokyo 104-8560 (Japan)
E-Mail koniwa@luke.or.jp

3 Chromosomal Disorders

Muenke M, Kruszka PS, Sable CA, Belmont JW (eds): Congenital Heart Disease: Molecular Genetics, Principles of Diagnosis and Treatment. Basel, Karger, 2015, pp 82–90
DOI: 10.1159/000375206

Down Syndrome

Paul S. Kruszka

National Human Genome Research Institutes, National Institutes of Health, Bethesda, Md., USA

Abstract

Down syndrome (DS) is the most common aneuploidy in live births and the most common cause of congenital heart disease (CHD) with almost half of all DS individuals being born with structural heart disease. The most prevalent heart defect is atrioventricular septal defect caused by improper development of the cardiac cushions during early embryogenesis. The prevailing theory is that one or more genes on chromosome 21 are overexpressed resulting in heart defects and other DS phenotypes. Partial trisomies and mouse models have been used to search for the putative genes causing CHD in DS, but the genetic etiology has not been fully elucidated. Although, most patients with DS did not survive childhood in the past, surgical repair of complex CHD has greatly contributed to extending the life span of individuals with DS to the 7th decade. As DS patients are living longer, understanding the molecular and genetic basis of the DS phenotype will be imperative to designing new treatments.

Down syndrome (DS) was first described by John Langdon Down in 1866 and nearly a century later, in 1959, Jerome Lejeune associated DS with trisomy 21. DS is caused by a third (whole or partial) chromosome 21 (*Homo sapiens* 21 or HSA21) and is the most common cause of intellectual disability and the most common genetic etiology of congenital heart disease (CHD), particularly atrioventricular (AV) septal defect (AVSD).There is a 1,000-fold increase in the incidence of AVSD in individuals with DS compared to non-DS individuals. AVSD is pathognomonic for DS as 65% of all AVSDs are found in DS patients [1, 2]. The infant mortality of DS is largely due to CHD; however, advances in cardiac surgery have greatly improved survival over the last 70 years from a median of 12 years to now 60 years [3, 4]. This chapter explores the genetic basis of CHD in DS with special emphasis on AVSD.

Epidemiology

The birth incidence of DS is 1 in 732, with increasing frequency in older mothers and potentially decreasing frequency in populations using prenatal screening [5]. Even with prenatal screening and elective terminations, in one European country DS has remained constant over the last 20 years, probably due to an increase in average maternal age [6]. Across multiple studies, the frequencies of overall CHD in DS and specific lesions are consistent (table 1). In a large study of 1,649 DS patients, 39% had AVSDs, 43% had ventricular septal defects (VSDs), 42% had atrial septal defects (ASDs), and

Table 1. Cardiac anomalies associated with DS

Cardiac anomalies	Irving and Chaudhari [6] (n = 821)	Torfs and Christianson [1] (n = 2,894)	Freeman et al. [7] (n = 1,469)
Congenital heart defects, %	42	56	44
AVSD, %	37	31	39
VSD, %	31	11	42
ASD, %	15	11	43
Tetralogy of Fallot, %	5	4	6
Patent ductus arteriosus, %	4	24	

6% had tetralogy of Fallot [7]. Supporting a genetic association with AVSDs, twice as many females compared to males (odds ratio, OR, 1.93; 95% confidence interval, CI, 1.40–2.67), twice as many blacks compared to whites (OR 2.06; 95% CI 1.32–3.21) and half as many Hispanics (OR 0.48; 95% CI 0.30–0.77) were affected with CHD in this study [7]. Even more interesting, using a panel of 164 polymorphic markers to estimate the admixture proportions, there was a significantly higher proportion ($p = 0.029$) of sub-Saharan African alleles among black infants with DS and AVSD (83.1%) than black infants with DS and no CHD (77.6%) [7]. This emphasizes the importance of genetic studies across multiple ethnicities, especially sub-Saharan Africa, which has been hindered in the past by lower levels of funding, poor infrastructure and public health systems, and the small pool of trained scientists [8].

Genetics

Most DS cases are caused by an extra HSA21 resulting from maternal nondisjunction during meiosis, but, less commonly, are also caused by Robertsonian translocations (translocation of the long arm of HSA21 onto another acrocentric chromosome, most commonly chromosome 14, but may also include another HSA21), or mosaic DS (only some cells have trisomy 21 and the others have a normal complement of 46 chromosomes). One large study of 29,000 cases of DS found 96% to be extra HAS21, 2.9% Robertsonian translocations, and 1% mosaic [9]. HSA21 is the smallest human chromosome (excluding sex chromosomes) with roughly 48 Mb (1.5% of the genome) and coding for 696 genes [10]. Risk factors for DS include advanced maternal age (greater than 35 years), either parent with a balanced Robertsonian translocation, and a previous child with DS. Currently, there are no known teratogenic agents that increase the risk of having a child with DS.

The consistent association of CHD with DS suggests increased gene dosage of one or more genes on chromosome 21 (HSA21) as a cause although this hypothesis remains to be proven [11]. Because CHD is one of the partially penetrant traits in DS, finding the genetic etiology is more complex. Two strategies have been used to elucidate the genetic basis of DS: partial trisomies with known breakpoints and gene content and animal models.

Initially, genotype-phenotype relationships of partial trisomies had been used to search for the putative gene responsible for CHDs; however, their rarity has limited the success of this approach. Using patients with partial trisomy 21, researchers isolated a 5.4-Mb region on HSA21 containing 50 genes thought to be responsible for the DS phenotype, including intellectual disability and CHD, termed the DS critical region [12, 13]. One group narrowed this region to a 2.82-Mb critical area using microarray technology, and, by further integrating their data with mouse model data [Dp (16)1Yu/– strain with regions on mouse chromosome 16 (Mus Musculus MMU16) orthologous to HSA21], a 1.77-Mb DS CHD critical region was proposed [14]. Genes of interest in this region include the cell adhesion molecule *DSCAM* gene, which is highly expressed in the developing heart, and thus it is a candidate for structural heart disease in DS [14].

However, some genes associated with CHD have been found outside this proposed 1.77-Mb critical region, including *COL6A1* [15]. *COL6A1* is expressed in the developing embryonic heart, is a major part of the extracellular matrix in the endocardial cushions [16], and has been connected to AVSD in gene association studies [15, 17, 18]. COL6A1 is part of the vascular endothelial growth factor (VEGF)-A pathway [19]. VEGF-A is a known regulator of AV septal formation, and changes in VEGF-A expression in animal models have been associated with AVSD [19].

Also part of the VEGF-A pathway but not on HSA21, *CRELD1* has been associated with AVSDs in both individuals with and without DS [20, 21]. Additionally, *CRELD1* and/or *CRELD2* mutations are thought to be the cause of AVSDs in 3p deletion syndrome [22]. In another pertinent pathway, genes of the folate pathway have been implemented in DS, specifically *SLC19A1* and *MTHFR* located on HSA21 and HSA1, respectively. These two genes were associated with DS and CHD using a 384-SNP, customized-assay, case-control study with 242 participants [23]. Previous studies that have associated CHD with both folate deficiency and genetic variation in folate pathway genes have excluded participants with DS; larger studies that include DS participants are needed [24].

In addition to partial trisomies, mouse models have contributed to our understanding of DS genetics. Mouse models are based on synteny with human chromosome HSA21, which is distributed across three mouse *(Mus musculus)* chromosomes, Mmu 16, 17, and 10, with most of the syntenic genes located on Mmu 16. The first mouse model studied was trisomy 16 developed from a spontaneous Robertsonian translocation; however, this model died in utero and had syntenies with other human chromosomes besides HSA21 [25]. The first viable mouse model was Ts65Dn, a partial Mmu 16 trisomy. A more complete model was developed by a transchromosomic or transspecies mouse strain in which mice carry an extra human chromosome; these mice transmit a freely segregating, human chromosome 21 (HSA21) which contains 92% of all known HSA21 genes [26]. In order to isolate disease-causing genes, the strains can be crossed with strains with small deletions to determine if reducing dosage of the trisomy genes to normal dosage can resolve the aberrant phenotype, implicating the genes in deletion as significant. And, lastly, extra copies of singles genes from HSA21 have been inserted into the mouse genome to generate single gene trisomy models [25].

Human partial trisomies and animal models have not elucidated the genetic etiology of CHD in DS as the genetic cause of CHD in DS is complex, considering that roughly three fourths of DS cases do not have AVSDs and half of DS patients have structurally normal hearts. CHD and AVSD is likely multifactorial with gene modifiers and environment playing an important role in addition to the gene dosage effects of trisomy 21 [27]. For AVSDs, there are a number of nonsyndromic gene associations, including *ALK2, BMP4, CRELD1, GATA4, NKX2–5*, and *TBX5,* that may also be involved in DS patients with CHD [22]. Environmental effects most likely play a role in AVSD, with the example of preconceptual maternal diabetes shown to increase the risk of AVSD (OR 22.8, 95% CI 7.4–70.5) in the Baltimore-Washington Infant study [28]. Noncoding DNA, such as microRNA, and epigenetic contributions must also be considered [29, 30].

Embryogenesis

The majority of CHD in DS result from abnormal septation, with AVSD being most common. AVSD is caused by an aberration in early embryonic development of the endocardial cushions (see chapter by Sylva and Moorman, pp. 11–25). The primitive heart tube is lined with endothelial cells, which is surrounded by myocardium. The myocardium induces the endocardial cells to delaminate and move into the extracellular matrix between the myocardium and endocardium, and transition into mesenchymal cells. The molecular signaling that induces the endocardial cells to migrate is not yet fully understood. A number of signaling pathways have been implicated, including VEGF, Notch,

Wnt/β-catenin, and bone morphogenetic signaling [31]. The superior and endocardial cushions then migrate towards each other and fuse, dividing the AV annuli into right and left tracts, which will go on to become the tricuspid and mitral valve annuli, respectively. Nonendothelial mesenchyme in the dorsal mesenchymal protrusion also plays a role in AV septation [32]. This protrusion arises from the venous pole of the heart, initially located at the posterior end of heart tube, and is derived from cells of the second heart field. Interestingly, in the mouse model, *Shh–/–* mutant embryos have been found to have AVSDs, implicating aberrant sonic hedgehog signaling in the second heart field [32, 33]. With contributions of the dorsal mesenchymal protrusion and sonic hedgehog signaling, it is now clear that more is involved in the development of AVSD than just abnormal endocardial cushion formation.

Clinical Presentation

DS is often diagnosed prenatally. Traditionally, prenatal screening has consisted of maternal serum screening for α-fetoprotein, unconjugated estriol, human β-chorionic gonadotropin, and inhibin-A, and a prenatal ultrasound concentrating on nuchal translucency and length of long bones. Maternal serum screening has a poor positive predictive value (high false-positive rate) and must be followed with an invasive test for confirmation, either chorionic villus sampling in the first trimester or amniocentesis in the second semester. In 2007, the American College of Obstetricians and Gynecologists recommended offering invasive testing to all women, including younger women without known risks [34]. Because these invasive tests have a small risk of procedure-related miscarriage, newer fetal cell-free DNA technologies have made DS screening more attractive. Cell-free DNA techniques use massively parallel shotgun sequencing techniques to count DNA fragments specific to HSA21, and have sensitivity and specificity rates greater than 98% for trisomy 21 [35]. Currently, cell-free fetal DNA testing is only recommended for screening high-risk women; however, this technology will most likely be applied to low-risk women and result in an increase in the prenatal diagnosis of DS [36, 37].

At birth, DS is recognizable on physical examination from the following signs: microcephaly, upslanting palpebral fissures, epicanthic folds, single transverse palmar crease, brachydactyly, clinodactyly of the fifth digit, a gap between first and second toes, hypotonia, and lymphedema. Intellectual disability becomes more apparent as the child ages. Other features seen in DS include flat nasal bridge, Brushfield spots, brachycephaly, and small mouth and ears (fig. 1) [38, 39]. Although this chapter focuses on the cardiac aspect of DS, noncardiac phenotypes must be considered given the multiple organ systems affected. Table 2 lists noncardiac diagnoses in DS.

Cardiac Phenotype

All children with DS should have an echocardiogram and consultation with a pediatric cardiologist in the newborn period due to the high incidence (>40%) of congenital heart malformations found in DS [38]. This section will focus on AVSD, which is pathognomonic for DS; the frequencies of the different CHDs are shown in table 1.

AVSDs comprise three defects: atrial septum primum defect, a membranous VSD and abnormal AV valve leaflets [33]. Normal hearts are divided into four separate chambers; however, the anatomy of the AVSD results in all four heart chambers being connected and the mixing of venous return blood with oxygenated blood from the lungs (fig. 2). AVSDs can be separated into two general subtypes: incomplete (or 'partial' AVSD, which consists of an ostium primum ASD with a cleft mitral valve) and the more severe complete AVSD [40]. Complete AVSD has a single AV valve and incomplete AVSD has distinct AV valves; there are usually five leaflets (anterior, inferior, left mural, right mural, and anterosuperior) that make up the AV valve, but in complete AVSD, two of the leaflets (inferior and anterior), called 'bridging leaflets', override the interventricular septum and stretch from the right to the left ventricle. In incomplete AVSD, the AV valves are divided by valvular tissue which connects the two

3

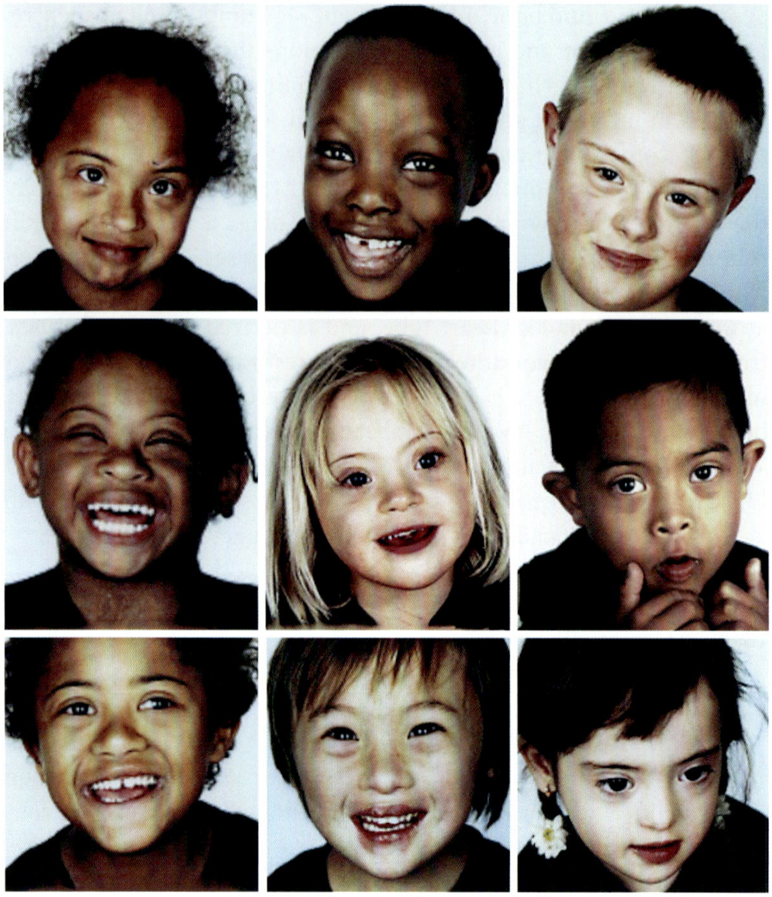

Fig. 1. Facial profiles of children of multiple ethnicities with DS. Note upslanting palpebral fissures, epicanthic folds, and mid-face hypoplasia. Photographs courtesy of Richard Bailey (richard@richard baileyphotography.co.uk)

bridging leaflets, and the left AV valve has a cleft which is the line of apposition between the anterior and inferior bridging leaflets. There is no connection of the bridging leaflets in complete AVSD, leaving a common AV valve. The aortic valve is in an unwedged position and located more anteriorly than normal making the inlet length approximately 0.7 less than the outlet length [41]. Another variable of AVSD is the degree of interatrial and interventricular communication. In complete AVSD, as shown in figure 2, there is both interatrial and interventricular communication in the form of an ostium primum ASD and an inlet-type VSD [42]. The interatrial communication is formed by the gap between the inferior atrial septum and the atrial surface of the common AV valve. The interventricular communication is a result of the large defect between the superior bridging leaflet and the septal crest [43].

Prenatally, an AVSD can be seen on an ultrasound four-chamber view of the heart, which shows the tricuspid valve with a slight apical displacement compared to normal hearts. The postnatal clinical course depends on AVSD severity and associated defects. In complete AVSD with interventricular shunting, infants develop congestive heart failure within months of birth when pulmonary resistance decreases. Associated findings such as coarctation of the aorta, significant valvular regurgitation, or ventricular imbalance will result in heart failure within days of birth. Depending on the degree of shunting, cyanosis may occur. Although a definitive diagnosis is made with two-dimensional echocardiography, the physical examination will show right ventricular impulse, an increased pulmonic component of the second heart sound, systolic ejection murmur, and apical mid-diastolic murmur in a large left-to-right

Table 2. Noncardiac DS manifestations

System	Disease
Eyes	Cataracts Strabismus
Ears, nose, throat	Hearing loss Otitis media Chronic sinus infections Tracheomalacia
Endocrine	Hypothyroidism Diabetes mellitus
Pulmonary	Pulmonary hypertension
Gastrointestinal	Celiac sprue Duodenal atresia Annular pancreas Imperforate anus Esophageal atresia with tracheoesophageal fistula
Immunologic	Cellular immune deficiency IgG subclass deficiency
Neurologic	Early onset Alzheimer disease Seizures Autism
Hematologic	Acute lymphoblastic leukemia Acute megakaryoblastic leukemia Transient myeloproliferative disorder
Orthopedic	Atlantooccipital instability Acetabular dysplasia Pes planus Ligamentous laxity
Growth and development	Short stature Obesity Delayed developmental milestones

shunt and pansystolic murmur with AV valve regurgitation [44]. ECG is significant for left axis deviation with a counterclockwise loop, indicating an inferiorly displaced conduction system. A chest X-ray may show cardiomegaly.

Treatment

CHD treatment in DS patients depends on the specific lesion and may consist only of observation in such cases as small VSDs. In the more severe cas-

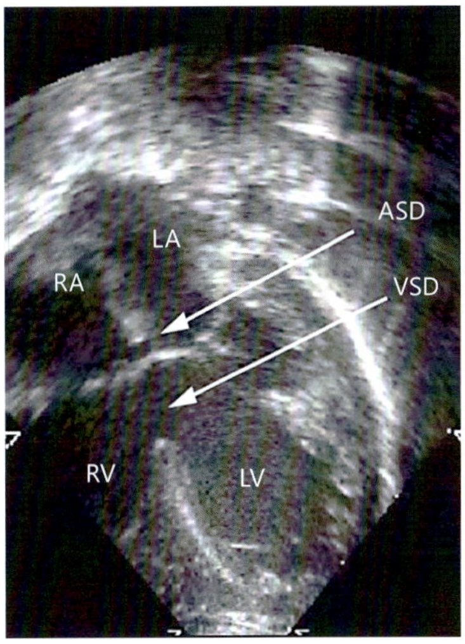

Fig. 2. This echocardiogram demonstrates the constellation of findings in complete AV canal defect including the primum-type ASD and the inlet-type VSD. LA = Left atrium; RA = right atrium; LV = left ventricle; RV = right ventricle (courtesy of Dr. Laura Olivieri).

es of AVSD, surgical treatment is needed for survival (see Costello et al. on Surgical Management of AVSD on p. 280). Because of its high frequency in DS and its severe presentation, this section will focus on AVSD. Once AVSD is diagnosed, medical treatment is a bridge to surgery and consists of typical therapy for heart failure: diuretics, calorie concentration, possibly afterload reduction, and digoxin. Lifelong medical therapy includes antibiotic prophylaxis for subacute bacterial endocarditis. The revised guidelines by the American Heart Association include the following indications pertinent to AVSD for prophylaxis: prosthetic cardiac valve, CHD, unrepaired cyanotic CHD (including palliative shunts and conduits), completely repaired congenital heart defect with prosthetic material or device during the first 6 months after the procedure, and repaired CHD with residual defects at the site or adjacent to the site of a prosthetic patch or prosthetic device (which inhibit endothelialization) [45].

For complete AVSD, surgical therapy is necessary and performed in the first few months of life, especially considering the early development of pulmonary vascular disease in DS [46]. Classical repair uses a single patch to repair atrial and ventricular defects or sometimes a two-patch approach is used. In a study of 476 patients with complete AVSD, of whom 71.6% had DS, there were no differences in the operative strategy, timing of repair, or survival between DS and non-DS patients [47]. This study demonstrates that DS patients with complete AVSD are not at higher risk for surgical therapy.

Continued genetic investigation will still be important for future researchers, as new genes are found that contribute to the pathogenicity to DS phenotypes, these genes may be amenable to therapeutic agents, such as new drugs or gene therapy.

Prognosis

With the advent of complex cardiac surgery, life expectancy for DS increased greatly. Without surgery of the most common cardiac DS malformation, complete AVSD, only 54% survive to 6 months of age and only 4% survive to age 5 years [48]. In a cohort of 363 patients with complete AVSD (65% of the participants with DS), 10-year survival was 83% following surgical repair [42]. The long-term survival for ostium primum (incomplete AVSD) after surgical repair was 40 years in a study of 334 patients, with death rates similar between DS and non-DS participants [49]. In a large US study of over 17,000 participants with DS, the median age at death was 25 years in 1983 and increased to 49 years in 1997, with the majority of patients dying from respiratory illness such as aspiration or pneumonia and congenital heart defects [50]. In another large population in Denmark's national register, using covariate analysis, mortality rates since 1968 only declined in the nonmosaic DS population with congenital heart defects, suggesting that advances in cardiac surgery are largely responsible for the increased life expectancy [51].

Gene Therapy for Future Directions

Even with well-developed mouse models, the genetic complexity and phenotypic variability of CHD in DS has made finding the pathogenetic mechanisms of gene dosage errors challenging. Until specific genes are known, newer therapies will be difficult to develop for cardiac and noncardiac phenotypes. Fortunately, genomic technology is advancing at a rapid rate and creative approaches to genetic diseases are emerging. One such creative idea uses epigenetic silencing of the third HSA21. Jiang et al. [52] used the concept that the XIST RNA molecule, which silences most of the X chromosomes in human females, could be inserted into a HSA21. Using induced pluripotent cells from a male individual with DS, they inserted the XIST gene into the *DYRK1A* locus on chromosome 21 thereby creating a 'chromosome 21 Barr body' which may be the first step towards chromosome therapy. Although this technology is not ready for therapeutic trials in humans, these types of advances give hope and promise for the future.

References

1 Torfs CP, Christianson RE: Anomalies in Down syndrome individuals in a large population-based registry. Am J Med Genet 1998;77:431–438.

2 Ferencz C, Neill CA, Boughman JA, Rubin JD, Brenner JI, Perry LW: Congenital cardiovascular malformations associated with chromosome abnormalities: an epidemiologic study. J Pediatr 1989;114:79–86.

3 Bittles AH, Bower C, Hussain R, Glasson EJ: The four ages of Down syndrome. Eur J Public Health 2007;17:221–225.

4 Weijerman ME, van Furth AM, Vonk Noordegraaf A, van Wouwe JP, Broers CJ, Gemke RJ: Prevalence, neonatal characteristics, and first-year mortality of Down syndrome: a national study. J Pediatr 2008;152: 15–19.

5 Sherman SL, Allen EG, Bean LH, Freeman SB: Epidemiology of Down syndrome. Ment Retard Dev Disabil Res Rev 2007;13:221–227.

6 Irving CA, Chaudhari MP: Cardiovascular abnormalities in Down's syndrome: spectrum, management and survival over 22 years. Arch Dis Child 2012;97:326–330.

7 Freeman SB, Bean LH, Allen EG, Tinker SW, Locke AE, Druschel C, Hobbs CA, Romitti PA, Royle MH, Torfs CP, Dooley KJ, Sherman SL: Ethnicity, sex, and the incidence of congenital heart defects: a report from the National Down Syndrome Project. Genet Med 2008;10:173–180.

8 Ramsay M: Africa: continent of genome contrasts with implications for biomedical research and health. FEBS Lett 2012;586: 2813–2819.

9 Morris JK, Alberman E, Mutton D, Jacobs P: Cytogenetic and epidemiological findings in Down syndrome: England and Wales 1989–2009. Am J Med Genet A 2012; 158A:1151–1157.

10 Sturgeon X, Gardiner KJ: Transcript catalogs of human chromosome 21 and orthologous chimpanzee and mouse regions. Mamm Genome 2011;22:261–271.

11 Lana-Elola E, Watson-Scales SD, Fisher EM, Tybulewicz VL: Down syndrome: searching for the genetic culprits. Dis Model Mech 2011;4:586–595.

12 Sinet PM, Théophile D, Rahmani Z, Chettouh Z, Blouin JL, Prieur M, Noel B, Delabar JM: Mapping of the Down syndrome phenotype on chromosome 21 at the molecular level. Biomed Pharmacother 1994;48:247–252.

13 Delabar JM, Theophile D, Rahmani Z, Chettouh Z, Blouin JL, Prieur M, Noel B, Sinet PM: Molecular mapping of twenty-four features of Down syndrome on chromosome 21. Eur J Hum Genet 1993;1:114–124.
14 Korbel JO, Tirosh-Wagner T, Urban AE, Chen XN, Kasowski M, Dai L, Grubert F, Erdman C, Gao MC, Lange K, Sobel EM, Barlow GM, Aylsworth AS, Carpenter NJ, Clark RD, Cohen MY, Doran E, Falik-Zaccai T, Lewin SO, Lott IT, McGillivray BC, Moeschler JB, Pettenati MJ, Pueschel SM, Rao KW, Shaffer LG, Shohat M, Van Riper AJ, Warburton D, Weissman S, Gerstein MB, Snyder M, Korenberg JR: The genetic architecture of Down syndrome phenotypes revealed by high-resolution analysis of human segmental trisomies. Proc Natl Acad Sci U S A 2009;106:12031–12036.
15 Davies GE, Howard CM, Farrer MJ, Coleman MM, Bennett LB, Cullen LM, Wyse RK, Burn J, Williamson R, Kessling AM: Genetic variation in the COL6A1 region is associated with congenital heart defects in trisomy 21 (Down's syndrome). Ann Hum Genet 1995;59(pt 3):253–269.
16 Klewer SE, Krob SL, Kolker SJ, Kitten GT: Expression of type VI collagen in the developing mouse heart. Dev Dyn 1998;211:248–255.
17 Davies GE, Howard CM, Farrer MJ, Coleman MM, Cullen LM, Williamson R, Wyse RK, Kessling AM: Unusual genotypes in the COL6A1 gene in parents of children with trisomy 21 and major congenital heart defects. Hum Genet 1994;93:443–446.
18 Davies GE, Howard CM, Gorman LM, Farrer MJ, Holland AJ, Williamson R, Kessling AM: Polymorphisms and linkage disequilibrium in the COL6A1 and COL6A2 gene cluster: novel DNA polymorphisms in the region of a candidate gene for congenital heart defects in Down's syndrome. Hum Genet 1993;90:521–525.
19 Ackerman C, Locke AE, Feingold E, Reshey B, Espana K, Thusberg J, Mooney S, Bean LJ, Dooley KJ, Cua CL, Reeves RH, Sherman SL, Maslen CL: An excess of deleterious variants in VEGF-A pathway genes in Down-syndrome-associated atrioventricular septal defects. Am J Hum Genet 2012;91:646–659.
20 Robinson SW, Morris CD, Goldmuntz E, Reller MD, Jones MA, Steiner RD, Maslen CL: Missense mutations in CRELD1 are associated with cardiac atrioventricular septal defects. Am J Hum Genet 2003;72:1047–1052.
21 Maslen CL, Babcock D, Robinson SW, Bean LJ, Dooley KJ, Willour VL, Sherman SL: CRELD1 mutations contribute to the occurrence of cardiac atrioventricular septal defects in Down syndrome. Am J Med Genet A 2006;140:2501–2505.
22 Briggs LE, Kakarla J, Wessels A: The pathogenesis of atrial and atrioventricular septal defects with special emphasis on the role of the dorsal mesenchymal protrusion. Differentiation 2012;84:117–130.
23 Locke AE, Dooley KJ, Tinker SW, Cheong SY, Feingold E, Allen EG, Freeman SB, Torfs CP, Cua CL, Epstein MP, Wu MC, Lin X, Capone G, Sherman SL, Bean LJ: Variation in folate pathway genes contributes to risk of congenital heart defects among individuals with Down syndrome. Genet Epidemiol 2010;34:613–623.
24 Huhta JC, Hernandez-Robles JA: Homocysteine, folate, and congenital heart defects. Fetal Pediatr Pathol 2005;24:71–79.
25 Sérégaza Z, Roubertoux PL, Jamon M, Soumireu-Mourat B: Mouse models of cognitive disorders in trisomy 21: a review. Behav Genet 2006;36:387–404.
26 O'Doherty A, Ruf S, Mulligan C, Hildreth V, Errington ML, Cooke S, Sesay A, Modino S, Vanes L, Hernandez D, Linehan JM, Sharpe PT, Brandner S, Bliss TV, Henderson DJ, Nizetic D, Tybulewicz VL, Fisher EM: An aneuploid mouse strain carrying human chromosome 21 with Down syndrome phenotypes. Science 2005;309:2033–2037.
27 Barlow GM, Chen XN, Shi ZY, Lyons GE, Kurnit DM, Celle L, Spinner NB, Zackai E, Pettenati MJ, Van Riper AJ, Vekemans MJ, Mjaatvedt CH, Korenberg JR: Down syndrome congenital heart disease: a narrowed region and a candidate gene. Genet Med 2001;3:91–101.
28 Loffredo CA, Wilson PD, Ferencz C: Maternal diabetes: an independent risk factor for major cardiovascular malformations with increased mortality of affected infants. Teratology 2001;64:98–106.
29 Elton TS, Sansom SE, Martin MM: Trisomy-21 gene dosage over-expression of miRNAs results in the haploinsufficiency of specific target proteins. RNA Biol 2010;7:540–547.
30 Griffiths-Jones S, Saini HK, van Dongen S, Enright AJ: miRBase: tools for microRNA genomics. Nucleic Acids Res 2008;36 (database issue):D154–D158, http://www.mirbase.org/index.shtml.
31 Smith KA, Joziasse IC, Chocron S, van Dinther M, Guryev V, Verhoeven MC, Rehmann H, van der Smagt JJ, Doevendans PA, Cuppen E, Mulder BJ, Ten Dijke P, Bakkers J: Dominant-negative ALK2 allele associates with congenital heart defects. Circulation 2009;119:3062–3069.
32 Benson DW, Sund KL: Looking down the atrioventricular canal. Cardiovasc Res 2010;88:205–206.
33 Goddeeris MM, Rho S, Petiet A, Davenport CL, Johnson GA, Meyers EN, Klingensmith J: Intracardiac septation requires hedgehog-dependent cellular contributions from outside the heart. Development 2008;135:1887–1895.
34 ACOG Committee on Practice Bulletins: ACOG Practice Bulletin No. 77: screening for fetal chromosomal abnormalities. Obstet Gynecol 2007;109:217–227.
35 Norwitz ER, Levy B: Noninvasive prenatal testing: the future is now. Rev Obstet Gynecol 2013;6:48–62.
36 American College of Obstetricians and Gynecologists Committee on Genetics: Committee Opinion No. 545: noninvasive prenatal testing for fetal aneuploidy. Obstet Gynecol 2012;120:1532–1534.
37 Bianchi DW, Parker RL, Wentworth J, Madankumar R, Saffer C, Das AF, Craig JA, Chudova DI, Devers PL, Jones KW, Oliver K, Rava RP, Sehnert AJ; CARE Study Group: DNA sequencing versus standard prenatal aneuploidy screening. N Engl J Med 2014;370:799–808.
38 Bull MJ; Committee on Genetics: Health supervision for children with Down syndrome. Pediatrics 2011;128:393–406.
39 Saenz RB: Primary care of infants and young children with Down syndrome. Am Fam Physician 1999;59:381–390, 392, 395–396.
40 Shuhaiber JH, Ho SY, Rigby M, Sethia B: Current options and outcomes for the management of atrioventricular septal defect. Eur J Cardiothorac Surg 2009;35:891–900.
41 Jacobs JP, Burke RP, Quintessenza JA, Mavroudis C: Congenital Heart Surgery Nomenclature and Database Project: atrioventricular canal defect. Ann Thorac Surg 2000;69(4 suppl):S36–S43.
42 Najm HK, Coles JG, Endo M, Stephens D, Rebeyka IM, Williams WG, Freedom RM: Complete atrioventricular septal defects: results of repair, risk factors, and freedom from reoperation. Circulation 1997;96(9 suppl):II-311–II-315.
43 Rastelli GC, Kirklin JW, Titus JL: Anatomic observations on complete form of common atrioventricular canal with special reference to atrioventricular valves. Mayo Clinic Proc 1966;41:296–308.
44 Craig B: Atrioventricular septal defect: from fetus to adult. Heart 2006;92:1879–1885.
45 Wilson W, Taubert KA, Gewitz M, Lockhart PB, Baddour LM, Levison M, Bolger A, Cabell CH, Takahashi M, Baltimore RS, Newburger JW, Strom BL, Tani LY, Gerber M, Bonow RO, Pallasch T, Shulman ST, Rowley AH, Burns JC, Ferrieri P, Gardner T, Goff D, Durack DT: Prevention of infective endocarditis: guidelines from the American Heart Association. Circulation 2007;116:1736–1754.
46 Saji T: Clinical characteristics of pulmonary arterial hypertension associated with Down syndrome. Pediatr Int 2014;56:297–303.

3

47 Lange R, Guenther T, Busch R, Hess J, Schreiber C: The presence of Down syndrome is not a risk factor in complete atrioventricular septal defect repair. J Thorac Cardiovasc Surg 2007;134:304–310.
48 Berger TJ, Blackstone EH, Kirklin JW, Bargeron LM Jr, Hazelrig JB, Turner ME Jr: Survival and probability of cure without and with operation in complete atrioventricular canal. Ann Thorac Surg 1979;27:104–111.
49 El-Najdawi EK, Driscoll DJ, Puga FJ, Dearani JA, Spotts BE, Mahoney DW, Danielson GK: Operation for partial atrioventricular septal defect: a forty-year review. J Thorac Cardiovasc Surg 2000;119:880–889.
50 Yang Q, Rasmussen SA, Friedman JM: Mortality associated with Down's syndrome in the USA from 1983 to 1997: a population-based study. Lancet 2002;359:1019–1025.
51 Zhu JL, Hasle H, Correa A, Schendel D, Friedman JM, Olsen J, Rasmussen SA: Survival among people with Down syndrome: a nationwide population-based study in Denmark. Genet Med 2013;15:64–69.
52 Jiang J, Jing Y, Cost GJ, Chiang JC, Kolpa HJ, Cotton AM, Carone DM, Carone BR, Shivak DA, Guschin DY, Pearl JR, Rebar EJ, Byron M, Gregory PD, Brown CJ, Urnov FD, Hall LL, Lawrence JB: Translating dosage compensation to trisomy 21. Nature 2013;500:296–300.

Dr. Paul S. Kruszka
National Human Genome Research Institute
National Institutes of Health
Bethesda, MD 20892 (USA)
E-Mail paul.kruszka@nih.gov

Muenke M, Kruszka PS, Sable CA, Belmont JW (eds): Congenital Heart Disease: Molecular Genetics, Principles of Diagnosis and Treatment. Basel, Karger, 2015, pp 91–99
DOI: 10.1159/000375207

Congenital Cardiovascular Defects in Monosomy X or Turner Syndrome

Carolyn Bondy

National Institute of Child Health and Human Development, National Institutes of Health, Bethesda, Md., USA

Abstract

Turner syndrome (TS) is due to haploinsufficiency for genes located on the sex chromosome short arms. There is a high rate of fetal demise in mid-late gestation resulting from aortic arch hypoplasia, and interruption and coarctation of the aorta, often associated with a bicuspid aortic valve (BAV) and left-heart hypoplasia. In fact, TS is the most common known genetic disorder associated with left-heart hypoplasia, coarctation of the aorta, and BAV. Surviving individuals with TS exhibit distinctive aortic arch abnormalities consistent with impaired development of 4th pharyngeal arch arteries. Aortic valve defects, ranging from partial fusion of the right and left coronary leaflets to BAV and unicuspid aortic valves, are common and associated with dilation of the ascending aorta. These abnormalities are associated with a high risk for aneurysms and dissection of both ascending and descending thoracic aortas in young adults with TS.

The Turner syndrome (TS) is a chromosomal disorder caused by complete or partial monosomy X and is found in approximately 1 in 2,500 live born females [1]. The most common karyotype associated with TS is 45,X, which appears to be due to loss of a sex chromosome during meiotic divisions in the process of gametogenesis. In 45,X patients, the ratio of maternally to paternally derived X chromosomes is slightly greater than 2:1 [2], consistent with a somewhat greater risk for loss of a paternal Y chromosome leading to monosomy X (monosomy Y is not viable). The 2nd most common karyotype found in TS is mosaicism for a 45,X cell line together with 46,XX, 47,XXX, or 46,XY cell lines, resulting from sex chromosome nondisjunction occurring in postzygotic mitotic cell divisions. The presence of cell lines with two or more sex chromosomes attenuates the Turner phenotype in most cases. The third major chromosomal source of TS arises from fragmentation of a sex chromosome commonly occurring during gametogenesis. The isochromosome is the most common sex chromosome abnormality formed by recombination errors involving highly repetitive often palindromic sequences near the X and Y chromosome centromeres. The resulting iso or isodicentric X or Y chromosomes share loss of most of the short arms, with duplication and end-to-end fusion of the long arms.

TS is also caused by deletion of the short arms of the X or Y chromosome, sometimes presenting as ring or marker chromosomes. The fragmentary sex chromosomes are mitotically unstable and thus are frequently lost in some cells during the course of embryonic development, resulting in individuals mosaic for the original 46,X,frag (X or Y) cell line and 45,X cells. This mosaic karyotype is not associated with moderation of the phenotype, since all cells are monosomic for the X chromosome short arm.

The common denominator of all karyotypes associated with TS is loss of terminal portions of short arms of the X or Y chromosome [3]. Since the male sex-determining gene SRY resides on the short arm of the Y chromosome, most patients are phenotypic females; in fact, the clinical diagnosis 'Turner syndrome' refers only to females. The much less common phenotypic male patient with the 45,X/46XY karyotype is classified under 'disorder of sexual development' [4].

Spectrum of Congenital Cardiovascular Malformations in Turner Syndrome

Aortic coarctation was a salient feature in the very first study linking TS to monosomy X [5]. Many Turner gestations end in 2nd–3rd trimesters due to left-heart and/or aortic hypoplasia [6]. Pathology studies of spontaneously aborted 45,X fetuses showed major left-ventricular outflow tract (LVOT) defects [6–8]. Miyabara et al. [9] examined 13 mid-trimester 45,X fetuses and found that all had abnormal aortic valve structure [11 had bicuspid aortic valves (BAV) and 2 unicuspid aortic valves] and tubular hypoplasia or interruption of the transverse aortic arch [9]. A significant number of newborns with TS present with lethal left-heart and aortic hypoplasia [10]. In fact, TS is the most common known genetic association underlying hypoplastic left-heart syndrome [11]. Thus, in fetal development, TS associates with a very distinctive profile of aortic arch, aortic valve, and left ventricular defects, which contribute to fetal demise of many if not most Turner gestations. The following sections describe the spectrum and prevalence of congenital cardiovascular defects determined by screening girls and women that have survived despite monosomy X (see chapter by Costello et al. on Surgical Management for discussion of treatment for Turner syndrome on p. 285).

Aortic Valve

More than 450 girls and women with karyotype-proven TS have undergone extensive cardiovascular screening in the context of the NIH Turner Syndrome Genotype-Phenotype Study (NCT00006334). This protocol is unique among clinical studies of TS in requiring a 50-cell karyotype with exclusion of any subjects with >30% normal cells [12]. In point of fact, the study cohort includes only 10% of subjects with evidence of a normal cell line on the peripheral blood karyotype. A 50-cell karyotype indicating 45,X excludes the presence of mosaicism with a certainty of 99% [13]. The prevalence of anatomic aortic valve abnormalities using most advanced MRI is 30–39% [12, 14, 15]. This prevalence is considerably higher than that estimated by studies using transthoracic echocardiography of 12–20% [16–18]. This lower prevalence may be explained by the inclusion of girls with a high proportion of normal cells and milder phenotype in these studies, and by the fact that echocardiography does not adequately visualize the aortic valve in 25% of TS patients [12, 14].

The valve defects illustrated by cardiac MRI range from unicuspid to bicuspid to partially fused to normal tricuspid morphology (fig. 1). The fusion pattern is similar to that seen in 'nonsyndromic' BAV in the general population, with the great majority exhibiting right-left coronary cusp fusion [12, 14]. Olivieri et al. [14] were the first to demonstrate that *partial* aortic valve fusion constitutes the mild end of a spectrum of aortic valve pathology seen in TS (fig. 1). This partial fusion entity was previously viewed as an acquired abnormality caused by atherosclerotic degeneration. In contrast, screening of a large group of relatively young (age range 7–67, median 29 years) and asymptomatic girls and women with TS shows that partial fusion is a congenital defect related to the more generalized LVOT spectrum

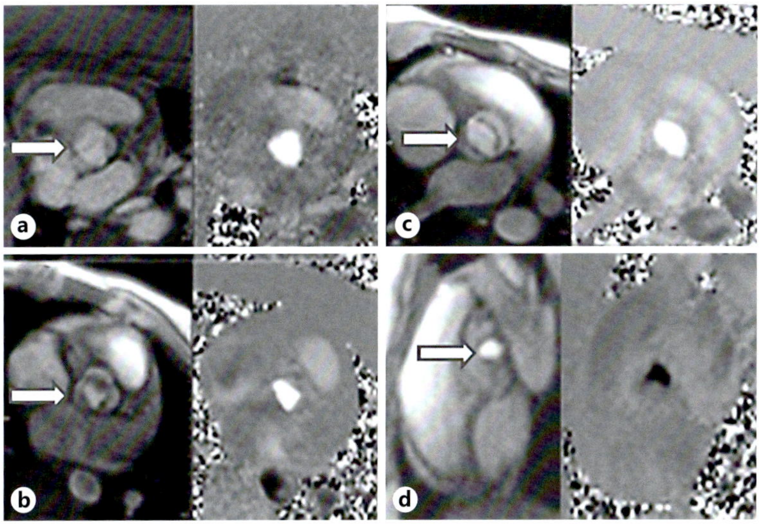

Fig. 1. Aortic valve structure in study subjects with TS demonstrated on cardiac MRI. Left panels are gradient-echo and right panels are phase-contrast images [adapted from Olivieri et al. [14]]. **a** Normal tricuspid valve structure. **b** Partial aortic valve fusion. **c** BAV. **d** Unicuspid aortic valve.

seen in TS. This entity was associated with mild but statistically significant acceleration of blood flow and an increased frequency of aortic valve insufficiency compared to those with normal tricuspid aortic valves, as well as mild dilation of the ascending aorta [14].

Aortic Dilation

BAV is associated with dilation of the ascending aorta in TS as in nonsyndromic BAV. Determination of aortic dilation in TS must account for the petite size of the affected individuals by normalization to the body surface area [19, 20]. The NIH data demonstrate that the ascending aortic diameter measured at the level of the pulmonary artery bifurcation is the most robust parameter distinguishing between TS patients with an aortic valve defect from those with normal tricuspid aortic valves [12, 14, 19]. The ascending aorta is the site of most significant dilation associated with BAV in the general population [21] and is also the site of progressive dilation at a rate of ~0.5 mm/year for BAV patients. This is in contrast to patients with the Marfan syndrome, who exhibit dilation primarily in the sinuses of Valsalva [22]. The rate of aortic dilation in TS has not been established. The only published study on this subject included just 80 adult TS subjects and did not separate results for women with BAV versus tricuspid aortic valves [23]. Aortic dilation rate (mm/year) was not statistically significant at any site, which may be related to the small sample size or may indicate that dilation is not rapidly progressive in this group [23].

Some TS patients with a normal aortic valve structure also show evidence of mild-moderate dilation of the ascending aorta [12, 20]. Likewise, family members of nonsyndromic BAV patients may demonstrate dilation of the ascending aorta despite normal valve structure [24]. These observations, together with well-documented associations of aortic valve abnormality and other aortic defects such as coarctation, support the view that the congenitally abnormal aortic valve is just one manifestation of a more extensive defect in aortic development and a risk for aneurysm and dissection [25].

Aortic Arch

As noted above, aortic arch defects, such as tubular hypoplasia and interruption, cause fetal demise in many if not most TS gestations. The use of MRI screening has revealed that aortic arch anomalies are found in more than 50% of girls and wom-

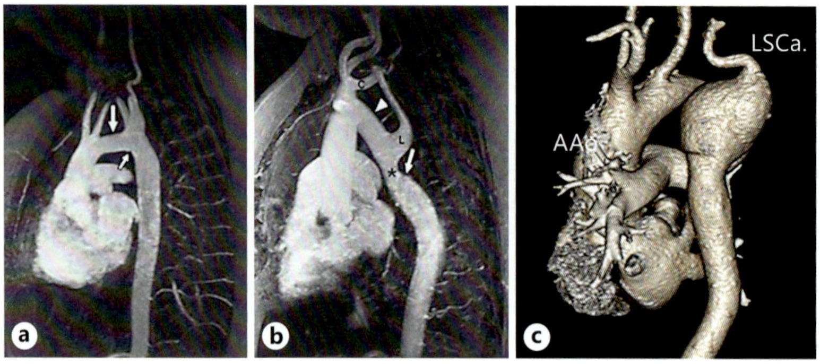

Fig. 2. Spectrum of aortic arch involvement in TS. **a** ETA (large arrow) associated with aberrant origin of the right subclavian (cf. additional images of this patient). The kink (small arrow) in the lesser curvature represents a form fruste of coarctation or pseudocoarctation. **b** ETA (arrowhead) associated with a coarctation (*) that was considered hemodynamically insignificant. There is prominent dilation of the left subclavian origin (L) and a poststenotic dilation of the descending aorta (arrow). **c** Left common carotid artery. 3D reconstruction of CT imaging shows large aneurysms of the ascending aorta (AAo, 4.5 cm) and descending aorta (6 cm) involving the origin of the left subclavian artery (LSCa). This completely asymptomatic young woman had been followed with cardiac ultrasound in the years preceding admission to the NIH TS protocol. During her teenage years, she was told there was a mild aortic coarctation that did not require treatment. Screening studies upon NIH admission showed BAV with mild regurgitation and the two aneurysms. The CT study was performed in preparation for surgical repair of the 6-cm aneurysm which was performed immediately; repair of the ascending aortic aneurysm was carried out 6 months later.

en with TS [15, 26–29]. Approximately 50% of girls and women with TS demonstrate an elongation of the transverse aortic arch (ETA) associated with coarctation or 'pseudocoarctation'. The latter is a kink in the lesser curvature of the descending aorta at the usual site of coarctation in TS. Pseudocoarctation is often associated with a bulb-like dilation of the takeoff of the left subclavian artery or with similar dilation of an aberrant right subclavian artery (fig. 2a). Pseudocoarctation is associated with type B dissection [30]. Aberrant origin of the right subclavian artery occurs in 6–15% of individuals with TS [15, 26, 31].

Partial Anomalous Pulmonary Venous Return

Partial anomalous pulmonary venous return has been noted in case reports [32] and studies of 45,X fetuses [9]. In asymptomatic girls and women with TS examined by contrast-enhanced MRI, prevalence is 13–15% [15, 26]. To date, the presence of partial anomalous pulmonary venous return has not been linked with any of the other cardiovascular defects in TS.

Other Cardiovascular Defects

Atrial septal defects (ASD) are not very common in TS. Among the 450 patients studied at NIH, 2 cases with a history of ASD that closed spontaneously were reported, and there was 1 complex case that presented in childhood with an incomplete atrioventricular canal, cleft mitral valve, primum ASD, and tubular hypoplasia of the transverse aorta [33]. In one echocardiography study, approximately 8% of the subjects had ASD [18]. Some early studies of the cardiovascular phenotype in TS included individuals with the Noonan syndrome (see chapter by Gelb et al. p. 122), which has a very different cardiac phenotype, e.g. pulmonic stenosis and hypertrophic cardiomyopathy [34].

Theories on the Cause of Congenital Cardiovascular Defects in Turner Syndrome

Association with Fetal Lymphedema

Pathology studies of 45,X fetuses often showed cystic hygroma (distended jugular lymphatics) together with major LVOT defects [6–8]. Prof. Clark hypothesized that obstruction of the developing lymphatic system could lead to impaired blood flow through the developing heart, resulting in the typical LVOT defects seen in TS [35]. In fact, BAV and coartation are significantly more common among TS girls with neck webbing, a residual of fetal cervical cystic hygroma [36, 37]. However, the two traits are not strictly convergent; a substantial number of patients showing evidence of fetal lymphedema have no detectable cardiovascular defects despite advanced cardiovascular screening, and others with typical LVOT defects lack evidence of fetal lymphedema [36]. Moreover, fetal cervical hygroma or lymphatic fluid collection also occurs in trisomies 21, 18 and 13 [38], and in the autosomal dominant Noonan and lymphedema-distichiasis syndromes, all of which have entirely different genetic origins and cardiovascular defects. These observations suggest that fetal lymphedema may be a nonspecific accompaniment of many developmental disorders involving the cardiovascular system. Finally, BAV is relatively common in the general population, often in kindred demonstrating left-heart hypoplasia or coarctation [39, 40], but not neck webbing or other evidence of fetal lymphedema.

Neural Crest

Miyabara et al. [9, 38] investigated lymphatic and cardiovascular anatomy in 45,X fetuses and found no evidence of a relationship between dilated lymphatics and the developing aortic valve or aorta. They suggested that the pattern of aortic arch defects in TS could be due to defective differentiation or migration of neural crest cells contributing to the 4th pharyngeal arch (see chapter by Sylva and Moorman p. 21). Cardiac neural crest cells populating the 4th pharyngeal arch are responsible for the differentiation of smooth muscle cells of the aortic arch and right subclavian artery (fig. 3). Figure 4 outlines a proposed pathogenetic sequence in which haploinsufficiency for unknown X:Y homologous gene(s) leads to cardiac neural crest cell impairment and consequent malformation of the aortic arch. The aortic arch defect is the most constant feature of the TS cardiovascular phenotype; this defect obstructs blood flow in the outflow tract, which may lead to left-heart hypoplasia and aortic valve defects as secondary effects.

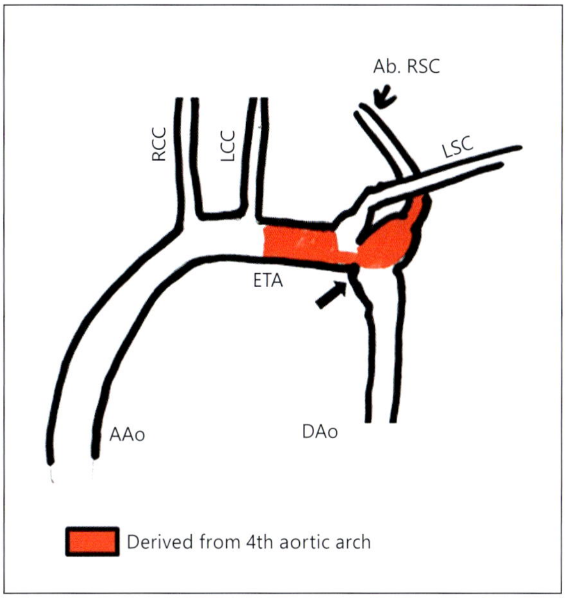

Fig. 3. Elongation of the transverse aortic arch (ETA) is the most common cardiovascular abnormality in TS. The arch is typically flattened and elongated between the left common carotid artery (LCC) and left subclavian (LSC) arteries. This malformation is associated with a distinct kink (arrow) in the lesser curvature of the descending aorta (DAo) at the usual site of aortic coarctation. ETA is often associated with aberrant (Ab.) origin of the right subclavian artery (RSC). This anomaly is frequently accompanied by a bulbous dilation of the takeoff of left and right subclavian arteries. The areas colored in red are derived from the 4th pharyngeal arch arteries. AAo = Ascending aorta; RCC = right common carotid.

Cardiac neural crest cells may also contribute directly to normal aortic valve development, and thus aortic valve abnormalities may represent a primary defect related to the neural crest deficit. Likewise, the high risk for aortic arch aneurysm/dissection in TS may result from abnormal blood flow patterns resulting from valve and arch malformation, or from an intrinsically abnormal aortic wall structure which is directly related to deficient or defective vascular smooth muscle cells.

Parallels with the 22q11.2 Deletion (DiGeorge Syndrome)

There are several notable similarities between these two syndromes (see Goldmuntz chapter p. 100). Type b interruption of the aortic arch is an important feature of both syndromes, although other cardiovascular defects are generally divergent. In ad-

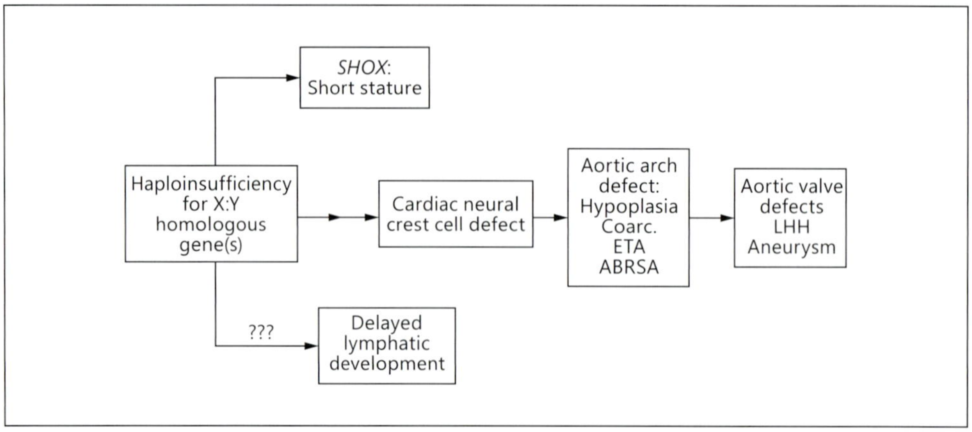

Fig. 4. Schematic outline of the hypothetical pathogenesis of LVOT abnormalities in TS. Haploinsufficiency for the pseudoautosomal gene SHOX causes short stature in TS patients and in male and female patients with mutations or microdeletions in this gene. Haploinsufficiency for unknown X:Y homologous gene(s) or noncoding RNA impairs the role of cardiac neural crest cells in promoting normal aortic arch development. An obstructed aortic arch impairs outflow tract blood flow resulting in defective development of the left heart and/or aortic valve. Disturbed blood flow through the aortic valve and arch contributes to an elevated risk for aortic aneurysm. Alternatively, the abnormality in cardiac neural crest cells may directly impair aortic valve formation and aortic arch structural integrity, independent of hydraulic effects. LHH = Left-heart hypoplasia; ABRSA = abberrant origin of the right subclavian artery.

dition, both syndromes demonstrate palatal abnormalities, micrognathia, hearing loss, and immunologic disorders. These observations suggest that there is overlap between pharyngeal arch developmental defects in TS and the DiGeorge syndrome.

Genes Implicated in Turner Syndrome

Monosomy for the X chromosome is the only monosomy compatible with life. This is likely due to the fact that the 2nd X chromosome is largely inactivated in normal females, and the Y chromosome has relatively few functional genes aside from those involved in male sex determination and spermiogenesis [41–43]. However, some important genes still exist on and are expressed from both sex chromosomes. The terminal regions of both the X and the Y chromosome exhibit homologous genes that promote pairing and recombination between the sex chromosomes [44]. These are termed pseudoautosomal regions (PAR1 located at short-arm termini) and PAR2 (located at the long-arm termini). Pseudoautosomal genes are expressed from both sex chromosomes in males and females. There are only a few genes in PAR2, and deletion of long-arm termini has little phenotypic effect; thus, investigations have focused on PAR1 to identify the haploinsufficiency for the gene which causes TS traits.

Haploinsufficiency for the PAR1 gene *SHOX* is responsible for the short stature and skeletal anomalies characteristic of TS [45, 46]. The genes related to cardiovascular and cognitive traits also map to the short arms of sex chromosomes [42, 43], but have not been identified. We recently showed that the locus for congenital heart defects in TS lies proximal to ChrX:41,500,000 [43]. In addition to candidate genes in PAR1, there are several Xp genes outside of PAR1 that escape X inactivation and have Y homologues, and thus may play a role in TS, as recently reviewed [47]. It is not feasible to nominate a candidate PAR1 gene based on putative function, since scores of transcriptional regulators and intra- and extracellular signaling pathways are implicated in cardiovascular development [48].

Male sex is an important risk factor for congenital LVOT defects that remains totally unexplained. For example, BAV affects ~2% of the general male population but less than 0.5% of (non-TS) females [21]. A similar male preponderance is observed for hypoplastic left-heart syndrome and aortic coarctation. To explain this epidemiology, one may suppose that an X:Y homologous gene must be expressed from both sex chromosomes for normal LVOT development, likely through the regulation of cardiac neural crest cell function (fig. 4). Haploinsufficiency for this locus occurs in TS due to loss of the distal portion of a sex chromosome short arm and results in a very high prevalence of the LVOT defect. It seems quite plausible that the excess prevalence in the general male population may be explained by the high rate of recombination errors between X and Y chromosomes, resulting in mutations/deletions in this putative locus, as previously suggested [49]. The recombination rate for PAR1 in male meiosis is 7-fold higher than that in females [50], substantially increasing the risk for gene disruption. There are several other X:Y homologues expressed from both sex chromosomes as recently reviewed. One of these is TBL1X and TBL1Y; mutation in the latter has been associated with aortic coarctation in 2/83 males [51]. This gene is also located in a Y-chromosome short-arm locus that is highly prone to rearrangements, which may contribute to an excess risk for LVOT-causing mutations on the Y chromosome.

X-Chromosome Genomic Imprinting

The parental origin of the single X chromosome may influence the expression of aspects of the TS phenotype that typically demonstrate sexual dimorphism in the general population [52], e.g. brain size, risk for autistic spectrum disorders, abdominal adiposity, and atherosclerosis. Thus, we investigated whether the parental origin of the single X chromosome influenced the expression of congenital heart defects in TS. We examined the prevalence of cardiovascular defects using echocardiography and MRI in groups separated on the basis of genotyping the parental origin of their single normal X chromosome [2]. BAV prevalence was equal in XM (n = 133) and XP (n = 50) groups. The prevalence of any cardiovascular anomaly, including BAV, coarctation, ETA, and partial anomalous pulmonary venous return, was 55% in the XM and 52% in the XP group, showing that X-chromosome imprinting is not implicated in TS cardiovascular defects.

Conclusion

Although haploinsufficiency of the short arm of the X chromosome is thought to be responsible for the cardiac phenotype in TS, the precise gene or genes has not been determined. There is still much work to be done in genetics, epigenetics, and gene expression studies in TS. Fortunately, there are active next-generation sequencing studies underway at the National Institutes of Health to answer this question, which will hopefully result in better patient outcomes in the future.

References

1 Nielsen J, Wohlert M: Chromosome abnormalities found among 34,910 newborn children: results from a 13-year incidence study in Arhus, Denmark. Hum Genet 1991;87:81–83.
2 Bondy C, Matura L, Wooten N, Troendle J, Zinn A, Bakalov V: The physical phenotype of girls and women with Turner syndrome is not X-imprinted. Hum Genet 2007;121:469–474.
3 Ferguson-Smith MA: Karyotype-phenotype correlations in gonadal dysgenesis and their bearing on the pathogenesis of malformations. J Med Genet 1965;2:142–155.
4 Bondy CA; Turner Syndrome Consensus Study Group: Care of girls and women with Turner syndrome: a guideline of the Turner Syndrome Study Group. J Clin Endocrinol Metab 2007;92:10–25.
5 Polani PE, Hunter WF, Lennox B: Chromosomal sex in Turner's syndrome with coarctation of the aorta. Lancet 1954;267:120–121.
6 Surerus E, Huggon IC, Allan LD: Turner's syndrome in fetal life. Ultrasound Obstet Gynecol 2003;22:264–267.
7 Lacro RV, Jones KL, Benirschke K: Coarctation of the aorta in Turner syndrome: a pathologic study of fetuses with nuchal cystic hygromas, hydrops fetalis, and female genitalia. Pediatrics 1988;81:445–451.
8 Barr M Jr, Oman-Ganes L: Turner syndrome morphology and morphometrics: cardiac hypoplasia as a cause of midgestation death. Teratology 2002;66:65–72.
9 Miyabara S, Nakayama M, Suzumori K, Yonemitsu N, Sugihara H: Developmental analysis of cardiovascular system of 45,X fetuses with cystic hygroma. Am J Med Genet 1997;68:135–141.
10 Sybert VP: Cardiovascular malformations and complications in Turner syndrome. Pediatrics 1998;101:e11.

11 Patel A, Hickey E, Mavroudis C, Jacobs JP, Jacobs ML, Backer CL, Gevitz M, Mavroudis CD: Impact of noncardiac congenital and genetic abnormalities on outcomes in hypoplastic left heart syndrome. Ann Thorac Surg 2010;89:1805–1814.
12 Sachdev V, Matura L, Sidenko S, Ho V, Arai A, Rosing D, Bondy C: Aortic valve disease in Turner syndrome. J Am Coll Cardiol 2008;51:1904–1909.
13 Hook EB: Exclusion of chromosomal mosaicism: tables of 90, 95 and 99% confidence limits and comments on use. Am J Hum Genet 1977;29:94–97.
14 Olivieri LJ, Baba RY, Arai AE, Bandettini WP, Rosing DR, Bakalov V, Sachdev V, Bondy CA: Spectrum of aortic valve abnormalities associated with aortic dilation across age groups in Turner syndrome. Circ Cardiovasc Imaging 2013;6:1018–1023.
15 Kim H, Gottliebson W, Hor K, Backeljauw P, Gutmark Little I, Salisbury S, Racadio J, Helton Skally K, Fleck R: Cardiovascular anomalies in Turner syndrome: spectrum, prevalence, and cardiac MRI findings in a pediatric and young adult population. AJR Am J Roentgenol 2011;196: 454–460.
16 Prandstraller D, Mazzanti L, Picchio F, Magnani C, Bergamaschi R, Perri A, Tsingos E, Cacciari E: Turner's syndrome: cardiologic profile according to the different chromosomal patterns and long-term clinical follow-up of 136 nonpreselected patients. Pediatr Cardiol 1999;20:108–112.
17 Gotzsche C, Krag-Olsen B: Prevalence of cardiovascular malformations and association with karyotypes in Turner's syndrome. Arch Dis Child 1994;71:433–436.
18 Volkl TM, Degenhardt K, Koch A, Simm D, Dorr HG, Singer H: Cardiovascular anomalies in children and young adults with Ullrich-Turner syndrome the Erlangen experience. Clin Cardiol 2005;28:88–92.
19 Matura L, Ho V, Rosing D, Bondy C: Aortic dilatation and dissection in Turner syndrome. Circulation 2007;116:1663–1670.
20 Lopez L, Arheart KL, Colan SD, Stein NS, Lopez-Mitnik G, Lin AE, Reller MD, Ventura R, Silberbach M: Turner syndrome is an independent risk factor for aortic dilation in the young. Pediatrics 2008;121: e1622–e1627.
21 Braverman AC, Güven H, Beardslee MA, Makan M, Kates AM, Moon MR: The bicuspid aortic valve. Curr Probl Cardiol 2005;30: 470–522.
22 Detaint D, Michelena HI, Nkomo VT, Vahanian A, Jondeau G, Sarano ME: Aortic dilatation patterns and rates in adults with bicuspid aortic valves: a comparative study with Marfan syndrome and degenerative aortopathy. Heart 2014;100:126–134.
23 Mortensen K, Hjerrild B, Stochholm K, Andersen N, Sorensen K, Lundorf E, Horlyck A, Pedersen E, Christiansen J, Gravholt C: Dilation of the ascending aorta in Turner syndrome – a prospective cardiovascular magnetic resonance study. J Cardiovasc Magn Reson 2011;13:24.
24 Biner S, Rafique A, Ray I, Cuk O, Siegel R, Tolstrup K: Aortopathy is prevalent in relatives of bicuspid aortic valve patients. J Am Coll Cardiol 2009;53:2288–2295.
25 Silberbach M: Bicuspid aortic valve and thoracic aortic aneurysm: toward a unified theory. J Am Coll Cardiol 2009;53:2296–2297.
26 Ho VB, Bakalov VK, Cooley M, Van PL, Hood MN, Burklow TR, Bondy CA: Major vascular anomalies in Turner syndrome: prevalence and magnetic resonance angiographic features. Circulation 2004;110: 1694–1700.
27 Ostberg JE, Brookes JAS, McCarthy C, Halcox J, Conway GS: A comparison of echocardiography and magnetic resonance imaging in cardiovascular screening of adults with Turner syndrome. J Clin Endocrinol Metab 2004;89:5966–5971.
28 Dawson-Falk KL, Wright AM, Bakker B, Pitlick PT, Wilson DM, Rosenfeld RG: Cardiovascular evaluation in Turner syndrome: utility of MR imaging. Australas Radiol 1992;36:204–209.
29 Hjerrild B, Mortensen K, Sorensen K, Pedersen E, Andersen N, Lundorf E, Hansen K, Horlyck A, Hager A, Christiansen J, et al: Thoracic aortopathy in Turner syndrome and the influence of bicuspid aortic valves and blood pressure: a CMR study. J Cardiovasc Magn Reson 2010;12:12.
30 Klein LW, Levin JL, Weintraub WS, Agarwal JB, Helfant RH: Pseudocoarctation of the aortic arch in a patient with Turner's syndrome. Clin Cardiol 1984;7:621–623.
31 Lee SH, Jung JM, Song MS, Choi SJ, Chung WY: Evaluation of cardiovascular anomalies in patients with asymptomatic Turner syndrome using multidetector computed tomography. J Korean Med Sci 2013;28: 1169–1173.
32 Bechtold SM, Dalla Pozza R, Becker A, Meidert A, Dohlemann C, Schwarz HP: Partial anomalous pulmonary vein connection: an underestimated cardiovascular defect in Ullrich-Turner syndrome. Eur J Pediatr 2004;163:158–162.
33 Oza NM, Siegenthaler M, Horvath K, Rosing DR, Chen MY, Arai A, Gould HN, Bakalov V, Bondy CA: Serious aortic complications in a patient with Turner syndrome. Eur J Pediatr 2013;172:703–705.
34 Nora JJ, Torres FG, Sinha AK, McNamara DG: Characteristic cardiovascular anomalies of XO Turner syndrome, XX and XY phenotype and XO-XX Turner mosaic. Am J Cardiol 1970;25:639–641.
35 Clark EB: Neck web and congenital heart defects: a pathogenic association in 45 X-O Turner syndrome. Teratology 1984;29: 355–361.
36 Loscalzo ML, Van PL, Ho VB, Bakalov VK, Rosing DR, Malone CA, Dietz HC, Bondy CA: Association between fetal lymphedema and congenital cardiovascular defects in Turner syndrome. Pediatrics 2005;115: 732–735.
37 Mazzanti L, Cacciari E: Congenital heart disease in patients with Turner's syndrome. Italian Study Group for Turner Syndrome (ISGTS). J Pediatr 1998;133:688–692.
38 Miyabara S, Sugihara H, Maehara N, Shouno H, Tasaki H, Yoshida K, Saito N, Kayama F, Ibara S, Suzumori K: Significance of cardiovascular malformations in cystic hygroma: a new interpretation of the pathogenesis. Am J Med Genet 1989;34:489–501.
39 Loffredo CA, Chokkalingam A, Sill AM, Boughman JA, Clark EB, Scheel J, Brenner JI: Prevalence of congenital cardiovascular malformations among relatives of infants with hypoplastic left heart, coarctation of the aorta, and d-transposition of the great arteries. Am J Med Genet A 2004;124A:225–230.
40 McBride K, Pignatelli R, Lewin M, Ho T, Fernbach S, Menesses A, Lam W, Leal S, Kaplan N, Schliekelman P, et al: Inheritance analysis of congenital left ventricular outflow tract obstruction malformations: segregation, multiplex relative risk, and heritability. Am J Med Genet A 2005;134A:180–186.
41 Blaschke RJ, Rappold GA: SHOX: growth, Leri-Weill and Turner syndromes. Trends Endocrinol Metab 2000;11:227–230.
42 Zinn A, Roeltgen D, Stefanatos G, Ramos P, Elder F, Kushner H, Kowal K, Ross J: A Turner syndrome neurocognitive phenotype maps to Xp22.3. Behav Brain Funct 2007;3:24.
43 Bondy C, Bakalov VK, Cheng C, Olivieri L, Rosing DR, Arai AE: Bicuspid aortic valve and aortic coarctation are linked to deletion of the X chromosome short arm in Turner syndrome. J Med Genet 2013;50: 662–665.
44 Rappold GA: The pseudoautosomal regions of the human sex chromosomes. Hum Genet 1993;92:315–324.
45 Rappold GA, Fukami M, Niesler B, Schiller S, Zumkeller W, Bettendorf M, Heinrich U, Vlachopapadoupoulou E, Reinehr T, Onigata K, et al: Deletions of the homeobox gene SHOX (short stature homeobox) are an important cause of growth failure in children with short stature. J Clin Endocrinol Metab 2002;87:1402–1406.

46 Rao E, Weiss B, Fukami M, Rump A, Niesler B, Mertz A, Muroya K, Binder G, Kirsch S, Winkelmann M, et al: Pseudoautosomal deletions encompassing a novel homeobox gene cause growth failure in idiopathic short stature and Turner syndrome. Nat Genet 1997;16:54–63.
47 Bondy C, Cheng C: Monosomy for the X chromosome. Chromosome Res 2009;17: 649–658.
48 Hickey EJ, Caldarone CA, McCrindle BW: Left ventricular hypoplasia: a spectrum of disease involving the left ventricular outflow tract, aortic valve, and aorta. J Am Coll Cardiol 2012;59(1 suppl):S43–S54.
49 Bondy CA: Aortic coarctation and coronary artery disease. Circulation 2012;126: 5–7.
50 Flaquer A, Rappold GA, Wienker TF, Fischer C: The human pseudoautosomal regions: a review for genetic epidemiologists. Eur J Hum Genet 2008;16:771–779.
51 Tagariello A, Breuer C, Birkner Y, Schmidt S, Koch AM, Cesnjevar R, Ruffer A, Dittrich S, Schneider H, Winterpacht A, et al: Functional null mutations in the gonosomal homologue gene TBL1Y are associated with non-syndromic coarctation of the aorta. Curr Mol Med 2012;12:199–205.
52 Bondy CA, Cheng C, Hougen HY, Zhou J: Genomic imprinting in Turner syndrome. Pediatr Endocrinol Rev 2012;2(suppl):728–732.

3

Dr. Carolyn Bondy
National Institute of Child Health and Human Development
National Institutes of Health
10 Center Drive
Bethesda, MD 20892 (USA)
E-Mail bondyc@mail.nih.gov

Muenke M, Kruszka PS, Sable CA, Belmont JW (eds): Congenital Heart Disease: Molecular Genetics, Principles of Diagnosis and Treatment. Basel, Karger, 2015, pp 100–111
DOI: 10.1159/000375208

The 22q11.2 Deletion Syndrome

Elizabeth Goldmuntz

Division of Cardiology, The Children's Hospital of Philadelphia, Philadelphia, Pa., USA

Abstract

The 22q11.2 deletion syndrome is most commonly characterized by facial dysmorphia, palate anomalies, immunodeficiency, hypocalcemia, conotruncal and related cardiac defects, as well as behavioral and psychiatric disorders. A patient may present with just a few features and only come to the diagnosis upon having a more severely affected child, or they can present at birth with extensive and severe manifestations. Approximately 6–10% of cases are familial, while most occur de novo. Nearly 75% of patients with a 22q11.2 deletion have a congenital heart malformation, including a subset of conotruncal and ventricular septal defects, as well as aortic arch anomalies. In the current era, most studies suggest that the cardiac patient with a 22q11.2 deletion does not suffer any increased risk of mortality but likely experiences a more complicated perioperative course. Given the clinical implications and difficulty identifying the minimally affected cardiac newborn with the 22q11.2 deletion syndrome, most advocate proactive genetic testing of the at-risk infant with typical cardiac manifestations of the deletion syndrome, particularly in the presence of an aortic arch anomaly. Identifying the cardiac patient with a 22q11.2 deletion allows for complete medical and reproductive counseling and, in the future world of personalized medicine, may dictate clinical management strategies.

DiGeorge syndrome was first described in 1968 as a rare developmental field defect affecting structures derived from the third and fourth embryonic pharyngeal arches [1, 2]. Characteristic features included distinct facial features, hypoplasia or aplasia of the thymus, hypoplasia or aplasia of the parathyroid glands, and conotruncal cardiac defects. Infants presented with hypocalcemia, immunodeficiency, and severe heart defects, which, at the time, were generally incompatible with life. The syndrome was observed to be etiologically heterogeneous occurring in the context of maternal diabetes or alcohol use, and in conjunction with a variety of chromosomal abnormalities identified by karyotyping. Studies subsequently found that approximately 10–20% of patients with the DiGeorge phenotype had a chromosomal alteration resulting in the loss of the proximal long arm of chromosome 22. Further molecular analysis revealed that nearly 90% of patients with the clinical features of DiGeorge syndrome had a microdeletion of a segment of chromosome 22, called a 22q11.2 deletion [3, 4].

Two patient populations that shared common features with that of DiGeorge syndrome, namely velocardiofacial (or Shprintzen) and conotruncal anomaly face syndromes, had also been described in different clinical settings. The velocardiofacial syndrome was characterized in 1978 by typical facial features, cleft palate, learning disabilities, and specific congenital heart defects [5]. The conotruncal anomaly face syndrome was originally described in Japan in 1976 and defined by conotruncal cardiac defects, hypernasal speech, mild mental retardation, neonatal tetany, thymic aplasia or hypoplasia, and facial dysmorphia [6]. Subsequent molecular investigations identified chromosome 22q11.2 deletions in 80–90% of patients with the clinical diagnosis of either velocardiofacial or conotruncal anomaly face syndrome [7–10]. Thus, the three clinical syndromes – DiGeorge, velocardiofacial and conotruncal anomaly face – were found to share a common genetic etiology in the majority of cases, namely a chromosome 22q11.2 deletion. These studies ultimately defined the most common deletion syndrome currently known, namely the 22q11.2 deletion syndrome, estimated to occur in approximately 1 in 4,000–6,000 live births [11, 12].

Molecular Characteristics of the 22q11.2 Deletion Syndrome

The 22q11.2 locus is flanked by chromosome-specific, low copy repeats that share greater than 97% sequence homology and render the region prone to misalignment of the low copy repeats during meiosis. Consequently, nonallelic homologous recombination events that result in either a deletion or a duplication of the region can occur. In those with a deletion, nearly 90% of patients share a common 3-Mb deletion, but approximately 8% have a smaller 1.5-Mb deletion, and rare patients have an even smaller (so-called 'nested') deletion within the disease locus [13]. Some of the smaller deletions were not detected by earlier clinical diagnostic tests as they surveyed only the most proximal segment of the common 3- or 1.5-Mb deletions, but current methods [multiplex ligation-dependent probe amplification (MLPA) and microarrays] evaluate the entire region for large or small deletions or duplications, such that patients with nested, variant deletions are now readily detected. Given that deletion size does not seem to explain the highly variable clinical presentation [14, 15], other currently undefined mechanisms must be invoked.

The commonly deleted region contains approximately 40 genes. As a consequence of the deletion, the affected patient is left with only one, rather than two copies of each deleted gene and presumably a decreased amount or dosage of the encoded gene product, a state otherwise known as haploinsufficiency. Several mouse models were developed to mirror the human syndrome given significant synteny of mouse chromosome 16 with the human chromosome 22 locus in an effort to identify which gene or genes might be directly related to the clinical phenotypes. Elegant experiments in the mouse suggested that *TBX1*, a T-box transcription factor, was an excellent candidate gene for the disorder [16–19]. Subsequent studies in humans that identified functionally significant missense mutations in *TBX1* in rare, non-deleted patients with typical features of the deletion syndrome support this hypothesis [20]. However, many questions remain as to whether other genes in the region contribute to the phenotype, particularly since some patients with classic features of the deletion syndrome have smaller deletions that do not include *TBX1*. Efforts to identify potential genetic modifiers of the cardiac phenotype are also underway [21, 22].

Clinical Characteristics of the 22q11.2 Deletion Syndrome

The clinical phenotype of the 22q11.2 deletion syndrome is highly variable among related and unrelated individuals. Most patients have a subset of the most common features (table 1). The presentation can be subtle and go unrecognized for decades, or more severe and easily recognized at birth. Approximately 6–10% of cases are familial, meaning the 22q11.2 deletion is inherited in an autosomal dominant fashion from an affected parent; frequently, the affected parent is only recognized to carry the 22q11.2 deletion upon their child's diagnosis.

Congenital Heart Disease in the 22q11.2 Deletion Syndrome

Hospital-based studies estimate that approximately 75–80% of patients with a 22q11.2 deletion have congenital heart disease [reviewed in ref. 23,

Table 1. Most common features of the 22q11.2 deletion syndrome

Congenital heart disease
Facial features
Palate anomalies
Feeding disorders
Hypocalcemia
Immunodeficiency
Renal anomalies
Skeletal anomalies
Speech disorders
Cognitive disabilities
Behavioral and/or psychiatric disorders

24–27]. These studies may overestimate the prevalence of cardiac defects in the deleted population given that children and adults without significant heart disease may escape diagnosis. As noted, many parents only learn of their own deletion status upon the delivery of a child with congenital heart disease who is diagnosed with a 22q11.2 deletion. By way of example, one report identified two families transmitting a 22q11.2 deletion over three generations, but the deletion was only identified with the delivery of children with heart defects [28]. On the other hand, subtle changes, such as clinically insignificant aortic arch anomalies (e.g. an aberrant right subclavian artery), often go unrecognized and thus the prevalence of cardiovascular manifestations may instead be underestimated.

The most common cardiac defects seen in the 22q11.2 deletion syndrome include: a subset of conotruncal defects (tetralogy of Fallot, interrupted aortic arch, or truncus arteriosus), a subset of ventricular septal defects (conoventricular, posterior malalignment and conoseptal hypoplasia), and less commonly atrial septal defects [reviewed in ref. 23, 24, 26, 27]. Aortic arch anomalies, either in isolation or in conjunction with intracardiac defects, are also commonly seen. The full range of aortic arch anomalies, including cervical aortic arch, double aortic arch, right-sided aortic arch, and abnormal origin of the subclavian arteries (both aberrant and isolated subclavian arteries), has been observed [23, 29–31]. In several patients, we have seen a left-sided aortic arch where a right-sided innominate artery branches in the neck and then the right subclavian artery courses inferiorly and to the right arm. On an echocardiogram, this branching pattern is not readily appreciated and may instead suggest abnormal branching of the head and neck vessels, which is later defined as unusual but essentially normal branching by cardiac MRI [unpubl. observation]. As many as 68% of patients with a 22q11.2 deletion and an intracardiac anomaly have a concurrent aortic arch anomaly [31]. Although conotruncal, ventricular septal, and aortic arch anomalies are by far the most common cardiac findings in the 22q11.2 deletion syndrome, patients with a wide variety of congenital heart defects have been reported, including those with hypoplastic left-heart syndrome, heterotaxy, valvar pulmonary stenosis, and bicuspid aortic valve, particularly in the setting of a concurrent aortic arch anomaly.

Many children present with noncardiac symptoms and are diagnosed with a 22q11.2 deletion later in infancy or childhood [32]. Although these patients are unlikely to have major intracardiac anomalies, isolated aortic arch anomalies are commonly identified in this subset of patients. In particular, 38% of the patients diagnosed with a 22q11.2 deletion after 6 months of age were found to have an aortic arch anomaly, of whom 27% had a symptomatic vascular ring [33]. As noted above, a remarkable variety of aortic arch anomalies has been seen in the 22q11.2-deleted population, including absent or isolated subclavian arteries where retrograde flow through the vertebral artery provides flow into the absent or isolated subclavian artery predisposing to a steal phenomenon [34]. Since respiratory symptoms including asthma and airway anomalies are commonly diagnosed in the 22q11.2-deleted population, it is important to identify which children have concurrent vascular rings contributing to or causing their respiratory symptoms, and therefore which should undergo surgical ligation.

In addition to cardiovascular malformations, a subset of patients with the 22q11.2 deletion syndrome develop aortic root dilation. In those without conotruncal defects, approximately 10% of cases had aortic root dilation in one study (11 of 94 cases) [35]. In this series, most patients with aortic root dilation

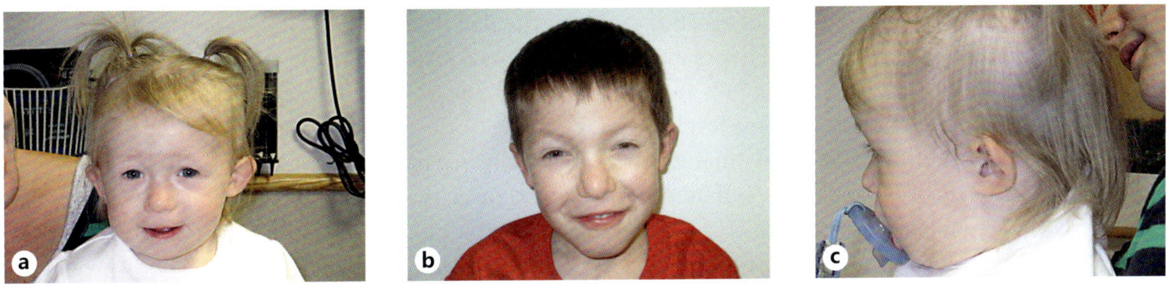

Fig. 1. Typical facial features of the 22q11.2 deletion syndrome. Children with typical facial features of the 22q11.2 deletion syndrome are pictured. Their features include hooded eyelids, a long tubular nose with a broad bulbous tip and hypoplastic nasal alae, long smooth philtrum, and thin vermillion border of the upper lip (**a**, **b**). Mild cupping and overfolding of the superior helix is also common (**c**).

(7 of 11) had additional minor cardiovascular anomalies, including bicuspid aortic valve (n = 3), repaired ventricular septal defect (n = 1), patent ductus arteriosus (n = 1), aortic arch anomaly (n = 1), and left pulmonary artery stenosis (n = 1), but 4 patients had only isolated aortic root dilation. Several patients developed aortic root dilation over time suggesting that this feature may be progressive. However, the clinical significance of this finding remains to be determined as there are no reports of aortic root dissection. In a separate study on patients aged 8–18 years with tetralogy of Fallot, those with a 22q11.2 deletion and concurrent aortic arch anomaly were at increased risk of aortic root dilation as compared to their nondeleted counterparts [36]. It remains to be seen whether the independent association between deletion status and aortic root dilation becomes more significant in an older cohort with tetralogy of Fallot in which aortic root dilation becomes more prevalent [37].

Noncardiac Manifestations of the 22q11.2 Deletion Syndrome

The most common noncardiac features of the 22q11.2 deletion syndrome encompass a wide range of systems (table 1) [24, 27]. Considering these features according to their age of presentation can assist with the diagnosis of the child who does not present with congenital heart disease, and assist with the proper counseling and management of the child with congenital heart disease.

Aside from congenital heart disease, the fetus with a 22q11.2 deletion may be noted to have an absent or aberrantly located thymus [38–40]. Less specific findings on a fetal ultrasound include polyhydramnios, intrauterine growth retardation, cleft palate, and renal anomalies [41, 42].

At delivery, dysmorphic features such as a long narrow face, malar flatness, hooded eyelids, long tubular nose with bulbous tip, hypoplastic nasal alae, nasal dimple or crease, small mouth, small protuberant ears with thick overfolded or crumpled helices, and asymmetric crying facies can be appreciated but are often unapparent at birth (fig. 1). Facial features can change over time and may be subtle in different racial groups [43, 44]. A cleft palate, reported in approximately 11% of 22q11.2-deleted patients, can be detected on examination as well [24, 27]. Feeding may prove to be challenging for the newborn with difficulty latching during breast-feeding and the majority (approximately 70%) experiencing nasal regurgitation due to velopharyngeal dysfunction. The nasopharyngeal reflux generally resolves by 1 year of age and does not predict the presence of hypernasal speech at a later age but is often an overlooked presenting feature of the 22q11.2 deletion syndrome. Feeding and growth may also be compromised by significant gastroesophageal reflux, dysmotility, and constipation [45, 46]. A subset of patients will undergo placement of a gastrostomy tube for feeding purposes. It is important to distinguish between such feeding issues and cardiac causes of poor feeding and growth in the cardiac patient with a 22q11.2 deletion.

On laboratory examination, at least half of the infants with a 22q11.2 deletion manifest hypocalcemia, which can result in hypocalcemic seizures if not recognized and treated appropriately. The hy-

3

pocalcemia usually resolves by 1 year of age, but can recur or present as seemingly isolated hypoparathyroidism for the first time at later ages [47, 48]. Approximately 80% also demonstrate some level of immunologic abnormality with most manifesting mild-to-moderate decrements in T-cell numbers due to thymic hypoplasia, and only a very rare minority (0.5%) manifesting severe immunodeficiency that requires immediate medical attention. Patients may also experience humoral defects (26%) and IgA deficiency (6%). Consequently, patients with the 22q11.2 deletion syndrome are at risk for recurrent, protracted infections, which later interfere with school attendance and continue into adulthood [reviewed in ref. 49]. Radiographic imaging may also identify renal [50] and skeletal anomalies (including butterfly vertebrae) in a minority of patients [51].

The toddler with a 22q11.2 deletion commonly manifests delayed emergence in speech and most will manifest hypernasal speech due to velopharyngeal dysfunction [52]. Articulation disorders may develop in compensation for palate abnormalities. Velopharyngeal function is assessed with the emergence of speech and pharyngoplasty is generally performed around 5 years of age if required [53].

The majority of school-aged children with a 22q11.2 deletion demonstrate neurocognitive deficits, though as with every other feature, the extent is highly variable and varies with development. Overall, only the minority tests at an average level of intellectual ability while the majority falls within the borderline range (full-scale IQ range 70–84), and approximately one third demonstrates mild intellectual disability. Only the rare individual demonstrates severe intellectual disabilities [reviewed in ref. 54–57]. In early childhood, nonverbal learning disabilities seem to be more significant, which is reflected by a lower performance than verbal IQ score. However, by adolescence, the difference is no longer detected. At this stage, reading skills are relatively stronger than arithmetic, which is a particular weakness. Rote memorization, word reading and phonics, and simple focused attention are relative strengths, whereas complex verbal learning, reading comprehension, visual perception and memory, visual-spatial processing, and executive function are particular weaknesses. As a consequence, most patients with a 22q11.2 deletion require assistance in school and many attend a special education classroom.

Behavioral and psychiatric disorders likewise become of increasing significance in school-aged children extending into adulthood [reviewed in 54, 55, 58, 59]. Attention deficit and anxiety disorders are relatively common in children with a 22q11.2 deletion, as are autistic spectrum features. Additional behavioral disorders include difficulty socializing, impulsivity, temper outbursts, perseverative speech, and repetitive behaviors. In adults, the specter of psychiatric disorders dominates with approximately 60% diagnosed with psychotic or nonpsychotic illnesses. There is a marked increase in generalized anxiety disorders, and approximately 20–25% of adult patients will be diagnosed with schizophrenia.

Thus, the presence of a 22q11.2 deletion confers multiple life-long challenges that are highly variable among individuals and change over time with development. These issues are often ironically of greater consequence than the congenital heart defect as they impact upon issues of daily living in the child (e.g. feeding, speech, recurrent infections, schooling, and behavior) and long-term achievement in the adult (e.g. academic achievement or psychiatric disorders).

The 22q11.2 Deletion Syndrome and Congenital Heart Disease

22q11.2 Deletions in Conotruncal Defects

Given the frequency of congenital heart disease in the 22q11.2 deletion syndrome, many have studied the corollary association, namely the prevalence of a 22q11.2 deletion in the cardiac population with conotruncal defects. Many studies have demonstrated that 22q11.2 deletions are common in patients with interrupted aortic arch type B (~50%), truncus arteriosus (~35%), tetralogy of Fallot (10–25%), isolated aortic arch anomalies (~5%), and conoventricular ventricular septal defects (~7%) [23, 31, 60, 61]. The presence of an aortic arch anomaly in conjunction with one of these intracardiac malformations increases the probability of finding a 22q11.2 deletion fivefold [31]. In particular, among patients with tetralogy of Fallot, although pulmonary valve atresia, absent pulmonary valve, aortic arch anomalies, and major aortopulmonary collaterals are more prevalent in the 22q11.2-deleted as compared to nondeleted subgroups [23], pulmonary valve atresia and particularly aortic arch anomaly are the strongest predictors of deletion status in multivariable logistic regression analysis [31]. A 22q11.2 deletion has been observed in all subtypes of truncus arteriosus (types I–IV) with no statistical difference in prevalence observed between them [31]. In our series, a 22q11.2 deletion was only observed in cases with type B but not type A interruption of the aortic arch regardless of other associated cardiac anomalies (i.e. simple or complex intracardiac anatomy), even though a 22q11.2 deletion in type A interruption has been reported [62]. We and others have identified a 22q11.2 deletion in rare patients with type C interruption of the aortic arch [unpubl. findings; 63, 64].

We recently reexamined the ventricular septal subtypes most commonly associated with a 22q11.2 deletion [31, 65]. Of those with a conoventricular septal defect, no one with coincident coarctation of the aorta had a 22q11.2 deletion. However, of those who did not have coarctation of the aorta, approximately 5% with normal arch anatomy (left sided with normal branching of the right innominate artery) and 29% with a concurrent aortic arch anomaly had a 22q11.2 deletion. Similarly, a 22q11.2 deletion was seen in patients with a posterior malalignment- or conoseptal hypoplasia-type ventricular septal defect only in the context of a concurrent aortic arch anomaly, whether or not there was a coarctation. Thus, a 22q11.2 deletion is relatively common in those cases with a conoventricular ventricular septal defect even in the presence of normal aortic arch anatomy, but in our series only present in the context of a concurrent aortic arch anomaly in other ventricular septal subtypes. While these results do not rule out the possibility of detecting a 22q11.2 deletion in posterior malalignment- or conoseptal hypoplasia-type ventricular septal defects with normal aortic arch anatomy, the risk appears to be low. Of note, the absence of 22q11.2 deletions in patients with a posterior malalignment-type ventricular septal defect, normal aortic arch anatomy and coarctation of the aorta is perhaps consistent with the observation that a 22q11.2 deletion is rarely seen in type A as compared to type B interruption of the aorta; these observations once again highlight the role that abnormal remodeling of the fourth embryonic pharyngeal arch artery likely plays in disease pathogenesis [66].

In contrast, a 22q11.2 deletion is rarely identified in patients with conotruncal defects characterized by abnormal great artery relationships and, in particular, is uncommon in patients with double-outlet right ventricle or D-transposition of the great arteries. A detailed evaluation of a large cohort with both defects found that only those patients with a concurrent aortic arch anomaly had a 22q11.2 deletion [31].

Identifying the Cardiac Patient with a 22q11.2 Deletion

Given that the 22q11.2 deletion syndrome is common among specific subsets of cardiac patients, debate has centered around detection strategies, some suggesting routine molecular genetic screening of patients with specific anatomic diagnoses and others relying on clinical detection by physical examination. Concern has focused in particular on the newborn and infant diagnosed with one of the high-risk cardiac lesions as facial features may be the only immediate and yet unappreciated feature at that age. However, the consequence of delayed diagnosis may be significant, including hypocalcemic seizures or a misinterpretation of reasons for poor feeding and growth in the context of congenital heart disease. Several investigators have approached this question by comparing the number of cases detected by clinical examination alone as compared to molecular genetic testing. Given the variable ages and patient populations, the results have not unexpectedly varied, with both false-positive and false-negative assignment of deletion status. Agergaard et al. [67] identified 14 such studies and reported that in a cumulative population of 1,458 cardiac patients, of whom 159 (11%) had a 22q11.2 deletion, clinicians identified 110 (69%) but did not identify 49 (31%) cases carrying a 22q11.2 deletion at various ages. Given the clinical implications associated with the 22q11.2 deletion syndrome, as well as the risk of re-

Table 2. Suggested screening strategy to identify the cardiac patient with a 22q11.2 deletion

Test the fetus/neonate/infant presenting with
Tetralogy of Fallot (with pulmonary valve stenosis, pulmonary valve atresia, or absent pulmonary valve)
Truncus arteriosus (all subtypes)
Interrupted aortic arch (particularly types B and C)
Ventricular septal defect (conoventricular, posterior malalignment, or conoseptal hypoplasia)
Isolated aortic arch anomaly
Consider testing the fetus/neonate/infant presenting with
Other cardiac defects with concurrent aortic arch anomaly
Cardiac defect(s) and other noncardiac feature(s) of the 22q11.2 deletion syndrome
Consider testing the child/adult with
Tetralogy of Fallot, truncus arteriosus, interrupted aortic arch, ventricular septal defect, or isolated aortic arch anomaly with concurrent feature(s) of the 22q11.2 deletion syndrome

currence if an affected parent is concurrently identified, most now advocate genetic testing for a 22q11.2 deletion in the newborn or infant with a typical cardiac anomaly when other syndromic features may not yet be apparent, as detailed in table 2 [68]. When the patient is older, one can call upon the presence or absence of associated syndromic features, such as delayed emergence of speech or learning disabilities to modify screening strategies, but a high index of suspicion should be held in those cardiac diagnoses most commonly seen in the context of the 22q11.2 deletion syndrome, and particularly so in the presence of a concurrent aortic arch anomaly. Still today, many adults with congenital heart disease remain undiagnosed, with obvious psychiatric and reproductive consequences [69, 70].

The molecular diagnosis of a 22q11.2 deletion was previously made using fluorescence in situ hybridization of test probes from the 22q11.2 locus hybridized with metaphase chromosomes. While this approach reliably identified the typical 3-Mb deletion and some smaller deletions, it failed to detect the less common 'nested' or atypical deletions [14, 15, 71]. Newer methods including MLPA and microarrays now identify both the common and atypical deletions in the region and are now the preferred methods of interrogation [72, 73]. Of note, MLPA, as a PCR-based assay, provides a rapid, focused, and generally less expensive approach to that of microarray analysis, but a microarray will identify other potentially disease-associated copy number variants (deletions or duplications) if the syndromic patient under evaluation does not carry a 22q11.2 deletion. Thus, different methods may be used based on need and institutional availability. Of interest, both methods have revealed the reciprocal finding of 22q11.2 duplications in a distinct, highly variable population whose characteristic phenotype is still under investigation [74].

Clinical Outcome

Early reports revealed a high rate of mortality for patients with DiGeorge syndrome on account of inoperable cardiac malformations and severe infections. With medical and surgical advances, survival has markedly improved for all patients with congenital heart disease, but numerous studies suggest that cases with a malformation syndrome suffer worse clinical outcomes than those with apparently isolated congenital heart disease. However, it is not clear that all syndromes suffer the same outcomes. Examining that question has been challenging given the anatomic and genetic heterogeneity of these disorders; in most series, each malformation syndrome is represented by a relatively small number of cases. An increasing number of studies have focused specifically on clinical outcomes in patients with congenital heart disease and 22q11.2 deletion, with variable results. Mahle et al. [75] first reported that patients with pulmonary atresia and ventricular septal defects (i.e. tetralogy of Fallot with pulmonary atresia) and a 22q11.2 deletion experienced significantly higher mortality by 5 years of age than their nondeleted counterparts (36 vs. 90%). Although the pulmonary arteries in patients with a 22q11.2 deletion appeared to be hypoplastic relative to those in the nondeleted subgroup and likely contributed to their poor outcome, deletion status was nonetheless an independent risk factor for mortality even after adjusting for the presence of major aortopulmonary collaterals (p = 0.004) and distinct from the Nakata index (a reflection of pulmonary artery size). This difference in survival was not explained by infectious complications, which occurred at similar frequencies in the 22q11.2-deleted and -nondeleted cohorts. Thus the presence of a 22q11.2 deletion placed this subset of patients at higher risk of mortality for reasons that were incompletely understood. Anaclerio et al. [76] also reported higher mortality rates in 22q11.2-deleted as compared to -nondeleted patients with tetralogy of Fallot and pulmonary atresia. Of interest, they also reported a higher mortality rate for patients with interrupted aortic arch and a 22q11.2 deletion compared to nonsyndromic patients.

The study by Michielon et al. [77] subsequently examined the association of genotype with surgical outcome in patients operated on for tetralogy of Fallot (with pulmonary stenosis). While actuarial survival at 10.4 years of age was better in the nonsyndromic compared to syndromic subset (94 vs. 84% respectively), and stratification in the presence of normal pulmonary arteries demonstrated similar findings, Cox proportional hazard multivariate analysis found that genetic syndrome and pulmonary hypoplasia were independent predictors of mortality. However, the syndromic patients with a 22q11.2 deletion (and trisomy 21) fared better than those with other genetic syndromes, approaching if not equating survival of the nonsyndromic cases. This study also demonstrated increased postoperative morbidity for those with a genetic syndrome, but they did not stratify by the specific syndrome. Thus, this report suggests that the presence of a syndrome itself does not always translate into higher mortality, but likely varies by the specific genotype. In a larger, subsequent study, Michielon et al. [78] reported similar results for a range of conotruncal defects (tetralogy of Fallot with or without pulmonary atresia, truncus arteriosus, and interrupted aortic arch), namely the presence of a genetic syndrome increased the risk of mortality and morbidity, but survival for those specifically with a 22q11.2 deletion was comparable to their nonsyndromic counterparts.

Subsequent studies have examined postoperative morbidity in the 22q11.2-deleted cardiac population in greater detail. In the subset of patients with tetralogy of Fallot/pulmonary atresia and truncus arteriosus, Ziolkowska et al. [79] reported increased postoperative surgical morbidity in those with compared to those without a 22q11.2 deletion. Those with tetralogy of Fallot/pulmonary atresia and a 22q11.2 deletion suffered more cardiopulmonary complications, including heart failure, respiratory failure with prolonged intubation/tracheostomy, laryngeal stridor, pneumonia, and sepsis. Those with truncus arteriosus and a 22q11.2 deletion underwent surgical intervention at an earlier age but still experienced more severe pulmonary hypertension than their nondeleted counterparts.

More recently, Mercer-Rosa et al. [80] studied the impact of 22q11.2 deletion status on the postoperative course in patients with tetralogy of Fallot (excluding those with complex-staged surgeries). While there was no difference in mortality between the two groups, those with a 22q11.2 deletion had undergone a modified Blalock-Taussig shunt prior to complete repair more commonly, and experienced a longer period of cardiopulmonary bypass, intensive care, and length of hospital stay as compared to the nondeleted cohort. In addition, those with a 22q11.2 deletion manifest increased resource use by way of more inhospital consultations and medications upon discharge. Similarly, O'Byrne et al. [81] found that patients with interrupted aortic arch and a 22q11.2 deletion experienced the same rate of mortality, but experienced a significantly longer length of hospital stay, period of ventilator support, period of intensive care, and increased resource utilization as compared to those without a deletion. The same trends were observed for the subset with truncus arteriosus. In the combined analysis of interrupted aortic arch and truncus arteriosus, cardiac reoperations were more frequent in those with a 22q11.2 deletion. In all three cohorts (tetralogy of Fallot, interrupted aortic arch, and truncus arteriosus), these differences in outcome were not explained by the presence of major additional congenital anomalies, frequency of infections, or use of nasogastric feeds,

3

as one might have predicted. Thus, it is clear that cardiac patients with a 22q11.2 deletion experience a more complicated postoperative course. The underlying mechanisms behind these complications are not well understood but worthy of further investigation. At the very least, such findings help inform physician counseling of families with a 22q11.2-deleted cardiac patient.

Clinical Management of the Cardiac Patient with a 22q11.2 Deletion

The most challenging yet most important step is to identify the cardiac patient with a 22q11.2 deletion so that appropriate counseling and anticipatory care can be provided. Given the highly variable phenotype associated with a 22q11.2 deletion, the clinical evaluation will by necessity vary both in extent and by age. Bassett et al. [82], representing the International 22q11.2 Deletion Consortium, provide guidelines on the management of the 22q11.2-deleted patient. In extensive tables, they detail the associated features as well as appropriate testing at diagnosis and by age. Specific precautions and issues to be considered are also reviewed. It is particularly important to note that features and symptoms, such as calcium homeostasis and neuropsychiatric issues, evolve over time and must be periodically reevaluated. Likewise, it is critical to screen parents for the 22q11.2 deletion in order to identify the previously undiagnosed adult as they have a 50% risk of recurrence in subsequent offspring and require clinical counseling to address their own clinical and neuropsychiatric needs. To date, the management of the associated congenital heart malformations follows standard approaches, but as our understanding of the 22q11.2-deleted patients' specific clinical challenges improve, care may soon be tailored to their specific needs. Such will mark the advent of personalized, or genotype-specific, clinical management (see Costello et al. chapter on Surgical Manangement for further discussion on management of 22q11.2 deletion p. 283).

References

1 Conley ME, Beckwith JB, Mancer JF, Tenckhoff L: The spectrum of the DiGeorge syndrome. J Pediatr 1979;94:883–890.

2 Kirkpatrick JA Jr, DiGeorge AM: Congenital absence of the thymus. Am J Roentgenol Radium Ther Nucl Med 1968;103:32–37.

3 Driscoll DA, Budarf ML, Emanuel BS: A genetic etiology for DiGeorge syndrome: consistent deletions and microdeletions of 22q11. Am J Hum Genet 1992;50:924–933.

4 Scambler PJ, Carey AH, Wyse RK, Roach S, Dumanski JP, Nordenskjold M, Williamson R: Microdeletions within 22q11 associated with sporadic and familial DiGeorge syndrome. Genomics 1991;10:201–206.

5 Shprintzen RJ, Goldberg RB, Lewin ML, Sidoti EJ, Berkman MD, Argamaso RV, Young D: A new syndrome involving cleft palate, cardiac anomalies, typical facies, and learning disabilities: velo-cardio-facial syndrome. Cleft Palate J 1978;15:56–62.

6 Kinouchi A, Mori K, Ando M, Takao A: Facial appearance of patients with conotruncal abnormalities. Pediatr Jpn 1976;17:84–89.

7 Burn J, Takao A, Wilson D, Cross I, Momma K, Wadey R, Scambler P, Goodship J: Conotruncal anomaly face syndrome is associated with a deletion within chromosome 22q11. J Med Genet 1993;30:822–824.

8 Driscoll DA, Spinner NB, Budarf ML, McDonald-McGinn DM, Zackai EH, Goldberg RB, Shprintzen RJ, Saal HM, Zonana J, Jones MC, et al: Deletions and microdeletions of 22q11.2 in velo-cardio-facial syndrome. Am J Med Genet 1992;44:261–268.

9 Kelly D, Goldberg R, Wilson D, Lindsay E, Carey A, Goodship J, Burn J, Cross I, Shprintzen RJ, Scambler PJ: Confirmation that the velo-cardio-facial syndrome is associated with haplo-insufficiency of genes at chromosome 22q11. Am J Med Genet 1993;45:308–312.

10 Matsuoka R, Takao A, Kimura M, Imamura S, Kondo C, Joh-o K, Ikeda K, Nishibatake M, Ando M, Momma K: Confirmation that the conotruncal anomaly face syndrome is associated with a deletion within 22q11.2. Am J Med Genet 1994;53:285–289.

11 Botto LD, May K, Fernhoff PM, Correa A, Coleman K, Rasmussen SA, Merritt RK, O'Leary LA, Wong LY, Elixson EM, Mahle WT, Campbell RM: A population-based study of the 22q11.2 deletion: phenotype, incidence, and contribution to major birth defects in the population. Pediatrics 2003;112:101–107.

12 Oskarsdottir S, Vujic M, Fasth A: Incidence and prevalence of the 22q11 deletion syndrome: a population-based study in Western Sweden. Arch Dis Child 2004;89:148–151.

13 Shaikh TH, Kurahashi H, Saitta SC, O'Hare AM, Hu P, Roe BA, Driscoll DA, McDonald-McGinn DM, Zackai EH, Budarf ML, Emanuel BS: Chromosome 22-specific low copy repeats and the 22q11.2 deletion syndrome: genomic organization and deletion endpoint analysis. Hum Mol Genet 2000;9:489–501.

14 Michaelovsky E, Frisch A, Carmel M, Patya M, Zarchi O, Green T, Basel-Vanagaite L, Weizman A, Gothelf D: Genotype-phenotype correlation in 22q11.2 deletion syndrome. BMC Med Genet 2012;13:122.

15 Verhagen JM, Diderich KE, Oudesluijs G, Mancini GM, Eggink AJ, Verkleij-Hagoort AC, Groenenberg IA, Willems PJ, du Plessis FA, de Man SA, Srebniak MI, van Opstal D, Hulsman LO, van Zutven LJ, Wessels MW: Phenotypic variability of atypical 22q11.2 deletions not including TBX1. Am J Med Genet A 2012;158A:2412–2420.

16 Baldini A: DiGeorge syndrome: the use of model organisms to dissect complex genetics. Hum Mol Genet 2002;11:2363–2369.

17 Baldini A: Dissecting contiguous gene defects: TBX1. Curr Opin Genet Dev 2005;15: 279–284.

18 Lindsay EA, Vitelli F, Su H, Morishima M, Huynh T, Pramparo T, Jurecic V, Ogunrinu G, Sutherland HF, Scambler PJ, Bradley A, Baldini A: Tbx1 haploinsufficieny in the DiGeorge syndrome region causes aortic arch defects in mice. Nature 2001;410:97–101.

19 Yamagishi H, Srivastava D: Unraveling the genetic and developmental mysteries of 22q11 deletion syndrome. Trends Mol Med 2003;9:383–389.

20 Yagi H, Furutani Y, Hamada H, Sasaki T, Asakawa S, Minoshima S, Ichida F, Joo K, Kimura M, Imamura S, Kamatani N, Momma K, Takao A, Nakazawa M, Shimizu N, Matsuoka R: Role of TBX1 in human del22q11.2 syndrome. Lancet 2003;362: 1366–1373.

21 Goldmuntz E, Driscoll DA, Emanuel BS, McDonald-McGinn D, Mei M, Zackai E, Mitchell LE: Evaluation of potential modifiers of the cardiac phenotype in the 22q11.2 deletion syndrome. Birth Defects Res A Clin Mol Teratol 2009;85:125–129.

22 Guo T, McDonald-McGinn D, Blonska A, Shanske A, Bassett AS, Chow E, Bowser M, Sheridan M, Beemer F, Devriendt K, Swillen A, Breckpot J, Digilio MC, Marino B, Dallapiccola B, Carpenter C, Zheng X, Johnson J, Chung J, Higgins AM, Philip N, Simon TJ, Coleman K, Heine-Suner D, Rosell J, Kates W, Devoto M, Goldmuntz E, Zackai E, Wang T, Shprintzen R, Emanuel B, Morrow B: Genotype and cardiovascular phenotype correlations with TBX1 in 1,022 velo-cardio-facial/DiGeorge/22q11.2 deletion syndrome patients. Hum Mutat 2011;32:1278–1289.

23 Momma K: Cardiovascular anomalies associated with chromosome 22q11.2 deletion syndrome. Am J Cardiol 2010;105:1617–1624.

24 McDonald-McGinn DM, LaRossa D, Goldmuntz E, Sullivan K, Eicher P, Gerdes M, Moss E, Wang P, Solot C, Schultz P, Lynch D, Bingham P, Keenan G, Weinzimer S, Ming JE, Driscoll D, Clark BJ 3rd, Markowitz R, Cohen A, Moshang T, Pasquariello P, Randall P, Emanuel BS, Zackai EH: The 22q11.2 deletion: screening, diagnostic workup, and outcome of results; report on 181 patients. Genet Test 1997;1:99–108.

25 Oskarsdottir S, Persson C, Eriksson BO, Fasth A: Presenting phenotype in 100 children with the 22q11 deletion syndrome. Eur J Pediatr 2005;164:146–153.

26 Park IS, Ko JK, Kim YH, Yoo HW, Seo EJ, Choi JY, Gil HY, Kim SJ: Cardiovascular anomalies in patients with chromosome 22q11.2 deletion: a Korean multicenter study. Int J Cardiol 2007;114:230–235.

27 Ryan AK, Goodship JA, Wilson DI, Philip N, Levy A, Seidel H, Schuffenhauer S, Oechsler H, Belohradsky B, Prieur M, Aurias A, Raymond FL, Clayton-Smith J, Hatchwell E, McKeown C, Beemer FA, Dallapiccola B, Novelli G, Hurst JA, Ignatius J, Green AJ, Winter RM, Brueton L, Brondum-Nielsen K, Scambler PJ, et al: Spectrum of clinical features associated with interstitial chromosome 22q11 deletions: a European collaborative study. J Med Genet 1997;34:798–804.

28 Shooner KA, Rope AF, Hopkin RJ, Andelfinger GU, Benson DW: Genetic analyses in two extended families with deletion 22q11 syndrome: importance of extracardiac manifestations. J Pediatr 2005;146: 382–387.

29 McElhinney DB, Clark BJ 3rd, Weinberg PM, Kenton ML, McDonald-McGinn D, Driscoll DA, Zackai EH, Goldmuntz E: Association of chromosome 22q11 deletion with isolated anomalies of aortic arch laterality and branching. J Am Coll Cardiol 2001; 37:2114–2119.

30 Momma K, Matsuoka R, Takao A: Aortic arch anomalies associated with chromosome 22q11 deletion (CATCH 22). Pediatr Cardiol 1999;20:97–102.

31 Peyvandi S, Lupo PJ, Garbarini J, Woyciechowski S, Edman S, Emanuel BS, Mitchell LE, Goldmuntz E: 22q11.2 deletions in patients with conotruncal defects: data from 1,610 consecutive cases. Pediatr Cardiol 2013;34:1687–1694.

32 Cancrini C, Puliafito P, Digilio MC, Soresina A, Martino S, Rondelli R, Consolini R, Ruga EM, Cardinale F, Finocchi A, Romiti ML, Martire B, Bacchetta R, Albano V, Carotti A, Specchia F, Montin D, Cirillo E, Cocchi G, Trizzino A, Bossi G, Milanesi O, Azzari C, Corsello G, Pignata C, Aiuti A, Pietrogrande MC, Marino B, Ugazio AG, Plebani A, Rossi P: Clinical features and follow-up in patients with 22q11.2 deletion syndrome. J Pediatr 2014;164:1475–1480.e2.

33 McElhinney DB, McDonald-McGinn D, Zackai EH, Goldmuntz E: Cardiovascular anomalies in patients diagnosed with a chromosome 22q11 deletion beyond 6 months of age. Pediatrics 2001;108:E104.

34 Johnson TR, Goldmuntz E, McDonald-McGinn DM, Zackai EH, Fogel MA: Cardiac magnetic resonance imaging for accurate diagnosis of aortic arch anomalies in patients with 22q11.2 deletion. Am J Cardiol 2005;96:1726–1730.

35 John AS, McDonald-McGinn DM, Zackai EH, Goldmuntz E: Aortic root dilation in patients with 22q11.2 deletion syndrome. Am J Med Genet A 2009;149A:939–942.

36 John AS, Rychik J, Khan M, Yang W, Goldmuntz E: 22q11.2 deletion syndrome as a risk factor for aortic root dilation in tetralogy of Fallot. Cardiol Young 2014;24:303–310.

37 Niwa K, Siu SC, Webb GD, Gatzoulis MA: Progressive aortic root dilatation in adults late after repair of tetralogy of Fallot. Circulation 2002;106:1374–1378.

38 Chaoui R, Kalache KD, Heling KS, Tennstedt C, Bommer C, Korner H: Absent or hypoplastic thymus on ultrasound: a marker for deletion 22q11.2 in fetal cardiac defects. Ultrasound Obstet Gynecol 2002;20:546–552.

39 Barrea C, Yoo SJ, Chitayat D, Valsangiacomo E, Winsor E, Smallhorn JF, Hornberger LK: Assessment of the thymus at echocardiography in fetuses at risk for 22q11.2 deletion. Prenat Diagn 2003;23:9–15.

40 Bataeva R, Bellsham-Revell H, Zidere V, Allan LD: Reliability of fetal thymus measurement in prediction of 22q11.2 deletion: a retrospective study using four-dimensional spatiotemporal image correlation volumes. Ultrasound Obstet Gynecol 2013;41:172–176.

41 Volpe P, Marasini M, Caruso G, Marzullo A, Buonadonna AL, Arciprete P, Di Paolo S, Volpe G, Gentile M: 22q11 deletions in fetuses with malformations of the outflow tracts or interruption of the aortic arch: impact of additional ultrasound signs. Prenat Diagn 2003;23:752–757.

42 Besseau-Ayasse J, Violle-Poirsier C, Bazin A, Gruchy N, Moncla A, Girard F, Till M, Mugneret F, Coussement A, Pelluard F, Jimenez M, Vago P, Portnoi MF, Dupont C, Beneteau C, Amblard F, Valduga M, Bresson JL, Carre-Pigeon F, Le Meur N, Tapia S, Yardin C, Receveur A, Lespinasse J, Pipiras E, Beaujard MP, Teboul P, Brisset S, Catty M, Nowak E, Douet Guilbert N, Lallaoui H, Bouquillon S, Gatinois V, Joly-Helas G, Prieur F, Cartault F, Martin D, Kleinfinger P, Molina Gomes D, Doco-Fenzy M, Vialard F: A French collaborative survey of 272 fetuses with 22q11.2 deletion: ultrasound findings, fetal autopsies and pregnancy outcomes. Prenat Diagn 2014;34:424–430.

43 Veerapandiyan A, Abdul-Rahman OA, Adam MP, Lyons MJ, Manning M, Coleman K, Kobrynski L, Taneja D, Schoch K, Zimmerman HH, Shashi V: Chromosome 22q11.2 deletion syndrome in African-American patients: a diagnostic challenge. Am J Med Genet A 2011;155A:2186–2195.

44 McDonald-McGinn DM, Minugh-Purvis N, Kirschner RE, Jawad A, Tonnesen MK, Catanzaro JR, Goldmuntz E, Driscoll D, Larossa D, Emanuel BS, Zackai EH: The 22q11.2 deletion in African-American patients: an underdiagnosed population? Am J Med Genet A 2005;134:242–246.

45 Eicher PS, McDonald-Mcginn DM, Fox CA, Driscoll DA, Emanuel BS, Zackai EH: Dysphagia in children with a 22q11.2 deletion: unusual pattern found on modified barium swallow. J Pediatr 2000;137:158–164.

46 Rommel N, Vantrappen G, Swillen A, Devriendt K, Feenstra L, Fryns JP: Retrospective analysis of feeding and speech disorders in 50 patients with velo-cardio-facial syndrome. Genet Couns 1999;10:71–78.
47 Greig F, Paul E, DiMartino-Nardi J, Saenger P: Transient congenital hypoparathyroidism: resolution and recurrence in chromosome 22q11 deletion. J Pediatr 1996;128: 563–567.
48 Hieronimus S, Bec-Roche M, Pedeutour F, Lambert JC, Wagner-Malher K, Mas JC, Sadoul JL, Fenichel P: The spectrum of parathyroid gland dysfunction associated with the microdeletion 22q11. Eur J Endocrinol 2006;155:47–52.
49 Maggadottir SM, Sullivan KE: The diverse clinical features of chromosome 22q11.2 deletion syndrome (DiGeorge syndrome). J Allergy Clin Immunol Pract 2013;1:589–594.
50 Wu HY, Rusnack SL, Bellah RD, Plachter N, McDonald-McGinn DM, Zackai EH, Canning DA: Genitourinary malformations in chromosome 22q11.2 deletion. J Urol 2002; 168:2564–2565.
51 Ming JE, McDonald-McGinn DM, Megerian TE, Driscoll DA, Elias ER, Russell BM, Irons M, Emanuel BS, Markowitz RI, Zackai EH: Skeletal anomalies and deformities in patients with deletions of 22q11. Am J Med Genet 1997;72:210–215.
52 Solot CB, Gerdes M, Kirschner RE, McDonald-McGinn DM, Moss E, Woodin M, Aleman D, Zackai EH, Wang PP: Communication issues in 22q11.2 deletion syndrome: children at risk. Genet Med 2001;3:67–71.
53 Kirschner RE, Baylis AL: Surgical considerations in 22q11.2 deletion syndrome. Clin Plast Surg 2014;41:271–282.
54 Philip N, Bassett A: Cognitive, behavioural and psychiatric phenotype in 22q11.2 deletion syndrome. Behav Genet 2011;41:403–412.
55 Duijff SN, Klaassen PW, de Veye HF, Beemer FA, Sinnema G, Vorstman JA: Cognitive development in children with 22q11.2 deletion syndrome. Br J Psychiatry 2012;200: 462–468.
56 Moss EM, Batshaw ML, Solot CB, Gerdes M, McDonald-McGinn DM, Driscoll DA, Emanuel BS, Zackai EH, Wang PP: Psychoeducational profile of the 22q11.2 microdeletion: a complex pattern. J Pediatr 1999; 134:193–198.
57 Woodin M, Wang PP, Aleman D, McDonald-McGinn D, Zackai E, Moss E: Neuropsychological profile of children and adolescents with the 22q11.2 microdeletion. Genet Med 2001;3:34–39.
58 Niarchou M, Zammit S, van Goozen SH, Thapar A, Tierling HM, Owen MJ, van den Bree MB: Psychopathology and cognition in children with 22q11.2 deletion syndrome. Br J Psychiatry 2014;204:46–54.
59 Schneider M, Debbane M, Bassett AS, Chow EW, Fung WL, van den Bree M, Owen M, Murphy KC, Niarchou M, Kates WR, Antshel KM, Fremont W, McDonald-McGinn DM, Gur RE, Zackai EH, Vorstman J, Duijff SN, Klaassen PW, Swillen A, Gothelf D, Green T, Weizman A, Van Amelsvoort T, Evers L, Boot E, Shashi V, Hooper SR, Bearden CE, Jalbrzikowski M, Armando M, Vicari S, Murphy DG, Ousley O, Campbell LE, Simon TJ, Eliez S: Psychiatric disorders from childhood to adulthood in 22q11.2 deletion syndrome: results from the International Consortium on Brain and Behavior in 22q11.2 Deletion Syndrome. Am J Psychiatry 2014;171:627–639.
60 Agergaard P, Olesen C, Ostergaard JR, Christiansen M, Sorensen KM: The prevalence of chromosome 22q11.2 deletions in 2,478 children with cardiovascular malformations. A population-based study. Am J Med Genet A 2012;158A:498–508.
61 Goldmuntz E, Clark BJ, Mitchell LE, Jawad AF, Cuneo BF, Reed L, McDonald-McGinn D, Chien P, Feuer J, Zackai EH, Emanuel BS, Driscoll DA: Frequency of 22q11 deletions in patients with conotruncal defects. J Am Coll Cardiol 1998;32:492–498.
62 Volpe P, Gentile M, Marasini M: Interrupted aortic arch type A with 22q11 deletion: prenatal detection of an unusual association. Prenat Diagn 2002;22:371–374.
63 Fujii I, Ueno Y, Kurano R, Goto Y: Interrupted aortic arch type C associated with DiGeorge syndrome in 22q11.2 deletion: first case detected in Japan. Pediatr Int 2005;47:698–700.
64 Cuturilo G, Drakulic D, Stevanovic M, Jovanovic I, Djukic M, Miletic-Grkovic S, Atanaskovic-Markovic M: A rare association of interrupted aortic arch type C and microdeletion 22q11.2. Eur J Pediatr 2008; 167:1195–1198.
65 McElhinney DB, Driscoll DA, Levin ER, Jawad AF, Emanuel BS, Goldmuntz E: Chromosome 22q11 deletion in patients with ventricular septal defect: frequency and associated cardiovascular anomalies. Pediatrics 2003;112:e472.
66 Scambler PJ: 22q11 deletion syndrome: a role for TBX1 in pharyngeal and cardiovascular development. Pediatr Cardiol 2010; 31:378–390.
67 Agergaard P, Hebert A, Sorensen KM, Ostergaard JR, Olesen C: Can clinical assessment detect 22q11.2 deletions in patients with cardiac malformations? A review. Eur J Med Genet 2011;54:3–8.
68 Pierpont ME, Basson CT, Benson DW Jr, Gelb BD, Giglia TM, Goldmuntz E, McGee G, Sable CA, Srivastava D, Webb CL: Genetic basis for congenital heart defects: current knowledge: a scientific statement from the American Heart Association Congenital Cardiac Defects Committee, Council on Cardiovascular Disease in the Young: endorsed by the American Academy of Pediatrics. Circulation 2007;115:3015–3038.
69 Liu AP, Chow PC, Lee PP, Mok GT, Tang WF, Lau ET, Lam ST, Chan KY, Kan AS, Chau AK, Cheung YF, Lau YL, Chung BH: Under-recognition of 22q11.2 deletion in adult Chinese patients with conotruncal anomalies: implications in transitional care. Eur J Med Genet 2014;57:306–311.
70 van Engelen K, Topf A, Keavney BD, Goodship JA, van der Velde ET, Baars MJ, Snijder S, Moorman AF, Postma AV, Mulder BJ: 22q11.2 deletion syndrome is under-recognised in adult patients with tetralogy of Fallot and pulmonary atresia. Heart 2010;96: 621–624.
71 Amati F, Conti E, Novelli A, Bengala M, Diglio MC, Marino B, Giannotti A, Gabrielli O, Novelli G, Dallapiccola B: Atypical deletions suggest five 22q11.2 critical regions related to the DiGeorge/velo-cardio-facial syndrome. Eur J Hum Genet 1999;7:903–909.
72 Jalali GR, Vorstman JA, Errami A, Vijzelaar R, Biegel J, Shaikh T, Emanuel BS: Detailed analysis of 22q11.2 with a high density MLPA probe set. Hum Mutat 2008;29:433–440.
73 Miller DT, Adam MP, Aradhya S, Biesecker LG, Brothman AR, Carter NP, Church DM, Crolla JA, Eichler EE, Epstein CJ, Faucett WA, Feuk L, Friedman JM, Hamosh A, Jackson L, Kaminsky EB, Kok K, Krantz ID, Kuhn RM, Lee C, Ostell JM, Rosenberg C, Scherer SW, Spinner NB, Stavropoulos DJ, Tepperberg JH, Thorland EC, Vermeesch JR, Waggoner DJ, Watson MS, Martin CL, Ledbetter DH: Consensus statement: chromosomal microarray is a first-tier clinical diagnostic test for individuals with developmental disabilities or congenital anomalies. Am J Hum Genet 2010;86:749–764.
74 Portnoi MF: Microduplication 22q11.2: a new chromosomal syndrome. Eur J Med Genet 2009;52:88–93.
75 Mahle WT, Crisalli J, Coleman K, Campbell RM, Tam VK, Vincent RN, Kanter KR: Deletion of chromosome 22q11.2 and outcome in patients with pulmonary atresia and ventricular septal defect. Ann Thorac Surg 2003;76:567–571.
76 Anaclerio S, Di Ciommo V, Michielon G, Digilio MC, Formigari R, Picchio FM, Gargiulo G, Di Donato R, De Ioris MA, Marino B: Conotruncal heart defects: impact of genetic syndromes on immediate operative mortality. Ital Heart J 2004;5:624–628.
77 Michielon G, Marino B, Formigari R, Gargiulo G, Picchio F, Digilio MC, Anaclerio S, Oricchio G, Sanders SP, Di Donato RM: Genetic syndromes and outcome after surgical correction of tetralogy of Fallot. Ann Thorac Surg 2006;81:968–975.

78 Michielon G, Marino B, Oricchio G, Digilio MC, Iorio F, Filippelli S, Placidi S, Di Donato RM: Impact of del22q11, trisomy 21, and other genetic syndromes on surgical outcome of conotruncal heart defects. J Thorac Cardiovasc Surg 2009;138:565–570.e2.
79 Ziolkowska L, Kawalec W, Turska-Kmiec A, Krajewska-Walasek M, Brzezinska-Rajszys G, Daszkowska J, Maruszewski B, Burczynski P: Chromosome 22q11.2 microdeletion in children with conotruncal heart defects: frequency, associated cardiovascular anomalies, and outcome following cardiac surgery. Eur J Pediatr 2008;167:1135–1140.
80 Mercer-Rosa L, Pinto N, Yang W, Tanel R, Goldmuntz E: 22q11.2 deletion syndrome is associated with perioperative outcome in tetralogy of Fallot. J Thorac Cardiovasc Surg 2013;146:868–873.
81 O'Byrne ML, Yang W, Mercer-Rosa L, Parnell AS, Oster ME, Levenbrown Y, Tanel RE, Goldmuntz E: 22q11.2 deletion syndrome is associated with increased perioperative events and more complicated postoperative course in infants undergoing infant operative correction of truncus arteriosus communis or interrupted aortic arch. J Thorac Cardiovasc Surg 2014;148:1597–1605.
82 Bassett AS, McDonald-McGinn DM, Devriendt K, Digilio MC, Goldenberg P, Habel A, Marino B, Oskarsdottir S, Philip N, Sullivan K, Swillen A, Vorstman J: Practical guidelines for managing patients with 22q11.2 deletion syndrome. J Pediatr 2011;159:332–339.e1.

Dr. Elizabeth Goldmuntz
Division of Cardiology, The Children's Hospital of Philadelphia
3615 Civic Center Boulevard
Philadelphia, PA 19104-4318 (USA)
E-Mail goldmuntz@email.chop.edu

Muenke M, Kruszka PS, Sable CA, Belmont JW (eds): Congenital Heart Disease: Molecular Genetics, Principles of Diagnosis and Treatment. Basel, Karger, 2015, pp 112–120
DOI: 10.1159/000375209

Other Genomic Disorders Causing Congenital Cardiovascular Malformations

Seema R. Lalani

Department of Molecular and Human Genetics, Baylor College of Medicine, Houston, Tex., USA

Abstract

Congenital cardiovascular malformations (CVM) are among the most common of all medically significant birth defects. Yet, the cause of these malformations is unknown in the majority of cases. In live-born infants, chromosomal abnormalities detected by conventional karyotyping account for approximately one tenth of all cardiac malformations. In addition, genomic disorders often resulting from instability of the regional genomic architecture, constitute a major fraction of CVM. These events are usually submicroscopic, and are observed as genomic deletions and/or duplications. The widespread use of array-comparative genomic hybridization has uncovered numerous DNA copy number variations, often encompassing important dosage-sensitive genes that are functionally relevant for CVM.

Congenital cardiovascular malformations (CVM) are one of the most common birth defects, affecting 0.5–0.7% of all live-born infants [1]. The incidence of prenatal cardiac anomalies is estimated to be about tenfold higher in the abortuses and stillborn infants [2]. Despite its recognized burden on public health, the etiology of the vast majority of cases is unknown. Cytogenetically visible abnormalities, including aneuploidies (trisomies 21, 18 and 13, and monosomy X) and 22q11.2 deletions, account for about 12% of all infants with CVMs [3]. Genomic disorders resulting from deletions or duplications of genomic segments due to genomic architecture are known to be an important cause of CVM, accounting for approximately 10% of all affected individuals (table 1). These submicroscopic events are often below the detection threshold of G-banded karyotype analysis and have been highlighted in the last decade due to the growing use of array-comparative genomic hybridization. Several genomic disorders are now recognized that are increasingly responsible for CVM. The 22q11.2 deletion syndrome is the most frequent genomic disorder associated with CVM, occurring in about 1 in 4,000 live births [4]. Other important genomic disorders known to cause CVM include 1p36 monosomy, Williams-Beuren syndrome (7q11.23 deletion), 8p23.1 deletion including *GATA4*, and 9q34 deletion encompassing *EHMT1* (Kleefstra syndrome). This review focuses on genomic disorders other than the 22q11.2 deletion syndrome that are major players in the etiology of human cardiac malformations.

Table 1. Genomic disorders known to cause CVM

Syndromes	OMIM No.	Cardiac lesions	Genes implicated in CVM
1p36 deletion	607872	Septal defects, PDA, valvular abnormalities, CoA, ToF, cardiomyopathy	*RERE, PRDM16*
1q21.1 deletion	612474	CoA, IAA-A, IAA-B, BAV, aortopathy, VSD, truncus arteriosus, TGA, CoA, PDA	*GJA5*
1q21.1 duplication	612475	ToF	*GJA5*
1q41-q42 deletion	612530	Septal defects, PDA	
3q29 deletion	609425	PDA, septal defects	
WHS (4p16.3 deletion)	194190	ASD, VSD, PS, ToF, PDA	*FGFRL1*
Cri-du-chat syndrome (5p15.2 deletion)	123450	VSD, ASD, PS, ToF, AS, PDA	
Sotos syndrome (5q35.2-q35.3 deletion)	117550	Septal defects, PDA	*NSD1*
6pter-p24 deletion	612582	ASD, ToF, PDA, mitral valve defect	*FOXC1*
6q24-q25 deletion	612863	VSD, ASD, mitral/aortic valve stenosis, hypoplastic aortic arch	*TAB2*
Williams-Beuren syndrome (7q11.23 deletion)	194050	SVAS, PPS	*ELN*
8p23.1 deletion	N/A	AVSD, ASD, PS, ToF	*GATA4, SOX7*
8p23.1 duplication	N/A	Septal defects, PS, ToF, AVSD	*GATA4, SOX7*
Kleefstra syndrome (9q34.3 deletion)	610253	Septal defects, PS, BAV, PDA	*EHMT1*
10q23 deletion	612242	AVSD	*BMPR1A*
10q26 deletion	609625	ASD, PDA	
Jacobsen syndrome (11qter deletion)	147791	VSD, ASD, TA, DORV, BAV, AS, HLHS, MS, CoA	*ETS1*
15q13.3 deletion	612001	ToF, AVSD, MVP	*KLF13*
15q26-qter deletion	612626	VSD, ASD, CoA, HLHS, AS	*COUP-TFII, MCTP2*
16p11.2 deletion	611913	PFO, aortic valve abnormalities	
16p13.3 deletion/Rubinstein-Taybi syndrome	610543	Septal defects, HLHS, dextrocardia, ToF	*CREBBP*
16p13.3 duplication	613458	ASD, ToF	*CREBBP*
16q24.3 deletion	N/A	Septal defects, cleft mitral valve, aortic root dilatation	*ANKRD11*
Miller-Dieker syndrome (17p13.3 deletion)	247200	Septal defects, ToF, PDA	
SMS (17p11.2 deletion)	182290	Septal defects, ToF, PS, PA, TAPVR	
PTLS (17p11.2 duplication)	610883	Dilated aortic root, septal defects, PFO, conduction abnormalities, BAV, HLHS	

Table 1. Continued

Syndromes	OMIM No.	Cardiac lesions	Genes implicated in CVM
Koolen-de Vries syndrome (17q21.31 deletion)	610443	Septal defects, PS, BAV	
17q23.1-q23.2 deletion	613355	PDA, ASD, pulmonary arterial hypertension	*TBX4*
18p deletion	146390	VSD, AS, HLHS, PDA, PS, heterotaxy	
18q deletion	601808	Pulmonary/aortic valve anomalies, septal defects, Ebstein's anomaly, AS, PDA	*GATA6*
DiGeorge/Velocardiofacial syndrome (22q11.2 deletion)	192430/ 188400	ToF, IAA-B, VSD, truncus arteriosus, DORV	*TBX1*
22q11.2 duplication	608363	ToF, HLHS, TGA	*TBX1*
Distal 22q11.2 deletion	611867	VSD, truncus arteriosus, PDA, ASD	*MAPK1*

AS = Aortic valve stenosis; DORV = double-outlet right ventricle; IAA-A/IAA-B = interruption of the aortic arch type A/B; MS = mitral stenosis; MVP = mitral valve prolapse; PFO = patent foramen ovale; PPS = peripheral pulmonary stenosis; SVAS = supravalvular aortic stenosis; TAPVR = total anomalous pulmonary venous return; TGA = transposition of the great arteries; ToF = tetralogy of Fallot; TA = truncus arteriosus; HLHS = hypoplastic left heart syndrome; AVSD = atrioventricular septal defect; CoA = coarctation of the aorta; PS = pulmonary valve stenosis.

Genomic Rearrangements

Genomic rearrangements not only cause Mendelian disorders, but also contribute to several complex diseases [5]. Often the disease mechanism relates to altered gene dosage of functionally relevant gene(s) within the deleted or duplicated intervals termed as copy number variations (CNVs). Low copy repeats (LCRs) or segmental duplications greater than 10 kb in length and with over ~97% sequence homology can cause local genomic instability and mediate genomic rearrangements. The LCRs can act as substrates for misalignment of chromosomes or chromatids during recombination and mediate nonallelic homologous recombination (NAHR) [6]. While recurrent rearrangements are frequently mediated by NAHR leading to reciprocal deletion and duplication, replication mechanisms are important contributors to nonrecurrent genomic rearrangements, where the breakpoints and event size can differ in the affected individuals.

Copy Number Variations in Congenital Cardiovascular Malformations

CNVs are reported in 3–20% of all CVM cases, depending on the classification of nonsyndromic or syndromic cardiac malformations, respectively [7–9]. Syndromic CVM is defined by accompanying extracardiac anomalies (ECA), such as developmental delay, and/or musculoskeletal, craniofacial, central nervous system, gastrointestinal, or genitourinary tract malformations. The burden of CNVs is significantly higher in syndromic CVM in comparison to non-syndromic cardiac malformations. To date, there are over 40 clinically delineated deletion and duplication syndromes with specific association to CVM. Genome-wide studies of rare CNVs have been accomplished in both isolated and syndromic cohorts [10], and the substantial contribution of segmental aneusomy in human congenital CVM is emphasized in several studies pertaining to tetralogy of Fallot (ToF) [11], heterotaxy [12], left-sided heart defects [13–15], single-ventricle heart defects [10, 16], and atrioventricular septal defects (AVSD) [17].

1p36 Deletion

Deletion of chromosome 1p36 (MIM 607872) is one of the most frequent subtelomeric rearrangements with an estimated incidence of 1 in 5,000 live births [18, 19]. The deletion is associated with cardiac abnormalities in up to 70% of the affected children [20, 21]. The structural heart defects include septal defects, patent ductus arteriosus (PDA), valvular abnormalities, coarctation of the aorta (CoA), and ToF. Cardiomyopathy, including left-ventricular noncompaction is observed in about 23–27% of all individuals with 1p36 deletion (see chapter by Towbin discussing Genetic Cardiomyothpathies on p. 210) [21]. ECA observed as characteristic dysmorphic features, senorineural hearing loss, seizures, intellectual disability, and structural brain abnormalities. Breakpoint analyses of genomic copy number alterations and cardiac-specific phenotypes have identified at least 5 critical regions underlying structural heart defects and two, characterizing the phenotype of left-ventricular noncompaction within the 1p36 region [22]. Deficiency of *Rere* in the murine model has been shown to recapitulate most features of the 1p36 monosomy syndrome [23]. RERE acts as a positive regulator of retinoic acid signaling. Homozygous mice with Rere deficiency have aortic arch abnormalities, double-outlet right ventricle, transposition of the great arteries, and perimembranous ventricular septal defect (VSD) [23]. *PRDM16* within this region has been implicated in cardiomyopathy [24]. Several other genes within the 1p36 region may be responsible for structural and functional abnormalities of the heart, as shown by extensive fine mapping studies in 1p36 monosomy. Increasing utilization of whole exome sequencing holds the promise of further defining the critical gene(s) responsible for human diseases within this region.

8p23.1 Deletion/Duplication

Recurrent deletions of 8p23.1 mediated by NAHR through local LCRs termed 8p-OR-REPD (REPeat distal) and 8p-OR-REPP (REPeat proximal) are frequently associated with CVM with high penetrance [10, 25]. This region includes at least two dosage sensitive genes: *GATA4* and *SOX7*. *GATA4* is a key cardiac transcription factor and has been known to cause isolated atrial septal defect (ASD), ToF, and AVSD [26, 27]. Congenital diaphragmatic hernia has been reported in some individuals with 8p23.1 deletion with incomplete penetrance. Structural cardiac defects include AVSD, ASD, pulmonary valve stenosis (PS), and ToF. Not surprisingly, the reciprocal duplication syndrome 8p23.1 mediated by NAHR is also linked to conotruncal and other cardiac defects, although with incomplete penetrance. ToF, septal defects, PS, and AVSD have all been reported [28–30].

Williams-Beuren Syndrome

Williams-Beuren syndrome (MIM 194050) resulting from recurrent deletion of 7q11.23 is another genomic disorder frequently characterized by cardiac defects. The syndrome is distinguished by typical facial features, social personality, and hypercalcemia. The estimated prevalence of this disorder is 1 in 7,500–10,000 newborns [31]. The recurrent deletion of ~1.55 Mb is mediated by unequal meiotic recombination between highly homologous regional segmental duplications. The classic cardiac lesion observed in Williams-Beuren syndrome is supravalvular aortic stenosis, which can be seen in approximately 75% of the affected individuals [32, 33]. Peripheral pulmonary stenosis is also encountered at a higher frequency [34]. Generalized arteriopathy leading to stenoses of medium and large arteries has been attributed to the haploinsufficiency of the elastin gene *(ELN)* within the commonly deleted interval [35]. Several *ELN* mutations have now been reported in both sporadic and familial cases of supravalvular aortic stenosis, categorically establishing the role of this gene in arteriopathy. Most of the described mutations are premature termination mutations, resulting in null alleles through the nonsense-mediated mRNA decay [36–38]. Mitral valve prolapse, aortic arch hypoplasia, aortic insufficiency, and VSD occur less frequently [39]. Rare reports of CoA and total anomalous pulmonary venous return have been described [40].

Kleefstra Syndrome

Kleefstra syndrome (MIM 610253), resulting from haploinsufficiency of euchromatin histone methyltransferase 1 (*EHMT1*), is reported in conjunction with CVM in about 40% of cases. The disorder is caused either by a submicroscopic deletion in the terminal region of chromosomal region 9q34.3 or point

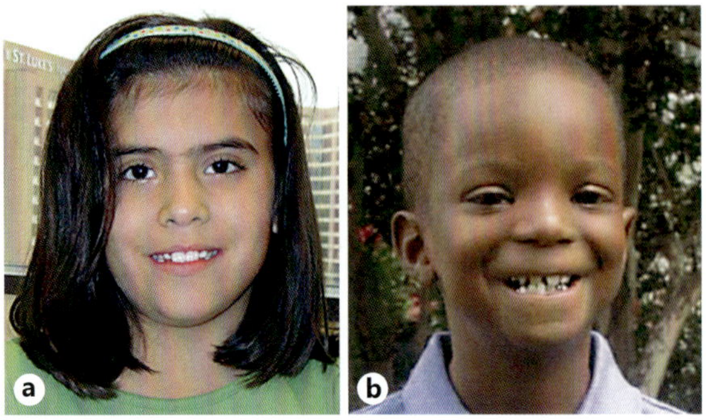

Fig. 1. **a** A 14-year-old female with the Smith-Magenis syndrome (17p11.2 deletion) is shown, with a diagnosis of partial anomalous pulmonary venous connection. **b** Photo of an 8-year-old male with the Potocki-Lupski syndrome (17p11.2 duplication) is illustrated. He has mild dilatation of aortic root and ascending aorta.

mutation of *EHMT1*. Haploinsufficiency of *EHMT1* results in a clinically recognizable disorder of distinctive facial features comprising brachycephaly, synophrys, cupid-bowed upper lip, and prominent jaw, hypotonia, intellectual disability, epilepsy, and behavior abnormalities [41]. The cardiac anomalies include septal defects, PS, bicuspid aortic valve (BAV), and PDA [42]. Cardiac arrhythmias, including atrial flutter, have also been described [43].

Smith-Magenis Syndrome/Potocki-Lupski Syndrome

Smith-Magenis syndrome (SMS; MIM 182290) caused by interstitial deletion of 17p11.2 is a well-recognized genomic disorder characterized by significant behavioral problems, sleep disturbances, and craniofacial, and skeletal anomalies (fig. 1). The common SMS deletion and the reciprocal Potocki-Lupski syndrome (PTLS; MIM 610883) duplication are caused by NAHR between the flanking distal and proximal LCRs called SMS-REPs [44], resulting in ~3.7-Mb segmental aneusomy. About one-third of individuals with SMS have cardiac lesions, observed as septal defects [45, 46] and ToF [47, 48]. Pulmonary atresia, pulmonic stenosis, and total anomalous pulmonary venous return have been described in a few reports. Cardiovascular abnormalities occur in about 40% of individuals with PTLS [49]. Dilated aortic root, septal defects, patent foramen ovale, conduction abnormalities, BAV, and hypoplastic left-heart syndrome (HLHS) have been described [49–51]. The extracardiac problems in PTLS include hypotonia, failure to thrive, and intellectual disability [52, 53]. It has been shown that cardiac lesions in SMS are less likely to be associated with haploinsufficiency of *RAI1*, since mutation carriers seldom have cardiac lesions [54]. It has been proposed that the cardiac phenotype in SMS and PTLS is likely due to altered copies of other dosage-sensitive genes within this region.

Koolen-de Vries Syndrome

Koolen-de Vries syndrome or 17q21.31 microdeletion syndrome (MIM 610443) is a recognizable syndrome associated with intellectual disability, with an estimated prevalence of approximately 1 in 16,000 individuals. The region on 17q21.31 contains a common inversion polymorphism (H2) of approximately 900 kb which is enriched in Europeans [55–57]. The carriers of the H2 ancestral haplotype in inverted orientation are predisposed to having offspring with the 17q21.31 microdeletion syndrome as a result of NAHR between directly oriented segmental duplications present on the inverted chromosome [56–58]. Distinctive facial features include a long face, upslanting palpebral fissures, epicanthic folds, tubular nose, and large prominent ears. Cardiac septal defects are noted in 30–40% of the affected individuals [59]. Other less common findings include PS and BAV [60]. Haploinsufficiency of *KANSL1* involved in histone acetylation within this region is now known to be the key disease mechanism in the deletion carriers [61, 62].

Wolf-Hirschhorn Syndrome

Structural heart defects occur in approximately 50% of individuals with Wolf-Hirschhorn syndrome (WHS/4p minus; MIM 194190) [63]. Children with WHS have deletions on chromosome 4p16.3 and have intellectual disability, multiple congenital anomalies, and characteristic 'Greek warrior helmet' craniofacial dysmorphism. ASDs are the most common cardiac defects reported in WHS. Other lesions include PS, ToF, VSD, and PDA [63]. Candidate gene analysis of phenotypic-specific defects in WHS has identified *FGFRL1* as an important player. The gene is distal to the critical regions 1 and 2 (WHSCR-1 and WHSCR-2). *Fgfrl1* null mice exhibit skeletal defects and cardiac abnormalities, including defects in the septation of ventricles, and thickened atrioventricular and semilunar valves [64].

Jacobsen Syndrome

The 11q terminal deletions between 5–16 Mb (Jacobsen syndrome; MIM 147791) are associated with CVM in about 56% of cases [65]. Affected individuals have growth retardation, thrombocytopenia, and multiple congenital anomalies [66]. Left-sided obstructive lesions are frequently reported in Jacobsen syndrome. HLHS occurs in about 5–10% of all patients with 11q deletion. A transcription factor (ETS1) encoded within this region has been implicated in cardiac defects [67]. *Ets1* deficient mice exhibit membranous VSDs and abnormal ventricular development [67]. Ets1 has been shown to be important for the formation of the interventricular septum and is required for the migration and differentiation of a subset of the cardiac neural crest [68].

Other Genomic Rearrangements

1q21.1. The recurrent 1q21.1 distal deletion (class I deletion; MIM 612474) mediated by NAHR and encompassing approximately 1.35 Mb is associated with CVM with incomplete penetrance (10–25% of cases). This deletion is 200 kb distal from the TAR (thrombocytopenia-absent radius syndrome) region. The larger deletion extending proximally to include the TAR region encompasses ~2.7 Mb and is designated as class II deletion. The spectrum of CVM in class I 1q21.1 deletion is relatively broad, including CoA, interruption of the aortic arch (types A and B) [69], BAV, aortopathy, PDA, truncus arteriosus, and transposition of the great arteries [70]. Within the deleted interval, GJA5 (gap junction α_5 protein), also known as connexin 40, has been implicated in cardiac defects. The reciprocal duplication of 1q21.1 (MIM 612475) is reported to be linked to ToF in several studies [11, 71, 72]. The recapitulation of conotruncal defects in connexin 40-deficient mice [73] and reports of small intragenic duplications of the gene in humans with nonsyndromic ToF [72] strengthen the role of this gene in cardiac morphogenesis in humans. It is noteworthy that several healthy carrier parents and unaffected individuals have been reported with genomic rearrangements of 1q21.1. The variable expressivity and incomplete penetrance related to this structural variation suggest that variation in other causative alleles on 1q21.1 may modulate disease susceptibility.

15q26. Deletions of 15q26 (MIM 612626) are frequently characterized by left-sided outflow tract lesions, including CoA and HLHS [74–80]. Within this region on 15q26.3, *NR2F2 (COUP-TFII)* encoding a transcription factor has been considered an important candidate gene for cardiac phenotype. Its important role has been established in angiogenesis, lymphatic development, and atrial malformations in animal models [81, 82]. In *Nr2f2* mutant mice, the sinus venosus and atria fail to develop past the primitive tube stage [81]. *MCTP2* is another gene in close proximity to *NR2F2* which has been shown to be important in the outflow tract formation in *Xenopus laevis* [83]. It is plausible that there are other dosage-sensitive genes within this region important for human cardiac morphogenesis.

16q24.3. Nonrecurrent deletions of 16q24.3 have been noted frequently and the phenotype associated with this genomic disorder has gradually evolved as more individuals have been ascertained [10, 43, 84, 85]. Initially identified in children with autism spectrum disorders, this deletion encompassing *ANKRD11* has now been linked to KBG syndrome, with common features of intellectual disability, facial dysmorphisms, macrodontia, and short stature [86]. Submicroscopic deletions involving *ANKRD11* have been described in patients with VSDs, cleft mitral valve, aortic root dilatation, and supravalvular pulmonic stenosis [10, 85, 87, 88]. Largely observed as de novo events, some of the smaller deletions within this region are familial. The penetrance of cardiac defects is uncertain at this time, as individuals with 16q24.3 deletion and normal cardiac examination seldom get follow-up echocardiograms for evaluation. The risk of aortic root dilatation has been shown in at least a few reports, suggesting careful echocardiographic evaluation of individuals with *ANKRD11* deletions or point mutations.

Less Frequent CVM-Associated Genomic Disorders

Several other genomic disorders that are less frequently observed in conjunction with cardiovascular defects are described in this section. Terminal deletion of 17p13.3 encompassing *PAFAH1B1* causes Miller-Dieker (MIM 247200) lissencephaly syndrome, characterized by cerebral agyria/pachygyria or type I lissencephaly, corpus callosum dysgenesis/agenesis, microcephaly, seizures, and distinctive facies. Septal defects and ToF are reported in both prenatal and postnatal cases in various studies [10, 89, 90]. The 17q23.1q23.2 deletion syndrome (MIM 613355), involving dosage-sensitive genes *TBX2* and *TBX4*, causes cardiovascular phenotypes, such as PDA, secundum ASD, and pulmonary hypertension [91–93]. As in most genomic disorders, this NAHR-mediated 2.2-Mb recurrent deletion has been shown to have extracardiac effects, including craniofacial dysmorphisms, musculoskeletal defects, growth retardation, and microcephaly. Recurrent deletions of 10q22q23 (MIM 612242) mediated by LCR3-LCR4 have been linked to congenital heart defects in a small fraction of cases. AVSDs have also been reported [94]. The deletion is rare in the population and encompasses *BMPR1A* (also known as *ALK3*) and *GRID1*. *BMPR1A* is an excellent candidate gene as tissue-specific disruptions of *Bmpr1a* result in defects of the endocardial cushions of the atrioventricular canal or malformation of the atrioventricular valves [95, 96].

Conclusion

Our understanding of the genetic basis of CVM has increased significantly in the last decade with the escalating use of array technologies to identify submicroscopic deletions and duplications in human CVM. While tremendous progress has been made in identifying regions of genomic instability causing recurrent and nonrecurrent rearrangements, considerable work remains in discerning smaller CNVs, especially involving single genes, likely functioning in an oligogenic model. Use of complete genome sequencing in large studies will be pivotal in ascertaining both rare sequence variants and copy number alterations of exons which may be major players in human CVM.

References

1 Hoffman JI, Kaplan S: The incidence of congenital heart disease. J Am Coll Cardiol 2002;39:1890–1900.
2 Hoffman JI: Incidence of congenital heart disease: II. Prenatal incidence. Pediatr Cardiol 1995;16:155–165.
3 Hartman RJ, Rasmussen SA, Botto LD, et al: The contribution of chromosomal abnormalities to congenital heart defects: a population-based study. Pediatr Cardiol 2011;32:1147–1157.
4 Burn J, Goodship J: Developmental genetics of the heart. Curr Opin Genet Dev 1996;6:322–325.
5 Girirajan S, Campbell CD, Eichler EE: Human copy number variation and complex genetic disease. Annu Rev Genet 2011;45:203–226.
6 Liu P, Carvalho CM, Hastings PJ, Lupski JR: Mechanisms for recurrent and complex human genomic rearrangements. Curr Opin Genet Dev 2012;22:211–220.
7 Thienpont B, Mertens L, de Ravel T, et al: Submicroscopic chromosomal imbalances detected by array-CGH are a frequent cause of congenital heart defects in selected patients. Eur Heart J 2007;28:2778–2784.
8 Derwinska K, Bartnik M, Wiśniowiecka-Kowalnik B, et al: Assessment of the role of copy-number variants in 150 patients with congenital heart defects. Med Wieku Rozwoj 2012;16:175–182.
9 Breckpot J, Thienpont B, Arens Y, Tranchevent LC, et al: Challenges of interpreting copy number variation in syndromic and non syndromic congenital heart defects. Cytogenet Genome Res 2011;135:251–259.
10 Lalani SR, Shaw C, Wang X, et al: Rare DNA copy number variants in cardiovascular malformations with extracardiac abnormalities. Eur J Hum Genet 2013;21:173–181.
11 Greenway SC, Pereira AC, Lin JC, et al: De novo copy number variants identify new genes and loci in isolated sporadic tetralogy of Fallot. Nat Genet 2009;41:931–935.
12 Fakhro KA, Choi M, Ware SM, et al: Rare copy number variations in congenital heart disease patients identify unique genes in left-right patterning. Proc Natl Acad Sci U S A 2011;108:2915–2920.
13 Iascone M, Ciccone R, Galletti L, et al: Identification of de novo mutations and rare variants in hypoplastic left heart syndrome. Clin Genet 2012;81:542–554.
14 Warburton D, Ronemus M, Kline J, et al: The contribution of de novo and rare inherited copy number changes to congenital heart disease in an unselected sample of children with conotruncal defects or hypoplastic left heart disease. Hum Genet 2014;133:11–27.
15 Hitz MP, Lemieux-Perreault LP, Marshall C, et al: Rare copy number variants contribute to congenital left-sided heart disease. PLoS Genet 2012;8:e1002903.
16 Carey AS, Liang L, Edwards J, et al: Effect of copy number variants on outcomes for infants with single ventricle heart defects. Circ Cardiovasc Genet 2013;6:444–451.
17 Priest JR, Girirajan S, Vu TH, et al: Rare copy number variants in isolated sporadic and syndromic atrioventricular septal defects. Am J Med Genet A 2012;158A:1279–1284.
18 Rosenfeld JA, Crolla JA, Tomkins S, et al: Refinement of causative genes in monosomy 1p36 through clinical and molecular cytogenetic characterization of small interstitial deletions. Am J Med Genet A 2010;152A:1951–1959.
19 Heilstedt HA, Ballif BC, Howard LA, et al: Physical map of 1p36, placement of breakpoints in monosomy 1p36, and clinical characterization of the syndrome. Am J Hum Genet 2003;72:1200–1212.
20 Gajecka M, Mackay KL, Shaffer LG: Monosomy 1p36 deletion syndrome. Am J Med Genet C Semin Med Genet 2007;145C:346–356.

21 Battaglia A, Hoyme HE, Dallapiccola B, et al: Further delineation of deletion 1p36 syndrome in 60 patients: a recognizable phenotype and common cause of developmental delay and mental retardation. Pediatrics 2008;121:404–410.
22 Zaveri HP, Beck TF, Hernández-García A, et al: Identification of critical regions and candidate genes for cardiovascular malformations and cardiomyopathy associated with deletions of chromosome 1p36. PLoS One 2014;9:e85600.
23 Kim BJ, Zaveri HP, Shchelochkov OA, et al: An allelic series of mice reveals a role for RERE in the development of multiple organs affected in chromosome 1p36 deletions. PLoS One 2013;8:e57460.
24 Arndt AK, Schafer S, Drenckhahn JD, et al: Fine mapping of the 1p36 deletion syndrome identifies mutation of PRDM16 as a cause of cardiomyopathy. Am J Hum Genet 2013;93:67–77.
25 Wat MJ, Shchelochkov OA, Holder AM, et al: Chromosome 8p23.1 deletions as a cause of complex congenital heart defects and diaphragmatic hernia. Am J Med Genet A 2009;149A:1661–1677.
26 Garg V, Kathiriya IS, Barnes R, et al: GATA4 mutations cause human congenital heart defects and reveal an interaction with TBX5. Nature 2003;424:443–447.
27 Nemer G, Fadlalah F, Usta J, et al: A novel mutation in the GATA4 gene in patients with tetralogy of Fallot. Hum Mutat 2006; 27:293–294.
28 Barber JC, Rosenfeld JA, Foulds N, et al: 8p23.1 duplication syndrome; common, confirmed, and novel features in six further patients. Am J Med Genet A 2013;161A:487–500.
29 Barber JC, Bunyan D, Curtis M, et al: 8p23.1 duplication syndrome differentiated from copy number variation of the defensin cluster at prenatal diagnosis in four new families. Mol Cytogenet 2010;3:3.
30 Zhang Y, Li Y, Wang Y, et al: 8p23.1 duplication detected by array-CGH with complete atrioventricular septal defect and unilateral hand preaxial hexadactyly. Am J Med Genet A 2013;161A:561–565.
31 Stromme P, Bjornstad PG, Ramstad K: Prevalence estimation of Williams syndrome. J Child Neurol 2002;17:269–271.
32 Keating MT: Genetic approaches to cardiovascular disease. Supravalvular aortic stenosis, Williams syndrome, and long-QT syndrome. Circulation 1995;92:142–147.
33 Eronen M, Peippo M, Hiippala A, et al: Cardiovascular manifestations in 75 patients with Williams syndrome. J Med Genet 2002; 39:554–558.
34 Collins RT 2nd, Kaplan P, Somes GW, Rome JJ: Long-term outcomes of patients with cardiovascular abnormalities and Williams syndrome. Am J Cardiol 2010; 105:874–878.
35 Merla G, Brunetti-Pierri N, Piccolo P, et al: Supravalvular aortic stenosis: elastin arteriopathy. Circ Cardiovasc Genet 2012;5:692–696.
36 Tassabehji M, Metcalfe K, Donnai D, et al: Elastin: genomic structure and point mutations in patients with supravalvular aortic stenosis. Hum Mol Genet 1997;6:1029–1036.
37 Metcalfe K, Rucka AK, Smoot L, et al: Elastin: mutational spectrum in supravalvular aortic stenosis. Eur J Hum Genet 2000;8: 955–963.
38 Micale L, Turturo MG, Fusco C, et al: Identification and characterization of seven novel mutations of elastin gene in a cohort of patients affected by supravalvular aortic stenosis. Eur J Hum Genet 2010;18:317–323.
39 Ergul Y, Nisli K, Kayserili H, et al: Cardiovascular abnormalities in Williams syndrome: 20 years' experience in Istanbul. Acta Cardiol 2012;67:649–655.
40 Ferrero GB, Biamino E, Sorasio L, et al: Presenting phenotype and clinical evaluation in a cohort of 22 Williams-Beuren syndrome patients. Eur J Med Genet 2007;50: 327–337.
41 Kleefstra T, Brunner HG, Amiel J, et al: Loss-of-function mutations in euchromatin histone methyl transferase 1 (EHMT1) cause the 9q34 subtelomeric deletion syndrome. Am J Hum Genet 2006;79:370–377.
42 Kleefstra T, van Zelst-Stams WA, Nillesen WM, et al: Further clinical and molecular delineation of the 9q subtelomeric deletion syndrome supports a major contribution of EHMT1 haploinsufficiency to the core phenotype. J Med Genet 2009;46:598–606.
43 Willemsen MH, Vulto-van Silfhout AT, Nillesen WM, et al: Update on Kleefstra syndrome. Mol Syndromol 2012;2:202–212.
44 Bi W, Park SS, Shaw CJ, et al: Reciprocal crossovers and a positional preference for strand exchange in recombination events resulting in deletion or duplication of chromosome 17p11.2. Am J Hum Genet 2003; 73:1302–1315.
45 Greenberg F, Lewis RA, Potocki L, et al: Multi-disciplinary clinical study of Smith-Magenis syndrome (deletion 17p11.2). Am J Med Genet 1996;62:247–254.
46 Smith AC, McGavran L, Robinson J, et al: Interstitial deletion of (17)(p11.2p11.2) in nine patients. Am J Med Genet 1986;24: 393–414.
47 Thomas DG, Jacques SM, Flore LA, et al: Prenatal diagnosis of Smith-Magenis syndrome (del 17p11.2). Fetal Diagn Ther 2000;15:335–337.
48 Sweeney E, Peart I, Tofeig M, Kerr B: Smith-Magenis syndrome and tetralogy of Fallot. J Med Genet 1999;36:501–502.
49 Jefferies JL, Pignatelli RH, Martinez HR, et al: Cardiovascular findings in duplication 17p11.2 syndrome. Genet Med 2012;14:90–94.
50 Sanchez-Valle A, Pierpont ME, Potocki L: The severe end of the spectrum: hypoplastic left heart in Potocki-Lupski syndrome. Am J Med Genet A 2011;155A:363–366.
51 Yusupov R, Roberts AE, Lacro RV, et al: Potocki-Lupski syndrome: an inherited dup(17)(p11.2p11.2) with hypoplastic left heart. Am J Med Genet A 2011;155A:367–371.
52 Wong JT, Chan DK, Wong KY, et al: Smith-Magenis syndrome and cyanotic congenital heart disease: a case report. Clin Dysmorphol 2003;12:73–74.
53 Myers SM, Challman TD: Congenital heart defects associated with Smith-Magenis syndrome: two cases of total anomalous pulmonary venous return. Am J Med Genet A 2004;131:99–100.
54 Edelman EA, Girirajan S, Finucane B, et al: Gender, genotype, and phenotype differences in Smith-Magenis syndrome: a meta-analysis of 105 cases. Clin Genet 2007;71: 540–550.
55 Stefansson H, Helgason A, Thorleifsson G, et al: A common inversion under selection in Europeans. Nat Genet 2005;37:129–137.
56 Koolen DA, Vissers LE, Pfundt R, et al: A new chromosome 17q21.31 microdeletion syndrome associated with a common inversion polymorphism. Nat Genet 2006;38:999–1001.
57 Steinberg KM, Antonacci F, Sudmant PH, et al: Structural diversity and African origin of the 17q21.31 inversion polymorphism. Nat Genet 2012;44:872–880.
58 Boettger LM, Handsaker RE, Zody MC, McCarroll SA: Structural haplotypes and recent evolution of the human 17q21.31 region. Nat Genet 2012;44:881–885.
59 Koolen DA, Sharp AJ, Hurst JA, et al: Clinical and molecular delineation of the 17q21.31 microdeletion syndrome. J Med Genet 2008;45:710–720.
60 Tan TY, Aftimos S, Worgan L, et al: Phenotypic expansion and further characterisation of the 17q21.31 microdeletion syndrome. J Med Genet 2009;46:480–489.
61 Koolen DA, Kramer JM, Neveling K, et al: Mutations in the chromatin modifier gene KANSL1 cause the 17q21.31 microdeletion syndrome. Nat Genet 2012;44:639–641.
62 Zollino M, Orteschi D, Murdolo M, et al: Mutations in KANSL1 cause the 17q21.31 microdeletion syndrome phenotype. Nat Genet 2012;44:636–638.
63 Battaglia A, Filippi T, Carey JC: Update on the clinical features and natural history of Wolf-Hirschhorn (4p-) syndrome: experience with 87 patients and recommendations for routine health supervision. Am J Med Genet C Semin Med Genet 2008;148C:246–251.

64 Catela C, Bilbao-Cortes D, Slonimsky E, et al: Multiple congenital malformations of Wolf-Hirschhorn syndrome are recapitulated in Fgfrl1 null mice. Dis Model Mech 2009;2:283–294.
65 Grossfeld PD, Mattina T, Lai Z, et al: The 11q terminal deletion disorder: a prospective study of 110 cases. Am J Med Genet A 2004;129A:51–61.
66 Mattina T, Perrotta CS, Grossfeld P: Jacobsen syndrome. Orphanet J Rare Dis 2009;4:9.
67 Ye M, Coldren C, Liang X, et al: Deletion of ETS-1, a gene in the Jacobsen syndrome critical region, causes ventricular septal defects and abnormal ventricular morphology in mice. Hum Mol Genet 2010;19:648–656.
68 Gao Z, Kim GH, Mackinnon AC, et al: Ets1 is required for proper migration and differentiation of the cardiac neural crest. Development 2010;137:1543–1551.
69 Christiansen J, Dyck JD, Elyas BG, et al: Chromosome 1q21.1 contiguous gene deletion is associated with congenital heart disease. Circ Res 2004;94:1429–1435.
70 Mefford HC, Sharp AJ, Baker C, et al: Recurrent rearrangements of chromosome 1q21.1 and variable pediatric phenotypes. N Engl J Med 2008;359:1685–1699.
71 Dolcetti A, Silversides CK, Marshall CR, et al: 1q21.1 microduplication expression in adults. Genet Med 2013;15:282–289.
72 Silversides CK, Lionel AC, Costain G, et al: Rare copy number variations in adults with tetralogy of Fallot implicate novel risk gene pathways. PLoS Genet 2012;8:e1002843.
73 Gu H, Smith FC, Taffet SM, et al: High incidence of cardiac malformations in connexin40-deficient mice. Circ Res 2003;93:201–206.
74 Baptista J, Mercer C, Prigmore E, et al: Breakpoint mapping and array CGH in translocations: comparison of a phenotypically normal and an abnormal cohort. Am J Hum Genet 2008;82:927–936.
75 Choi JH, Kang M, Kim GH, et al: Clinical and functional characteristics of a novel heterozygous mutation of the IGF1R gene and IGF1R haploinsufficiency due to terminal 15q26.2->qter deletion in patients with intrauterine growth retardation and postnatal catch-up growth failure. J Clin Endocrinol Metab 2011;96:E130–E134.
76 Davidsson J, Collin A, Björkhem G, Soller M: Array based characterization of a terminal deletion involving chromosome subband 15q26.2: an emerging syndrome associated with growth retardation, cardiac defects and developmental delay. BMC Med Genet 2008;9:2.
77 Klaassens M, Galjaard RJ, Scott DA, et al: Prenatal detection and outcome of congenital diaphragmatic hernia (CDH) associated with deletion of chromosome 15q26: two patients and review of the literature. Am J Med Genet A 2007;143A:2204–2212.
78 Scott DA, Klaassens M, Holder AM, et al: Genome-wide oligonucleotide-based array comparative genome hybridization analysis of non-isolated congenital diaphragmatic hernia. Hum Mol Genet 2007;16:424–430.
79 Slavotinek AM, Moshrefi A, Davis R, et al: Array comparative genomic hybridization in patients with congenital diaphragmatic hernia: mapping of four CDH-critical regions and sequencing of candidate genes at 15q26.1–15q26.2. Eur J Hum Genet 2006;14:999–1008.
80 Tumer Z, Harboe TL, Blennow E, et al: Molecular cytogenetic characterization of ring chromosome 15 in three unrelated patients. Am J Med Genet A 2004;130A:340–344.
81 Pereira FA, Qiu Y, Zhou G, et al: The orphan nuclear receptor COUP-TFII is required for angiogenesis and heart development. Genes Dev 1999;13:1037–1049.
82 Aranguren XL, Beerens M, Vandevelde W, et al: Transcription factor COUP-TFII is indispensable for venous and lymphatic development in zebrafish and Xenopus laevis. Biochem Biophys Res Commun 2011;410:121–126.
83 Lalani SR, Ware SM, Wang X, et al: MCTP2 is a dosage-sensitive gene required for cardiac outflow tract development. Hum Mol Genet 2013;22:4339–4348.
84 Willemsen MH, Fernandez BA, Bacino CA, et al: Identification of ANKRD11 and ZNF778 as candidate genes for autism and variable cognitive impairment in the novel 16q24.3 microdeletion syndrome. Eur J Hum Genet 2010;18:429–435.
85 Sacharow S, Li D, Fan YS, Tekin M: Familial 16q24.3 microdeletion involving ANKRD11 causes a KBG-like syndrome. Am J Med Genet A 2012;158A:547–552.
86 Sirmaci A, Spiliopoulos M, Brancati F, et al: Mutations in ANKRD11 cause KBG syndrome, characterized by intellectual disability, skeletal malformations, and macrodontia. Am J Hum Genet 2011;89:289–294.
87 Devriendt K, Holvoet M, Fryns JP: Further delineation of the KBG syndrome. Genet Couns 1998;9:191–194.
88 Nicolini F, Beghi C, Gherli T: Aortic valve regurgitation in a patient affected by KBG syndrome. J Heart Valve Dis 2009;18:122–124.
89 Chen CP, Liu YP, Lin SP, et al: Ventriculomegaly, intrauterine growth restriction, and congenital heart defects as salient prenatal sonographic findings of Miller-Dieker lissencephaly syndrome associated with monosomy 17p (17p13.2 -> pter) in a fetus. Taiwan J Obstet Gynecol 2010;49:81–86.
90 Kowase K, Nakamura T, Okumura W, et al: Novel deletion on the short arm of chromosome 17 in a patient with multiple cardiac anomalies. Jpn Circ J 1997;61:882–885.
91 Ballif BC, Theisen A, Rosenfeld JA, et al: Identification of a recurrent microdeletion at 17q23.1q23.2 flanked by segmental duplications associated with heart defects and limb abnormalities. Am J Hum Genet 2010;86:454–461.
92 Kerstjens-Frederikse WS, Bongers EM, Roofthooft MT, et al: TBX4 mutations (small patella syndrome) are associated with childhood-onset pulmonary arterial hypertension. J Med Genet 2013;50:500–506.
93 Nimmakayalu M, Major H, Sheffield V, et al: Microdeletion of 17q22q23.2 encompassing TBX2 and TBX4 in a patient with congenital microcephaly, thyroid duct cyst, sensorineural hearing loss, and pulmonary hypertension. Am J Med Genet A 2011;155A:418–423.
94 van Bon BW, Balciuniene J, Fruhman G, et al: The phenotype of recurrent 10q22q23 deletions and duplications. Eur J Hum Genet 2011;19:400–408.
95 Gaussin V, Morley GE, Cox L, et al: Alk3/Bmpr1a receptor is required for development of the atrioventricular canal into valves and annulus fibrosus. Circ Res 2005;97:219–226.
96 Song L, Fässler R, Mishina Y, et al: Essential functions of Alk3 during AV cushion morphogenesis in mouse embryonic hearts. Dev Biol 2007;301:276–286.

Dr. Seema R. Lalani
Department of Molecular and Human Genetics, Baylor College of Medicine
6701 Fannin Street
Houston, TX 77030 (USA)
E-Mail seemal@bcm.edu

4 Single Gene Disorders

Muenke M, Kruszka PS, Sable CA, Belmont JW (eds): Congenital Heart Disease: Molecular Genetics, Principles of Diagnosis and Treatment. Basel, Karger, 2015, pp 122–130
DOI: 10.1159/000375210

Noonan Syndrome and Other RAS/ MAPK Pathway Syndromes

Bruce D. Gelb[a] · Amy E. Roberts[b] · Marco Tartaglia[c]

[a]Mindich Child Health and Development Institute, Departments of Pediatrics, and Genetics and Genomic Sciences, Icahn School of Medicine at Mount Sinai, New York, N.Y., and [b]Department of Cardiology and Division of Genetics, Boston Children's Hospital, Boston, Mass., USA; [c]Dipartimento di Ematologia, Oncologia e Medicina Molecolare, Istituto Superiore di Sanità, Rome, Italy

Abstract

The Noonan syndrome and its related disorders, now collectively called RASopathies, are autosomal dominant traits with pleiomorphic features, including cardiovascular involvement at high prevalence. The cardiovascular abnormalities include congenital heart defects, with valve stenosis and atrial septal defects being commonest, and an early-onset form of hypertrophic cardiomyopathy. The mutations underlying the RASopathies alter genes encoding proteins with roles in signal transduction through the RAS/MAPK pathway. Nearly all lesions are missense variants and generally have gain-of-function effects. Mutations in several genes underlie the Noonan syndrome, the commonest of these disorders, with well-established genotype-phenotype correlations. Disease pathogenesis for the RASopathies is being elucidated using mouse models, which generally recapitulate the associated cardiovascular defects. It appears that certain phenotypes may be amenable to drug therapies, but gene/mutation-specific approaches may be necessary.

The Noonan syndrome (NS) is an autosomal dominant disorder described by two pediatric cardiologists, Jacqueline Noonan and Dorothy Ehmke [1, 2]. They based their description of this putatively novel syndrome on observations made in 9 patients with pulmonary valve stenosis (PS) and distinctive dysmorphic features, including hypertelorism, ptosis, low-set ears, webbed neck, and chest deformities (fig. 1). Since then, the pleiomorphic extent of the phenotype has been delineated, including recognition of a broader range of congenital heart defects (CHD) as well as early-onset hypertrophic cardiomyopathy (HCM) (see chapter by Towbin for discussion of hypertophic cardiomyopathy on p. 216).

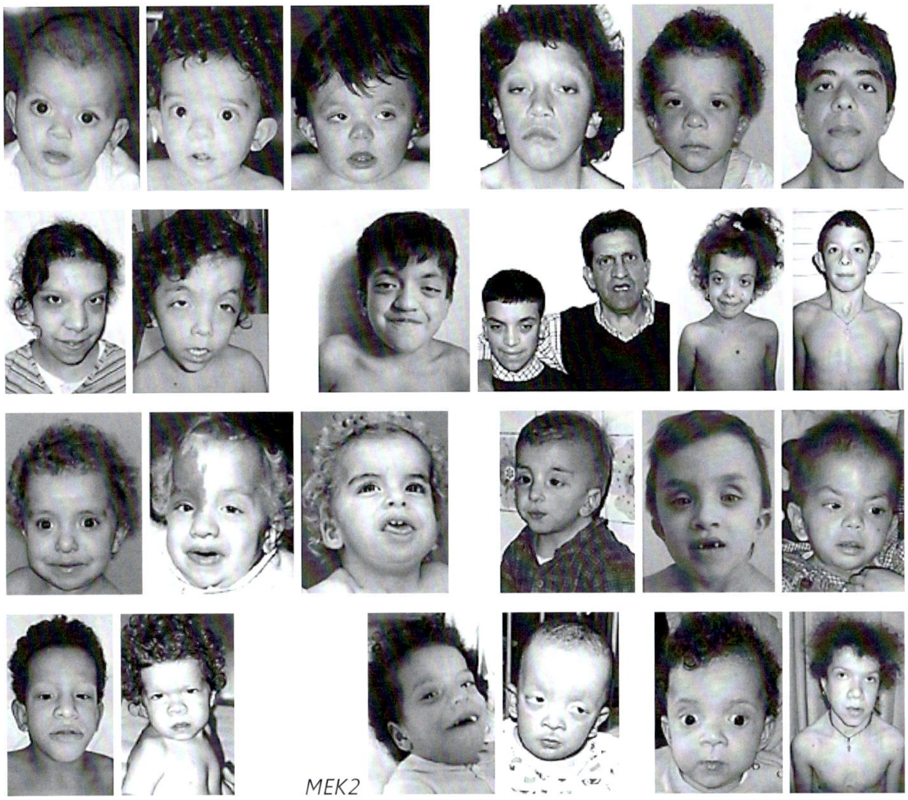

Fig. 1. Facial features in the RASopathies. Series of affected individuals heterozygous for mutations in different RASopathy genes are shown (kindly provided by G. Zampino, M.C. Digilio, B. Dallapiccola, L. Mazzanti, and G.B. Ferrero).

Several additional autosomal dominant disorders with phenotypic overlap with the NS have been described subsequently, including the NS with multiple lentigines (NSML; formerly, LEOPARD syndrome), cardiofaciocutaneous syndrome (CFCS), the Costello syndrome (CS), and Noonan-like syndrome with loose anagen hair (NSLAH).

While the NS and the related disorders were grouped based on their overlapping phenotypic features, the discoveries that the causative genes all encode proteins relevant for signal transduction through the RAS/MAPK (mitogen-activated protein kinase) pathway have provided biological coherence to them being classified together as RASopathies (fig. 2). Moreover, identification of these genes has enabled the establishment of strong genotype-phenotype correlations, including several relevant for the cardiovascular involvement in these disorders.

The RASopathies are complex multisystem disorders. Herein, we will focus on the cardiovascular manifestations and issues important to cardiovascular and surgical management.

RASopathy-Associated Cardiovascular Involvement

The Noonan Syndrome

For the NS, ~90% of affected individuals have cardiovascular involvement, with various forms of CHD predominating. The commonest is PS, often with dysplastic valve leaflets, which is present in

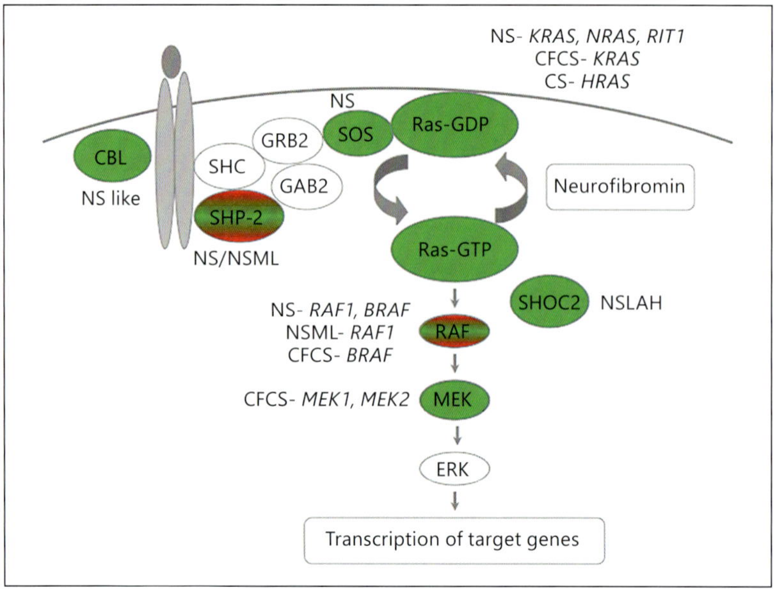

Fig. 2. The RAS/MAPK pathway. RASopathy-associated mutant proteins with gain and loss of function are indicated in green and red, respectively. The specific genes and phenotypes resulting from mutations are indicated. The gray ovals at the top left represent a receptor tyrosine kinase with its ligand.

~60% of cases. Among those with PS, a long-term history study suggested that 40% will require intervention [3]. Aside from the proclivity for requiring surgical intervention due to the dysplastic valve leaflets, which are often not amenable to successful balloon valvuloplasty, progression appears to depend on the degree of stenosis at presentation: mild PS may not progress whereas moderate PS can require intervention many years later [4] (see Costello et al. chapter on Surgical Management for more information on surgical therapy for Noonan syndorme on p. 285). Other forms of CHD associated with the NS include secundum atrial septal defects (ASD; found in 6–10% of affected individuals) as well as numerous others listed in table 1. Aside from the aforementioned challenges in addressing PS with dysplastic valve leaflets when that is required, the therapeutic strategies for the other forms of CHD are standard.

Table 1. Congenital heart defects in Noonan syndrome [adapted from ref. 42]

Defect	Frequency, %
Pulmonary valve stenosis	43
Partial atrioventricular canal	17
Aortic coarctation	10
Secundum atrial septal defect	9
Mitral valve anomalies	7
Tetralogy of Fallot	5
Ventricular septal defect	5
Patent ductus arteriosus	2
Pulmonary atresia/intact ventricular septum	2

Two comorbidities associated with the NS are worth noting: a bleeding diathesis, attributable to coagulation factor deficiencies and/or platelet dysfunction, and lymphatic dysgenesis. The former can result in significant hemorrhaging perioperatively for cardiac surgery, generally necessitating hematological evaluation prior to major procedures. The latter can first manifest during fetal life with cystic hygroma or increased nuchal translucency. Patients with the NS are more prone to develop chylothorax after cardiac surgery. A small percentage develops peripheral lymphedema, which can be readily mistaken for congestive heart failure, particularly if there is a history of CHD.

Approximately 20% of individuals with the NS will develop HCM [3]. More than half of the patients with the NS and HCM will also have CHD. The natural history of HCM in the context of the NS is unusual in several respects [5, 6]. NS-associated HCM presents early in life with more than half being diagnosed by 6 months of age. The mortality from NS-associated HCM is higher than that observed in other children with HCM, with a particularly high mortality among those presenting congestive heart failure at age <6 months (1-year survival of 31%) [6]. Longer-term follow-up also suggests increased late mortality in NS-associated HCM compared to sarcomeric HCM [5]. The primary cause of death for NS-associated HCM is congestive heart failure [3, 5, 6].

In the NS, the electrocardiogram often displays a wide QRS complex with a predominantly negative pattern in the left precordial leads and left-axis deviation with giant Q waves [7]. This may be the case even when the heart and chest wall are structurally normal.

Cardiovascular disease in the NS that is not congenital includes arterial aneurysm, most prevalently of the aortic root, but it can also involve the coronary or intracranial arteries. A recent retrospective cohort study of the ascending aorta in the NS concluded that onset of dilation at the aortic annulus and root was early in childhood and that the aortopathy appeared to be progressive, with more than 20% of individuals having abnormal root dimensions (*Z* score >2) [8]. The clinical implications of these observations, particularly with respect to therapy and intervention, remain to be determined.

The Noonan Syndrome with Multiple Lentigines

NSML is the RASopathy that most closely resembles the NS. In fact, the two disorders can be difficult to distinguish in infancy and early childhood. The distinctive feature of NSML is the presence of lentigines, small hyperpigmented skin lesions that resemble freckles and typically arise in the thousands on the face, trunk, and extremities by age 5 years. Café-au-lait spots are more common in NSML than in the NS. Sensorineural deafness is commoner in NSML but is present in a minority of patients (~20%).

HCM is observed in roughly 80% of those with NSML, which is the highest rate among the RASopathies [9]. Left-ventricular outflow tract obstruction from hypertrophy is present in about half of those with HCM. Rare cases of HCM that presents in early infancy and progresses rapidly have been described. Nonetheless, the clinical course of HCM in most individuals with NSML is relatively benign.

As with the NS, the commonest CHD are valvulopathies [9]. PS is observed in about one quarter of patients, but the valve leaflets are usually not dysplastic. Aortic stenosis is rarely observed. As with the NS, CHD can accompany HCM.

ECG abnormalities are common in NSML. Aside from findings such as left-ventricular hypertrophy that are typically associated with HCM, nearly one quarter of patients have conduction defects, including bundle branch blocks and hemiblocks.

The Cardiofaciocutaneous Syndrome

CFCS is a RASopathy distinguishable by the severity of the ectodermal findings (skin and hair) and neurocognitive impairment, sometimes with underlying structural brain abnormalities [10]. The facial dysmorphia is often striking with macrocephaly, prominent forehead and bitemporal narrowing (fig. 1). CFCS almost invariably arises sporadically due to poor reproductive fitness.

As with the other RASopathies, cardiovascular involvement in CFCS is prevalent (~75%) [10]. Among CHD, PS is the most common abnormality, present in 45% of the patients. The degree of PS is often mild, but minimal natural history data are available. Nearly one quarter have an ASD, some requiring intervention. HCM is diagnosed in 40% of CFCS patients. Severity varies widely from localized subaortic involvement to severe global hypertrophy with obstruction.

The Costello Syndrome

CS is a RASopathy with features overlapping with the NS. Distinctive noncardiac features include coarse features (fig. 1), papillomata, splayed finger with ulnar deviation, and increased prevalence of certain cancers such as rhabdomyosarcoma and neuroblastoma.

Less than half of CS cases have CHD [11]. The rate of PS is the same as involvement of one or more other valves (aortic/mitral), each being 20%. Different from the NS, ASD, particular those requiring intervention, are rare.

The prevalence of HCM in CS is roughly 65%, notably higher than for the NS [11]. Among individuals with CS and HCM, the pattern is asymmetric in more than 60%. The natural history of CS-

4

associated HCM is variable but includes severe or progressive disease in 40% of cases and nearly 25% of patients undergoing septal myectomy. The histology of this HCM is indistinguishable from sarcomeric HCM with myocardial fiber disarray [11, 12].

Atrial arrhythmias are prevalent in CS, affecting about 50% of patients. Two relatively unusual forms of atrial tachyarrhythmia, multifocal atrial tachycardia and ectopic atrial tachycardia, are observed in one quarter of those with CS. The association between CS and multifocal atrial tachycardia is so striking that it is the diagnosis of exclusion for any infant presenting with this difficult-to-treat tachyarrhythmia.

The Noonan Syndrome with Loose Anagen Hair

NSLAH, a RASopathy first described in 2003, is characterized by ectodermal features including darkly pigmented skin with eczema or ichthyosis and loose anagen hair [13]. While a limited number of individuals with NSLAH have been described in publications, it appears that a high percentage of affected individuals have cardiovascular involvement [14–17]. HCM prevalence is 25%, but its natural history has not been delineated well. The types of CHD observed to date are typical for those observed in RASopathies in general, but there is a relative excess of mitral valve dysplasia.

RASopathy Genetics

Not long after its description, the NS was recognized to be an autosomal dominant disorder based on transmission patterns in familial cases.

In 2001, Tartaglia et al. [18] identified mutations in *PTPN11* as a cause of the NS, and study of a number of unrelated individuals with the disorder showed that *PTPN11* mutations cause approximately one half of cases. *PTPN11* encodes the protein tyrosine phosphatase, SHP2, which has a largely positive role in promoting signal transduction, particularly through the MAPK and PI3K/AKT cascades. The causative mutations, which were all missense defects, altered SHP2 in a manner predicted to result in increased and prolonged phosphatase activity, i.e. gain of function. Biochemical characterization of NS-associated SHP2 mutants confirmed this [19]. Genes subsequently found to also cause the NS (*KRAS, SOS1, RAF1, NRAS*, and *RIT1*) also encode proteins that, when mutated, variably promote signal transduction through RAS and downstream cascades [20]. Specific *PTPN11* missense mutations, not observed in NS, were found in 90% of individuals with NSML [21, 22]. Biochemical studies of the NSML-associated SHP2 mutants showed perturbations notably different from those for NS [23–25]. Specifically, those mutant SHP2 proteins had reduced catalytic function.

Table 2. Genes mutated in the RASopathies

	NS	NSML	CFCS	CS	NSLAH
PTPN11	X	X			
RAF1	X	X			
SOS1	X				
RIT1	X				
CBL[1]	X				
NRAS	X				
KRAS	X		X		
BRAF	X		X		
MEK1			X		
MEK2			X		
HRAS				X	
SHOC2					X

[1] *CBL* mutations underlie a previously unrecognized RASopathy with features that overlap NS in a minority of subjects.

Given the phenotypic overlap, it is not surprising that genes encoding additional proteins involved in the RAS/MAPK signaling pathway were discovered to underlie the other RASopathies. Indeed, *HRAS* mutations are the sole cause of CS [26], *MEK1, MEK2,* and *BRAF* mutations cause CFCS, and a recurrent missense mutation in *SHOC2* underlies NSLAH (table 2; fig. 2). Aside from the NSML-associated *PTPN11* mutations, the other defects for the assorted RASopathies can be generalized as gain-of-function perturbations of signal transduction.

Most recently, new mutations causing the NS were found in *RIT1* using whole exome sequencing

[27]. The use of next-generation DNA sequencing, either whole exome, transcriptome or genome sequencing, is likely to yield the remaining genes for the NS and other RASopathies in the near future.

Genotype-Phenotype Associations

The identification of gene mutations underlying the RASopathies has enabled the establishment of genotype-phenotype correlations, which are useful for prognosticating about patients who are diagnosed early in life. Here, we will focus on the cardiovascular genotype-phenotype correlations [see ref. 28 for discussion of noncardiac genotype phenotype correlations].

For the NS, there are clear differences in the cardiovascular involvement that depend upon the gene mutation. Patients harboring NS-causing *PTPN11* mutations are more likely than all individuals with the NS to have PS and are less likely to have an ASD or develop HCM [29]. Similarly, HCM prevalence among those with *SOS1* mutations is less than one third of that in the NS overall [30]. In contrast, individuals with the NS due to *RAF1* mutations are very likely to develop HCM (~85%) [31, 32]. For patients harboring *RIT1* mutations, the prevalence of PS is typical (65%), but HCM occurs more frequently than in NS in general (70%) [27]. As a result, the combination of PS and HCM is more frequent among individuals with the NS due to *RIT1* mutations. For the remaining genes underlying the NS, whose mutation frequencies are low in the disorder, the numbers of individuals is too small to support meaningful analysis of genotype-phenotype associations.

For CFCS, two studies contained adequate numbers of individuals with *BRAF* mutations or *MEK* defects (either *MEK1* or *MEK2)* to permit a comparison of PS and HCM [33, 34]. Taken together, the prevalence of PS was 47% *(BRAF)* and 20% *(MEK)*, which was significantly different. The prevalence of HCM was not different (*BRAF* 35% and *MEK* 21%). The number of individuals with CFCS due to *KRAS* mutations is too small to allow meaningful comparison.

Pathogenesis of Cardiovascular Disease in the RASopathies

The Noonan Syndrome

A mouse bearing the *PTPN11* D61G mutation was generated using homologous recombination in embryonic stem cells [35]. The heterozygous mice recapitulated several aspects of the NS phenotype including CHD. Approximately one half of the *Ptpn11*$^{D61G/+}$ embryos had ventricular septal defects, double-outlet right ventricle and increased valve primordia size. Myocardial development was grossly normal. The other half of these embryos had mitral valve enlargement. The endocardial cushion cells had increased proliferation, decreased apoptosis and increased activation of the Mapks Erk1/2.

A second NS mouse model bearing a conditional *Ptpn11* D61Y allele was generated [36]. When expressed ubiquitously, the *Ptpn11* D61Y allele was embryonic lethal with enlarged developing valve cushions. Expression in the developing endocardium alone recapitulated the cardiac phenotype. In contrast, expression in the developing neural crest or myocardium did not alter cardiovascular development. Thus, expression in the developing endocardium appears to be crucial for the CHD observed in NS.

A mouse bearing the L613V mutation in the *Raf1* gene was generated using homologous recombination in embryonic stem cells [37]. This mouse model faithfully recapitulated the major phenotypic features of NS associated with *RAF1* mutations including HCM, evident as early as 2 weeks of age. Increased signaling through the RAS-MAPK pathway was apparent with increased activation of Mek and Erk in neonatal cardiomyocytes and cardiac fibroblasts with the L613V mutation. Treatment of *Raf1*$^{L613V/+}$ mice with a MEK inhibitor from 4 weeks of age resulted in reversal of HCM [34].

A mouse bearing the E846K mutation in the *SOS1* gene was generated using homologous recombination in embryonic stem cells [38]. This mouse model recapitulated phenotypic features of RASopathies, including aortic valve leaflet thickening that became apparent after age 8.5 months in 40% of the animals. In addition, 20% of the mice exhibited

4

HCM with increased signaling through RAS/Mapk and also the Rho GTPase Rac. As HCM is negatively associated with *SOS1* mutations in humans, these latter findings in this mouse model may be less informative.

The Noonan Syndrome with Multiple Lentigines

A mouse model of NSML was generated by introducing the Y279C mutation into the *Ptpn11* gene using homologous recombination in embryonic stem cells [39]. The phenotype of the *Ptpn11*$^{Y279C/+}$ mice recapitulated several aspects of the NSML phenotype, particularly HCM with postnatal onset. Consistent with prior biochemical analyses of NSML-associated SHP-2 mutant proteins, the Y279C Shp-2 in mouse hearts had diminished phosphatase activity. Impaired agonist-induced activation of the Mapks Erk1/2 was also observed. In contrast, Akt activation was significantly increased, which was consistent with previous findings obtained in vitro [40], as was its downstream target, the mTor pathway. Treatment of the *Ptpn11*$^{Y279C/+}$ mice with rapamycin, an mTor inhibitor, prevented or reversed HCM depending on the timing of the therapy.

The Costello Syndrome

A mouse model with the *HRAS* G12V mutation was generated through homologous recombination in embryonic stem cells [41]. The phenotype of the heterozygous mice recapitulates some aspects of CS, but the cardiovascular aspects are difficult to interpret. Specifically, these mice exhibited cardiac hyper trophy with fibrosis evident by 4 months of age, but systemic hypertension was also present. Treatment of the latter with the angiotensin-converting enzyme inhibitor captopril partially reversed the cardiac hypertrophy. Of interest, these mice also had aortic valve leaflet thickening, which was ameliorated through the captopril treatment. A conditional *Hras* allele may be needed to dissect the direct effects on the myocardium from the indirect ones.

Concluding Remarks

The RASopathies comprise several autosomal dominant disorders, NS being the most common, with overlapping cardiac and noncardiac features. While CHD and HCM are observed for all of these diagnoses, there are important differences in their relative prevalence as well as the distribution of CHD types. The elucidation of the genetic mutations for NS in particular has made clear that prognosis for important aspects, including the cardiovascular involvement, is dependent upon the genotype. Therefore, diagnostic genetic testing may be useful, particularly in an infant suspected of having a RASopathy. Ongoing studies of animal models suggest that treatment of RASopathy-associated HCM is possible, but will likely need to be gene/mutation specific. In addition, prevention of progression of valve stenosis using small molecules may also be plausible.

Acknowledgments

This manuscript was prepared with grant support from the National Institutes of Health (R01 HL071207) to B.D.G. and Telethon-Italy (GGP13107) to M.T.

References

1 Noonan J, Ehmke D: Associated non cardiac malformations in children with congenital heart disease. J Pediatr 1963;63:468–470.
2 Noonan JA: Hypertelorism with Turner phenotype. A new syndrome with associated congenital heart disease. Am J Dis Child 1968;116:373–380.
3 Shaw AC, Kalidas K, Crosby AH, Jeffery S, Patton MA: The natural history of Noonan syndrome: a long-term follow-up study. Arch Dis Child 2007;92:128–132.
4 Colquitt JL, Noonan JA: Cardiac findings in Noonan syndrome on long-term follow-up. Congenit Heart Dis 2014;9:144–150.
5 Hickey EJ, Mehta R, Elmi M, Asoh K, McCrindle BW, Williams WG, Manlhiot C, Benson L: Survival implications: hypertrophic cardiomyopathy in Noonan syndrome. Congenit Heart Dis 2011;6:41–47.
6 Wilkinson JD, Lowe AM, Salbert BA, Sleeper LA, Colan SD, Cox GF, Towbin JA, Connuck DM, Messere JE, Lipshultz SE: Outcomes in children with Noonan syndrome and hypertrophic cardiomyopathy: a study from the Pediatric Cardiomyopathy Registry. Am Heart J 2012;164:442–448.
7 Sanchez-Cascos A: The Noonan syndrome. Eur Heart J 1983;4:223–229.
8 Cornwall JW, Green RS, Nielsen JC, Gelb BD: Frequency of aortic dilation in Noonan syndrome. Am J Cardiol 2014;113:368–371.

9 Limongelli G, Pacileo G, Marino B, Digilio MC, Sarkozy A, Elliott P, Versacci P, Calabro P, De Zorzi A, Di Salvo G, Syrris P, Patton M, McKenna WJ, Dallapiccola B, Calabro R: Prevalence and clinical significance of cardiovascular abnormalities in patients with the LEOPARD syndrome. Am J Cardiol 2007;100:736–741.
10 Roberts A, Allanson J, Jadico SK, Kavamura MI, Noonan J, Opitz JM, Young T, Neri G: The cardiofaciocutaneous syndrome. J Med Genet 2006;43:833–842.
11 Lin AE, Alexander ME, Colan SD, Kerr B, Rauen KA, Noonan J, Baffa J, Hopkins E, Sol-Church K, Limongelli G, Digilio MC, Marino B, Innes AM, Aoki Y, Silberbach M, Delrue MA, White SM, Hamilton RM, O'Connor W, Grossfeld PD, Smoot LB, Padera RF, Gripp KW: Clinical, pathological, and molecular analyses of cardiovascular abnormalities in Costello syndrome: a Ras/MAPK pathway syndrome. Am J Med Genet A 2011;155A:486–507.
12 Tomita H, Fuse S, Ikeda K, Matsuda K, Chiba S: An infant with Costello syndrome complicated with fatal hypertrophic obstructive cardiomyopathy. Acta Paediatr Jpn 1998;40:608–611.
13 Mazzanti L, Cacciari E, Cicognani A, Bergamaschi R, Scarano E, Forabosco A: Noonan-like syndrome with loose anagen hair: a new syndrome? Am J Med Genet A 2003; 118A:279–286.
14 Gripp KW, Zand DJ, Demmer L, Anderson CE, Dobyns WB, Zackai EH, Denenberg E, Jenny K, Stabley DL, Sol-Church K: Expanding the SHOC2 mutation associated phenotype of Noonan syndrome with loose anagen hair: structural brain anomalies and myelofibrosis. Am J Med Genet A 2013;161: 2420–2430.
15 Komatsuzaki S, Aoki Y, Niihori T, Okamoto N, Hennekam RC, Hopman S, Ohashi H, Mizuno S, Watanabe Y, Kamasaki H, Kondo I, Moriyama N, Kurosawa K, Kawame H, Okuyama R, Imaizumi M, Rikiishi T, Tsuchiya S, Kure S, Matsubara Y: Mutation analysis of the SHOC2 gene in Noonan-like syndrome and in hematologic malignancies. J Hum Genet 2010;55:801–809.
16 Mazzanti L, Tamburrino F, Scarano E, Perri A, Vestrucci B, Guidetti M, Rossi C, Tartaglia M: GH therapy and first final height data in Noonan-like syndrome with loose anagen hair (Mazzanti syndrome). Am J Med Genet A 2013;161A:2756–2761.
17 Cordeddu V, Di Schiavi E, Pennacchio LA, Ma'ayan A, Sarkozy A, Fodale V, Cecchetti S, Cardinale A, Martin J, Schackwitz W, Lipzen A, Zampino G, Mazzanti L, Digilio MC, Martinelli S, Flex E, Lepri F, Bartholdi D, Kutsche K, Ferrero GB, Anichini C, Selicorni A, Rossi C, Tenconi R, Zenker M, Merlo D, Dallapiccola B, Iyengar R, Bazzicalupo P, Gelb BD, Tartaglia M: Mutation of SHOC2 promotes aberrant protein N-myristoylation and causes Noonan-like syndrome with loose anagen hair. Nat Genet 2009;41:1022–1026.
18 Tartaglia M, Mehler EL, Goldberg R, Zampino G, Brunner HG, Kremer H, van der Burgt I, Crosby AH, Ion A, Jeffery S, Kalidas K, Patton MA, Kucherlapati RS, Gelb BD: Mutations in PTPN11, encoding the protein tyrosine phosphatase SHP-2, cause Noonan syndrome. Nat Genet 2001;29:465–468.
19 Fragale A, Tartaglia M, Wu J, Gelb BD: Noonan syndrome-associated SHP2/PTPN11 mutants cause EGF-dependent prolonged GAB1 binding and sustained ERK2/MAPK1 activation. Hum Mutat 2004;23:267–277.
20 Tartaglia M, Gelb BD: Disorders of dysregulated signal traffic through the RAS-MAPK pathway: phenotypic spectrum and molecular mechanisms. Ann NY Acad Sci 2010; 1214:99–121.
21 Digilio MC, Conti E, Sarkozy A, Mingarelli R, Dottorini T, Marino B, Pizzuti A, Dallapiccola B: Grouping of multiple-lentigines/LEOPARD and Noonan syndromes on the PTPN11 gene. Am J Hum Genet 2002; 71:389–394.
22 Legius E, Schrander-Stumpel C, Schollen E, Pulles-Heintzberger C, Gewillig M, Fryns JP: PTPN11 mutations in LEOPARD syndrome. J Med Genet 2002;39:571–574.
23 Tartaglia M, Martinelli S, Stella L, Bocchinfuso G, Flex E, Cordeddu V, Zampino G, Burgt I, Palleschi A, Petrucci TC, Sorcini M, Schoch C, Foa R, Emanuel PD, Gelb BD: Diversity and functional consequences of germline and somatic PTPN11 mutations in human disease. Am J Hum Genet 2006; 78:279–290.
24 Kontaridis MI, Swanson KD, David FS, Barford D, Neel BG: PTPN11 (Shp2) mutations in LEOPARD syndrome have dominant negative, not activating, effects. J Biol Chem 2006;281:6785–6792.
25 Hanna N, Montagner A, Lee WH, Miteva M, Vidal M, Vidaud M, Parfait B, Raynal P: Reduced phosphatase activity of SHP-2 in LEOPARD syndrome: consequences for PI3K binding on Gab1. FEBS Lett 2006;580: 2477–2482.
26 Aoki Y, Niihori T, Kawame H, Kurosawa K, Ohashi H, Tanaka Y, Filocamo M, Kato K, Suzuki Y, Kure S, Matsubara Y: Germline mutations in HRAS proto-oncogene cause Costello syndrome. Nat Genet 2005;37: 1038–1040.
27 Aoki Y, Niihori T, Banjo T, Okamoto N, Mizuno S, Kurosawa K, Ogata T, Takada F, Yano M, Ando T, Hoshika T, Barnett C, Ohashi H, Kawame H, Hasegawa T, Okutani T, Nagashima T, Hasegawa S, Funayama R, Nakayama K, Inoue S, Watanabe Y, Ogura T, Matsubara Y: Gain-of-function mutations in RIT1 cause Noonan syndrome, a RAS/MAPK pathway syndrome. Am J Hum Genet 2013;93:173–180.
28 Roberts AE, Allanson JE, Tartaglia M, Gelb BD: Noonan syndrome. Lancet 2013;381: 333–342.
29 Tartaglia M, Kalidas K, Shaw A, Song X, Musat DL, van der Burgt I, Brunner HG, Bertola DR, Crosby A, Ion A, Kucherlapati RS, Jeffery S, Patton MA, Gelb BD: PTPN11 mutations in Noonan syndrome: molecular spectrum, genotype-phenotype correlation, and phenotypic heterogeneity. Am J Hum Genet 2002;70:1555–1563.
30 Lepri F, De Luca A, Stella L, Rossi C, Baldassarre G, Pantaleoni F, Cordeddu V, Williams BJ, Dentici ML, Caputo V, Venanzi S, Bonaguro M, Kavamura I, Faienza MF, Pilotta A, Stanzial F, Faravelli F, Gabrielli O, Marino B, Neri G, Silengo MC, Ferrero GB, Torrrente I, Selicorni A, Mazzanti L, Digilio MC, Zampino G, Dallapiccola B, Gelb BD, Tartaglia M: SOS1 mutations in Noonan syndrome: molecular spectrum, structural insights on pathogenic effects, and genotype-phenotype correlations. Hum Mutat 2011;32:760–772.
31 Pandit B, Sarkozy A, Pennacchio LA, Carta C, Oishi K, Martinelli S, Pogna EA, Schackwitz W, Ustaszewska A, Landstrom A, Bos JM, Ommen SR, Esposito G, Lepri F, Faul C, Mundel P, Lopez Siguero JP, Tenconi R, Selicorni A, Rossi C, Mazzanti L, Torrente I, Marino B, Digilio MC, Zampino G, Ackerman MJ, Dallapiccola B, Tartaglia M, Gelb BD: Gain-of-function RAF1 mutations cause Noonan and LEOPARD syndromes with hypertrophic cardiomyopathy. Nat Genet 2007;39:1007–1012.
32 Razzaque MA, Nishizawa T, Komoike Y, Yagi H, Furutani M, Amo R, Kamisago M, Momma K, Katayama H, Nakagawa M, Fujiwara Y, Matsushima M, Mizuno K, Tokuyama M, Hirota H, Muneuchi J, Higashinakagawa T, Matsuoka R: Germline gain-of-function mutations in RAF1 cause Noonan syndrome. Nat Genet 2007;39: 1013–1017.
33 Allanson JE, Anneren G, Aoki Y, Armour CM, Bondeson ML, Cave H, Gripp KW, Kerr B, Nystrom AM, Sol-Church K, Verloes A, Zenker M: Cardio-facio-cutaneous syndrome: does genotype predict phenotype? Am J Med Genet C Semin Med Genet 2011; 157C:129–135.
34 Abe Y, Aoki Y, Kuriyama S, Kawame H, Okamoto N, Kurosawa K, Ohashi H, Mizuno S, Ogata T, Kure S, Niihori T, Matsubara Y: Prevalence and clinical features of Costello syndrome and cardio-facio-cutaneous syndrome in Japan: findings from a nationwide epidemiological survey. Am J Med Genet A 2012;158A:1083–1094.

35 Araki T, Mohi MG, Ismat FA, Bronson RT, Williams IR, Kutok JL, Yang W, Pao LI, Gilliland DG, Epstein JA, Neel BG: Mouse model of Noonan syndrome reveals cell type- and gene dosage-dependent effects of Ptpn11 mutation. Nat Med 2004;10:849–857.
36 Araki T, Chan G, Newbigging S, Morikawa L, Bronson RT, Neel BG: Noonan syndrome cardiac defects are caused by PTPN11 acting in endocardium to enhance endocardial-mesenchymal transformation. Proc Natl Acad Sci U S A 2009;106:4736–4741.
37 Wu X, Simpson J, Hong JH, Kim KH, Thavarajah NK, Backx PH, Neel BG, Araki T: MEK-ERK pathway modulation ameliorates disease phenotypes in a mouse model of Noonan syndrome associated with the Raf1(L613V) mutation. J Clin Invest 2011;121:1009–1025.
38 Chen PC, Wakimoto H, Conner D, Araki T, Yuan T, Roberts A, Seidman CE, Bronson R, Neel BG, Seidman JG, Kucherlapati R: Activation of multiple signaling pathways causes developmental defects in mice with a Noonan syndrome-associated Sos1 mutation. J Clin Invest 2010;120:4353–4365.
39 Marin TM, Keith K, Davies B, Conner DA, Guha P, Kalaitzidis D, Wu X, Lauriol J, Wang B, Bauer M, Bronson R, Franchini KG, Neel BG, Kontaridis MI: Rapamycin reverses hypertrophic cardiomyopathy in a mouse model of LEOPARD syndrome-associated PTPN11 mutation. J Clin Invest 2011;121:1026–1043.
40 Edouard T, Combier JP, Nedelec A, Bel-Vialar S, Metrich M, Conte-Auriol F, Lyonnet S, Parfait B, Tauber M, Salles JP, Lezoualc'h F, Yart A, Raynal P: Functional effects of PTPN11 (SHP2) mutations causing LEOPARD syndrome on epidermal growth factor-induced phosphoinositide 3-kinase/AKT/glycogen synthase kinase 3beta signaling. Mol Cell Biol 2010;30:2498–2507.
41 Schuhmacher AJ, Guerra C, Sauzeau V, Canamero M, Bustelo XR, Barbacid M: A mouse model for Costello syndrome reveals an Ang II-mediated hypertensive condition. J Clin Invest 2008;118:2169–2179.
42 Marino B, Digilio MC, Toscano A, Giannotti A, Dallapiccola B: Congenital heart diseases in children with Noonan syndrome: an expanded cardiac spectrum with high prevalence of atrioventricular canal. J Pediatr 1999;135:703–706.

Dr. Bruce D. Gelb
Mindich Child Health and Development Institute
Departments of Pediatrics, and Genetics and Genomic Sciences
Icahn School of Medicine at Mount Sinai
One Gustave Levy Place
New York, NY, 10029 (USA)
E-Mail bruce.gelb@mssm.edu

Muenke M, Kruszka PS, Sable CA, Belmont JW (eds): Congenital Heart Disease: Molecular Genetics, Principles of Diagnosis and Treatment. Basel, Karger, 2015, pp 131–144
DOI: 10.1159/000375211

The Holt-Oram Syndrome and Other Transcription Factor-Related Heart Diseases

Jürgen Borlak[a] · Yari Ciribilli[b]

[a]Center for Pharmacology and Toxicology, Hannover Medical School, Hannover, Germany;
[b]Center for Integrative Biology, University of Trento, Mattarello, Italy

4

Abstract

The genetic basis of congenital heart diseases is largely unknown, and much of what we do know involves mutations in transcription factors expressed in the developing heart. In this chapter, we start with the first-described human cardiac transcription factor, *TBX5,* which is associated with the Holt-Oram syndrome. Although the Holt-Oram syndrome is a rare genetic disorder, occurring in 1 per 100,000 individuals, the cardiac malformations associated with this syndrome are common in the general population. Therefore, *TBX5* and other transcription factors involved in heart malformations are an important area of investigation. After introducing the Holt-Oram syndrome, we discuss the range of known transcriptions factors involved in congenital heart diseases, both germline and somatic ones. We conclude this chapter with a discussion evaluating the functional importance of the mutations identified in transcriptional factors.

The Holt-Oram Syndrome

The genetic basis for most congenital heart diseases (CHD) remains unknown, and much of our present knowledge is based on the role of transcription factors (TF), which regulate cardiac gene expression. The first autosomal dominant TF found to be associated with CHD was *TBX5*, which causes the Holt-Oram syndrome (HOS), a syndrome affecting heart and limb development [1, 2]. *TBX5* is a member of the T-box family of TF [1, 2]. The highly conserved T-box domain is the DNA binding region. TBX5 is discussed in detail below. Although the HOS is a rare genetic disorder, occurring in 1 per 100,000 individuals [1], the cardiac malformations associated with this syndrome are common in the general population, making *TBX5* and other TF involved in heart malformation an important research topic.

HOS, a multiple congenital anomaly characterized by limb and heart defects, was first described in

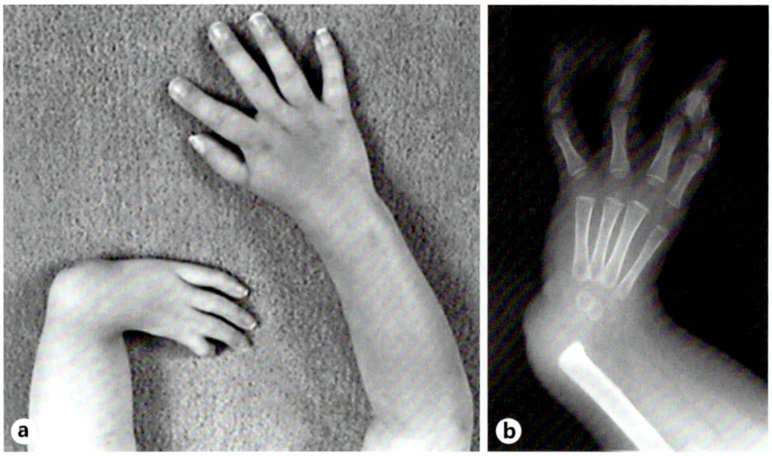

Fig. 1. **a** Clinical photograph of left radial longitudinal deficiency. Note the partial syndactyly between the index and middle fingers. **b** Radiograph of the same patient's left hand. The index ray is hypoplastic. Reprinted from Goldfarb und Wall [73] with permission from Elsevier.

1960 by Holt and Oram [3]. Heart anomalies include ostium secundum atrial septal defects (ASD) and ventricular septal defects (VSD), especially muscular-type VSD. Other heart lesions, including mitral valve prolapse, hypoplastic left-heart syndrome and persistent superior vena cava, have also been reported [4]. Approximately 75% of individuals with the HOS have cardiac malformations [1]. Cardiac conduction disease, including atrioventricular (AV) block and atrial fibrillation, may occur with or without heart malformations.

Limb defects include carpal, thenar, and radial bone malformations. The HOS has variable expression, with all individuals having carpal bone malformations with or without the other anomalies listed above [4]. Limb abnormalities may only be apparent radiographically, such as carpal bone malformations, or more severe thumb anomalies, such as triphalangism, aplasia, or phocomelia (fig. 1).

The management of the disease includes a multidisciplinary team of geneticists, cardiologists, and orthopedic specialists.

Transcription Factors and Embryogenesis

In the developing heart, two distinct sources of myocardial progenitor cells contribute to different parts of the heart, and this process is governed by a network and combinatorial interactions of TF. Essentially, within 8 weeks of embryogenesis, human heart development is complete. In a short span of time, the heart undergoes several stages of development, involving cardiac crescent formation, linear heart tube formation, cardiac looping, chamber formation and maturation, septation and valve formation (see chapter by Sylva and Moorman on the Normal Development of the Heart on p. 11). Independent studies have revealed that two distinct sources of myocardial progenitor cells, instead of one as was previously assumed, contribute to different parts of the heart [5]. The primary heart field contributes to the ventricles, the AV canal, and both atria, while the secondary heart field contributes to the outflow tract and all other heart regions, except for the left ventricle. The existence of these two distinct populations of cardiac progenitors may explain cardiac abnormalities in which specific segments of the heart are underdeveloped, while the remainder of the heart remains unaffected. Furthermore, organogenesis of the heart requires the sequential and timely interplay of regulatory master proteins, notably distinct TF [6, 7]. Such a network of TF connects signaling pathways with genes for muscle growth, patterning, and contractility.

A core set of evolutionarily conserved TF (NK2, MEF2, GATA, TBX, HRT, and HAND) controls cardiac cell fate, the expression of genes encoding contractile proteins, and the morphogenesis of cardiac structures (fig. 2) [8]. Hence, animal models help to define pathomechanisms of CHD. Notably, these TF also regulate each other's expression, serving to sta-

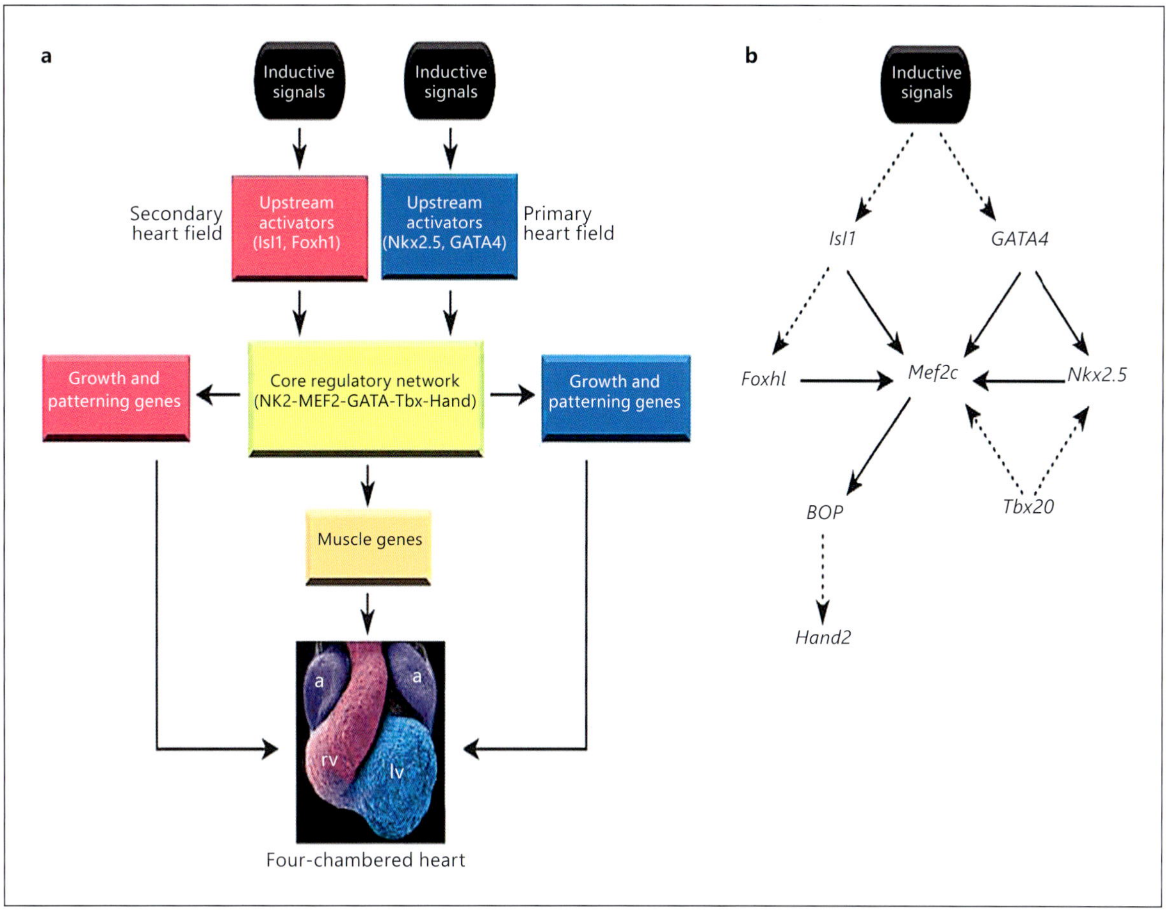

Fig. 2. Schematic of transcriptional networks involved in mammalian heart development. **a** Inductive signals activate a set of upstream regulatory genes encoding TF in the primary and secondary heart fields. The products of these genes activate the genes in the core cardiac network (NK2-MEF2-GATA-TBX-HAND). Some components of the network, such as Nkx2.5, are also activated in the primary heart field in response to inductive signals. The core network genes cross- and autoregulate their expression and serve as the central regulatory network for the activation of muscle-specific genes and genes that control the growth and patterning of derivatives of the primary and secondary heart fields. The primary heart field gives rise to the left ventricle (lv) and portions of the atria (a), whereas the secondary heart field gives rise to the right ventricle (rv), portions of the atria, and the outflow tract. A scanning electron micrograph of a mouse heart on embryonic day 14.5 is shown at the bottom. Derivatives of primary and secondary heart fields are shown in blue and pink, respectively. The atria, which are derived from the primary and secondary heart fields, are shown in purple (see online version for colors). **b** Regulatory interactions among cardiac TF in the secondary heart field. Solid lines indicate direct transcriptional connections and dotted lines indicate connections not yet shown to be direct. Source: Olson [8].

bilize and reinforce the cardiac gene program. Dozens of other TF contribute to cardiogenesis, and in many cases they serve as accessory factors for these core regulators. Different cardiac malformation phenotypes can be observed after knockout of TF genes in animal models [8, 9]. In mice lacking Nkx2.5, the initial events of heart formation occur normally, but embryos die from abnormal morphogenesis of the heart tube and failure in left-ventricular development. Mice lacking Hand2 do not form a right ventricle, and Hand1-mutant embryonic stem cells are unable to contribute to the outer curvature of the heart that gives rise to the left ventricle. Deletion of Hand2 and Nkx2.5 eliminates both ventricular chambers, leaving only an atrial remnant. Mice lacking Tbx5 display defects in the posterior region of the heart tube from which the atria are derived. Adding to complexity, combinatorial interactions of TF are

Table 1. Mutations in cardiac TF and structural proteins in CHD cases

Gene name	OMIM	Germline mutations, n	Disease classification	Mutations in sporadic CHD cases
NKX2.5	*600584	34, private	ASD, VSD, ToF	≤3%
GATA4	*600576	7	ASD, ToF	≤2%
TBX5	*601620	At least 49	HOS	
NKX2.6	NA	1	CAT	No info
ZIC3	*300265	3	TGA	
TBX20	*606061	2	Complex	No info
CRELD1	*607170	3	AVSD	~3–5%
NOTCH1	*190198	3	AVD	
MYH6	+160710	1	ASD	No info
CITED2	*602937	No info	ASD, VSD	~4%

CAT = Common arterial trunk; TGA = transposition of the great arteries; ToF = tetralogy of Fallot.

necessary in regulating cardiac gene expressions during this process [10, 11]. For example, the zinc finger TF Gata4 networks with other TF including Nkx2.5, Nf-At3, Mef2c, Hand2, and Fog2 to regulate cardiac gene expression [12, 13]. Recently, it has been shown that *TBX20* interacts physically, functionally, and genetically with other cardiac TF, including NKX2.5, GATA4, and TBX5 [14].

Germline Mutations

Germline mutations in cardiac TF genes have been identified in patients with CHD (fig. 3; table 1). Most mutations are heterozygous alleles, and the lack of individuals with homozygous mutations is suggestive of embryonic lethality associated with this genotype [15]. Mutations demonstrate variable expression, in which varied phenotypes even from the same mutation have been observed, suggesting further that other factors including coregulatory elements and epigenetic effects also play a role in disease manifestation.

In the case of *NKX2.5*, 34 different germline mutations in ASD and/or conduction defects have been reported in 13 studies [16–20], 33 of which are located in the coding region. But mutations so far identified are mostly familial, and individual families have unique mutations. No mutation has been associated with a specific clinical phenotype. Germline mutations are rare in sporadic cases of CHD [21, 22], and in the case of *NKX2.5* occur only in 3% of cases. Furthermore, many cases of CHD come from unaffected family members. For instance, 16 of 18 individuals with *NKX2.5* mutations had no family history of cardiac anomalies [21]. A population-

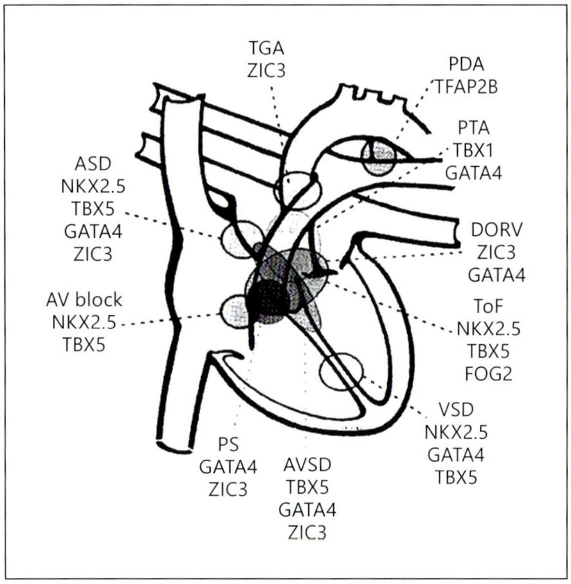

Fig. 3. Sites of structural anomalies associated with cardiac TF gene mutations. DORV = Double-outlet right ventricle; PDA = patent ductus arteriosus; PS = pulmonary stenosis; PTA = persistent truncus arteriosus; TGA = transposition of the great arteries; ToF = tetralogy of Fallot. Source: Clark et al. [15].

based study investigated the genotypes of five known germline *NKX2.5* mutations in 227 babies with CHD, but did not find any evidence of these germline mutations [23].

Five *GATA4* mutations have been identified in families with CHD, notably ASD [18, 24, 25], but *GATA4* germline mutations are also rather rare. Two studies analyzed 16 families each, but only 2 of the 16 families with multiply affected members carried *GATA4* mutations [17, 18]. In 42 patients with nonsyndromic AV septal defects (AVSD; familial as well as sporadic), no *GATA4* mutations have been detected [26]. Further studies on unrelated patients found similar results. Screening of 99 Danish patients with different CHD phenotypes did not identify *GATA4* mutations [27]. Analysis of 157 unrelated patients with nonsyndromic CHD of variable ethnicity (76 European Americans, 53 Hispanics, 21 African-Americans, and 7 Asians) did not identify disease-associated mutations [28]. In sporadic cases of CHD from a Lebanese population, a search for mutations affecting the zinc finger and basic region of *GATA4* were analyzed [29]. A mutation (p.E216D) in the N-terminal zinc finger was detected in 2 of 26 patients with tetralogy of Fallot, and this mutation resulted in reduced transcriptional activity without affecting the ability of GATA4 to bind to DNA or its interaction with ZFPM2 (FOG2). However, none of the other 94 patients with various CHD phenotypes carried a *GATA4* mutation.

As discussed above, mutations in the human *TBX5* gene cause HOS, a disorder characterized by heart and upper limb deformities. Although at least 49 sequence alterations leading to a truncated or nontruncated TBX5 protein have been found in familial and sporadic cases of HOS (http://www.medizin.uni-leipzig.de/~genetik/TBX5) [30, 31], the mutation detection rate can be as low as 22–35% [32]. These alterations include single-base substitutions, additions, deletions, translocations as well as exonic deletions. Hand and heart malformations in HOS vary considerably, even among affected family members who share an identical *TBX5* mutation.

Mutations in other cardiac TF genes have been identified, too. For instance, gene linkage analysis in a family of 6 individuals affected by a common arterial trunk identified an amino acid substitution, p.F151L, at position 20 of the homeodomain of the TF NKX2.6 [33]. Functional analysis of this mutation revealed diminished transcriptional activation, and the corresponding mutation in NKX2.5 reduced DNA binding to target promoters in conjunction with GATA4 and TBX5.

Several mutations in the zinc finger TF *ZIC3* have been identified in heterotaxy as well as isolated CHD [34–36]. In a recent study, the frequency of *ZIC3* mutations in 42 transpositions of the great arteries has been investigated [37]. A mutation in the X chromosome at the *ZIC3* gene was found in 2 affected siblings (1 male and 1 female) and their unaffected mother. In this family, the missense mutation (p.W255G) was found in the first zinc finger of *ZIC3*, a domain that is relatively specific to each of the five human ZIC genes. A second factor, a skewed X-inactivation pattern, explained the discrepancy between the daughter/mother phenotype.

Nonsense (p.Q195X) and missense (p.I152M) germline mutations within the T-box DNA binding domain of human *TBX20* were associated with a family history of CHD and a complex spectrum of developmental anomalies, including defects in septation, chamber growth, and valvulogenesis [14]. Biophysical characterization of wild-type and mutant proteins indicated how the missense mutation disrupts the structure and function of the TBX20 T-box. These findings firstly link *TBX20* mutations to human pathology.

In addition to cardiac TF genes, mutations in other genes have been identified, such as in *CRELD1*, a gene expressed in the development of AV endocardial cushions, which encodes a cell surface protein that likely functions as a cell adhesion molecule. A study investigating 50 individuals with AVSD identified three missense mutations in *CRELD1* that are specifically associated with AVSD [38]. Analysis of the DNA from family members of one of the patients with a partial AVSD in which a missense mutation (p.R329C) was identified showed that the mutation was inherited from the father. The sister of this patient also carried the mutation. Two-dimensional echocardiography and color Doppler studies indicated that the father and sister had structurally and functionally normal hearts, demonstrating incomplete penetrance of this *CRELD1* variant. In a later study, another missense mutation in an individual with a partial AVSD that was also incompletely penetrant was identified [39]. Together these results suggest that *CRELD1* mutations act in a dominant manner with incomplete penetrance and that *CRELD1* is an AVSD susceptibility gene that may act in concert with additional modifier genes at other loci. No pathogenic mutations in an additional 31 individuals with isolated AVSD were observed [26]. Collectively, patient studies indicate that *CRELD1* mutations occur in about 3% of euploid individuals with AVSD, most frequently in cases of partial AVSD. About 4.5% of individuals with partial AVSD have a *CRELD1* mutation. Furthermore, two heterozygous missense mutations in 2 unrelated subjects with Down syndrome and AVSD have been identified [40]. Identification of *CRELD1* mutations in 2 of 39 individuals (5.1%) with Down syndrome and complete AVSD suggests that defects in *CRELD1* may contribute to the pathogenesis of AVSD in the context of trisomy 21.

It is also of considerable importance that mutations in the signaling and transcriptional regulator NOTCH1 cause a spectrum of developmental anomalies and severe valve calcification in nonsyndromic autosomal-dominant human pedigrees. A large family with autosomal-dominant aortic valve disease consisting of bicuspid aortic valve and aortic valve calcification was studied using genome-wide linkage analysis. This led to the identification of a nonsense mutation in NOTCH1 in affected individuals. This finding was supported by the discovery of a NOTCH1 frameshift mutation in an unrelated family with similar aortic valve disease, suggesting that NOTCH1 haploinsufficiency was a genetic cause of aortic valve malformations and calcification [41, 42]. A further study detected two novel missense mutations (p.T596M and p.P1797H) in *NOTCH1* in patients with bicuspid aortic valve [43].

In a large family with dominantly inherited ASD, a missense substitution (I820N) was identified in an α-myosin heavy chain (MYH6), a structural protein expressed at high levels in the developing atria, which affects the binding of the heavy chain to its regulatory light chain [44]. The cardiac TF TBX5 strongly regulates MYH6 expression, but mutant forms of TBX5, which cause HOS, do not. Morpholino knock-down of the expression of the chick Myh6 homologue eliminates the formation of the atrial septum without overtly affecting atrial chamber formation. These data provide evidence for a link between a TF, a structural protein, and CHD.

Functionally relevant mutations in *CITED2* have been identified in patients with CHD [45]. *CITED2* encodes a CREBBP/EP300 interacting transcriptional modulator of HIF1A and TFAP2. Analysis of 392 well-characterized patients and 192 control individuals using denaturing high-performance liquid chromatography, sequencing, and Amplifluor genotyping techniques, 15 *CITED2* nucleotide alterations were identified. Seven of these alterations were found only in CHD patients and were not detected in controls, including three mutations leading to amino acid sequence alterations (p.Ser170_Gly178del, p.Gly178_Ser179ins9, and p.Ser198_Gly199del). These mutations significantly reduced the capacity of CITED2 to transrepress HIF1A, and that the p.Ser170_Gly178del mutation significantly diminished TFAP2C coactivation.

In summary, germline gene mutations have been identified in CHD, but the detection level is low and mutations are mostly familial cases. So far, no germline mutations have been detected in *HEY2* [46–48], and *PTPN11* mutations play a minor role in isolated CHD [49].

Somatic Mutations

Usually genetic studies on CHD are based on blood samples (lymphocytic DNA), and this type of analysis may not reveal complete genetic alterations leading to the disease, as has been shown in the autoimmune lymphoproliferative syndrome (ALPS), a disease of the immune system [50]. ALPS is characterized by lymphoproliferation, autoimmunity, and abundant double-negative T cells, and this disease has been associated with germline mutations in the gene that encodes the FAS protein, a cell surface receptor and a mediator of programmed cell death or apoptosis. Most patients with ALPS have heterozygous *FAS* mutations leading to a defective protein, but others lack mutations in the DNA from whole blood lymphocytes. In this latter type of ALPS patients (ALPS type III), analysis of *FAS* in double-negative T cells revealed mutations which were absent in hair or mucosal epithelial cells. This study clearly demonstrates that somatic mutations can cause an autoimmune disease, and that cells within the site of the defect should be examined for genetic alterations.

Notably, somatic mutations are well known in cancer, but there is now evidence that such mutations can cause disease in nonmalignant settings as well [51–53]. Examples of disorders due to somatic mutations include, besides ALPS, neurofibromatosis 1 and 2, and the McCune-Albright syndrome. Somatic mutations can arise in discrete cell lineages early in embryonic development or during postnatal life, and their implications for disease depend on the stage they arise. Somatic mutations that arise early during embryogenesis may affect the structure, function, and survival of tissues derived from that cell lineage. Furthermore, somatic mutations and mosaicism in congenital heart anomalies is a possible molecular rationale, since many cases of CHD are sporadic. Somatic mosaicism refers to the condition in which a mutation arises after fertilization such that only a subset of cells or tissues harbors the defects. The review of Weismann and Gelb [54] pointed out that many of the genes that control cardiac development also play critical roles in the development of other organ systems. As such, germline inheritance of mutations for these genes may not be compatible with the survival of the developing embryo and, in any case, would not likely cause only CHD. Moreover, mutations in relevant genes are found in a very small percentage of isolated CHD, suggesting that investigators might be examining the wrong portions of genes (i.e. the coding region) or the wrong tissue (the vast majority using DNA obtained from peripheral blood).

To elucidate genetic alterations in the malformed heart, genetic analysis of cardiac TF genes, such as *NKX2.5, TBX5, GATA4, MEF2C, HEY2, HAND1,* and *HAND2,* was performed on 68 formalin-fixed hearts of patients with CHD, the so called 'Leipzig collection of malformed hearts' (fig. 4). These hearts were obtained from the Institute of Anatomy, University of Leipzig, and from part of the collection made by Dr. F. Spreer from 1954 to 1982 at the Institute of Pathology, University of Leipzig, and the District Hospital Borna, Germany. The explanted malformed hearts were classified by sequential segmental analysis according to their septal defects into 29 VSD, 16 ASD and 23 AVSD, but they were also affected with other complex malformations [55]. Most patients died at birth or in early infancy. Four patients within VSD and 14 patients with AVSD had the Down syndrome. Surprisingly, direct sequencing of genes such as *NKX2.5* [55, 56], *TBX5* [57], and *GATA4* [58] revealed mutations in diseased heart tissues, which were mainly absent in normal heart tissues of the same CHD patients. Even more unexpected was the frequent appearance of multiple mutations and different haplotypes. Altogether, these results suggest a somatic origin of mutations and genomic instability in the diseased cardiac tissues of patients with CHD. The detection of multiple mutations may be explained by a mixed population of cardiomyocytes carrying different mutations or de novo chromosomal rearrangements and gene duplications. However, the frequency and the occurrence of multiple mutations (i.e. haplotypes) suggest novel mechanisms of genetic changes such as gene conversion from a pseudogene.

Through collaborative efforts, the functional consequences of single and multiple somatic mutations of *NKX2.5* have been investigated [59]. An assay was developed to determine the clinical significance in the budding yeast *Saccharomyces cerevisiae* that could determine the transactivation capacity and specificity of the patient's *NKX2.5* alleles expressed towards targeted response element (RE) sequences (for description of the assay see Inga [59]). This research focused on mutants of the third helix, which provides DNA binding specificity, and characterized mutations that were highly associated with either VSD or AVSD. Individual mutants exhibited partial to complete loss of function as well as differences in the transactivation capacity between the various RE. The mutants also exhibited gene dosage rather than dominant effects on transcription. Surprisingly, nearly all AVSD patients (22/23)

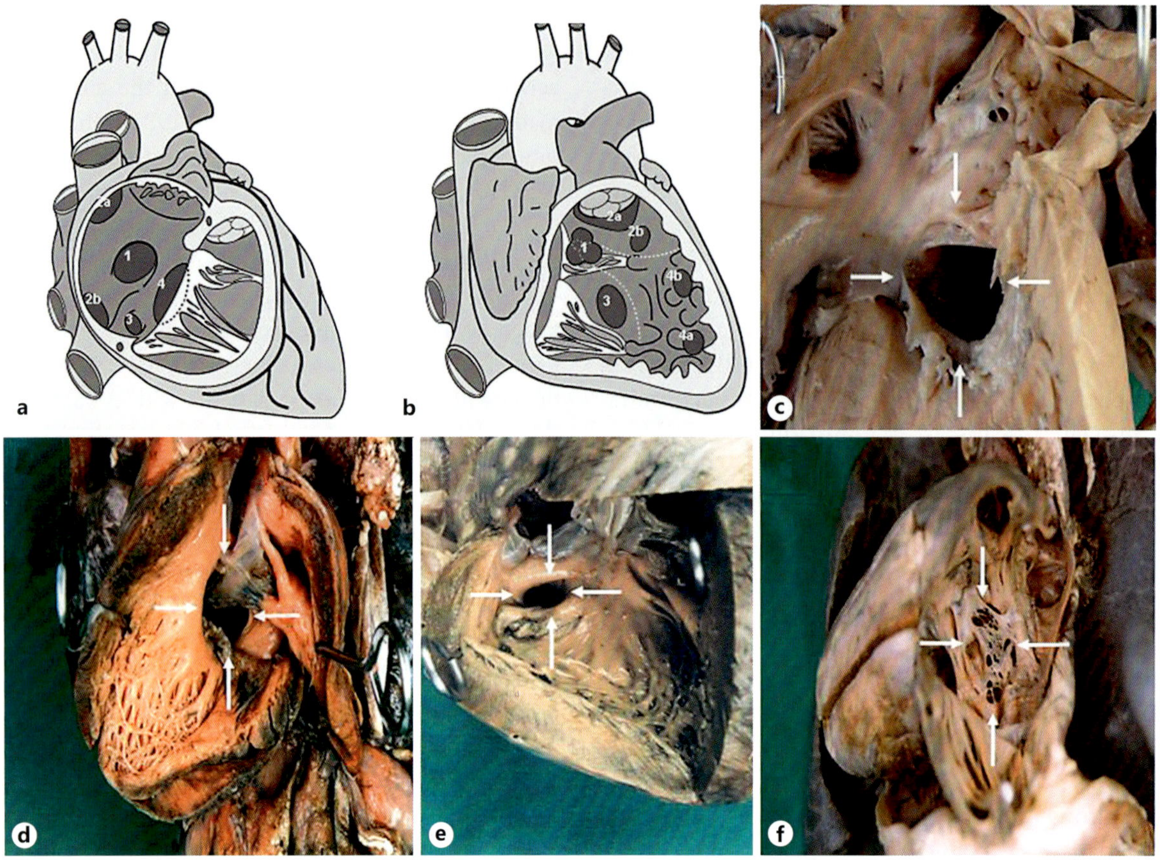

Fig. 4. Examples from the Leipzig collection of malformed hearts. Source: Reamon-Buettner et al. [55]. **a** Diagram showing the classification of defects with interatrial shunt. 1 = ASD at fossa ovalis (ostium secundum type); 2a = ASD at superior vena cava ostium (sinus venosus type); 2b = ASD at inferior vena cava ostium (sinus venosus type); 3 = ASD at coronary sinus ostium (sinus coronarius type); 4 = AVSD (ostium primum type). **b** Diagram showing the classification of defects with interventricular shunt. Inlet, trabecular, and infundibular septal components are separated by dotted lines. 1 = VSD at the membranous septum – subaortic (perimembranous septal defect); 2a = VSD of the outlet septum – subarterial/subvalvar; 2b = VSD of the outlet septum not related to arterial valves; 3 = VSD of the inlet septum (central muscular septal defect); 4a = VSD of the apical septum – central (centroapical muscular septal defect); 4b = VSD of apical septum – marginal. **c, d** Large AVSD (arrows). **e** Muscular VSD (arrows). **f** Arrows: ASD (ostium secundum type). Copyright information: http://www.ncbl.nlm.nih.gov/pmc/articles/PMC1615780/figure/F1-4116/.

had a single K183E mutation that resulted in transcriptional inactivation. None of the VSD patients had this mutation; yet 14 of 29 patients had at least one mutation in the third helix leading to either inactivation of or reduction in *NKX2.5* transactivation. Therefore, mutations in the binding domains of NKX2.5 were associated specifically with AVSD or VSD and resulted in loss of protein function. Furthermore, patients were found who had combined mutations in different binding domains of TF. For instance, Reamon-Buettner et al. [60] identified 21 patients with combined mutations in the *GATA4* zinc fingers and the homeodomain of *NKX2.5*. Breakdown of TF cross talks is a likely cause of complex CHD.

Gene Reporter Assays to Evaluate the Clinical Significance of Mutations

Next to genetic analysis, it is important to evaluate the functional importance of the mutation identified. In the past, we reported the functional dissection of sequence-specific *NKX2.5* DNA bind-

Table 2. Comparison of yeast and mammalian reporter assay systems

Gene/ mutant allele	Results in yeast	Study, year	Results in human cell models/ predictions	Study, year
NKX2.5				
T178M	Loss of function	Reamon-Buettner et al. [58], 2005	Loss of function	Kasahara [75], 2000
K183E	Loss of function	Reamon-Buettner et al. [58], 2005	Loss of function	Leng et al. [76], 2011
Q187X	Loss of function	Reamon-Buettner et al. [58], 2005	Loss of function	Ouyang and Xin [77], 2011
K194R	Partial function	Reamon-Buettner et al. [58], 2005	No effect	SNPeffect Database [78]
A219V	Partial function	Reamon-Buettner et al. [58], 2005	No effect	SNPeffect dababase [78]
HAND1				
L28H	Wt like	Reamon-Buettner et al. [74], 2010	Wt like/neutral	Reamon-Buettner et al. [74], 2010
A126Fs	Loss of function	Reamon-Buettner et al. [74], 2010	Loss of function	Reamon-Buettner et al. [74], 2010
L138P	Loss of function	Reamon-Buettner et al. [74], 2010	Loss of function	Reamon-Buettner et al. [74], 2010
TP63				
G134D	Partial function	Monti et al. [79], 2013	Partial function	Monti et al. [79], 2013
G134V	Partial function	Monti et al. [79], 2013	Partial function	Monti et al. [79], 2013
R204W	Loss of function	Monti et al. [79], 2013	Loss of function	Monti et al. [79], 2013
TP53				
>100 alleles tested in yeast and in mammalian cell assays with a very high correlation of results.			IARC TP53 Database [80]	

ing domain mutations associated with human heart septation defects using a yeast-based system. Notably, the budding yeast *S. cerevisiae* has been successfully employed to investigate transcriptional responses. For its simplicity in genetic manipulation and cultivation, this single-cell lower eukaryotic organism gained popularity in the scientific community and was rightly considered to be a 'honorary mammalian' [61]. The similarities between yeast and mammalian cells are striking, and examples of findings obtained with mutant alleles in yeast and mammalian reporter systems are given in table 2.

The yeast transcriptional assay system is versatile and particularly recommended for the analysis of genetic defects targeting TF. Many basal transcription-associated factors are highly conserved, and the yeast and human TBP (TATA-box binding proteins) share >80% sequence identity and can therefore be considered interchangeable in function when RNA polymerase II-dependent transcription is investigated [62]. Even the large subunit of RNA polymerase II is highly conserved [63]. Moreover, chromatin remodelers are conserved and both the yeast and mammalian systems share analogous complexes with histone acetyl-transferase function, for example [64]. However, TAF (TATA-box associated factors) are conserved to a lesser extent [65]. With the aid of the yeast functional assay, mutations identified in *NKX2.5* [59, 66], HAND1 [67, 68], and *GATA4* were investigated by taking advantage of the following system attributes.

'Isogenic Nature'

The isogenic nature of the system can minimize the variability in results. Studying TF capabilities and specificities in yeast cells is generally achieved through the cloning of the TF binding site or TF-RE upstream a of particular reporter gene (the luciferase gene for example). In this way, a vast group of yeast strains, which differ only in the DNA sequence they would bind, can be easily generated, using a well-defined genetic engineering technique called *'Delitto Perfetto'* approach [69, 70]. The name of this experimental approach came from the Italian translation of 'perfect murder', since the method does not leave evidence and can be considered synonymous for 'perfect deletion.' The process is dependent on RAD52 (a protein that shares similarity to the *S. cerevisiae* protein Rad52 and is important for DNA double-strand break repair) and exploits the homologous recombination DNA repair machine of yeast cells using integrative oligonucleotides containing the desired response sequence flanked by regions that will find homology with the target selection cassette on the yeast genome. The yeast strains that the researcher obtains are genetically equal except for the DNA that regulates the reporter gene expression. This enables researchers to understand the transcriptional features of the studied TF. With the aim to elucidate the transcriptional capabilities of cardiac-specific TF, we have generated many isogenic yeast reporter strains where the RE are present within target gene promoters, placed immediately upstream the reporter gene, i.e. ANF (atrial natriuretic factor) or ECE (endothelin-converting enzyme). When appropriate, ad hoc generated artificial RE (or superresponse sequence) can be obtained as well (i.e. a sequence that perfectly matches the consensus site of the studied TF or a multimeric consensus site to increase the responsiveness to the TF).

'Chromatin Environment'

The chromatin environment where the functionality of a particular TF is analyzed can be considered constant. This reflects the nature of the characteristic described in the isogenic section. Since the TF-RE is located in a specific genomic location, the organization of chromatin will be at least very similar among different isogenic strains. This characteristic will strengthen the importance of subtle modifications in the intrinsic responsiveness of the DNA sequence that guides the expression of the reporter gene. The mammalian endogenous genomic location can be very different among different RE sites, at least in terms of chromatin accessibility and nucleosome repositioning. In the yeast system, the researcher is able to register the specific effect on direct DNA binding.

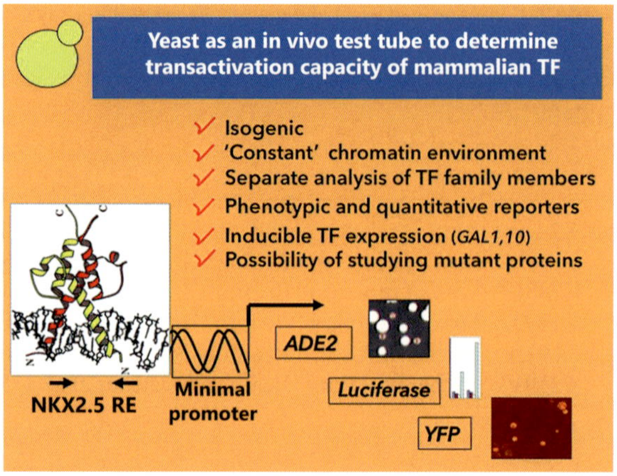

Fig. 5. Different versions of the reporter gene have been developed. ADE2 (i), luciferase (ii), and GFP or YFP.

'Reporter Constructs'

Many different versions of the reporter gene have been developed (fig. 5). We need to distinguish between qualitative (also known as phenotypic, where the differences can be seen directly) and quantitative reporters (where the researcher can measure and therefore quantitate the effects observed). Different examples of reporters include: (i) ADE2, (ii) luciferase (LUC), and (iii) fluorescent proteins, e.g. GFP (green fluorescent protein) or YFP (yellow fluorescent proteins. In (i) ADE2, the first historical version of the assay, the studied TF-RE is placed upstream of a gene involved in the biosynthesis of adenine. Yeast cells transformed with an expression plasmid harboring the wild-type cDNA of the studied TF will generate normal-shaped white colonies on selective plates containing a limited amount of adenine. When TF is not able to transactivate the reporter gene, the ADE2 protein is not produced and yeast colonies will turn red, since a red-colored intermediate within the adenine biosynthetic pathway will accumulate. Nowadays, the luciferase gene from the firefly *Photinus pyralis* (ii) is the most used reporter gene. In this case, the transactivation of the luciferase gene will produce a protein that when added to the correct substrates (luciferin with hydrogen peroxide and ATP) will trigger a chemoluminescent reaction generating light that can be measured by readers (luminometers). We have recently miniaturized the yeast luciferase assay to make it amenable for high-throughput screening of molecules and cofactors that modify the transcriptional capacity of TF [71]. (iii) Beyond luciferase, the production of fluorescent proteins such as GFP or YFP can be registered using fluorimeters.

Furthermore, the yeast system allows for separate analysis of different TF or TF family members. Since many mammalian (or human) TF do not have yeast homologues, the effect of their expression can be analyzed in a cleaner cellular model, avoiding the confusing impact of endogenously expressed proteins of the same family.

'Rheostatable Promoters'

In the yeast system, the expression of a TF can be inducible through the cloning of TF cDNA under the control of the rheostatable *GAL1* promoter that provides for highly controlled expression of the desired proteins. When the yeast cells are grown in a glucose-containing medium, the *GAL1* promoter is repressed. In raffinose medium, the *GAL1* promoter is de-repressed but still not induced, resulting in basal levels of expression. Variable expression is then achieved by the addition of increasing amounts of galactose. Depending on the concentration of galactose, the expression can be varied over a big fold range. This characteristic provides for the possibility to study the TF transactivation potential at various levels of expression. This can also enable the detection of even subtle differences that can be visible if the TF is expressed only at very low levels, something that could not be determined with a constitutive promoter (i.e. *ADH1* promoter).

'Mutant Protein Assays'

The yeast system is particularly amenable for studying mutant proteins. Since the most powerful feature is the ability to study wild-type TF in a clean model, the impact of point mutations on the binding, multimerization, or recruitment of basal transcriptional machinery capacities can be easily achieved. With this approach, we have studied some mutants affecting the NKX2.5 gene (more extensively the K183E mutant) associated with the HOS syndrome as well as other diseases that affect the correct development of cardiac muscle such as AVSD and VSD. The system has enabled us to detect even subtle defects of particular mutants or single nucleotide polymorphisms or even nonsynonymous changes in a family affected by both AVSD and hypoplastic left-heart syndrome [66].

However, some caveats in the use of the yeast system need to be considered:

New Transactivation Motifs. In the yeast system, TF with transactivation domains (TAD) that are relatively new, evolutionary speaking, do not work. However, acidic TAD, such as the ones present in some TF like the tumor suppressor p53 or estrogen receptors, can easily activate transcription in yeast. Usually, this weakness is overcome using chimeras. For example cardiac TF such as NKX2.5, HAND1, and GATA4 containing proline- or glutamine-rich TAD are less active or completely inactive, and for this reason do not function in the yeast system [72]. We solved this problem through the generation of chimeras where the TAD from p53 (an acidic TAD – known to effectively induce transcription activation in yeast) was fused at the N terminus of all these cardiac TF, stimulating the transactivation potential.

Artificial Design. The yeast system is normally designed for relative short promoter- or enhancer-containing sequences; often only the TF binding sites are placed upstream of the reporter gene. This might affect the responsiveness of certain target sequences where the flanking regions or the co-presence of adjacent regulatory elements play important roles.

Cofactors. Critical cofactors important for the transcriptional regulation may be absent. In the physiologic environment, most of the TF recruit critical co-activator or co-repressor complexes able to influence the final outcome. This cannot be observed with the yeast functional assay unless ectopically expressed.

Permeability. The yeast system can be used relatively easily as a high-throughput screening technology for testing small molecules able to stimulate or repress the function of a TF. However, the permeability of yeast cells to different compounds can be variable due to the presence of the cell wall that is surrounding the plasma membrane, an additional barrier to molecules coming from outside the

4

cell. Indeed, bulky compounds can be excluded from the target cells. This can be bypassed by generating yeast cells lacking the cell wall, called 'spheroplasts', through enzymatic digestion (achieved by lyticase or zymolase enzymes), that are more vulnerable but still viable. Moreover, the effectiveness of a particular compound can be reduced by the presence of efficient outflow pumps, such as the ABC transporter PDR5 and the regulator of its expression PDR1. We bypassed this problem through the generation of yeast strains lacking these nonessential genes [71].

Conclusion

TF have provided much of the understanding of the genetic basis of congenital heart malformations. However, germline mutations in TF such as *TBX5* only explain a small fraction of CHD. Our research in somatic mutations and emerging research in epigenetics and noncoding regions of the genome along with the risk of gene-environment interactions will supply more answers to this puzzle.

References

1 Basson CT, Bachinsky DR, Lin RC, et al: Mutations in human TBX5 [corrected] cause limb and cardiac malformation in Holt-Oram syndrome. Nat Genet 1997;15:30–35, erratum 411.

2 Li QY, Newbury-Ecob RA, Terrett JA, et al: Holt-Oram syndrome is caused by mutations in TBX5, a member of the Brachyury (T) gene family. Nat Genet 1997;15:21–29.

3 Holt M, Oram S: Familial heart disease with skeletal malformations. Br Heart J 1960;22:236–242.

4 Basson CT, Cowley GS, Solomon SD, et al: The clinical and genetic spectrum of the Holt-Oram syndrome (heart-hand syndrome). N Engl J Med 1994;330:885–891.

5 Buckingham M, Meilhac S, Zaffran S: Building the mammalian heart from two sources of myocardial cells. Nat Rev Genet 2005;6:826–835.

6 Bruneau BG: Transcriptional regulation of vertebrate cardiac morphogenesis. Circ Res 2002;90.509–519.

7 Harvey RP: Patterning the vertebrate heart. Nat Rev Genet 2002;3:544–556.

8 Olson EN: Gene regulatory networks in the evolution and development of the heart. Science 2006;313:1922–1927.

9 Gruber PJ, Epstein JA: Development gone awry: congenital heart disease. Circ Res 2004;94:273–283.

10 Nemer G, Nemer M: Regulation of heart development and function through combinatorial interactions of transcription factors. Ann Med 2001;33:604–610.

11 Sepulveda JL, Vlahopoulos S, Iyer D, et al: Combinatorial expression of GATA4, Nkx2-5, and serum response factor directs early cardiac gene activity. J Biol Chem 2002;277:25775–25782.

12 Molkentin JD: The zinc finger-containing transcription factors GATA-4, -5, and -6. Ubiquitously expressed regulators of tissue-specific gene expression. J Biol Chem 2000;275:38949–38952.

13 Pikkarainen S, Tokola H, Kerkelä R, Ruskoaho H: GATA transcription factors in the developing and adult heart. Cardiovasc Res 2004;63:196–207.

14 Kirk EP, Sunde M, Costa MW, et al: Mutations in cardiac T-box factor gene *TBX20* are associated with diverse cardiac pathologies, including defects of septation and valvulogenesis and cardiomyopathy. Am J Hum Genet 2007;81:280–291.

15 Clark KL, Yutzey KE, Benson DW: Transcription factors and congenital heart defects. Annu Rev Physiol 2006;68:97–121.

16 Kasahara H, Benson DW: Biochemical analyses of eight NKX2.5 homeodomain missense mutations causing atrioventricular block and cardiac anomalies. Cardiovasc Res 2004;64:40–51.

17 Hirayama-Yamada K, Kamisago M, Akimoto K, et al: Phenotypes with GATA4 or NKX2.5 mutations in familial atrial septal defect. Am J Med Genet A 2005;135:47–52.

18 Sarkozy A, Conti E, Neri C, et al: Spectrum of atrial septal defects associated with mutations of NKX2.5 and GATA4 transcription factors. J Med Genet 2005;42:e16.

19 Gutierrez-Roelens I, De Roy L, Ovaert C, et al: A novel CSX/NKX2-5 mutation causes autosomal-dominant AV block: are atrial fibrillation and syncopes part of the phenotype? Eur J Hum Genet 2006;14:1313–1316.

20 Rifai L, Maazouzi W, Sefiani A: Novel point mutation in the NKX2-5 gene in a Moroccan family with atrioventricular conduction disturbance and an atrial septal defect in the oval fossa. Cardiol Young 2006;17:107–109.

21 McElhinney DB, Geiger E, Blinder J, et al: NKX2.5 mutations in patients with congenital heart disease. J Am Coll Cardiol 2003;42:1650–1655.

22 Elliott DA, Kirk EP, Yeoh T, et al: Cardiac homeobox gene NKX2-5 mutations and congenital heart disease: associations with atrial septal defect and hypoplastic left heart syndrome. J Am Coll Cardiol 2003;41:2072–2076.

23 Hobbs CA, Cleves MA, Keith C, et al: NKX2.5 and congenital heart defects: a population-based study. Am J Med Genet A 2005;134:223–225.

24 Garg V, Kathiriya IS, Barnes R, et al: GATA4 mutations cause human congenital heart defects and reveal an interaction with TBX5. Nature 2003;424:443–447.

25 Okubo A, Miyoshi O, Baba K, et al: A novel GATA4 mutation completely segregated with atrial septal defect in a large Japanese family. J Med Genet 2004;41:e97.

26 Sarkozy A, Esposito G, Conti E, et al: CRELD1 and GATA4 gene analysis in patients with nonsyndromic atrioventricular canal defects. Am J Med Genet A 2005;139:236–238.

27 Zhang L, Tümer Z, Jacobsen JR, et al: Screening of 99 Danish patients with congenital heart disease for GATA4 mutations. Genet Test 2006;10:277–280.

28 Schluterman MK, Krysiak AE, Kathiriya IS, et al: Screening and biochemical analysis of GATA4 sequence variations identified in patients with congenital heart disease. Am J Med Genet A 2007;143:817–823.

29 Nemer G, Fadlalah F, Usta J, et al: A novel mutation in the GATA4 gene in patients with tetralogy of Fallot. Hum Mutat 2006;27:293–294.

30 Mori AD, Bruneau BG: TBX5 mutations and congenital heart disease: Holt-Oram syndrome revealed. Curr Opin Cardiol 2004;19:211–215.

31 Borozdin W, Bravo Ferrer Acosta AM, Bamshad MJ, et al: Expanding the spectrum of TBX5 mutations in Holt-Oram syndrome: detection of two intragenic deletions by quantitative real time PCR, and report of eight novel point mutations. Hum Mutat 2006;27:975–976.
32 Debeer P, Race V, Gewillig M, et al: Novel TBX5 mutations in patients with Holt-Oram syndrome. Clin Orthop Relat Res 2007;462:20–26.
33 Heathcote K, Braybrook C, Abushaban L, et al: Common arterial trunk associated with a homeodomain mutation of NKX2.6. Hum Mol Genet 2005;14:585–593.
34 Gebbia M, Ferrero GB, Pilia G, et al: X-linked situs abnormalities result from mutations in ZIC3. Nat Genet 1997;17:305–308.
35 Megarbane A, Salem N, Stephan E, et al: X-linked transposition of the great arteries and incomplete penetrance among males with a nonsense mutation in ZIC3. Eur J Hum Genet 2000;8:704–708.
36 Ware SM, Peng J, Zhu L, et al: Identification and functional analysis of ZIC3 mutations in heterotaxy and related congenital heart defects. Am J Hum Genet 2004;74:93–105.
37 Chhin B, Hatayama M, Bozon D, et al: Elucidation of penetrance variability of a ZIC3 mutation in a family with complex heart defects and functional analysis of ZIC3 mutations in the first zinc finger domain. Hum Mutat 2007;28:563–570.
38 Robinson SW, Morris CD, Goldmuntz E, et al: Missense mutations in CRELD1 are associated with cardiac atrioventricular septal defects. Am J Hum Genet 2003;72:1047–1052.
39 Zatyka M, Priestley M, Ladusans EJ, et al: Analysis of CRELD1 as a candidate 3p25 atrioventicular septal defect locus (AVSD2). Clin Genet 2005;67:526–528.
40 Maslen CL, Babcock D, Robinson SW, et al: CRELD1 mutations contribute to the occurrence of cardiac atrioventricular septal defects in Down syndrome. Am J Med Genet A 2006;140:2501–2505.
41 Garg V, Muth AN, Ransom JF, et al: Mutations in NOTCH1 cause aortic valve disease. Nature 2005;437:270–274.
42 Garg V: Molecular genetics of aortic valve disease. Curr Opin Cardiol 2006;21:180–184.
43 Mohamed SA, Aherrahrou Z, Liptau H, et al: Novel missense mutations (p.T596M and p.P1797H) in NOTCH1 in patients with bicuspid aortic valve. Biochem Biophys Res Commun 2006;345:1460–1465.
44 Ching YH, Ghosh TK, Cross SJ, et al: Mutation in myosin heavy chain 6 causes atrial septal defect. Nat Genet 2005;37:423–428.
45 Sperling S, Grimm CH, Dunkel I, et al: Identification and functional analysis of CITED2 mutations in patients with congenital heart defects. Hum Mutat 2005;26:575–582.
46 Fischer A, Klamt B, Schumacher N, et al: Phenotypic variability in Hey2–/– mice and absence of HEY2 mutations in patients with congenital heart defects or Alagille syndrome. Mamm Genome 2004;15:711–716.
47 Sarkozy A, Conti E, D'Agostino R, et al: ZFPM2/FOG2 and HEY2 genes analysis in nonsyndromic tricuspid atresia. Am J Med Genet A 2005;133:68–70.
48 Reamon-Buettner SM, Borlak J: HEY2 mutations in malformed hearts. Hum Mutat 2006;27:118.
49 Weismann CG, Hager A, Kaemmerer H, et al: PTPN11 mutations play a minor role in isolated congenital heart disease. Am J Med Genet A 2005;136:146–151.
50 Holzelova E, Vonarbourg C, Stolzenberg MC, et al: Autoimmune lymphoproliferative syndrome with somatic Fas mutations. N Engl J Med 2004;351:1409–1418.
51 Erickson RP: Somatic gene mutation and human disease other than cancer. Mutat Res 2003;543:125–136.
52 Puck JM, Straus SE: Somatic mutations – not just for cancer anymore. N Engl J Med 2004;351:1388–1390.
53 Weiss KM: Cryptic causation of human disease: reading between the (germ) lines. Trends Genet 2005;21:82–88.
54 Weismann CG, Gelb BD: The genetics of congenital heart disease: a review of recent developments. Curr Opin Cardiol 2007;22:200–206.
55 Reamon-Buettner SM, Hecker H, Spanel-Borowski K, et al: Novel NKX2-5 mutations in diseased heart tissues of patients with cardiac malformations. Am J Pathol 2004;164:2117–2125.
56 Reamon-Buettner SM, Borlak J: Somatic NKX2-5 mutations as a novel mechanism of disease in complex congenital heart disease. J Med Genet 2004;41:684–690.
57 Reamon-Buettner SM, Borlak J: TBX5 mutations in non-Holt-Oram syndrome (HOS) malformed hearts. Hum Mutat 2004;24:104.
58 Reamon-Buettner SM, Borlak J: GATA4 zinc finger mutations as a molecular rationale for septation defects of the human heart. J Med Genet 2005;42:e32.
59 Inga A, Reamon-Buettner SM, Borlak J, Resnick MA: Functional dissection of sequence-specific NKX2-5 DNA binding domain mutations associated with human heart septation defects using a yeast-based system. Hum Mol Genet 2005;14:1965–1975.
60 Reamon-Buettner SM, Cho SH, Borlak J: Mutations in the 3′-untranslated region of GATA4 as molecular hotspots for congenital heart disease (CHD). BMC Med Genet 2007;8:38.
61 Resnick MA, Cox BS: Yeast as an honorary mammal (review). Mutat Res 2000;451:1–11.
62 Strubin M, Struhl K: Yeast and human TFIID with altered DNA-binding specificity for TATA elements. Cell 1992;68:721–730.
63 Sweetser D, Nonet M, Young RA: Prokaryotic and eukaryotic RNA polymerases have homologous core subunits. Proc Natl Acad Sci USA 1987;84:1192–1196.
64 Candau R, Moore PA, Wang L, et al: Identification of human proteins functionally conserved with the yeast putative adaptors ADA2 and GCN5. Mol Cell Biol 1996;16:593–602.
65 Cormack BP, Strubin M, Stargell LA, Struhl K: Conserved and nonconserved functions of the yeast and human TATA-binding proteins. Genes Dev 1994;8:1335–1343.
66 Reamon-Buettner SM, Sattlegger E, Ciribilli Y et al: Transcriptional defect of an inherited NKX2-5 haplotype comprising a SNP, a nonsynonymous and a synonymous mutation, associated with human congenital heart disease. PLoS One 2013;8:e83295.
67 Reamon-Buettner SM, Ciribilli Y, Inga A, Borlak J: A loss-of-function mutation in the binding domain of HAND1 predicts hypoplasia of the human hearts. Hum Mol Genet 2008;17:1397–1405.
68 Reamon-Buettner SM, Ciribilli Y, Traverso I, et al: A functional genetic study identifies HAND1 mutations in septation defects of the human heart. Hum Mol Genet 2009;18:3567–3578.
69 Storici F, Lewis LK, Resnick MA: In vivo site-directed mutagenesis using oligonucleotides. Nat Biotechnol 2001;19:773–776.
70 Storici F, Durham CL, Gordenin DA, Resnick MA: Chromosomal site-specific double-strand breaks are efficiently targeted for repair by oligonucleotides in yeast. Proc Natl Acad Sci U S A 2003;100:14994–14999.
71 Andreotti V, Ciribilli Y, Monti P, et al: p53 transactivation and the impact of mutations, cofactors and small molecules using a simplified yeast-based screening system. PLoS One 2011;6:e20643.
72 Kennedy BK: Mammalian transcription factors in yeast: strangers in a familiar land. Nat Rev Mol Cell Biol 2002;3:41–49.
73 Goldfarb CA, Wall LB: Holt-Oram syndrome. J Hand Surg Am 2014;39:1646–1648.
74 Reamon-Buettner SM, Borlak J: NKX2-5: an update on this hypermutable homeodomain protein and its role in human congenital heart disease (CHD) (review). Hum Mutat 2010;31:1185–1194.

75 Kasahara H: Loss of function and inhibitory effects of human CSX/NKX2.5 homeoprotein mutations associated with congenital heart disease. J Clin Invest 2000;106:299–308.
76 Leng S, Bernauer AM, Zhai R, et al: Discovery of common SNPs in the miR-205/200 family-regulated epithelial to mesenchymal transition pathway and their association with risk for non-small cell lung cancer. Int J Mol Epidemiol Genet 2011;2:145–155.
77 Ouyang P, Xin WQ: Identification and functional analysis of a de novo NKX2.5 mutation and translational readthrough analysis of NKX2.5 nonsense mutations by aminoglycosides; PhD thesis, Huazhong University of Science and Technology, 2011, http://www.dissertationtopic.net/doc/1507805.
78 SNPeffect Database for phenotyping human single nucleotide polymorphisms (SNPs). http://snpeffect.switchlab.org (accessed March 5, 2015).
79 Monti P, Russo D, Bocciardi R, et al: EEC- and ADULT-associated TP63 mutations exhibit functional heterogeneity toward P63 responsive sequences. Hum Mutat 2013;34: 894–904.
80 International Agency for Research on Cancer. IARC TP53 Database. http://p53.iarc.fr/TP53GeneVariations.aspx (accessed March 5, 2015).

Prof. Jürgen Borlak
Center for Pharmacology and Toxicology, Hannover Medical School
Carl-Neuberg-Strasse 1
DE–30625 Hannover (Germany)
E-Mail borlak.juergen@mh-hannover.de

Muenke M, Kruszka PS, Sable CA, Belmont JW (eds): Congenital Heart Disease: Molecular Genetics, Principles of Diagnosis and Treatment. Basel, Karger, 2015, pp 145–154
DOI: 10.1159/000375212

CHARGE Syndrome

Nicole Corsten-Janssen · Conny M.A. van Ravenswaaij-Arts

Department of Genetics, University Medical Center Groningen, University of Groningen, Groningen, The Netherlands

Abstract

The CHARGE syndrome is a multiple congenital malformation syndrome occurring in 6–7 per 100,000 live births and presenting with a variable combination of coloboma, choanal atresia, cranial nerve defects, specific ear anomalies, and semicircular canal defects as its major features. In most patients, a de novo loss-of-function mutation in the *CHD7* gene can be identified. The CHARGE syndrome can be diagnosed using clinical criteria, but 17% of the patients with a proven *CHD7* mutation do not fulfill these criteria. Identifying a *CHD7* mutation in a suspected patient confirms the diagnosis and assures appropriate clinical follow-up and genetic counseling. Heart defects occur in approximately 75% of patients with a pathogenic *CHD7* mutation. The types of heart defects are variable, but atrioventricular septal defects and conotruncal defects are relatively overrepresented. CHD7 is a member of the chromodomain helicase DNA-binding protein family that regulates transcription by chromatin remodeling. CHD7 has been shown to have a cell-type-specific and stage-dependent function in enhancer-mediated transcription. In the heart, CHD7 is emerging as an important epigenetic factor, but further research is needed to fully understand the function of CHD7 and the broad spectrum of clinical features that is caused by haploinsufficiency of CHD7.

The CHARGE syndrome (OMIM 214800) is a multiple congenital malformation syndrome that is highly variable and has an estimated birth prevalence of 6–7 per 100,000 [1]. The acronym CHARGE was introduced in 1981 and summarizes some of the cardinal features: ocular coloboma, congenital heart defects, choanal atresia, retardation of growth and development, genital hypoplasia, and ear anomalies with or without deafness [2]. The first patients with what we now call the CHARGE syndrome were described in 1961 [3, 4], but it was not until 1979 that the association between coloboma, congenital heart defects, and choanal atresia was recognized by an ophthalmologist as well as by a pediatrician [5, 6]. In 2004, loss-of-function mutations in the *CHD7* (chromodomain helicase DNA-binding protein 7) gene (OMIM *608892) were identified as the major cause of the CHARGE syndrome [7].

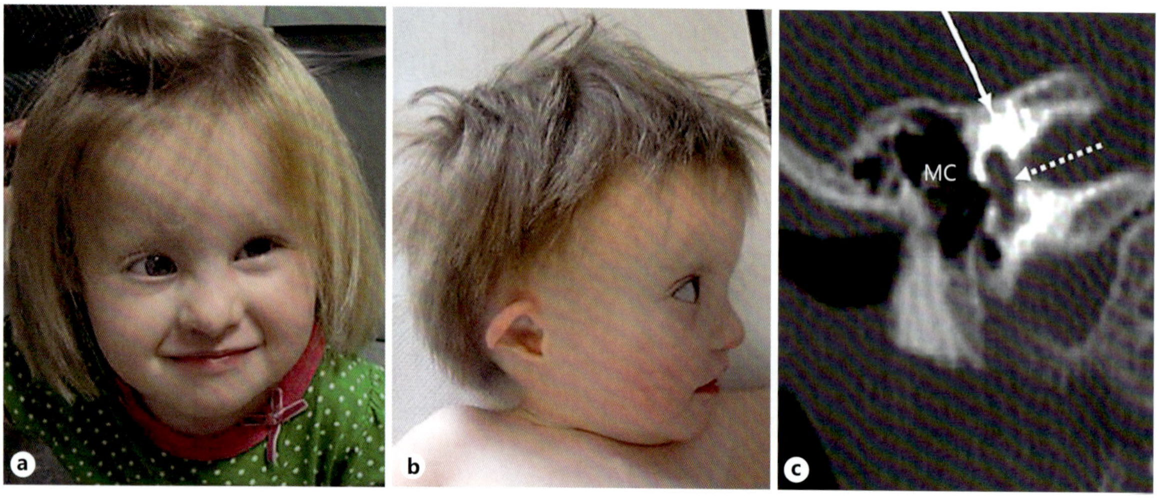

Fig. 1. Female patient with the CHARGE syndrome due to a nonsense mutation in the *CHD7* gene (c.7879C→T; p.Arg2627*) at the age of 4.5 years (**a**; frontal view) and 3.5 years (**b**; lateral view). She was born with a complex heart defect (double-outlet right ventricle, atrial and ventricular septal defects, pulmonary stenosis, and right descending aorta), diaphragmatic hernia, bilateral intraocular coloboma, mild right-sided facial palsy (**a**), and dysmorphic ears (**b**). She did not have a choanal atresia or cleft lip/palate. Her right ear is deaf and she has bilateral absence of the semicircular canals (**c**; MC = Middle ear cavity; dashed arrow indicates the basal curve of the cochlea; arrow indicates absence of semicircular canals). The hernia and cardiac defect were surgically treated (Blalock-Taussig shunt, followed by complete correction at the age of 19 months). She had percutaneous gastric tube feeding until the age of 2 years. Her speech development was normal at the age of 4.5 years. Because of growth deficiency, she was treated with growth hormone with good response (1.16 m, –3.5 standard deviation score (SDS) at the age of 9 years and –5 SDS before treatment). At the age of 9 years she was attending a mainstream school. She had some problems with mathematics, but her IQ was within the normal range.

The *CHD7* gene is located at chromosome 8q12, has a genomic size of 188 kb, and consists of 38 exons, of which the first is noncoding [7]. The encoded protein has 2,997 amino acids and belongs to the third subfamiliy of a group of CHD proteins that play a role in regulating the transcription of genes by chromatin remodeling [7, 8]. For this function, all CHD members have two N-terminal tandem chromo (chromatin organization modifier) domains and a centrally located SNF2-like ATPase domain, which uses the energy from ATP hydrolysis to alter the histone-DNA contact with the nucleosome. In addition, the third subfamily, which includes CHD7, has a C-terminal paired BRK (Brahma and Kismet) domain and a SANT-like (switching-defective protein 3, adaptor 2, nuclear receptor corepressor, transcription factor IIIB-like) domain [8]. CHD7 probably plays a role in controlling gene expression by ATP-dependent chromatin remodeling in embryonic stem cells and in other cell types [9, 10].

The CHARGE syndrome is usually a sporadic condition caused by de novo mutations, although, rarely, it can be transmitted as an autosomal dominant disease [11]. The full clinical spectrum of the CHARGE syndrome has gradually expanded since the *CHD7* gene was recognized as its major cause in 2004 [11].

Diagnosis

Clinical Diagnosis

Before the discovery of the *CHD7* gene, the CHARGE syndrome could only be diagnosed using the major clinical criteria [12, 13]: coloboma, choanal atresia, cranial nerve dysfunction, ear anomalies, and semicircular canal anomalies (fig. 1). In both sets of clinical criteria that are currently used (Blakes and Verloes), the clinical diagnosis of the CHARGE syndrome can only be made if a patient has at least coloboma or choanal atresia (table 1). However, since the discovery of the *CHD7* gene, patients with a *CHD7* mutation have been identified who do not fulfill the clinical criteria and have a

Table 1. Clinical criteria for the CHARGE syndrome

	Blake	Verloes
Major criteria	(1) Ocular coloboma, microphthalmia (2) Choanal atresia or stenosis[1] (3) Characteristic external ear anomaly, middle/inner ear malformations, mixed deafness (4) Cranial nerve dysfunction	(1) Ocular coloboma (2) Choanal atresia (3) Hypoplastic semicircular canals
Minor criteria	(1) Cardiovascular malformations (2) Tracheoesophageal defects (3) Genital hypoplasia or delayed pubertal development (4) Cleft lip and/or palate (5) Developmental delay (6) Growth retardation (7) Characteristic face	(1) Heart or esophagus malformation (2) Malformation of the middle or external ear (3) Rhombencephalic dysfunction including sensorineural deafness (4) Hypothalamohypophyseal dysfunction (gonadotropin or growth hormone deficiency) (5) Mental retardation
Inclusion rule	Typical CHARGE: 4 major criteria or 3 major + 3 minor	Typical CHARGE: 3 major criteria or 2 major + 2 minor Partial CHARGE: 2 major + 1 minor criteria Atypical CHARGE: 2 major + 0 minor criteria or 1 major + 3 minor

There are currently two clinical systems in use to diagnose the CHARGE syndrome: Blake's, updated by a consortium in 2006 and 2009 [13], and Verloes' criteria [12].

[1] Choanal atresia can be substituted by cleft palate, since these anomalies rarely occur in combination.

milder clinical phenotype [11]. *CHD7* analysis now makes a major contribution to the diagnosis of the CHARGE syndrome, although there is some discussion on the naming of patients with only a few of its clinical features. In contrast, no *CHD7* mutations can be identified in 5–10% of the patients who do fulfill the clinical diagnostic criteria [11, 14, 15]. These patients are still registered as having the CHARGE syndrome on clinical grounds as long as other diagnoses have been excluded, such as chromosomal defects and clinically overlapping syndromes.

Molecular Diagnosis

Molecular genetic analysis of *CHD7* comprises the sequencing of all the coding exons and intron-exon boundaries of the gene. If no mutation is identified, a partial or whole gene deletion should be excluded by multiplex ligation-dependent probe amplification (MLPA) [16]. The analysis of *CHD7* helps clinicians make the diagnosis of the CHARGE syndrome, anticipate problems, assure appropriate clinical surveillance, and give accurate genetic counseling. There is a guideline to help clinicians decide when to perform *CHD7* analysis (table 2) based on the clinical features seen in 280 patients with a proven *CHD7* mutation [11]. In addition to the features that are part of the clinical diagnostic criteria (table 1), the *CHD7* guideline includes features seen in family members as supporting information. The guideline also indicates when imaging of the semicircular canals is an appropriate next diagnostic step.

CHD7 analysis in a clinical setting reveals mutations in 32–41% of the patients suspected of having the CHARGE syndrome [1, 17]. Whereas in a re-

Table 2. Guidelines for *CHD7* analysis

Cardinal features	Supportive features
– Coloboma – Choanal atresia or stenosis – Characteristic external ear anomaly (triangular conchae or cup ear) – Cranial nerve dysfunction (facial palsy, sensorineural hearing loss, or hypoplasia of cranial nerves on imaging) – Vestibular phenotype[1]	– Cleft lip/palate – Hypogonadotropic hypogonadism or anosmia – Congenital heart defect or tracheoesophageal malformation – Mental retardation (IQ <70) – Growth retardation (length –2.5 SDS) – Family member with 1 cardinal or 2 supportive features
Perform temporal bone CT scan when patient has: 2 cardinal features or 1 cardinal + 1 supportive feature	
Perform CHD7 *analysis including MLPA when patient has:* 3 cardinal or 2 cardinal + 1 supportive feature or 2 cardinal + typical SCC abnormalities on temporal bone CT scan or 1 cardinal + 1 supportive feature + typical SCC abnormalities on temporal bone CT scan	
Perform genome-wide array analysis when patient has: CHD7 analysis with no mutation or deletion or 2 cardinal + no typical SCC abnormalities on temporal bone CT scan or 1 cardinal + 1 supportive feature + no typical SCC abnormalities on temporal bone CT scan	

[1] A convincing history of vestibular problems (e.g. five-point crawl) or abnormal vestibular test or semicircular canal (SCC) hypoplasia [adapted from ref. 11].

search setting, the detection rates range from 33 to 100% depending on the patient inclusion criteria and the techniques used for *CHD7* analysis [reviewed in ref. 1], in patients fulfilling the clinical diagnostic criteria, the mutation detection rate is over 90%.

Over 500 different pathogenic *CHD7* mutations have been identified (www.CHD7.org), of which 97% are intragenic mutations spread throughout the coding region of the *CHD7* gene. Most are truncating frameshifts (44%) or nonsense alterations (34%), while splice site and missense mutations occur in 11 and 8%, respectively. Complete and partial deletions of the *CHD7* gene and translocations including *CHD7* rarely occur. Mutations are often unique for a patient or a family, but recurrent mutations do occur, especially arginine to stop codon alterations are overrepresented at codons 494 and 2,627 [1, 17].

The interpretation of the effect of missense variations is often difficult, especially in rare syndromes like the CHARGE syndrome, where most variations are unique and no functional assay is available. The correct interpretation is essential for adequate genetic counseling and a classification system was therefore proposed to predict the effect of missense variations. The prediction is based on the combination of results from computational algorithms, a structural model, segregation data, and phenotypic data [18]. For the correct interpretation of missense variations, it is essential to collect the segregation and phenotypic information in patients.

Other Causes of the CHARGE Syndrome

CHD7 mutations are the major cause of the CHARGE syndrome, but its cause is unclear in 5–10% of the clinically typical CHARGE patients, and in an even higher percentage of the patients who are suspected of the CHARGE syndrome but who do not have the full clinical presentation. Nondetectable rearrangements of *CHD7* might partly explain the CHARGE syndrome features in these patients, but there might also be other genes involved. Besides the *SEMA3E* gene that was found to be disrupted in 2 patients with the clinical diagnosis of the CHARGE syndrome, no other genes have been identified [1, 19]. Different chromosomal imbalances which cause phenocopies of the CHARGE syndrome have been described [reviewed in ref. 1] and a recurring phenotypic overlap has been reported for 22q11.2 deletions [20, 21]. When patients suspected of the CHARGE syndrome do not harbor a *CHD7* mutation, a genome-wide array analysis should be performed to exclude chromosomal alterations. Besides the 22q11.2 deletion syndrome (see chapter by Goldmuntz on 22q11.2 deletion on p. 100), other syndromes may also mimic the CHARGE syndrome, such as the branchiootorenal syndrome, Kabuki syndrome (see Russell and Hannibal p. 187 for information on Kabuki syndrome), and mandibulofacial dysostosis (Treacher Collins syndrome) caused by *EFTUD2* mutations [13, 22].

Broad Phenotypic Spectrum of *CHD7* Mutations

Clinical Features of Patients with a CHD7 Mutation

A study of clinical features in 280 patients with a proven *CHD7* mutation showed that three features are almost always present: external ear anomalies, cranial nerve dysfunction, and semicircular canal defects (fig. 1). Therefore, when a patient is suspected of having the CHARGE syndrome, a clinician needs to pay special attention to these features – indicated by cup-shaped ears with triangular conchae, facial palsy, or sensorineural deafness, and delayed motor milestones [11]. Other features that occur in more than 75% of the patients are coloboma, genital hypoplasia, congenital heart defects, and intellectual disability. However, it is important to realize that around 20% of the patients with a *CHD7* mutation have a normal level of intelligence (fig. 1) [11, 23].

Since the identification of the *CHD7* gene, several studies have focused on the mild end of the phenotypic spectrum and shown that up to 17% of the patients do not fulfill the clinical criteria [11, 14]. The clinical variability is nicely demonstrated in the 18 familial cases reported thus far [reviewed in ref. 1, 11]. Additionally, monozygotic twins may have different features of the CHARGE syndrome.

CHD7 Mutations in Other Syndromes

CHD7 mutations have also been identified in patients diagnosed with two other syndromes: the Kallmann and 22q11.2 deletion syndromes. The Kallmann syndrome is the combination of hypogonadotropic hypogonadism and anosmia. Both features also occur in roughly 80% of the patients with the CHARGE syndrome [24]. Other features found in both syndromes are cleft lip and/or palate, and hearing loss. The Kallmann syndrome is heterogeneous with mutations identified in the genes *CHD7, FGF8, FGFR1, KAL1, PROKR2,* and *PROK2*; together these mutations explain 30–45% of the patients [25]. Mutational analysis of *CHD7* has been performed in patients with hypogonadotropic hypogonadism with or without anosmia in four studies, and mutations were identified in 13 of 319 patients [26–29]. The chance of finding a *CHD7* mutation is highest if at least anosmia or one other feature of the CHARGE syndrome is present. Heart defects are not a common feature of the Kallmann syndrome, but a bicuspid aortic valve was present in 1 of the 13 patients with a *CHD7* mutation.

In contrast, the 22q11.2 deletion syndrome does share heart defects as a common feature with the CHARGE syndrome, in addition to cleft palate, deafness, and immunodeficiency [20, 21]. In most patients with the 22q11.2 deletion syndrome, a common 3-Mb deletion including the *TBX1* gene has been identified. *CHD7* analysis in 20 patients clinically suspected of having the 22q11.2 deletion syndrome but without a deletion or mutation of *TBX1* revealed truncating mutations in 5 patients [30]. Therefore, *CHD7* analysis should also be performed in patients suspected of having the 22q11.2 deletion syndrome without a TBX1 mutation or deletion.

Genotype-Phenotype Associations

There is no clear genotype-phenotype association for *CHD7* mutations but, in general, missense mutations are associated with a milder phenotype.

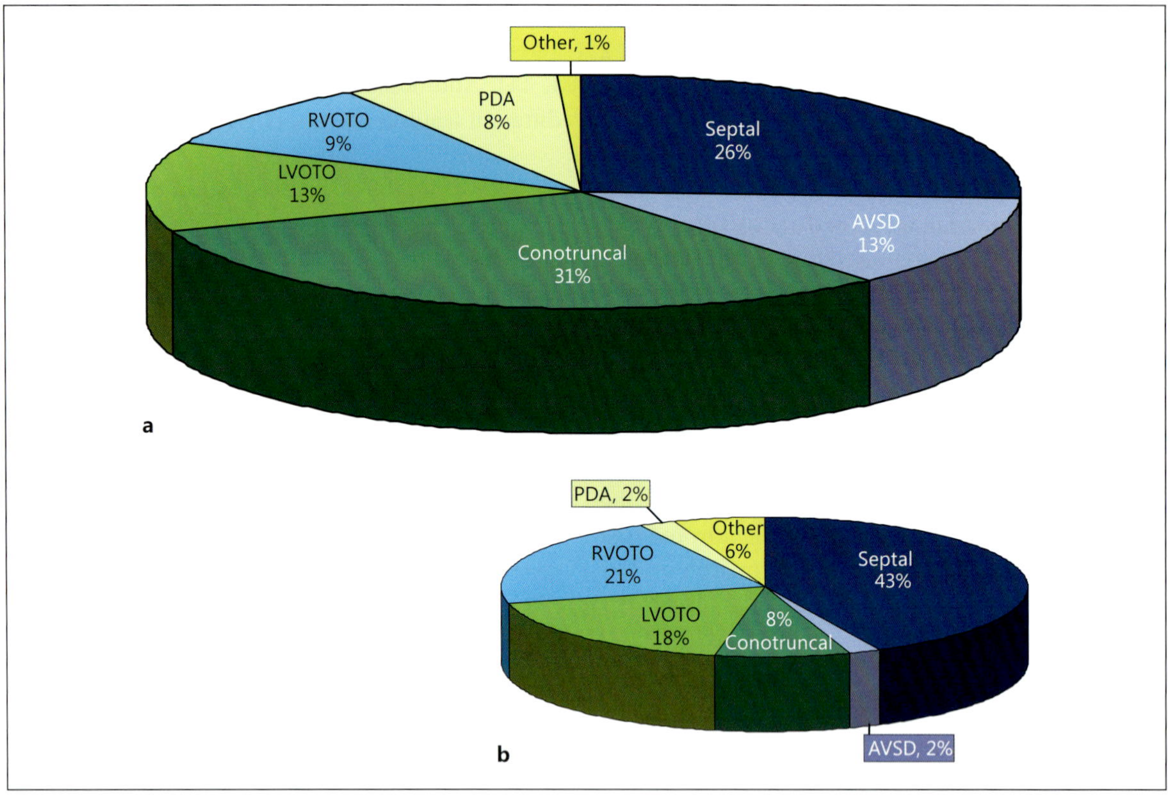

Fig. 2. The distribution of congenital heart defects in a group of 202 patients with a *CHD7* mutation (**a**) and in 1,007 patients with non-syndromic congenital heart defects (**b**) [adapted from ref. 30]. The types of heart defects differ significantly between these two groups; especially conotruncal heart defects and atrioventricular septal defects (AVSD) are overrepresented in patients with *CHD7* mutations. LVOTO = Left-ventricular outflow tract obstruction; PDA = patent ductus arteriosus; RVOTO = right-ventricular outflow tract obstruction.

Especially, cleft lip/palate, choanal atresia, and congenital heart defects are seen less often in patients with a missense mutation.

Heart Defects in the CHARGE Syndrome

Before the identification of mutations in the *CHD7* gene as the major cause of the CHARGE syndrome, two studies had focused on congenital heart defects in the CHARGE syndrome in 83 and 59 patients, respectively [31, 32]. Both studies identified that conotruncal heart defects often occur in the CHARGE syndrome. More recently, a study was performed specifically on congenital heart defects in 299 patients with a proven *CHD7* mutation [30], and congenital heart defects were present in 74% of these patients. The type of heart defect was variable, but compared to a group of patients with nonsyndromic congenital heart defects, atrioventricular septal defects and conotruncal defects were overrepresented (fig. 2). In the group of conotruncal heart defects, there was a remarkable overrepresentation of aortic arch anomalies such as aberrant subclavian artery. Heart defects occurred equally in males and females, but were significantly more frequent in patients with truncating mutations than splice site or missense mutations.

When looking at congenital heart defects, it is worth remembering the overlap already mentioned between the CHARGE and 22q11.2 deletion syndromes. Both syndromes show an overrepresentation of conotruncal heart defects, and, in mice, *Tbx1* and *Chd7* are the only genes known to cause anomalies of the fourth pharyngeal arch arteries that can result in an interrupted aortic arch [20, 33, 34].

Based on the high frequency of congenital heart defects and the observation that *CHD7* mutations may be found in patients with only a few features of the CHARGE syndrome, it was thought that *CHD7* mutations might also be found in patients with isolated heart defects. However, *CHD7* analysis in 67 patients with isolated congenital heart defects did not reveal any pathogenic mutations [35]. Also in 46 patients selected for atrioventricular or conotruncal heart defects and one other feature within the spectrum of the CHARGE syndrome, no pathogenic *CHD7* variants could be identified [36]. In a recent exome sequencing study of 362 parent-offspring trios with a child with a severe congenital heart defect, a truncating *CHD7* mutation in a patient with tetralogy of Fallot and pulmonary atresia was identified [37]. This patient also had other features of the CHARGE syndrome, namely a cleft lip and palate, inguinal hernia, micropenis, sensorineural hearing loss, and abnormal neurodevelopment. However, the patient did not fulfill the clinical criteria of the CHARGE syndrome. This case exemplifies why one should be aware of other features of the CHARGE syndrome in patients with congenital heart defects, such as hearing loss, external ear anomalies, cranial nerve dysfunction, and semicircular canal defects, especially if they have an atrioventricular septal defect or conotruncal heart defects including aortic arch anomalies. In addition, if patients are suspected of having the 22q11.2 deletion syndrome and the 22q11.2 deletion is absent, they should be examined carefully for CHARGE features [20, 30]. Furthermore, *CHD7* should be included in gene panels that screen patients with syndromic congenital heart defects.

CHD7 Function in the Heart

CHD7 expression has been studied in human, mouse and chick embryos, for example. Mouse embryo in situ hybridization on embryonic day 10.5 showed expression of Chd7 in the cardiac outflow tract and truncus arteriosus in one study, while in another study Chd7 expression did not appear to be above background in the myocardium and conotruncal region of the heart on embryonic day 12.5 [15, 38]. In a heterozygous Chd7-deficient mouse (due to a gene-trapped lacZ reporter embryonic stem cell line), expression was seen in the heart at several embryonic stages [38–40]. In chicken embryos, no expression in the heart was seen at any stage in one study, while another study reported expression in the branchial arches that form the cardiac outflow tract at Hamburger and Hamilton stage 20 [41, 42]. In situ hybridization of normal human fetal and embryonic tissue showed expression of CHD7 at the mesenchyme of the pharyngeal arches on days 26 and 33, but no expression in the heart was observed at any stage [43].

Heart defects have been studied in different animal models with heterozygous *Chd7* mutations, including mice and the African clawed frog (*Xenopus laevis*). In some mouse embryos, edema, ventricular septal defects, and pharyngeal arch defects were noticed [34, 38, 44]. In *X. laevis,* heart defects, including abnormal positioning of the truncus arteriosus and cardiac outflow tract, were identified [9]. These findings together with the high prevalence of heart defects in patients with a *CHD7* mutation suggest that CHD7 is important in embryonic cardiac development. Although the function of CHD7 is gradually becoming clear, it is still not known exactly how CHD7 haploinsufficiency causes heart defects.

CHD7 has been shown to regulate gene expression by enhancer-mediated transcription and ribosomal RNA biogenesis in the nucleolus [10, 45]. CHD7 also binds to different sites on the DNA with protein complexes in a time- and tissue-specific manner, thereby regulating various target genes (fig. 3) [10, 45]. The clinical variability seen in different organ systems of individuals with the CHARGE syndrome, including the variety of heart defects, is probably caused by the continuum of influence of CHD7 in different cell types [46, 47]. CHD7 probably regulates the expression of important cardiac development genes by chromatin remodeling [48, 49]. A recent study in mouse embryos showed Chd7 interacts with intracellular BMP-activated SMADs (SMAD1, SMAD5, and SMAD8) to specifically regulate transcription of important cardiac development genes like *Nkx2.5* [40]. Other proteins that are known to be important in cardiac development and that have been associated with CHD7 are the ATP-dependent chromatin-remodeling protein complex PBAF (polybromo- and BRGI-associated factor)

4

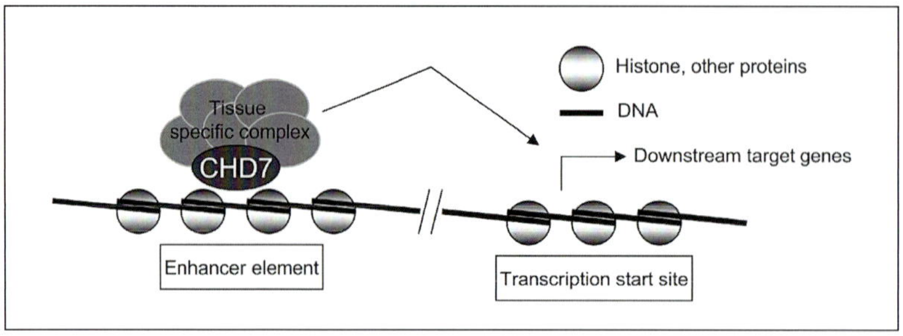

Fig. 3. Based on current studies, CHD7 has been shown to bind to different sites on the DNA with various protein complexes in a time- and tissue-specific manner, regulating various target genes [adapted from ref. 46].

and the histone acetyl transferase p300 [9, 10, 48, 49]. Furthermore, CHD7 has been shown to be important for the formation of multipotent migratory neural crest cells, which play a major role in cardiac development [9]. It has also been shown that Chd7 is required in the ectoderm of the pharyngeal arch during embryogenesis for normal great vessel development in mice [35]; therefore, the heart defects seen in the CHARGE syndrome cannot be explained by the effect of CHD7 on neural crest cells alone.

Further research is necessary to fully understand how CHD7 affects cardiac development and to identify other genes involved in this pathway. Since monozygotic twins can have different cardiac phenotypes, environmental factors cannot be ignored in this respect.

Clinical Surveillance and Genetic Counseling

The CHARGE syndrome is a complex disorder involving different organ systems and, therefore, follow-up is recommended in a multidisciplinary expert setting. Fortunately, guidelines for the clinical surveillance of patients are available to clinicians [11, 13]. In all patients with the CHARGE syndrome, the heart and kidneys should be screened, since mild congenital anomalies may remain undetected, but can have clinical consequences. Cranial nerve evaluation is important, since dysfunction may contribute to respiratory aspiration, postoperative complications, and sudden death. Evaluation of hypogonadotropic hypogonadism should also be done at an appropriate age allowing for induction of pubertal development at a natural age and prevention of osteoporosis. Evaluation of hearing loss and visual impairment should be done early on, so that hearing devices can be used and communication can be adapted to the child's capabilities. An individualized educational program is also important to fully stimulate the child's intellectual potential and to manage behavioral problems.

Heart defects in patients with the CHARGE syndrome should be treated just as in other patients with heart defects. However, one should be aware that anesthetic complications can arise and procedures that need anesthetics should, therefore, be combined whenever possible [11, 13].

Identifying a *CHD7* mutation provides a basis for genetic counseling. The CHARGE syndrome is a sporadic condition, but familial recurrence has been described due to germline mosaicism and in mildly affected parents. Parents of a patient should, therefore, be screened for the *CHD7* mutation found in their child. If a mutation is found de novo in a patient, the recurrence risk for another child is 2–3% due to germline mosaicism. CHARGE patients, if they are fertile, have a 50% risk of having a child with the CHARGE syndrome. Prenatal diagnosis (molecular analysis and/or ultrasound) should be discussed with the parents of affected children and patients. However, the degree of severity of the CHARGE syndrome cannot be predicted by the mutation found, and the prognostic value of prenatal ultrasound is limited.

Concluding Remarks

The CHARGE syndrome is an extremely variable and multiple congenital malformation syndrome that is caused by mutations in the chromodomain gene *CHD7* in the majority of patients. The diagnosis of the CHARGE syndrome can be made using clinical criteria, but *CHD7* mutational analysis can be helpful to confirm the diagnosis in suspect cases. A diagnosis allows for more accurate clinical surveillance and genetic counseling.

Heart defects are present in the majority of patients with a *CHD7* mutation, although the type of heart defect can be variable, with an overrepresentation of conotruncal heart defects and atrioventricular septal defects.

The function of CHD7 and its interaction with other genes are slowly being unraveled, indicating a role in embryonic stage- and tissue-specific gene expression. In the heart, CHD7 has also been shown to be an important epigenetic factor regulating the genes involved in cardiac development, but further research is needed to fully understand why patients with the CHARGE syndrome show so much clinical variability.

References

1 Janssen N, Bergman JE, Swertz MA, Tranebjaerg L, Lodahl M, Schoots J, Hofstra RM, van Ravenswaaij-Arts CM, Hoefsloot LH: Mutation update on the CHD7 gene involved in CHARGE syndrome. Hum Mutat 2012;33:1149–1160.

2 Pagon RA, Graham JM Jr, Zonana J, Yong SL: Coloboma, congenital heart disease, and choanal atresia with multiple anomalies: CHARGE association. J Pediatr 1981;99: 223–227.

3 Angelman H: Syndrome of coloboma with multiple congenital abnormalities in infancy. Br Med J 1961;i:1212–1214.

4 Edwards JH, Finlay HVL, Young RB: Coloboma with multiple congenital anomalies. Br Med J 1961;ii:586–587.

5 Hall BD: Choanal atresia and associated multiple anomalies. J Pediatr 1979;95:395–398.

6 Hittner HM, Hirsch NJ, Kreh GM, Rudolph AJ: Colobomatous microphthalmia, heart disease, hearing loss, and mental retardation – a syndrome. J Pediatr Ophthalmol Strabismus 1979;16:122–128.

7 Vissers LE, van Ravenswaaij CM, Admiraal R, Hurst JA, De Vries BB, Janssen IM, van der Vliet WA, Huys EH, de Jong PJ, Hamel BC, Schoenmakers EF, Brunner HG, Veltman JA, van Kessel AG: Mutations in a new member of the chromodomain gene family cause CHARGE syndrome. Nat Genet 2004; 36:955–957.

8 Marfella CG, Imbalzano AN: The Chd family of chromatin remodelers. Mutat Res 2007;618:30–40.

9 Bajpai R, Chen DA, Rada-Iglesias A, Zhang J, Xiong Y, Helms J, Chang CP, Zhao Y, Swigut T, Wysocka J: CHD7 cooperates with PBAF to control multipotent neural crest formation. Nature 2010;463:958–962.

10 Schnetz MP, Handoko L, Akhtar-Zaidi B, Bartels CF, Pereira CF, Fisher AG, Adams DJ, Flicek P, Crawford GE, LaFramboise T, Tesar P, Wei CL, Scacheri PC: CHD7 targets active gene enhancer elements to modulate ES cell-specific gene expression. PLoS Genet 2010;6:e1001023.

11 Bergman JE, Janssen N, Hoefsloot LH, Jongmans MC, Hofstra RM, van Ravenswaaij-Arts CM: CHD7 mutations and CHARGE syndrome: the clinical implications of an expanding phenotype. J Med Genet 2011; 48:334–342.

12 Verloes A: Updated diagnostic criteria for CHARGE syndrome: a proposal. Am J Med Genet A 2005;133:306–308.

13 Lalani SR, Hefner MA, Belmont JW, Davenport SLH: CHARGE syndrome (2006; updated 2012); in Pagon RA, Adam MP, Ardinger HH, et al (eds): GeneReviews [Internet]. Seattle, University of Washington, 1993–2015, http://www.ncbi.nlm.nih.gov/books/NBK1117/.

14 Jongmans MC, Admiraal RJ, van der Donk KP, Vissers LE, Baas AF, Kapusta L, van Hagen JM, Donnai D, de Ravel TJ, Veltman JA, Geurts van Kessel A, De Vries BB, Brunner HG, Hoefsloot LH, van Ravenswaaij CM: CHARGE syndrome: the phenotypic spectrum of mutations in the CHD7 gene. J Med Genet 2006;43:306–314.

15 Lalani SR, Safiullah AM, Fernbach SD, Harutyunyan KG, Thaller C, Peterson LE, McPherson JD, Gibbs RA, White LD, Hefner M, Davenport SL, Graham JM, Bacino CA, Glass NL, Towbin JA, et al: Spectrum of CHD7 mutations in 110 individuals with CHARGE syndrome and genotype-phenotype correlation. Am J Hum Genet 2006;78: 303–314.

16 Bergman JE, de Wijs I, Jongmans MC, Admiraal RJ, Hoefsloot LH, Ravenswaaij-Arts CM: Exon copy number alterations of the CHD7 gene are not a major cause of CHARGE and CHARGE-like syndrome. Eur J Med Genet 2008;51:417–425.

17 Bartels CF, Scacheri C, White L, Scacheri PC, Bale S: Mutations in the CHD7 gene: the experience of a commercial laboratory. Genet Test Mol Biomarkers 2010;14:881–891.

18 Bergman JE, Janssen N, van der Sloot AM, de Walle HE, Schoots J, Rendtorff ND, Tranebjaerg L, Hoefsloot LH, van Ravenswaaij-Arts CM, Hofstra RM: A novel classification system to predict the pathogenic effects of CHD7 missense variants in CHARGE syndrome. Hum Mutat 2012;33: 1251–1260.

19 Lalani SR, Safiullah AM, Molinari LM, Fernbach SD, Martin DM, Belmont JW: SEMA3E mutation in a patient with CHARGE syndrome. J Med Genet 2004;41:e94.

20 Corsten-Janssen N, Saitta SC, Hoefsloot LH, McDonald-McGinn DM, Driscoll DA, Derks R, Dickinson KA, Kerstjens-Frederikse WS, Emanuel BS, Zackai EH, van Ravenswaaij-Arts CMA: More clinical overlap between 22q11.2 deletion syndrome and CHARGE syndrome than often anticipated. Mol Syndromol 2012;4:235–245.

21 Jyonouchi S, McDonald-Mcginn DM, Bale S, Zackai EH, Sullivan KE: CHARGE (coloboma, heart defect, atresia choanae, retarded growth and development, genital hypoplasia, ear anomalies/deafness) syndrome and chromosome 22q11.2 deletion syndrome: a comparison of immunologic and nonimmunologic phenotypic features. Pediatrics 2009;123:e871–e877.

22 Luquetti DV, Hing AV, Rieder MJ, Nickerson DA, Turner EH, Smith J, Park S, Cunningham ML: 'Mandibulofacial dysostosis with microcephaly' caused by EFTUD2 mutations: expanding the phenotype. Am J Med Genet A 2013;161A:108–113.

23 Zentner GE, Layman WS, Martin DM, Scacheri PC: Molecular and phenotypic aspects of CHD7 mutation in CHARGE syndrome. Am J Med Genet A 2010;152A:674–686.

24 Bergman JE, Bocca G, Hoefsloot LH, Meiners LC, Ravenswaaij-Arts CM: Anosmia predicts hypogonadotropic hypogonadism in CHARGE syndrome. J Pediatr 2011;158: 474–479.

25 Buck C, Balasubramanian R, Crowley WF: Isolated gonadotropin-releasing hormone (GnRH) deficiency (2007; updated 2013); in Pagon RA, Adam MP, Ardinger HH, et al (eds): GeneReviews [Internet]. Seattle, University of Washington, 1993–2015, http://www.ncbi.nlm.nih.gov/books/NBK1334/.
26 Bergman JE, de Ronde W, Jongmans MC, Wolffenbuttel BH, Drop SL, Hermus A, Bocca G, Hoefsloot LH, van Ravenswaaij-Arts CM: The results of CHD7 analysis in clinically well-characterized patients with Kallmann syndrome. J Clin Endocrinol Metab 2012;97:e858–e862.
27 Jongmans MC, Ravenswaaij-Arts CM, Pitteloud N, Ogata T, Sato N, Claahsen-van der Grinten HL, van der Donk K, Seminara S, Bergman JE, Brunner HG, Crowley WF Jr, Hoefsloot LH: CHD7 mutations in patients initially diagnosed with Kallmann syndrome – the clinical overlap with CHARGE syndrome. Clin Genet 2009;75:65–71.
28 Kim HG, Kurth I, Lan F, Meliciani I, Wenzel W, Eom SH, Kang GB, Rosenberger G, Tekin M, Ozata M, Bick DP, Sherins RJ, Walker SL, Shi Y, Gusella JF, et al: Mutations in CHD7, encoding a chromatin-remodeling protein, cause idiopathic hypogonadotropic hypogonadism and Kallmann syndrome. Am J Hum Genet 2008;83:511–519.
29 Laitinen EM, Vaaralahti K, Tommiska J, Eklund E, Tervaniemi M, Valanne L, Raivio T: Incidence, phenotypic features and molecular genetics of Kallmann syndrome in Finland. Orphanet J Rare Dis 2011;6:41.
30 Corsten-Janssen N, Kerstjens-Frederikse WS, du Marchie Sarvaas GJ, Baardman ME, Bakker MK, Bergman JE, Hove HD, Heimdal KR, Rustad CF, Hennekam RC, Hofstra RM, Hoefsloot LH, Van Ravenswaaij-Arts CM, Kapusta L: The cardiac phenotype in patients with a CHD7 mutation. Circ Cardiovasc Genet 2013;6:248–254.
31 Wyse RK, al-Mahdawi S, Burn J, Blake K: Congenital heart disease in CHARGE association. Pediatr Cardiol 1993;14:75–81.
32 Lin AE, Chin AJ, Devine W, Park SC, Zackai E: The pattern of cardiovascular malformation in the CHARGE association. Am J Dis Child 1987;141:1010–1013.
33 McDonald-McGinn DM, Emanuel BS, Zackai EH: 22q11.2 deletion syndrome (1999; updated 2013); in Pagon RA, Adam MP, Ardinger HH, et al (eds): GeneReviews [Internet]. Seattle, University of Washington, 1993–2015, http://www.ncbi.nlm.nih.gov/books/NBK1523/.
34 Randall V, McCue K, Roberts C, Kyriakopoulou V, Beddow S, Barrett AN, Vitelli F, Prescott K, Shaw-Smith C, Devriendt K, Bosman E, Steffes G, Steel KP, Simrick S, Basson MA, et al: Great vessel development requires biallelic expression of Chd7 and Tbx1 in pharyngeal ectoderm in mice. J Clin Invest 2009;119:3301–3310.
35 Qi Q, Yi L, Yang C, Chen H, Shen L, Mo X, Hu Y, Wang Y: Mutation analysis of the CHD7 gene in patients with congenital heart disease (in Chinese). Zhonghua Yi Xue Yi Chuan Xue Za Zhi 2008;25:637–641.
36 Corsten-Janssen N, du Marchie Sarvaas GJ, Kerstjens-Frederikse WS, Hoefsloot LH, van Beynum IM, Kapusta L, van Ravenswaaij-Arts CM: CHD7 mutations are not a major cause of atrioventricular septal and conotruncal heart defects. Am J Med Genet Part A 2014;164A:3003–3009
37 Zaidi S, Choi M, Wakimoto H, Ma L, Jiang J, Overton JD, Romano-Adesman A, Bjornson RD, Breitbart RE, Brown KK, Carriero NJ, Cheung YH, Deanfield J, DePalma S, Fakhro KA, et al: De novo mutations in histone-modifying genes in congenital heart disease. Nature 2013;498:220–223.
38 Bosman EA, Penn AC, Ambrose JC, Kettleborough R, Stemple DL, Steel KP: Multiple mutations in mouse Chd7 provide models for CHARGE syndrome. Hum Mol Genet 2005;14:3463–3476.
39 Hurd EA, Capers PL, Blauwkamp MN, Adams ME, Raphael Y, Poucher HK, Martin DM: Loss of Chd7 function in gene-trapped reporter mice is embryonic lethal and associated with severe defects in multiple developing tissues. Mamm Genome 2007;18:94–104.
40 Liu Y, Harmelink C, Peng Y, Chen Y, Wang Q, Jiao K: CHD7 interacts with BMP R-SMADs to epigenetically regulate cardiogenesis in mice. Hum Mol Genet 2014;23:2145–2156.
41 Aramaki M, Kimura T, Udaka T, Kosaki R, Mitsuhashi T, Okada Y, Takahashi T, Kosaki K: Embryonic expression profile of chicken CHD7, the ortholog of the causative gene for CHARGE syndrome. Birth Defects Res A Clin Mol Teratol 2007;79:50–57.
42 Kosaki K: Role of rare cases in deciphering the mechanisms of congenital anomalies: CHARGE syndrome research. Congenit Anom (Kyoto) 2011;51:12–15.
43 Sanlaville D, Etchevers HC, Gonzales M, Martinovic J, Clement-Ziza M, Delezoide AL, Aubry MC, Pelet A, Chemouny S, Cruaud C, Audollent S, Esculpavit C, Goudefroye G, Ozilou C, Fredouille C, et al: Phenotypic spectrum of CHARGE syndrome in fetuses with CHD7 truncating mutations correlates with expression during human development. J Med Genet 2006;43:211–217.
44 Cleary JO, Price AN, Thomas DL, Scambler PJ, Kyriakopoulou V, McCue K, Schneider JE, Ordidge RJ, Lythgoe MF: Cardiac phenotyping in ex vivo murine embryos using microMRI. NMR Biomed 2009;22:857–866.
45 Zentner GE, Hurd EA, Schnetz MP, Handoko L, Wang C, Wang Z, Wei C, Tesar PJ, Hatzoglou M, Martin DM, Scacheri PC: CHD7 functions in the nucleolus as a positive regulator of ribosomal RNA biogenesis. Hum Mol Genet 2010;19:3491–3501.
46 Layman WS, Hurd EA, Martin DM: Chromodomain proteins in development: lessons from CHARGE syndrome. Clin Genet 2010;78:11–20.
47 Martin DM: Chromatin remodeling in development and disease: focus on CHD7. PLoS Genet 2010;6:e1001010.
48 Han P, Hang CT, Yang J, Chang C: Chromatin remodeling in cardiovascular development and physiology. Circ Res 2011;108:378–396.
49 Bruneau BG: Chromatin remodeling in heart development. Curr Opin Genet Dev 2010;20:505–511.

Professor Conny M.A. van Ravenswaaij-Arts
Department of Genetics
University Medical Center Groningen
PO Box 30 001, NL–9700 RB Groningen (The Netherlands)
E-Mail c.m.a.van.ravenswaaij@umcg.nl

Muenke M, Kruszka PS, Sable CA, Belmont JW (eds): Congenital Heart Disease: Molecular Genetics, Principles of Diagnosis and Treatment. Basel, Karger, 2015, pp 155–165
DOI: 10.1159/000375213

Alagille Syndrome

Henry C. Lin[a] · Alexandra Falsey[b] · Ian Krantz[c] · Nancy Spinner[b]

[a]Division of Pediatric Gastroenterology, Hepatology, and Nutrition, Department of Pediatrics, The Children's Hospital of Philadelphia, and [b]Department of Pathology and Laboratory Medicine and [c]Division of Human Genetics and Molecular Biology, Department of Pediatrics, The Children's Hospital of Philadelphia and The Perelman School of Medicine, University of Pennsylvania, Philadelphia, Pa., USA

Abstract

The Alagille syndrome (ALGS) is a complex, multisystem, autosomal dominant disorder characterized by variable expressivity of developmental abnormalities in multiple organ systems, including the hepatic, cardiac, ophthalmologic, skeletal, craniofacial, renal, and vascular systems. ALGS is caused by haploinsufficiency of one of two genes in the Notch signaling pathway: Jagged 1 *(JAG1)* and Notch 2 *(NOTCH2)*. *JAG1* encodes for a cell surface protein that acts as one of five Notch receptor ligands, and mutations in *JAG1* are found in approximately 95% of clinically diagnosed probands. ALGS is classically defined by the presence of intrahepatic bile duct paucity via liver biopsy in association with at least three of the major clinical features: chronic cholestasis, cardiac disease, skeletal abnormalities, ocular abnormalities, and characteristic facial features; however, with the availability of genetic testing, liver biopsy is no longer required for the diagnosis of ALGS as the presence of a known *JAG1* or *NOTCH2* mutation in association with one main clinical feature is now considered diagnostic. The management of ALGS is focused on identifying all affected organ systems and supportive care with emphasis on nutrition and growth. Genetic counseling is an important part of the interdisciplinary management of ALGS as approximately 50% of individuals have an inherited mutation. As cardiac disease contributes to the majority of early deaths in ALGS, early detection and directed management of cardiovascular malformations are important.

The Alagille syndrome (ALGS, OMIM 118450) is a complex, multisystem, autosomal dominant disorder. It is characterized by variable expressivity of developmental abnormalities in multiple organ systems, including the hepatic, cardiac, ophthalmologic, skeletal, craniofacial, renal, and vascular systems [1–4]. ALGS was first described in 1969 when Alagille et al. [1] recognized a pattern of clinical features involving cardiac and vertebral anomalies in patients with idiopathic bile duct paucity [1, 5, 6]. Watson and Miller [7] independently reported cases of familial pulmonary valvular stenosis in association with neonatal liver disease characterized by obstructive jaundice in 1973 and Alagille et al. [2] furthered these observations in 1975 when describing several patients with hepatic ductular hypoplasia associated with characteristic facies, and cardiac and vertebral anomalies. This amalgam of clinical features highlighted by bile duct paucity was named Alagille syndrome and is also known as syndromic paucity or arteriohepatic dysplasia.

ALGS is classically defined by the presence of intrahepatic bile duct paucity via liver biopsy in association with at least three of the major clinical features: chronic cholestasis, cardiac disease, skeletal abnormalities, ocular abnormalities, and characteristic facial features [8–10]. Historically, the incomplete penetrance of and variability in clinical features made it difficult to estimate the overall incidence of ALGS. However, the advent of molecular testing has allowed for identification of individuals with mild disease phenotypes. The current estimated incidence of ALGS is between 1: 30,000 and 1:45,000 with no difference in gender [11].

ALGS is the second most common cause of intrahepatic cholestasis in infancy. Chronic cholestatic liver disease is a main cause of morbidity in ALGS. Overall mortality is approximately 10%, with liver disease, cardiac disease, and vascular accidents as the main contributors [12, 13]. As cholestasis is a central and ongoing clinical feature, ALGS has historically been managed by gastroenterologists. However, the extent of *JAG1*-associated disease with the potential of multiorgan system involvement often benefits from an interdisciplinary team to help in the diagnosis, management, and genetic counseling of ALGS [14, 15].

Pathophysiology

ALGS is an autosomal dominant disease caused by haploinsufficiency of one of two genes in the Notch signaling pathway: Jagged 1 *(JAG1)* and Notch 2 *(NOTCH2)* [16–21]. *JAG1*, which is located on chromosome 20, encodes for a cell surface protein that acts as one of five Notch receptor ligands, and mutations are found in approximately 95% of clinically diagnosed probands [16, 17]. Mutations in *NOTCH2*, which encodes for one of four human Notch receptors, are found in <1% of probands [20, 21]. Approximately half of the JAG1 Mutations in ALGS occur de novo. For the inherited *JAG1* mutations, the variable expressivity in ALGS is evident, as >40% of *JAG1* mutations were found in relatively healthy parents who underwent genetic analysis following the diagnosis of a family member [4, 22]. In most cases, no genotype-phenotype correlation between mutation type or origin and clinical manifestations has been reported. One exception to this appears to be a JAG1 missense mutation found segregating with isolated cardiac disease in a large family [23].

The Notch signaling pathway is an evolutionarily conserved intercellular signaling mechanism, which plays a key role in cell fate determination. Binding between the Notch receptor and ligand results in the cleavage and release of the Notch intracellular domain, which activates transcription factors that play a role in cell differentiation and morphogenesis [24–26]. *JAG1* is highly expressed in many of the affected organ systems in ALGS [22], but the penetrance and expressivity of ALGS are not uniform across patients or organ systems [27]. In addition, there exists a subset of patients with features similar to ALGS but no identified mutation on *JAG1* or *NOTCH2*.

Clinical Features

Over 500 patients with ALGS have been reported in the literature. The major clinical manifestations of ALGS can be attributed to structural or functional defects during embryogenesis and include cholestasis characterized by bile duct paucity, cardiac defects, vertebral anomalies, ocular anomalies, and characteristic facies. Renal and vascular anomalies are also well described [12, 28]. There is variable expressivity for each of the affected organ systems, ranging from no apparent involvement to severe disease. In addition, clinical complications can arise from long-standing biochemical or anatomic abnormalities, which lead to management challenges. The overall frequency of

Table 1. Summary of clinical features in ALGS

Feature	Alagille [3] 1987	Deprettere [6] 1987	Hoffenberg [5] 1995	Emerick [9] 1999	Quiros-Tejeira [29] 1999	Weighted, %
Patients, n	80	27	26	92	43	
Bile duct paucity, %	100	81	80	85	83	89
Cholestasis, %	91	93	100	96	100	95
Murmur, %	85	96	96	97	98	94
Vertebral anomalies, %	87	33	48	51	38	61
Ocular findings, %	88	56	85	78	73	80
Facies, %	95	70	92	96	98	92
Renal disease, %	73	–	19	40	50	44
Intracranial event or vascular anomaly, %	–	–	15	14	12	14

the clinical features of ALGS is difficult to ascertain; table 1 lists the frequencies of these clinical features published in large patient series [3, 5, 6, 9, 29].

Hepatic Manifestations

Hepatic involvement of ALGS ranges from mild to severe cholestasis, with a small subset of patients having no obvious hepatic manifestations. The most common clinical presentation of ALGS is neonatal cholestasis, which is biochemically characterized by conjugated hyperbilirubinemia with high γ-glutamyl transpeptidase and alkaline phosphatase, mildly elevated liver enzymes, and increased serum bile acids. Hepatomegaly is almost universally recognized, and clinical sequelae of chronic cholestasis include pruritus, xanthomas, coagulopathy, and poor growth – all of which are targets of management strategies. Pruritus has been reported to be out of proportion to the degree of cholestasis and is present even in anicteric individuals. Formation of xanthomas is related to the severity of cholestasis and often seen with serum cholesterol levels >500 mg/dl [3, 9, 30, 31]. Growth failure, characterized by height and weight below the 5th percentile for age, is common, and is compounded by fat-soluble vitamin deficiencies, which can lead to complications such as rickets and fractures [9, 32]. Delayed puberty and hypogonadism have also been reported, possibly as a consequence of poor nutrition [3, 30].

Neonatal cholestatic liver disease is typically indicative of more severe liver involvement in ALGS. Infants presenting with neonatal jaundice are more likely to remain jaundiced and have persistent pruritus and xanthomas compared to ALGS patients who present with liver disease during childhood [33]. The initial evaluation of neonatal cholestasis may involve nuclear scintigraphy, cholangiogram, and liver biopsy. With the availability of genetic testing, liver biopsy is no longer required for the diagnosis of ALGS as presence of a known *JAG1* or *NOTCH2* mutation in association with one main clinical feature is now considered diagnostic [30]. Timing of the liver biopsy is integral as paucity is progressive and may not be noted on initial biopsy. In a study by Emerick et al. [9] in 1999, bile duct paucity was present in only 60% of infants under 6 months of age, but in 95% older than 6 months. Bile duct paucity is defined as a ratio of bile ducts to portal tracts <0.5 in a liver biopsy specimen with at least 10 portal tracts for evaluation [30].

Liver histopathology in ALGS can show a range of bile duct involvement from paucity to proliferation, depending on the timing of the biopsy. In addition, there is a spectrum of extrahepatic biliary involvement in ALGS with cases of hypoplastic extrahepatic biliary ducts. An intraoperative cholangiogram, which is used to detect large duct obstruction that is typically seen in biliary atresia and not typical of ALGS, can be misleading in ALGS patients with a hypoplastic extrahepatic biliary

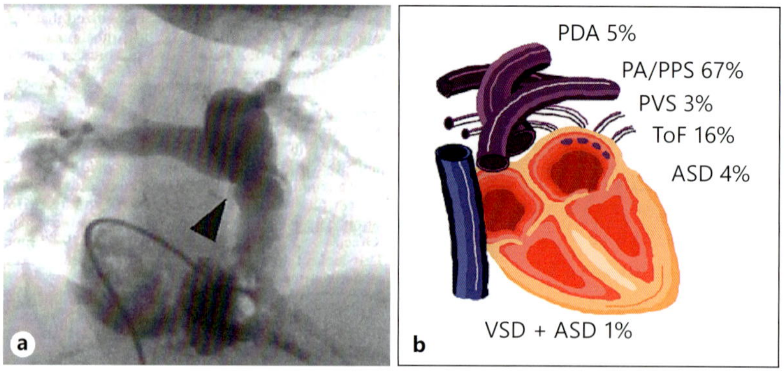

Fig. 1. Cardiac involvement in ALGS. **a** Angiogram of a patient with valvular pulmonic stenosis with diffuse branch pulmonary artery hypoplasia: catheter in the right ventricle for contrast injection. Arrowhead points to the thickened valve leaflets that do not open completely in systole. **b** Schematic of the heart: the frequencies of varying cardiac complications in the ALGS patient population are given. ASD = Atrial septal defect; PA/PPS = pulmonary atresia/peripheral pulmonary stenosis; PDA = patent ductus arteriosus; PVS = pulmonary valve stenosis; VSD = ventricular septal defect.

tree. In these instances, there may not appear to be an extrahepatic biliary tree, thus raising concern for biliary atresia and a subsequent need for a hepatoportoenterostomy. This differentiation of the etiology of biliary duct obstruction underscores a key management challenge of neonatal cholestasis as studies have shown that a hepatoportoenterostomy is not beneficial in ALGS [9, 30, 34]. These difficulties in interpreting the various diagnostic tests suggest a role for genetic testing of ALGS mutations and highlight the importance of looking for clinical features outside of those involving the liver [4].

Cardiac Manifestations

Cardiovascular anomalies are noted in 81–100% of individuals with ALGS [3, 9]. There is a spectrum of cardiac involvement, ranging from peripheral pulmonary artery stenosis to more complex malformations including tetralogy of Fallot (ToF), truncus arteriosus, anomalous pulmonary venous return, ventricular septal defect, atrial septal defect, aortic stenosis, pulmonary valve stenosis, and single right ventricle with pulmonary valve atresia (fig. 1). Extracardiac vascular lesions, including coarctation of the aorta and patent ductus arteriosus, are also seen in ALGS [35, 36].

Peripheral pulmonary stenosis is the most common cardiac manifestation in ALGS and obstruction at multiple levels in the pulmonary arterial vasculature or diffuse hypoplasia are common [36]. ToF is the most common congenital defect in ALGS and occurs in 7–12% of individuals with ALGS. The frequency of more clinically severe forms of ToF is greater in ALGS as 40% of patients with ALGS and ToF have pulmonary atresia [35, 36]. Mutations in *JAG1* have also been described in congenital heart disease in the absence of ALGS. *JAG1* mutations were first reported in an individual with pulmonary stenosis and ToF [37].

In addition, *JAG1* mutations have been identified in all forms of nonsyndromic ToF, including classic ToF, as well as ToF variants with pulmonic atresia, pulmonic stenosis, and absent pulmonary valve [23, 38, 39]. Eldadah et al. [23] reported their findings of a mutation in *JAG1* that segregates with isolated cardiac disease within a large family. Phenotypic findings include classic ToF, ventricular septal defect with aortic dextroposition and isolated peripheral pulmonic stenosis as well as characteristic facial features (distinct from unaffected family members and classic ALGS). Le Caignec et al. [40] have also described a cohort with familial deafness, congenital heart defects, and posterior embryotoxon (PE) who share a mutation in the first epidermal growth factor-like domain of *JAG1*. These findings prompted Bauer et al. [38] to hypothesize that *JAG1* may be a candidate gene for additional cardiac findings and that the wider utility of whole genome analysis may reveal modifying factors contributing to the development of isolated cardiac disease in *JAG1* mutation-positive individuals.

The Notch signaling pathway clearly plays a role in the development of cardiac defects. *JAG1* mediates cell-cell interactions during early cardiac embryogenesis [41–43] and Notch signaling has been shown to be involved in ventricular septum formation as well as the development of heart valves and cardiac outflow tracts [36, 44, 45]. Mutations resulting in haploinsuffiency of JAG1 lead to abnormal development of the heart, as cardiogenesis requires a higher dosage of JAG1 [43]. In animal models, *JAG1* expression has been shown to correlate with the spectrum of cardiac disease in ALGS [46]. Specifically, cardiac defects, including ventricular septal defects and pulmonary artery stenosis, are seen in mice with attenuated Notch signaling (Jag1/+; Notch2/+). These mice also develop multisystem defects similar to those seen in ALGS [47]. In addition, *HEY2*, a downstream transcription factor induced by Notch signaling, is integral in the development of the aorta. Deficiency in *HEY2* leads to arterial maturation defects [48, 49] as *HEY2*-deficient mice have been shown to develop ventricular septal defects, right ventricular hypertrophy, and pulmonic stenosis. Some mice also develop cardiac anomalies similar to ToF [50], suggesting that inhibition of Notch signal propagation and downstream *HEY2* inactivation may be the basis of the cardiac defects in ALGS.

Overall, cardiac disease is the main cause of early mortality in ALGS as patients with intracardiac lesions have a 40% 6-year survival rate compared to 95% in patients without cardiac lesions [9]. The Notch signaling pathway seems to be involved in the development of cardiac disease in ALGS and leads to a variety of phenotypes. While the identified *JAG1* mutations in nonsyndromic ToF have not been associated with ALGS, the clinical implications of finding a *JAG1* mutation carrier could help identify people with subclinical ALGS features [38, 39]. It is also possible that these individuals with nonsyndromic ToF could have a variant of ALGS without liver dysfunction.

Musculoskeletal Manifestations

Vertebral anomalies have been described in up to 80% of people with ALGS. Butterfly vertebrae or sagittal vertebral clefts, which are due to failure of fusion of the anterior vertebral arches, are the most commonly described anomaly (fig. 2) [5, 6, 29, 51–53]. Butterfly vertebrae are frequently an incidental

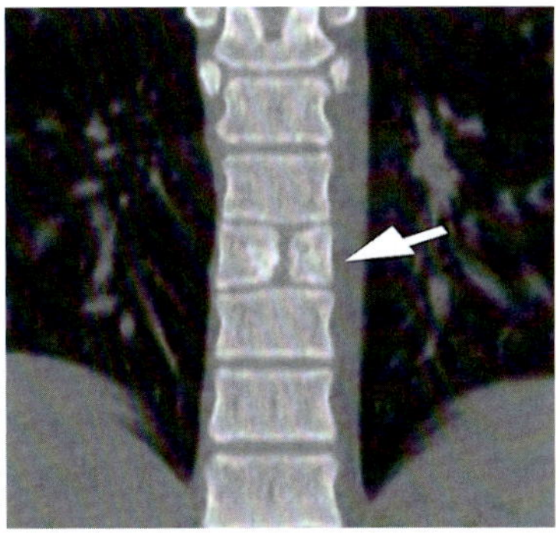

Fig. 2. Skeletal involvement in ALGS. The arrow points to an anterior-posterior radiograph of a thoracic butterfly vertebra, with a MR cross-sectional view demonstrating the midline defect in the vertebral body.

finding that carries no structural significance and patients are generally asymptomatic. Although relatively uncommon, butterfly vertebrae are also seen in a wide range of disorders including Crouzon syndrome, 22q11 deletion syndrome, and VATER syndrome (vertebral defects, anal atresia, tracheoesophageal fistula with esophageal atresia, and radial or renal dysplasia) [30, 54]. Other skeletal findings in ALGS patients include spina bifida occulta, pointed anterior process of C1, narrowing of the adjusted interpedicular spaces of the lumbar spine [55], vertebral fusions [27], and hemivertebrae [56]. In addition, shortened distal phalanges and supernumerary digital flexion creases are also noted with increased frequency in ALGS.

Metabolic bone disease characterized by osteoporosis and fractures are a significant source of morbidity in ALGS [33]. A myriad of factors contribute to metabolic bone disease, including malnutrition, vitamin D deficiency, magnesium deficiency, and chronic liver and renal disease [30, 31, 57]. As a consequence, pathologic fractures occur with increased frequency as one study reports a 50 times greater incidence of femur fractures in people with ALGS [58].

Ocular Manifestations

Ocular abnormalities in ALGS include structural anomalies of the cornea, iris, retina, and optic disc, as well as being secondary to vitamin deficien-

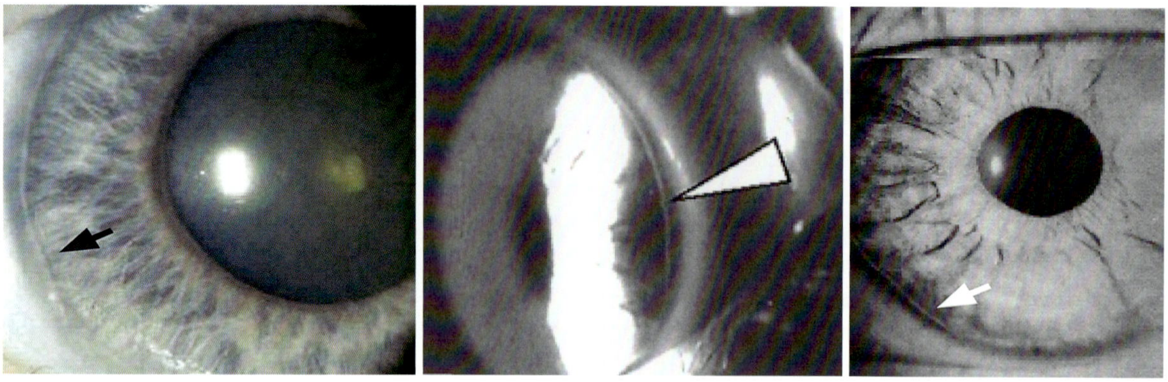

Fig. 3. Ophthalmologic involvement in ALGS. Arrow(head)s point to the prominent Schwalbe's ring in 3 ALGS patients with PE.

cies. The most common ophthalmologic finding is PE, which is seen in up to 90% of patients with ALGS [59]. PE is a prominence of the Schwalbe's ring where the corneal endothelium and the uveal trabecular meshwork join (fig. 3). PE also has a 8–15% prevalence in the general population [30]. This characteristic finding is clinically of no significance, but is a highly useful diagnostic sign for ALGS.

Axenfeld anomaly, which is characterized by a prominent Schwalbe's ring and peripheral iris strands that span the anterior chamber of the eye, is found in 13% of ALGS patients [60]. Other ophthalmologic findings in ALGS include Rieger anomaly, anterior segment dysgenesis marked by atrophy of the iris stroma, microcornea, keratoconus, congenital macular dystrophy, shallow anterior chambers, exotropia, ectopic pupil, band keratopathy, choroidal folds, and anomalous optic discs including optic disc drusen [51, 61, 62]. Despite these findings, the overall, visual prognosis is good.

Facial Features

Characteristic facial features of ALGS include a broad forehead, deep-set eyes that are hyperteloric, a straight nose with a flattened tip, and a prominent, pointed chin, which gives the face an overall triangular appearance (fig. 4) [61, 63]. These facial features typically become more prominent with age. The diagnostic specificity of ALGS facial features as evaluated by clinical dysmorphologists has been demonstrated to be over 80% in a Caucasian cohort [63] and the prevalence of the facial phenotype in *JAG1*-mutation-positive individuals is >90% [9]. A similar prevalence has been noted in several population-based studies in Italian, Australian, and Polish ALGS populations [64–68] as well as among non-Caucasian cohorts, including Japanese, Korean, Chinese, and Vietnamese populations [69–75]. Notably, ALGS patients with *NOTCH2* mutations appear to have different facial features, as in one report, only 20% of these children have the classic ALGS facies [21].

Renal Manifestations

Renal abnormalities, which can be categorized as structural, functional, and acquired renal disorders, are found in approximately 40% of ALGS patients [28]. Structural anomalies found in ALGS are numerous and include small, solitary, or ectopic kidneys as well as renal cysts and ureteropelvic obstruction. In addition, renovascular hypertension occurs secondary to renal artery stenosis. Functional renal disorders include renal tubular acidosis, tubulointerstitial nephropathy, IgA nephritis, mesangiolipidosis, and fatal juvenile nephronophthisis [15, 51, 76]. Renal insufficiency is common and has been reported in all age groups from infancy to adulthood, either as a primary disorder or secondary to end-stage liver disease with some patients requiring renal transplantation [28, 77]. Initial studies suggested a greater prevalence of renal disease in individuals with *NOTCH2* mutations.

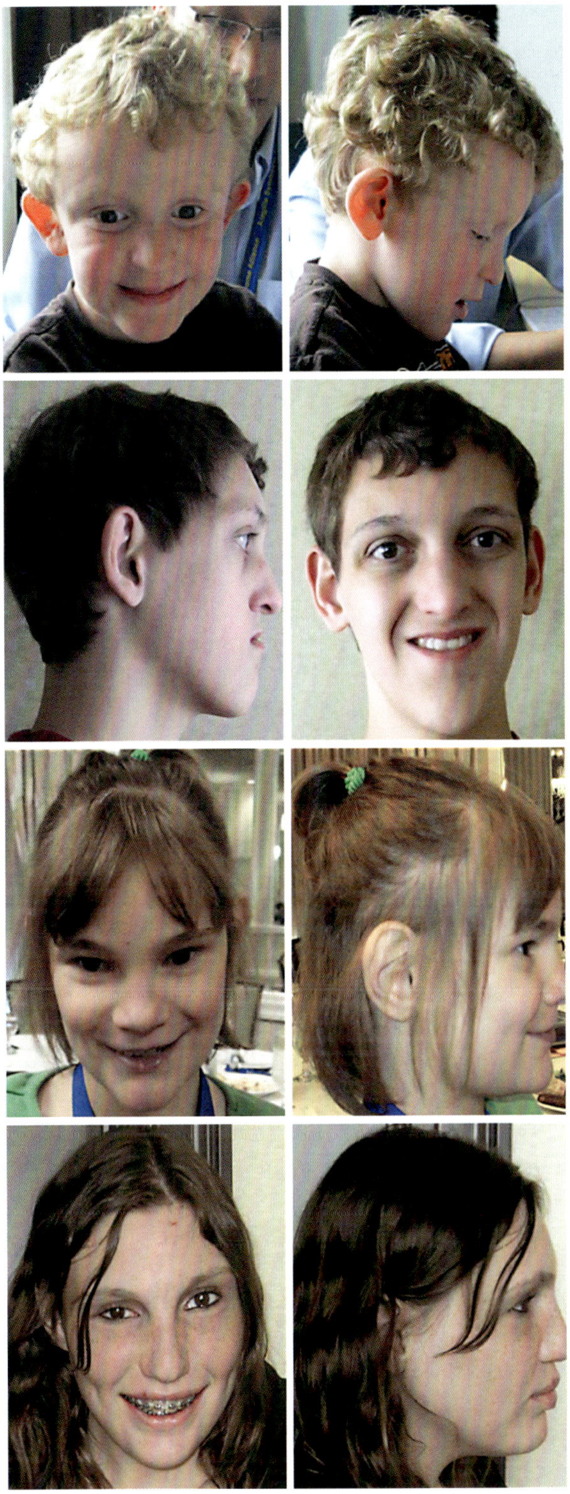

Fig. 4. Representative facial features of 4 individuals with ALGS, shown in profile and frontal view.

The first report of *NOTCH2* mutations in ALGS described 3 mutation-positive relatives without a clinical diagnosis of ALGS, but significant renal disease [20].

Vascular Manifestations

Vascular anomalies in ALGS have been noted since the earliest descriptions, and pulmonary artery involvement is one of the most common manifestations. Other structural vascular anomalies seen in ALGS are renal artery stenosis, coarctation of the aorta, aortic aneurysms, and cerebral vasculature problems, which include aneurysms of the basilar, carotid, and middle cerebral arteries. Moyamoya disease, a progressive intracranial arterial occlusive disease, has also been described [9, 12, 78]. Magnetic resonance angiography (MRA) can detect these vascular lesions, and the current recommendation for all ALGS patients is to have a baseline screening MRA.

Vascular accidents have been reported in up to 15% of cases and are a significant cause of mortality in ALGS [5, 9, 12, 78]. These episodes of intracranial bleeding may occur spontaneously or as a consequence of relatively minor head trauma, and involve a spectrum of diseases from asymptomatic cerebral infarcts to fatal events. Epidural, subdural, subarachnoid, and intraparenchymal bleeding has also been reported [12].

Cognitive Function

Early reports of the syndrome included description of significant intellectual disability (IQ 60–80) in 9 of 30 individuals [2]. Later studies reported mild delays in gross motor skills in 16% of patients studied and mild intellectual impairment in only 2% of patients [9]. This discrepancy in accounts may be linked to earlier disease recognition and increased medical, surgical and nutritional management and intervention.

Diagnosis

Traditionally, the diagnosis of ALGS is based on a combination of the presence of intrahepatic bile duct paucity on liver biopsy in association with at least three of the major clinical features [8–10]. ALGS remains a clinical diagnosis, but the identification of the genetic basis of ALGS has demonstrated that not all people with disease causing *JAG1* or *NOTCH2* mutations may present with the entire spectrum of clinical features due to the variability in expressivity. The availability of molecular testing now allows for a genotypic diagnosis and has consequently led to the suggestion of accounting for family history and genetics in the diagnosis of ALGS. Specifically, the proposed revised diagnostic criteria for ALGS include the presence of a disease-causing mutation in addition to only one major clinical feature [11].

Management

Following the diagnosis of ALGS, it is important to complete the evaluation for involvement of other organ systems. Specifically, the following assessments should be considered:

(1) assessment of liver function by a gastroenterologist to include liver function tests, liver synthetic function tests (coagulation studies), serum bile acids, serum cholesterol, ultrasound of the liver, and a liver biopsy;

(2) cardiac evaluation including an echocardiogram;

(3) anteroposterior X-ray of the spine;

(4) ophthalmologic examination;

(5) assessment of characteristic ALGS facial features by a clinician;

(6) laboratory evaluation of renal function and renal ultrasound, and

(7) MRA of the brain.

As liver disease is often the primary clinical feature, management of ALGS often focuses on cholestatic liver disease with close monitoring of growth, development, and nutritional status. Management of cardiac and renal manifestations is dependent on the underlying malformation. Vertebral and ophthalmic anomalies generally do not require interventions. Overall, the prognosis of ALGS is highly variable and is primarily related to the severity of hepatic and cardiac diseases [14, 30, 51].

As cardiac disease contributes to the majority of early deaths in ALGS, early detection and directed management is important. Patients presenting with cardiac disease and features that are not typical of ALGS should have formal genetic evaluation. The velocardiofacial syndrome (22q deletion) should be considered as these patients may have cardiac disease including ToF in association with PE, butterfly vertebrae, and a characteristic facies. Genetic evaluation may include fluorescence in situ hybridization for 22q deletion [54]. Therapeutic interventions are directed at the underlying cardiac lesion and patients with ToF will require eventual surgical correction. Regarding peripheral pulmonary stenosis, most patients are asymptomatic and require no intervention, but nonsurgical invasive techniques such as balloon dilation and stent placement have been successfully used [79, 80]. While cardiac function can deteriorate, heart transplant is not typically performed, but there has been a case report of a combined heart-lung-liver transplant in a child with ALGS [81].

Maximizing the growth potential is important with a focus on adequate nutrition via a high-calorie diet with a large proportion of fat from medium-chain triglycerides during the neonatal period. In addition, fat-soluble vitamin levels should be checked and supplemented as necessary. Symptomatic management of pruritus involves the use of cholerectic agents, such as ursodeoxycholic acid as well as cholestyramine, rifampin, and naltrexone. In select instances, external biliary diversion has offered some symptomatic relief, but pruritus can be refractory to treatment [82]. Management does not impact the natural history of liver disease, and 21–47% of individuals with ALGS-associated liver disease ultimately require a liver transplant [5, 9, 29]. Overall, the estimated survival with native liver in ALGS has been reported to be 51% at 10 years and 38% at 20 years [33]. Patients with ALGS do well after transplantation, and transplant outcomes are comparable to other diseases with 1-year patient and graft survival rates of 87.5 and 91.7%, respectively [33]. Living related donors should be considered with caution in this genetic disease, as candidates for living donation should undergo genetic testing for ALGS to rule out the gene carrier status [14, 51].

Genetic Counseling

Genetic counseling is an important part of the interdisciplinary management of ALGS. Approximately 50% of individuals have an inherited mutation, and screening individuals within an affected family can help to identify clinically asymptomatic individuals and help with family planning. As ALGS is an autosomal dominant disease, children of an individual with ALGS have a 50% chance of inheriting ALGS. Prenatal testing for at-risk pregnancies is possible if the disease-causing mutation is known, but this genetic testing cannot predict the occurrence or severity of clinical manifestations [13].

Conclusion

ALGS affects multiple organ systems with varying severity and typically involves the hepatic, cardiac, musculoskeletal, ophthalmic, renal, and vascular systems. There are multiple examples of individuals with JAG1 or NOTCH2 mutations who present with apparently isolated clinical features limited to the heart, and knowledge of the other syndromic features is important to arrive at the correct diagnosis. Diagnosis can be difficult in asymptomatic individuals and molecular testing now allows for genetic diagnosis in suspected individuals. Once identified, management of ALGS is focused on identifying all affected organ systems and supportive care with emphasis on nutrition and growth.

References

1 Alagille D, Habib E, Thomassin N: L'atrésie des voies biliaires extrahépatiques perméables chez l'enfant. J Par Pediatr 1969, pp 301–318.

2 Alagille D, Odièvre M, Gautier M, Dommergues JP: Hepatic ductular hypoplasia associated with characteristic facies, vertebral malformations, retarded physical, mental, and sexual development, and cardiac murmur. J Pediatr 1975;86:63–71.

3 Alagille D, Estrada A, Hadchouel M, Gautier M, Odièvre M, Dommergues JP: Syndromic paucity of interlobular bile ducts (Alagille syndrome or arteriohepatic dysplasia): review of 80 cases. J Pediatr 1987;110:195–200.

4 Krantz ID, Piccoli DA, Spinner NB: Alagille syndrome. J Med Genet 1997;34:152–157.

5 Hoffenberg EJ, Narkewicz MR, Sondheimer JM, Smith DJ, Silverman A, Sokol RJ: Outcome of syndromic paucity of interlobular bile ducts (Alagille syndrome) with onset of cholestasis in infancy. J Pediatr 1995;127: 220–224.

6 Deprettere A, Portmann B, Mowat AP: Syndromic paucity of the intrahepatic bile ducts: diagnostic difficulty; severe morbidity throughout early childhood. J Pediatr Gastroenterol Nutr 1987;6:865–871.

7 Watson GH, Miller V: Arteriohepatic dysplasia: familial pulmonary arterial stenosis with neonatal liver disease. Arch Dis Child 1973;48:459–466.

8 Elmslie FV, Vivian AJ, Gardiner H, et al: Alagille syndrome: family studies. J Med Genet 1995;32:264–268.

9 Emerick KM, Rand EB, Goldmuntz E, Krantz ID, Spinner NB, Piccoli DA: Features of Alagille syndrome in 92 patients: frequency and relation to prognosis. Hepatology 1999;29:822–829.

10 Krantz ID, Piccoli DA, Spinner NB: Clinical and molecular genetics of Alagille syndrome. Curr Opin Pediatr 1999;11:558–564.

11 Kamath BM, Bason L, Piccoli DA, et al: Consequences of JAG1 mutations. J Med Genet 2003;40:891–895.

12 Kamath BM, Spinner NB, Emerick KM, et al: Vascular anomalies in Alagille syndrome: a significant cause of morbidity and mortality. Circulation 2004;109:1354–1358.

13 Spinner NB, Leonard LD, Krantz ID: Alagille syndrome (2000; updated 2013); in Pagon RA, Adam MP, Ardinger HH, Bird TD, Dolan CR, Fong CT, Smith RJH, Stephens K (eds): GeneReviews [Internet]. Seattle, University of Washington, 1993–2015.

14 Kamath BM, Loomes KM, Piccoli DA: Medical management of Alagille syndrome. J Pediatr Gastroenterol Nutr 2010;50:580–586.

15 Tsai E: Genomic Approaches to Understanding Variable Expressivity in Alagille Syndrome and Genetic Susceptibility to Biliary Atresia; thesis, University of Pennsylvania, Philadelphia, 2013.

16 Oda T, Elkahloun AG, Pike BL, et al: Mutations in the human Jagged1 gene are responsible for Alagille syndrome. Nat Genet 1997;16:235–242.

17 Li L, Krantz ID, Deng Y, et al: Alagille syndrome is caused by mutations in human Jagged1, which encodes a ligand for Notch1. Nat Genet 1997;16:243–251.

18 Morrissette JD, Colliton RP, Spinner NB: Defective intracellular transport and processing of JAG1 missense mutations in Alagille syndrome. Hum Mol Genet 2001;10: 405–413.

19 Boyer-Di Ponio J, Wright-Crosnier C, Groyer-Picard MT, et al: Biological function of mutant forms of JAGGED1 proteins in Alagille syndrome: inhibitory effect on Notch signaling. Hum Mol Genet 2007;16:2683–2692.

20 McDaniell R, Warthen DM, Sanchez-Lara PA, et al: NOTCH2 mutations cause Alagille syndrome, a heterogeneous disorder of the notch signaling pathway. Am J Hum Genet 2006;79:169–173.

21 Kamath BM, Bauer RC, Loomes KM, et al: NOTCH2 mutations in Alagille syndrome. J Med Genet 2012;49:138–144.

22 Crosnier C, Lykavieris P, Meunier-Rotival M, Hadchouel M: Alagille syndrome. The widening spectrum of arteriohepatic dysplasia. Clin Liver Dis 2000;4:765–778.

23 Eldadah ZA, Hamosh A, Biery NJ, et al: Familial tetralogy of Fallot caused by mutation in the jagged1 gene. Hum Mol Genet 2001; 10:163–169.

24 Artavanis-Tsakonas S, Rand MD, Lake RJ: Notch signaling: cell fate control and signal integration in development. Science 1999; 284:770–776.

25 Gridley T: Notch signaling and inherited disease syndromes. Hum Mol Genet 2003; 12(spec No 1):R9–R13.

26 Hori K, Sen A, Artavanis-Tsakonas S: Notch signaling at a glance. J Cell Sci 2013;126(pt 10):2135–2140.

27 Shulman SA, Hyams JS, Gunta R, et al: Arteriohepatic dysplasia (Alagille syndrome): extreme variability among affected family members. Am J Med Genet 1984;19:325–332.
28 Kamath BM, Spinner NB, Rosenblum ND: Renal involvement and the role of Notch signalling in Alagille syndrome. Nat Rev Nephrol 2013;9:409–418.
29 Quiros-Tejeira RE, Ament ME, Heyman MB, et al: Variable morbidity in Alagille syndrome: a review of 43 cases. J Pediatr Gastroenterol Nutr 1999;29:431–437.
30 Kamath BM, Spinner N, Piccoli DA: Alagille syndrome; in Suchy FJ, Balistreri WF, Sokol J (eds): Liver Disease in Children. Cambridge, Cambridge University Press, 2007, pp 326–345.
31 Loomes KM, Emerick KM: Pediatric cholestatic liver disease with genetic etiology; in Wyllie R, Hyams JS, Kay M (eds): Pediatric Gastrointestinal and Liver Disease. Philadelphia, Elsevier, 2011, pp 752–766.
32 Rovner AJ, Schall JI, Jawad AF, et al: Rethinking growth failure in Alagille syndrome: the role of dietary intake and steatorrhea. J Pediatr Gastroenterol Nutr 2002;35:495–502.
33 Lykavieris P, Hadchouel M, Chardot C, Bernard O: Outcome of liver disease in children with Alagille syndrome: a study of 163 patients. Gut 2001;49:431–435.
34 Kaye AJ, Rand EB, Munoz PS, et al: Effect of Kasai procedure on hepatic outcome in Alagille syndrome. J Pediatr Gastroenterol Nutr 2010;51:319–321.
35 Silberbach M, Lashley D, Reller MD, et al: Arteriohepatic dysplasia and cardiovascular malformations. Am Heart J 1994;127:695–699.
36 McElhinney DB, Krantz ID, Bason L, et al: Analysis of cardiovascular phenotype and genotype-phenotype correlation in individuals with a JAG1 mutation and/or Alagille syndrome. Circulation 2002;106:2567–2574.
37 Krantz ID, Smith R, Colliton RP, et al: Jagged1 mutations in patients ascertained with isolated congenital heart defects. Am J Med Genet 1999;84:56–60.
38 Bauer RC, Laney AO, Smith R, et al: Jagged1 (JAG1) mutations in patients with tetralogy of Fallot or pulmonic stenosis. Hum Mutat 2010;31:594–601.
39 Guida V, Chiappe F, Ferese R, et al: Novel and recurrent JAG1 mutations in patients with tetralogy of Fallot. Clin Genet 2011;80:591–594.
40 Le Caignec C, Lefevre M, Schott JJ, et al: Familial deafness, congenital heart defects, and posterior embryotoxon caused by cysteine substitution in the first epidermal-growth-factor-like domain of jagged 1. Am J Hum Genet 2002;71:180–186.
41 Lai EC: Notch signaling: control of cell communication and cell fate. Development 2004;131:965–973.
42 Lu F, Morrissette JJ, Spinner NB: Conditional JAG1 mutation shows the developing heart is more sensitive than developing liver to JAG1 dosage. Am J Hum Genet 2003;72:1065–1070.
43 Kola S, Koneti NR, Golla JP, et al: Mutational analysis of JAG1 gene in non-syndromic tetralogy of Fallot children. Clin Chim Acta 2011;412:2232–2236.
44 MacGrogan D, Nus M, de la Pompa JL: Notch signaling in cardiac development and disease. Curr Top Dev Biol 2010;92:333–365.
45 Penton AL, Leonard LD, Spinner NB: Notch signaling in human development and disease. Semin Cell Dev Biol 2012;23:450–457.
46 Loomes KM, Underkoffler LA, Morabito J, et al: The expression of Jagged1 in the developing mammalian heart correlates with cardiovascular disease in Alagille syndrome. Hum Mol Genet 1999;8:2443–2449.
47 McCright B, Lozier J, Gridley T: A mouse model of Alagille syndrome: Notch2 as a genetic modifier of Jag1 haploinsufficiency. Development 2002;129:1075–1082.
48 Zhong TP, Rosenberg M, Mohideen MA, Weinstein B, Fishman MC: Gridlock, an HLH gene required for assembly of the aorta in zebrafish. Science 2000;287:1820–1824.
49 Gessler M, Knobeloch KP, Helisch A, et al: Mouse gridlock: no aortic coarctation or deficiency, but fatal cardiac defects in Hey2–/– mice. Curr Biol 2002;12:1601–1604.
50 Donovan J, Kordylewska A, Jan YN, Utset MF: Tetralogy of Fallot and other congenital heart defects in Hey2 mutant mice. Curr Biol 2002;12:1605–1610.
51 Turnpenny PD, Ellard S: Alagille syndrome: pathogenesis, diagnosis and management. Eur J Hum Genet 2012;20:251–257.
52 Muller F, O'Rahilly R, Benson DR: The early origin of vertebral anomalies, as illustrated by a 'butterfly vertebra'. J Anat 1986;149:157–169.
53 Sanderson E, Newman V, Haigh SF, et al: Vertebral anomalies in children with Alagille syndrome: an analysis of 50 consecutive patients. Pediatr Radiol 2002;32:114–119.
54 McDonald-McGinn DM, Kirschner R, Goldmuntz E, et al: The Philadelphia story: the 22q11.2 deletion: report on 250 patients. Genet Couns 1999;10:11–24.
55 Rosenfield NS, Kelley MJ, Jensen PS, et al: Arteriohepatic dysplasia: radiologic features of a new syndrome. AJR Am J Roentgenol 1980;135:1217–1223.
56 Greenwood RD, Rosenthal A, Crocker AC, Nadas AS: Syndrome of intrahepatic biliary dysgenesis and cardiovascular malformations. Pediatrics 1976;58:243–247.
57 Heubi JE, Higgins JV, Argao EA, et al: The role of magnesium in the pathogenesis of bone disease in childhood cholestatic liver disease: a preliminary report. J Pediatr Gastroenterol Nutr 1997;25:301–306.
58 Bales CB, Kamath BM, Munoz PS, et al: Pathologic lower extremity fractures in children with Alagille syndrome. J Pediatr Gastroenterol Nutr 2010;51:66–70.
59 Hingorani M, Nischal KK, Davies A, et al: Ocular abnormalities in Alagille syndrome. Ophthalmology 1999;106:330–337.
60 Brodsky MC, Cunniff C: Ocular anomalies in the Alagille syndrome (arteriohepatic dysplasia). Ophthalmology 1993;100:1767–1774.
61 Krantz ID, Rand EB, Genin A, et al: Deletions of 20p12 in Alagille syndrome: frequency and molecular characterization. Am J Med Genet 1997;70:80–86.
62 Johnson BL: Ocular pathologic features of arteriohepatic dysplasia (Alagille's syndrome). Am J Ophthalmol 1990;110:504–512.
63 Kamath BM, Loomes KM, Oakey RJ, et al: Facial features in Alagille syndrome: specific or cholestasis facies? Am J Med Genet 2002;112:163–170.
64 Pilia G, Uda M, Macis D, et al: Jagged-1 mutation analysis in Italian Alagille syndrome patients. Hum Mutat 1999;14:394–400.
65 Heritage ML, MacMillan JC, Colliton RP, et al: Jagged1 (JAG1) mutation detection in an Australian Alagille syndrome population. Hum Mutat 2000;16:408–416.
66 Heritage ML, MacMillan JC, Anderson GJ: DHPLC mutation analysis of Jagged1 (JAG1) reveals six novel mutations in Australian Alagille syndrome patients. Hum Mutat 2002;20:481.
67 Ropke A, Kujat A, Gräber M, et al: Identification of 36 novel Jagged1 (JAG1) mutations in patients with Alagille syndrome. Hum Mutat 2003;21:100.
68 Jurkiewicz D, Popowska E, Gläser C, et al: Twelve novel JAG1 gene mutations in Polish Alagille syndrome patients. Hum Mutat 2005;25:321.
69 Yuan ZR, Kohsaka T, Ikegaya T, et al: Mutational analysis of the Jagged 1 gene in Alagille syndrome families. Hum Mol Genet 1998;7:1363–1369.
70 Yuan ZR, Okaniwa M, Nagata I, et al: The DSL domain in mutant JAG1 ligand is essential for the severity of the liver defect in Alagille syndrome. Clin Genet 2001;59:330–337.
71 Onouchi Y, Kurahashi H, Tajiri H, et al: Genetic alterations in the JAG1 gene in Japanese patients with Alagille syndrome. J Hum Genet 1999;44:235–239.

72 Kasahara M, Kiuchi T, Inomata Y, et al: Living-related liver transplantation for Alagille syndrome. Transplantation 2003;75:2147–2150.
73 Kim B, Park SH, Yang HR, et al: Hepatocellular carcinoma occurring in Alagille syndrome. Pathol Res Pract 2005;201:55–60.
74 Wang JS, Wang XH, Zhu QR, et al: Clinical and pathological characteristics of Alagille syndrome in Chinese children. World J Pediatr 2008;4:283–288.
75 Lin HC, Le Hoang P, Hutchinson A, et al: Alagille syndrome in a Vietnamese cohort: mutation analysis and assessment of facial features. Am J Med Genet A 2012;158A:1005–10013.
76 Tolia V, Dubois RS, Watts FB Jr, Perrin E: Renal abnormalities in paucity of interlobular bile ducts. J Pediatr Gastroenterol Nutr 1987;6:971–976.
77 Schonck M, Hoorntje S, van Hooff J: Renal transplantation in Alagille syndrome. Nephrol Dial Transplant 1998;13:197–199.
78 Connor SE, Hewes D, Ball C, Jarosz JM: Alagille syndrome associated with angiographic moyamoya. Childs Nerv Syst 2002;18:186–190.
79 Saidi AS, Kovalchin JP, Fisher DJ, et al: Balloon pulmonary valvuloplasty and stent implantation. For peripheral pulmonary artery stenosis in Alagille syndrome. Tex Heart Inst J 1998;25:79–82.
80 Sugiyama H, Veldtman GR, Norgard G, et al: Bladed balloon angioplasty for peripheral pulmonary artery stenosis. Catheter Cardiovasc Interv 2004;62:71–77.
81 Gandhi SK, Reyes J, Webber SA, et al: Case report of combined pediatric heart-lung-liver transplantation. Transplantation 2002; 73:1968–1969.
82 Mattei P, von Allmen D, Piccoli D, Rand E: Relief of intractable pruritus in Alagille syndrome by partial external biliary diversion. J Pediatr Surg 2006;41:104–107; discussion 104–107.

Dr. Henry C. Lin
Division of Gastroenterology, Hepatology, and Nutrition
Department of Pediatrics, The Children's Hospital of Philadelphia
34th Street and Civic Center Boulevard, Philadelphia, PA 19104 (USA)
E-Mail linhc@email.chop.edu

Muenke M, Kruszka PS, Sable CA, Belmont JW (eds): Congenital Heart Disease: Molecular Genetics, Principles of Diagnosis and Treatment. Basel, Karger, 2015, pp 166–177
DOI: 10.1159/000375214

Heterotaxy

Cecilia Lo[a] · You Li[a] · Hisato Yagi[a] · George Gabriel[a] · Nikolai Klena[a] · Kristi Lemke[a] · Linda Leatherbury[b]

[a]Department of Developmental Biology, University of Pittsburgh School of Medicine, Pittsburgh, Pa., and [b]Children's National Heart Institute, Children's National Medical Center, Washington, D.C., USA

Abstract

Heterotaxy, a birth defect associated with randomization of left-right visceral organ asymmetry, is highly associated with complex congenital heart disease (CHD). This reflects the essential role of left-right patterning in the formation of the four-chamber heart required for the systemic/pulmonary circulation. Clinically, a narrow spectrum of heterotaxy patients with CHD is classified as either having left (LAI) or right atrial isomerism (RAI). The most common CHD observed with heterotaxy is atrioventricular (AV) septal defect, with RAI having a worse prognosis due to more complex CHD involving AV or ventriculoarterial discordance; those with LAI may suffer from conduction abnormalities, but with less serious structural heart defects. While heterotaxy may have a genetically heterogeneous etiology with a male bias, recent studies suggest some heterotaxy patients may share a common genetic etiology with primary ciliary dyskinesia (PCD) involving motile cilium defects. Similar to PCD, patients with heterotaxy secondary to ciliary dysfunction (CD) may have respiratory disease, more postsurgical respiratory complications and a trend towards increased morbidity/mortality. Together these findings suggest heterotaxy patients may benefit from presurgical screening for airway CD and potential pulmonary therapy to improve postsurgical outcome.

Heterotaxy is a birth defect characterized by randomized left-right patterning of visceral organ situs in the thoracic or abdominal cavity. Left-right patterning plays an essential role in cardiovascular development, as the heart is the most left-right asymmetric organ in the body. This asymmetry is essential for partitioning the left versus right sides of the heart and separating the systemic versus the pulmonary circulation, which allows for efficient oxygenation of blood. With normal left-right visceral organ situs, referred to as situs solitus, the asymmetric placement of organs comprises levocardia with the heart apex pointing to the left, three lung lobes on the right and two on the left, eparte-

Fig. 1. Three distinct laterality phenotypes and congenital heart defects in Sharpei mutant mice with Dyx1c1 PCD gene mutation. **a–c** Homozygous *Sharpei* mutants can exhibit situs solitus with normal visceral organ positioning (**a**), heterotaxy with randomized left-right patterning of visceral organ situs (**b**) or situs inversus totalis with mirror-symmetric visceral organ situs (**c**). While both the heterotaxy and situs inversus mutants shown have mirror-symmetric organ placement in the chest cavity with dextrocardia (situs denoted by white arrow), left-sided inferior vena cava (IVC), and inverted lung lobation (numbered 1–5), the heterotaxy mutant (**b**) exhibited left-sided pancreas (Pan) and spleen (Sp) with right-sided stomach (S) and inverted liver lobation (Lv), while the situs inversus mutant (**c**) exhibited malpositioning of the great arteries (**d**). Right (R)/left (L) orientation is the same (**a–c**). **d–f** Analysis of intracardiac anatomy by histopathology revealed complex congenital heart defects in *Sharpei* mutants with heterotaxy. The heterotaxy mutant (**b**) was observed to have dextrocardia with transposition of the great arteries (**d**, **e**). The aorta (Ao) is connected to the morphological right ventricle (mRV; **e**) and the pulmonary artery (PA) to the morphological left ventricle (mLV; **e**). A ventricular septal defect (VSD) and coronary fistula (denoted by arrowhead) were also observed (**f**). DA = ductus arteriosus; mRA = morphological right atrium. **g–i** Another *Sharpei* mutant with heterotaxy exhibited dextrocardia (**g**) with double-outlet right ventricle, which is indicated by the pulmonary artery (PA) and aorta (Ao) emerging from the mRV (**h**). This mutant also exhibited AV septal defect (AVSD), muscular VSD (**i**: arrow), and RAI. White double arrows denote right (R)/left (L) orientation, which is the same for all panels. Reproduced from Tarkar et al. [67].

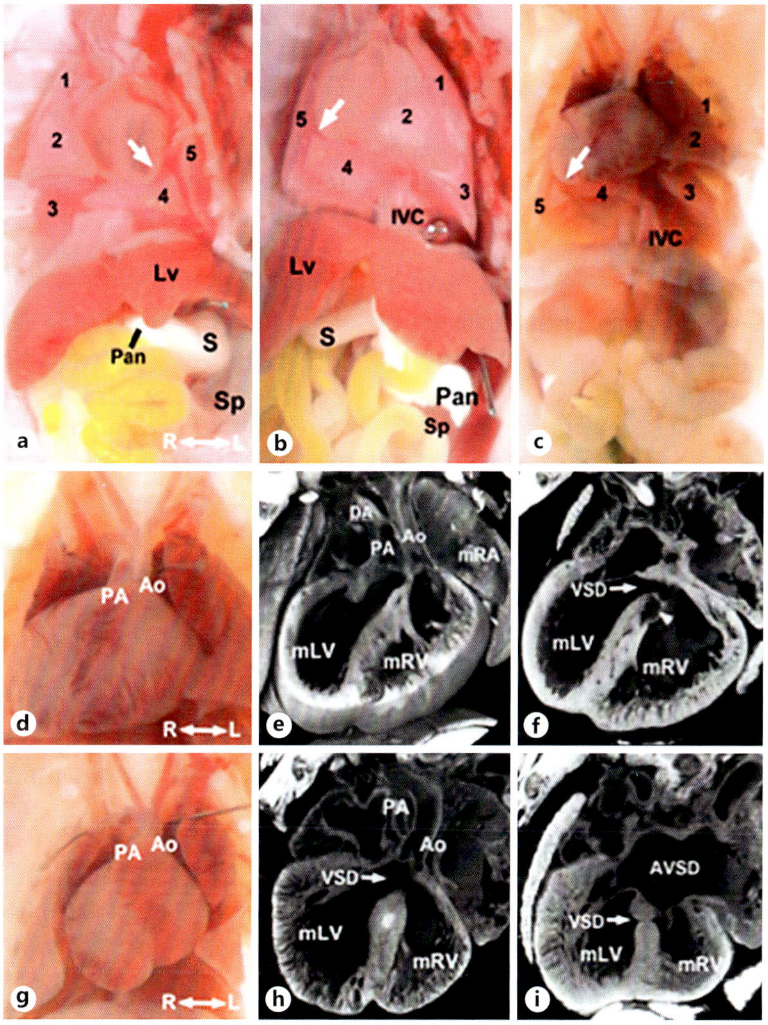

rial branching of the right bronchus, and right-dominant liver with left-sided placement of the stomach and spleen (fig. 1a: newborn mouse with situs solitus). With heterotaxy, also referred to as situs ambiguous, the asymmetric patterning and positioning of the visceral organs are randomized (fig. 1b: mouse heterotaxy mutant). Structures that are unilateral, such as the superior or inferior vena cava, can be misplaced or duplicated, and the gut may be malrotated. In some patients with laterality defects, there can be complete mirror-symmetric placement of organs, referred to as situs inversus totalis (fig. 1c: mouse mutant with situs inversus). In contrast to heterotaxy patients, such individuals are usually without cardiac defects.

The clinical diagnosis of heterotaxy requires assessment by multiple imaging modalities. This typically includes echocardiography for evaluating structural heart defects, chest X-ray for the assessment of bronchus-branching patterns, abdominal ultrasound for visualization of the liver, gallbladder, stomach and spleen, upper gastrointestinal series for the detection of gut malrotation, and hepatobiliary scintigraphy to assess biliary duct abnormalities. Many different combinations of visceral organ situs defects can be observed through imaging, and heterotaxy patients with congenital heart disease (CHD) associated with ambiguous atria are typically classified into two broad categories known as right (RAI) or left atrial isomerism (LAI). Typically with RAI, not only are both atrial appendages anatomically right sided, there is often also asplenia or absence of the spleen. Conversely, LAI is associated with bilateral left-sided atrial appendages and multiple spleens or polysplenia. In conjunction with identity differences in the atrial appendages, other structural perturbations may be found, such as interruption of the inferior vena cava or duplication of the superior vena cava. Patients with heterotaxy may exhibit other malformations, including CNS, genitourinary, and axial skeletal defects. Additional imaging, such as brain MRI, should be considered based on clinical criteria.

Classification of Heterotaxy: Atrial Isomerisms and Other Laterality Defects

The classification of CHD patients with heterotaxy into those with RAI or LAI is largely driven by their differing structural malformations and the resulting clinical exigencies. While atrioventricular (AV) septal defects are commonly observed in both LAI and RAI (fig. 1g–i), complex CHD is frequently observed with RAI, often associated with AV and/or ventriculoarterial discordance disrupting the normal systemic/pulmonary circulation. RAI infants typically present with a single atrium, single right ventricle, and a single AV connection. Additionally, RAI may have D-transposition of the great arteries (D-TGA), bilateral superior vena cavae, total anomalous pulmonary venous connection, pulmonary outflow obstruction, coronary sinus unroofing, bilateral trilobed lungs, right-sided stomach, asplenia, mid-line liver, and malrotation of intestines. Approximately 60–80% of patients with RAI have D-TGA [1]. D-TGA is characterized by AV concordance and ventriculoarterial discordance, where the aorta arises from the right ventricle and the pulmonary artery arises from the left ventricle. Thus, heterotaxy patients with RAI typically require palliation with complex cardiac surgeries. Despite surgical advances and advances in critical care medicine, prognosis is significantly worse for heterotaxy patients with RAI, with one study showing a 5-year survival of only 35% after palliative surgery and none surviving biventricular repair [2]. In contrast, patients with LAI have less severe cardiac malformations and a high prevalence of AV septal defects and AV discordance with less pulmonary stenosis requiring immediate neonatal surgery. Also prevalent are interrupted inferior vena cava, AV block, and more extracardiac anomalies [2, 3]. Patients with LAI typically require either no surgical intervention or often are effectively treated with biventricular cardiac surgery [2].

While the stratification of heterotaxy-CHD patients as having LAI or RAI is clinically driven, heterotaxy-CHD patients can have laterality disturbance other than RAI or LAI. This may include patients with isolated dextrocardia or mesocardia, or AV discordance and/or L-TGA. L-TGA of the great arteries is when both the great arteries and the ventricles (L-looping) are inverted, thus systemic venous return from the right atrium is directed through the morphologic left ventricle and into the pulmonary artery, and pulmonary venous return is directed through the morphologic right ventricle and into the aorta. L-TGA is commonly referred to as congenitally corrected transposition of the great arteries. Heterotaxy-CHD patients also may have normal cardiac situs, but exhibit an abnormal or discordant situs in any organ system typically implicated in laterality disorders, such as the pulmonary, gastrointestinal, splenic, and/or hepatobiliary system.

Overall, CHD patients with heterotaxy, especially those with RAI, have more postsurgical complications and worse outcomes. Regardless of the stratification of CHD patients with heterotaxy, insights into the clinical sequelae of heterotaxy patients will require a better understanding of the developmental and genetic etiology of CHD. Only with such mechanistic insights can we hope to develop more effective surgical and therapeutic interventions to improve outcome for these highly vulnerable CHD patients.

Association of Complex Congenital Heart Disease with Heterotaxy

Clinically, heterotaxy is relatively rare with a prevalence of 1 in 10,000, but it is highly associated with CHD – comprising approximately 3% of CHD cases [4, 5]. This suggests left-right patterning may play an important role in the etiology of complex CHD. In recent studies involving large-scale mouse forward genetic screening for CHD-causing mutations, we have confirmed the essential role of left-right patterning in complex CHD. Using fetal echocardiography, we conducted a prenatal fetal ultrasound screen of chemically mutagenized mice to recover mutants with CHD [6]. This phenotype-driven non-gene-biased approach yielded more than 200 mutant lines with a wide array of complex CHD (http://www.informatics.jax.org/searchtool/Search.do?query=b2b&submit=Quick%0D%0ASearch). We found more than half of the CHD mutant lines with complex CHD also had laterality defects.

Our analysis revealed an interesting characteristic of mutations causing laterality defects – a single pathogenic mutation in genes required for left-right patterning can elicit mutants with a wide spectrum of complex CHD in conjunction with heterotaxy [7, 8]. Some examples of the complex CHD types observed in heterotaxy mutants recovered from our screen are shown in figure 2, and include hypoplastic right heart syndrome (fig. 2a), univentricular heart (fig. 2b), ventricular dextroversion (fig. 2c), and superior-inferior ventricles (fig. 2c, d). These complex CHD types and the resulting AV and/or ventriculoarterial discordance are challenging to palliate, with many not amenable to biventricular repair. From our use of fetal ultrasound imaging to interrogate CHD mutant mouse models, we noted fetal mice with complex structural heart defects often expired prenatally, and it is only with the capability of conducting prenatal fetal ultrasound that we were successful in discovering such mutants. Thus, clinically, it is likely that many of the most severe complex CHD types associated with heterotaxy are subject to loss in utero. Indeed, previous clinical studies of CHD associated with fetal deaths showed a markedly higher prenatal incidence of CHD compared to live-born infants [9, 10].

Left-Right Patterning and Regulation of Cardiac Looping

To understand the etiology of complex CHD associated with heterotaxy, it is necessary to consider how left-right patterning is established during embryonic development. Left-right axis specification in the early embryo is initiated with early left-sided expression of Nodal and right-sided expression of its inhibitor Dand5 in the embryonic node. This differential activation of Nodal expression at the node is one of the early signs of laterality in the mouse embryo, and is initiated via signaling mediated by motile and sensory cilium function at the node. Monociliated cells at the node have motile cilia that exhibit clockwise rotation generating a leftward flow. Such flow is thought to impinge on cilia in the crown cells at the edge of the node, causing left-sided propagation of calcium signaling [11, 12]. Experimental evidence has led to three models for how the nodal flow generated by the motile cilia is perceived by the nodal and perinodal crown cells: (1) the accumulation of extracellular morphogens on the left side of the embryo; (2) asymmetric distribution of node vesicular parcels containing hedgehog proteins and retinoic acid regulated by FGF8 [13, 14], and (3) detection of fluid flow by mechanosensory cilia leading to an asymmetrical influx of Ca^{2+} via Pkd2 and Pkd1l1 in the nonmotile primary cilia of the perinodal crown cells [14–23].

Nodal signaling at the node is propagated to the left lateral plate mesoderm, where Nodal expression is also activated. This left-sided Nodal activation requires the EGF-CFC coreceptor and activin receptors (ALK4/7 and Acvr2b) [24–30], and results in the downstream activation of *Lefty1/Lefty2* and

4

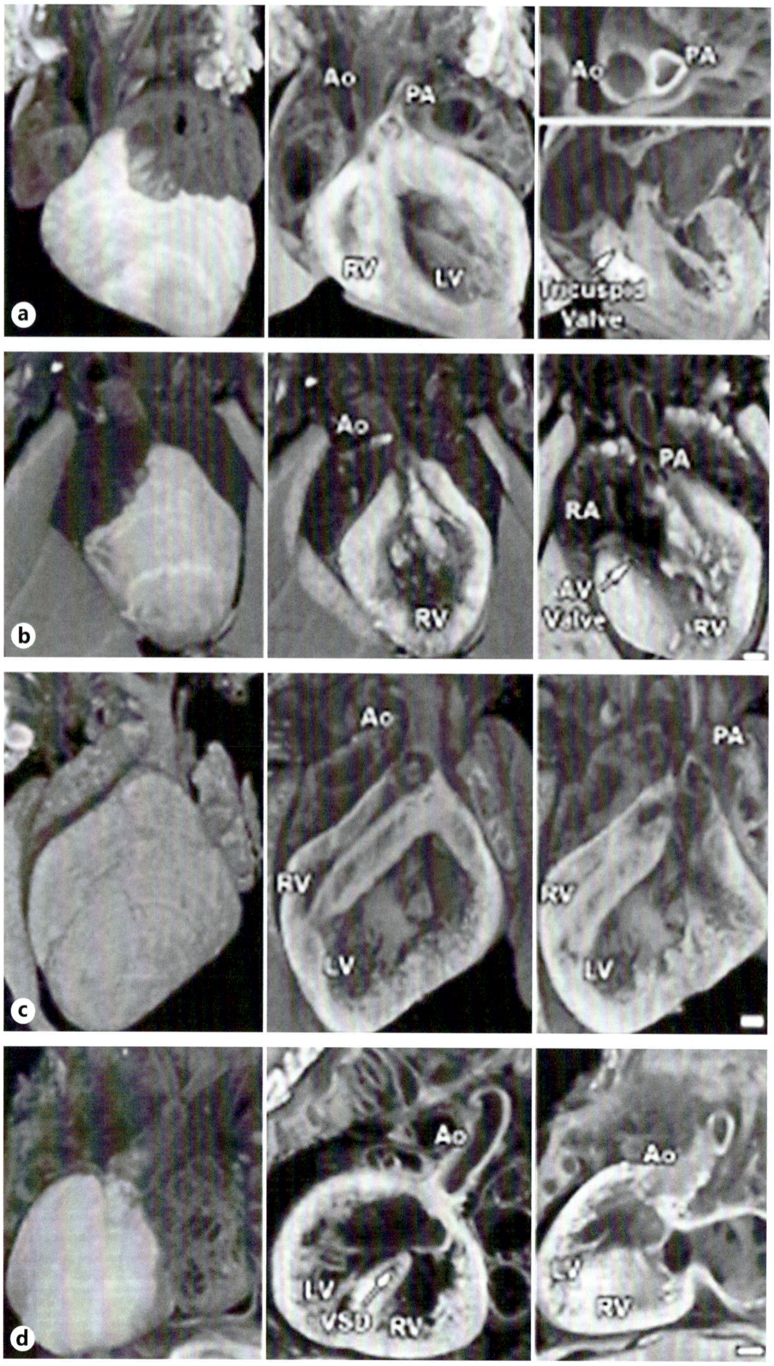

Fig. 2. Wide spectrum of complex congenital heart defects associated with heterotaxy. Histological analysis by episcopic confocal microscopy of mouse hearts in mutants exhibiting heterotaxy reveals a wide spectrum of complex congenital heart defects. **a** Hypoplastic right heart syndrome consisting of a hypoplastic right ventricle (RV) with small tricuspid valve and hypoplastic main pulmonary artery (PA) trunk. **b** Single RV with TGA {A, A, D}, a common AV valve, and a common atrium. **c** Dextroversion comprising ventricular inversion with TGA {A, D, D}, hypoplastic RV, an unbalanced AV septal defect, and superior-inferior ventricles. **d** Dextrocardia with pulmonary atresia, ventricular septal defect (VSD) and superior-inferior ventricules {A, L, A}. Scale bars = 0.2 mm. Ao = Aorta; PA = pulmonary artery; RV = right ventricle; LV = left ventricle; RA = right atrium, { } = Van Pragh classification.

Pitx2. Ultimately, the left-right patterning of visceral organ situs is thought to arise from the left-sided expression of *Pitx2* in organ primordia [31–33]. Studies in zebrafish model systems suggest the activation of Nodal signaling in the left lateral plate mesoderm drives the direction of heart looping via modulation of the directional migration of cardiac progenitors [34]. This is mediated by left-sided BMP inhibition causing a reduction in nonmuscle myosin II expression and concomitant higher cell motility on the embryo's left side. This left versus right difference in cell motility is proposed to drive the asymmetric looping of the heart tube in zebrafish embryos [35]. As the asymmetric expression of nonmuscle myosin II was actually first reported in mouse embryos, this mechanism regulating the orientation of heart looping is likely conserved in mammals [36–38]. How this initial asymmetric looping of the heart tube is integrated with Pitx2 signaling and the subsequent AV and outflow tract septation events driving cardiac morphogenesis are critical outstanding questions, questions that can only be fully addressed with further studies using animal models with four-chamber hearts.

Genetic Etiology of Heterotaxy

Various studies have suggested the involvement of both genetic and environmental risk factors in heterotaxy [39]. Family history of heterotaxy, maternal diabetes, and environmental pollutants have been associated with heterotaxy [39–41]. Genetic studies have shown that heterotaxy is genetically heterogeneous, and may involve autosomal recessive, autosomal dominant, and X-linked modes of inheritance [42]. X-linked inheritance is suggested by a 2:1 ratio of male to females with heterotaxy and the identification of *ZIC3*, a gene encoding a transcription factor on the X chromosome, as being required for left-right patterning [43]. However, most cases of heterotaxy occur sporadically and their genetic etiology remains largely unknown. Clinical studies have identified several genes as likely playing a role in heterotaxy, including *NODAL* [44, 45], *ZIC3* [43], *LEFTY2* [46], *CFC1* [47], *ACVR2B* [48], *FOXH1* [49], *GDF1* [49, 50], *GALNT11* [51], *SESN1* [52, 53], and *SHROOM3* [54]. Most of these genes play a role either directly or indirectly in modulating Nodal signaling. Mutations in *NKX2.5* [55], *CRELD1* [56], and *GLI2* [57] also have been implicated in heterotaxy.

Studies of mutant and knockout animal models have identified many other genes that can cause laterality defects. Some examples include *Bicc1* [58], *Epb4.1l5* [59], *Tbx6* [60], *Sept6* [61], *Trb3* [62], and *Lamb1a* [63]. The role of these genes in human heterotaxy remains to be investigated. Mutations in *Bicc1*, an RNA binding protein known to have a role in microRNA regulation, causes heterotaxy with CHD in conjunction with polycystic kidney disease [58], an indication of the disruption of primary cilium function. Analysis of laterality mutants recovered from our mouse mutagenesis screen with complex CHD and heterotaxy revealed many of the disease-causing pathogenic mutations are in fact in cilium-related or ciliome genes, including *Mks1* [64], *Wdpcp* [65], *Dnah5* [7], *Dnai1* [8, 66], *Dnah11, Dyx1c1* [67], and *Armc4* [68]. While *Mks1* encodes a centrosomal/basal protein associated with the ciliopathy Meckel syndrome, *Dnah5, Dnai1*, and *Dnah11* mutations are well-described causes of motile cilium defects associated with primary ciliary dyskinesia (PCD). PCD is a sinopulmonary disease associated with mucociliary transport defects due to immotile or dyskinetic cilia in the respiratory epithelia. PCD patients can exhibit male infertility due to sperm motility defects and situs inversus, also known as Kartagener syndrome. Recent clinical studies also showed mutations in *Dyx1c1* and *Armc4* can cause PCD, findings confirmed by our recovery of *Dyx1c1* and *Armc4* mouse mutations causing laterality defects, including heterotaxy and complex CHD (fig. 1) [67, 68]. Together these findings suggest a common etiology for heterotaxy and PCD, with PCD mutations contributing to complex CHD associated with heterotaxy.

Ciliopathies and Heterotaxy

Laterality defects including heterotaxy have been reported for a number of human diseases known as ciliopathies, including Meckel syndrome, Bardet-Biedl syndromes, renal hepatic pancreatic dysplasia, Ellis-van Creveld syndrome, oral-facial-digital syndrome type 1, Jeune syndrome/asphyxiating thoracic dystrophy and short rib-polydactyly syndromes [4, 61, 69, 70]. Ciliopathies are a class of heritable human diseases arising from mutations that cause sensory or primary cilium defects. They are often associated with a wide spectrum of structural birth defects, and can also be associated with mental retardation, blindness, deafness, or obesity. The finding of laterality defects amongst patients with ciliopathies suggests that cilium-related genes may play an important role in the genetic etiology of heterotaxy, consistent with embryological studies showing the essential role of cilia in the developmental specification of the left-right body axis. The finding of heterotaxy with PCD [7, 71] is of particular importance, given that PCD and heterotaxy are both rare disorders with a prevalence of 1 in 10,000. In a recent study of PCD patients, a >6% incidence of heterotaxy was observed [71], confirming a mechanistic link involving cilium defects in the developmental etiology of both PCD and heterotaxy. We also conducted a clinical study of heterotaxy patients, which showed a high prevalence of respiratory ciliary dysfunction (CD) in patients with CHD that is similar to that of PCD [72]. These heterotaxy patients also had a high prevalence of mutations in PCD genes, suggesting PCD-related ciliome mutations may contribute to respiratory disease in heterotaxy patients [72].

Airway Cilium Dysfunction Associated with Primary Ciliary Dyskinesia and Heterotaxy

Unlike other ciliopathies, which are largely thought of as affecting only nonmotile sensory or primary cilia, PCD involves the disruption of motile cilium function. Recent studies of mutant mouse models harboring pathogenic mutations in genes known to cause PCD confirmed that heterotaxy can arise from PCD mutations [7, 71]. Interestingly, such studies showed mice with pathogenic mutations or knockout alleles in PCD genes, such as *Dnah5, Dnai1, Dyx1c1*, or *Armc4*, can have three distinct laterality phenotypes. Approximately half of the mutants exhibit either normal situs solitus or situs inversus, while the remaining 50% exhibit heterotaxy (fig. 1). While almost all heterotaxy mutants will have complex CHD and show pre- or neonatal lethality, those with situs solitus or situs inversus are usually postnatally viable and typically will have only an occasional ventricular septal defect or interrupted inferior vena cava with azygous or hemiazygous continuation.

Similar to PCD patients, mice with PCD mutations exhibit immotile or slow/dyskinetic ciliary motion in the tracheal respiratory epithelia. In the embryonic node, cilia are usually immotile. These observations led to the surprising conclusion that motile cilia are not essential for either breaking bilateral symmetry or the concordant specification of normal left-right visceral organ situs. Nevertheless, without motile cilium function, half of the mutant embryos will develop heterotaxy and CHD. Thus perhaps motile cilium function at the node evolved as a protective mechanism to ensure consistent specification of situs solitus required for normal cardiac morphogenesis.

Respiratory Symptoms and Disease in Ciliopathy and Heterotaxy Patients

Ciliopathies are considered to arise from sensory or primary cilium defects (except for PCD), but a study of patients with nonsyndromic Leber's congenital amaurosis, a severe inherited retinal degenerative disorder, revealed both abnormal ciliary motion and short and sparse ciliation in the airway epithelia [73]. These patients showed moderate but recurrent inflammatory disease in the upper and lower airways [73]. Similarly, a study of patients with Usher syndrome, a common cause of combined blindness and deafness due to sensorineural hearing defect and retinitis pigmentosa, showed a reduction in ciliary beat frequency [74, 75]. Also notable, patients with autosomal dominant polycystic kidney disease exhibit an increased prevalence of bronchiectasis [76]. While cystic kidney disease is well described to involve primary cilium defects, the concomitant finding of bronchiectasis, which is highly associated with PCD and defects in mucociliary clearance, would suggest there is a functional overlap in motile and primary cilium defects. Such overlap between sensory versus motile cilium defects is not entirely unexpected, since the same ciliary axoneme comprising nine microtubule doublets built on a basal body template is conserved in both primary and motile cilia.

The finding that heterotaxy patients can have a high prevalence of respiratory CD suggests CHD patients with heterotaxy may be at increased risk for respiratory complications. Perhaps this might contribute to the worse outcome known to be associated with this cohort of CHD patients. The study of heterotaxy patients for airway CD utilized two tests normally used for PCD assessments. This included analysis of ciliary motion in nasal tissue biopsies using high-resolution videomicroscopy, and the measurement of nasal NO (typically very low with PCD). Based on this dual assessment, we observed 18 of 43 (42%) CHD patients with heterotaxy had CD characterized by both abnormal ciliary motion and low nasal NO (fig. 3) [72]. We then showed that heterotaxy patients with CD had increased respiratory symptoms and disease, including a higher incidence of chronic wet cough, otitis media, newborn respiratory distress, and bronchiectasis, all features associated with PCD [72]. Exome sequencing again showed an increase in the incidence of mutations in cilium genes known to cause PCD [72], suggesting cilium-related genes may contribute to the airway CD associated with heterotaxy. A more complex polygenic model of disease for heterotaxy involving mutations in multiple laterality genes has been suggested previously [77]. This is compatible with the known complexity of the cilium, a highly conserved microtubule-based organelle comprising more than 500 proteins [78].

Respiratory Complications and Worse Outcome in Heterotaxy Patients

The finding of airway CD in CHD patients with heterotaxy is of significant clinical interest [79], as heterotaxy patients with CHD have disproportionately higher morbidity and mortality despite significant advances in palliative surgeries and critical care medicine. Several clinical studies have shown heterotaxy patients with CHD have a prolonged clinical course and a worse postsurgical outcome [80]. In one retrospective study at the Children's Hospital in Boston, 11 of 16 heterotaxy patients died during the 1-month postoperative follow-up period [81]. In another study of surgical outcomes, CHD patients with heterotaxy had twice the rate of postoperative mortality compared to CHD patients without heterotaxy (4.8 vs. 2.4%) [82]. Our own retrospective review of CHD patients undergoing cardiac surgery at the Children's National Medical Center showed 84 heterotaxy patients had a higher postsurgical mortality, increased postsurgical respiratory complications, and a more complicated postsurgical course as compared to 634 CHD patients without heterotaxy. As these two patient cohorts were matched for RACHS-1 scores, the differences were not related to surgical complexity [83].

It is significant to note that respiratory complications in CHD patients are usually attributed to the heart disease and airway CD is usually not considered. In light of our finding of a high prevalence of CD in heterotaxy patients, we propose that undiagnosed PCD-like airway ciliary defects could be a significant factor contributing to the increased respiratory complications in this patient population. If this is not preemptively managed, it could contribute to the worse outcome. Indeed our prospective analysis of CHD patients with heterotaxy undergoing cardiac surgery revealed those with CD had significantly more postsurgical and respiratory complications than those without CD, and they used more inhaled β-agonists [84]. These findings provide independent confirmation that airway clearance function is markedly compromised in heterotaxy patients secondary to CD. In this initial study, a trend towards increased mortality was also noted [84], a finding that will require further validation with the analysis of a larger patient cohort. Nevertheless, the findings from this study provide strong evidence of a role for airway CD in the complicated clinical sequelae and poor outcome of CHD patients with heterotaxy.

Summary and Future Prospects for Improving Clinical Care and Outcome

Heterotaxy patients have some of the most complex CHD types. They show an overlapping molecular etiology with PCD involving motile cilium defects. Studies in mouse models show mutations in genes known to cause PCD and three distinct

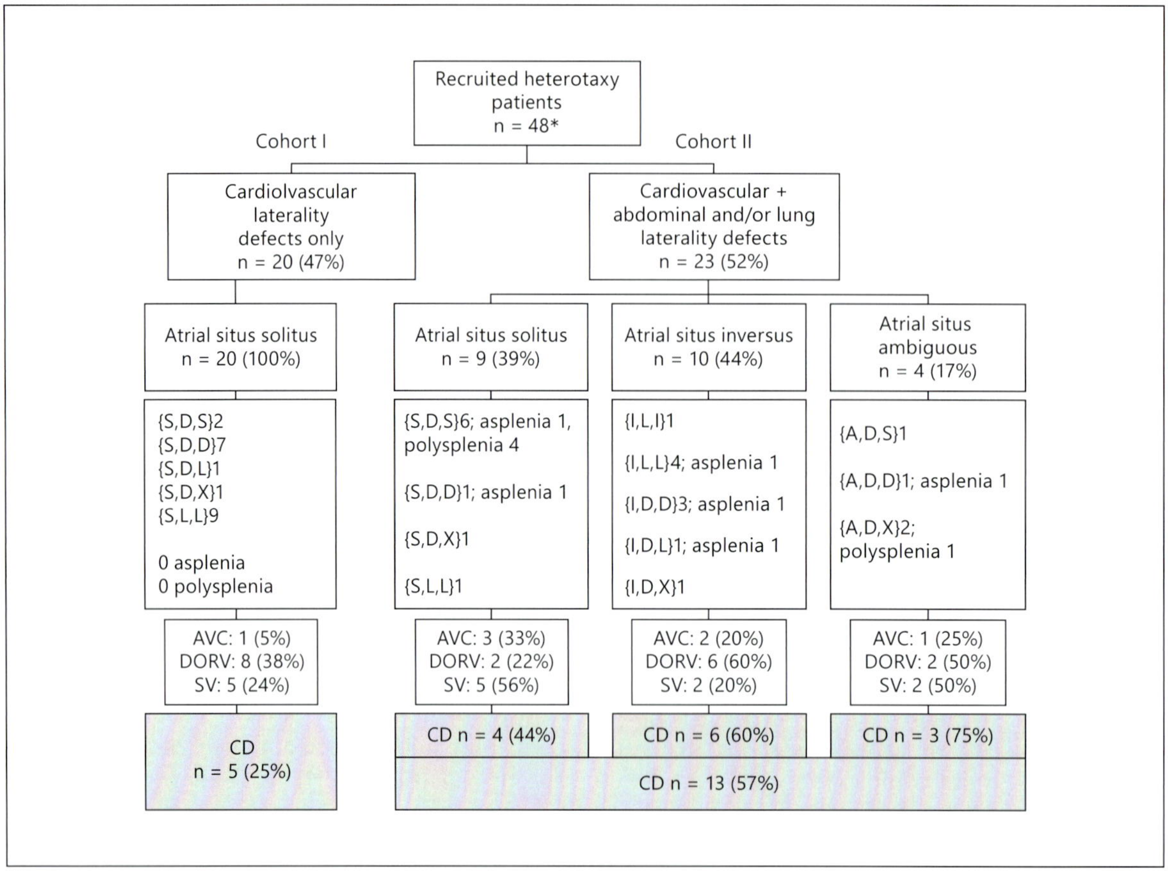

Fig. 3. Prevalence of airway CD in heterotaxy patients stratified by laterality and cardiovascular defect phenotypes. Heterotaxy patients were recruited to assess for airway CD. These patients were stratified by laterality and cardiovascular defect phenotypes, with the cardiac AV/ventriculoarterial alignment delineated using the Van Praagh classification. Included among the patients with atrial situs ambiguous are those with LAI and RAI. Of the 48 patients recruited, 43 completed the studies, and of these, 18 (42%) showed respiratory CD*. This comprised 25% of the heterotaxy patients with cardiovascular laterality defects only and 57% of heterotaxy patients with both cardiac and abdominal/lung laterality defects, showing patients with more severe laterality disturbance had greater risk of having airway CD (p = 0.037). AVC = AV canal; DORV = double-outlet right ventricle; SV = single ventricle. Reproduced from Nakhleh et al. [72].

phenotypes have been reported: situs solitus, situs inversus, or heterotaxy. With either situs solitus or situs inversus, there is generally no structural heart defect except for the infrequent simple ventricular septal defect or azygous continuation. In contrast, heterotaxy mutant mice invariably die prenatally or neonatally from complex CHD. In heterotaxy patients with CHD, clinical studies have shown high morbidity and mortality rates, and increased respiratory and other postsurgical complications. We observed a high prevalence of airway CD in a broad spectrum of heterotaxy patients and propose their poor outcome may reflect undiagnosed and therefore untreated respiratory airway CD. Consistent with this, heterotaxy patients exhibit an increased incidence of PCD gene mutations. However, as these PCD mutations were found only in heterozygosity and PCD is a recessive disorder, perhaps heterotaxy patients with airway CD are distinct from PCD. Nevertheless, heterotaxy patients with CD show a substantial increase in the risk for postsurgical respiratory complications, and as such this may contribute to increased morbidity and mortality, and a worse outcome. Therefore, we propose there could be significant benefit in screening heterotaxy patients presurgically for respiratory CD and providing pulmonary therapy to heterotaxy patients with CD to enhance airway clearance. This change in the standard of care could minimize the risk for respiratory infections and other respiratory complications, and could help improve the prognosis for these high-risk cardiac-surgery patients who continue to suffer some of the highest morbidity and mortality amongst all CHD patients.

Acknowledgments

This work was supported by funding from NIH grants HL098180 and OD010340.

References

1 Marino B, Capolino R, Digilio MC, et al: Transposition of the great arteries in asplenia and polysplenia phenotypes. Am J Med Genet 2002;110:292–294.

2 Lim JS, McCrindle BW, Smallhorn JF, et al: Clinical features, management, and outcome of children with fetal and postnatal diagnoses of isomerism syndromes. Circulation 2005;112:2454–2461.

3 Rose V, Izukawa T, Moes CA: Syndromes of asplenia and polysplenia. A review of cardiac and non-cardiac malformations in 60 cases with special reference to diagnosis and prognosis. Br Heart J 1975;37:840–852.

4 Ware SM, Aygun MG, Hildebrandt F: Spectrum of clinical diseases caused by disorders of primary cilia. Proc Am Thorac Soc 2011;8:444–450.

5 Lin AE, Krikov S, Riehle-Colarusso T, et al: Laterality defects in the National Birth Defects Prevention Study (1998–2007): birth prevalence and descriptive epidemiology. Am J Med Genet A 2014;164A:2581–2591.

6 Liu X, Francis R, Kim AJ, et al: Interrogating congenital heart defects with noninvasive fetal echocardiography in a mouse forward genetic screen. Circ Cardiovasc Imaging 2014;7:31–42.

7 Tan SY, Rosenthal J, Zhao XQ, et al: Heterotaxy and complex structural heart defects in a mutant mouse model of primary ciliary dyskinesia. J Clin Invest 2007;117:3742–3752.

8 Francis RJ, Christopher A, Devine WA, et al: Congenital heart disease and the specification of left-right asymmetry. Am J Physiol Heart Circ Physiol 2012;302:H2102–H2111.

9 Hoffman JI: Incidence of congenital heart disease: II. Prenatal incidence. Pediatr Cardiol 1995;16:155–165.

10 Hoffman JI: Incidence of congenital heart disease: I. Postnatal incidence. Pediatr Cardiol 1995;16:103–113.

11 Hirokawa N, Tanaka Y, Okada Y: Cilia, KIF3 molecular motor and nodal flow. Curr Opin Cell Biol 2012;24:31–39.

12 Nonaka S, Tanaka Y, Okada Y, et al: Randomization of left-right asymmetry due to loss of nodal cilia generating leftward flow of extraembryonic fluid in mice lacking KIF3B motor protein. Cell 1998;95:829–837.

13 Takeda S, Yonekawa Y, Tanaka Y, et al: Left-right asymmetry and kinesin superfamily protein KIF3A: new insights in determination of laterality and mesoderm induction by kif3A–/– mice analysis. J Cell Biol 1999;145:825–836.

14 Tanaka Y, Okada Y, Hirokawa N: FGF-induced vesicular release of Sonic hedgehog and retinoic acid in leftward nodal flow is critical for left-right determination. Nature 2005;435:172–177.

15 Basu B, Brueckner M: Cilia multifunctional organelles at the center of vertebrate left-right asymmetry. Curr Top Dev Biol 2008;85:151–174.

16 Field S, Riley KL, Grimes DT, et al: Pkd1l1 establishes left-right asymmetry and physically interacts with Pkd2. Development 2011;138:1131–1142.

17 Kamura K, Kobayashi D, Uehara Y, et al: Pkd1l1 complexes with Pkd2 on motile cilia and functions to establish the left-right axis. Development 2011;138:1121–1129.

18 McGrath J, Brueckner M: Cilia are at the heart of vertebrate left-right asymmetry. Curr Opin Genet Dev 2003;13:385–392.

19 McGrath J, Somlo S, Makova S, et al: Two populations of node monocilia initiate left-right asymmetry in the mouse. Cell 2003;114:61–73.

20 Norris DP: Cilia, calcium and the basis of left-right asymmetry. BMC Biol 2012;10:102.

21 Pennekamp P, Karcher C, Fischer A, et al: The ion channel polycystin-2 is required for left-right axis determination in mice. Curr Biol 2002;12:938–943.

22 Tabin CJ, Vogan KJ: A two-cilia model for vertebrate left-right axis specification. Genes Dev 2003;17:1–6.

23 Yost HJ: Left-right asymmetry: nodal cilia make and catch a wave. Curr Biol 2003;13:R808–R809.

24 Cheng SK, Olale F, Bennett JT, et al: EGF-CFC proteins are essential coreceptors for the TGF-beta signals Vg1 and GDF1. Genes Dev 2003;17:31–36.

25 Cheng SK, Olale F, Brivanlou AH, Schier AF: Lefty blocks a subset of TGFbeta signals by antagonizing EGF-CFC coreceptors. PLoS Biol 2004;2:E30.

26 Chu J, Ding J, Jeays-Ward K, et al: Non-cell-autonomous role for Cripto in axial midline formation during vertebrate embryogenesis. Development 2005;132:5539–5551.

27 Minchiotti G: Nodal-dependant Cripto signaling in ES cells: from stem cells to tumor biology. Oncogene 2005;24:5668–5675.

28 Reissmann E, Jörnvall H, Blokzijl A, et al: The orphan receptor ALK7 and the Activin receptor ALK4 mediate signaling by Nodal proteins during vertebrate development. Genes Dev 2001;15:2010–2022.

29 Yan YT, Liu JJ, Luo Y, et al: Dual roles of Cripto as a ligand and coreceptor in the nodal signaling pathway. Mol Cell Biol 2002;22:4439–4449.

30 Yeo C, Whitman M: Nodal signals to Smads through Cripto-dependent and Cripto-independent mechanisms. Mol Cell 2001;7:949–957.

31 Franco D, Campione M: The role of Pitx2 during cardiac development. Linking left-right signaling and congenital heart diseases. Trends Cardiovasc Med 2003;13:157–163.

32 Kitamura K, Miura H, Miyagawa-Tomita S, et al: Mouse Pitx2 deficiency leads to anomalies of the ventral body wall, heart, extra- and periocular mesoderm and right pulmonary isomerism. Development 1999;126:5749–5758.

33 Martin JF, Brown NA: Pitx2 in cardiac left-right asymmetry and human disease. In Heart Development and Regeneration. 2010. Vol. 1. London, Academic Press. Edited by Nadia Rosenthal and Richard P. Harvey.

34 Smith KA, Chocron S, von der Hardt S, et al: Rotation and asymmetric development of the zebrafish heart requires directed migration of cardiac progenitor cells. Dev Cell 2008;14:287–297.

35 Veerkamp J, Rudolph F, Cseresnyes Z, et al: Unilateral dampening of Bmp activity by nodal generates cardiac left-right asymmetry. Dev Cell 2013;24:660–667.
36 Tsuda T, Philp N, Zile MH, Linask KK: Left-right asymmetric localization of flectin in the extracellular matrix during heart looping. Dev Biol 1996;173:39–50.
37 Tsuda T, Majumder K, Linask KK: Differential expression of flectin in the extracellular matrix and left-right asymmetry in mouse embryonic heart during looping stages. Dev Genet 1998;23:203–214.
38 Lu W, Seeholzer SH, Han M, et al: Cellular nonmuscle myosins NMHC-IIA and NMHC-IIB and vertebrate heart looping. Dev Dyn 2008;237:3577–3590.
39 Kuehl KS, Loffredo C: Risk factors for heart disease associated with abnormal sidedness. Teratology 2002;66:242–248.
40 Kuehl KS, Loffredo CA: Population-based study of l-transposition of the great arteries: possible associations with environmental factors. Birth Defects Res A Clin Mol Teratol 2003;67:162–167.
41 Lin AE, Ticho BS, Houde K, et al: Heterotaxy: associated conditions and hospital-based prevalence in newborns. Genet Med 2000;2:157–172.
42 Belmont JW, Mohapatra B, Towbin JA, Ware SM: Molecular genetics of heterotaxy syndromes. Curr Opin Cardiol 2004;19:216–220.
43 Ware SM, Peng J, Zhu L, et al: Identification and functional analysis of ZIC3 mutations in heterotaxy and related congenital heart defects. Am J Hum Genet 2004;74:93–105.
44 Mohapatra B, Casey B, Li H, et al: Identification and functional characterization of NODAL rare variants in heterotaxy and isolated cardiovascular malformations. Hum Mol Genet 2009;18:861–871.
45 Sutherland MJ, Ware SM: Disorders of left-right asymmetry: heterotaxy and situs inversus. Am J Med Genet C Semin Med Genet 2009;151C:307–317.
46 Kosaki K, Bassi MT, Kosaki R, et al: Characterization and mutation analysis of human LEFTY A and LEFTY B, homologues of murine genes implicated in left-right axis development. Am J Hum Genet 1999;64:712–721.
47 Bamford RN, Roessler E, Burdine RD, et al: Loss-of-function mutations in the EGF-CFC gene CFC1 are associated with human left-right laterality defects. Nat Genet 2000;26:365–369.
48 Kosaki R, Gebbia M, Kosaki K, et al: Left-right axis malformations associated with mutations in ACVR2B, the gene for human activin receptor type IIB. Am J Med Genet 1999;82:70–76.
49 Roessler E, Ouspenskaia MV, Karkera JD, et al: Reduced NODAL signaling strength via mutation of several pathway members including FOXH1 is linked to human heart defects and holoprosencephaly. Am J Hum Genet 2008;83:18–29.
50 Karkera JD, Lee JS, Roessler E, et al: Loss-of-function mutations in growth differentiation factor-1 (GDF1) are associated with congenital heart defects in humans. Am J Hum Genet 2007;81:987–994.
51 Boskovski MT, Yuan S, Pedersen NB, et al: The heterotaxy gene GALNT11 glycosylates Notch to orchestrate cilia type and laterality. Nature 2013;504:456–459.
52 Peeters H, Debeer P, Bairoch A, et al: PA26 is a candidate gene for heterotaxia in humans: identification of a novel PA26-related gene family in human and mouse. Hum Genet 2003;112:573–580.
53 Peeters H, Voz ML, Verschueren K, et al: Sesn1 is a novel gene for left-right asymmetry and mediating nodal signaling. Hum Mol Genet 2006;15:3369–3377.
54 Tariq M, Belmont JW, Lalani S, et al: SHROOM3 is a novel candidate for heterotaxy identified by whole exome sequencing. Genome Biol 2011;12:R91.
55 Watanabe Y, Benson DW, Yano S, et al: Two novel frameshift mutations in NKX2.5 result in novel features including visceral inversus and sinus venosus type ASD. J Med Genet 2002;39:807–811.
56 Robinson SW, Morris CD, Goldmuntz E, et al: Missense mutations in CRELD1 are associated with cardiac atrioventricular septal defects. Am J Hum Genet 2003;72:1047–1052.
57 Kevelam SH, van Harssel JJ, van der Zwaag B, et al: A patient with a mild holoprosencephaly spectrum phenotype and heterotaxy and a 1.3 Mb deletion encompassing GLI2. Am J Med Genet A 2012;158A:166–173.
58 Cogswell C, Price SJ, Hou X, et al: Positional cloning of jcpk/bpk locus of the mouse. Mamm Genome 2003;14:242–249.
59 Lee JD, Migeotte I, Anderson KV: Left-right patterning in the mouse requires Epb4.1l5-dependent morphogenesis of the node and midline. Dev Biol 2010;346:237–246.
60 Hadjantonakis AK, Pisano E, Papaioannou VE: Tbx6 regulates left/right patterning in mouse embryos through effects on nodal cilia and perinodal signaling. PLoS One 2008;3:e2511.
61 Zhai G, Gu Q, He J, et al: Sept6 is required for ciliogenesis in Kupffer's vesicle, the pronephros, and the neural tube during early embryonic development. Mol Cell Biol 2014;34:1310–1321.
62 Anuppalle M, Maddirevula S, Huh TL, Rhee M: Trb3 regulates LR axis formation in zebrafish embryos. Mol Cells 2013;36:542–547.
63 Hochgreb-Hägele T, Yin C, Koo DE, et al: Laminin β1a controls distinct steps during the establishment of digestive organ laterality. Development 2013;140:2734–2745.
64 Cui C, Chatterjee B, Francis D, et al: Disruption of Mks1 localization to the mother centriole causes cilia defects and developmental malformations in Meckel-Gruber syndrome. Dis Model Mech 2011;4:43–56.
65 Cui C, Chatterjee B, Lozito TP, et al: Wdpcp, a PCP protein required for ciliogenesis, regulates directional cell migration and cell polarity by direct modulation of the actin cytoskeleton. PLoS Biol 2013;11:e1001720.
66 Damerla RR, Chatterjee B, Li Y, et al: Ion Torrent sequencing for conducting genome-wide scans for mutation mapping analysis. Mamm Genome 2014;25:120–128.
67 Tarkar A, Loges NT, Slagle CE, et al: DYX1C1 is required for axonemal dynein assembly and ciliary motility. Nat Genet 2013;45:995–1003.
68 Hjeij R, Lindstrand A, Francis R, et al: ARMC4 mutations cause primary ciliary dyskinesia with randomization of left/right body asymmetry. Am J Hum Genet 2013;93:357–367.
69 Huber C, Cormier-Daire V: Ciliary disorder of the skeleton. Am J Med Genet C Semin Med Genet 2012;160C:165–174.
70 Fliegauf M, Benzing T, Omran H: When cilia go bad: cilia defects and ciliopathies. Nat Rev Mol Cell Biol 2007;8:880–893.
71 Kennedy MP, Omran H, Leigh MW, et al: Congenital heart disease and other heterotaxic defects in a large cohort of patients with primary ciliary dyskinesia. Circulation 2007;115:2814–2821.
72 Nakhleh N, Francis R, Giese RA, et al: High prevalence of respiratory ciliary dysfunction in congenital heart disease patients with heterotaxy. Circulation 2012;125:2232–2242.
73 Papon JF, Perrault I, Coste A, et al: Abnormal respiratory cilia in non-syndromic Leber congenital amaurosis with CEP290 mutations. J Med Genet 2010;47:829–834.
74 Armengot M, Salom D, Diaz-Llopis M, et al: Nasal ciliary beat frequency and beat pattern in retinal ciliopathies. Invest Ophthalmol Vis Sci 2012;53:2076–2079.
75 Piatti G, De Santi MM, Brogi M, et al: Emerging ciliopathies: are respiratory cilia compromised in Usher syndrome? Am J Otolaryngol 2014;35:340–346.
76 Driscoll JA, Bhalla S, Liapis H, et al: Autosomal dominant polycystic kidney disease is associated with an increased prevalence of radiographic bronchiectasis. Chest 2008;133:1181–1188.
77 De Luca A, Sarkozy A, Consoli F, et al: Familial transposition of the great arteries caused by multiple mutations in laterality genes. Heart 2010;96:673–677.

78 Pazour GJ, Agrin N, Leszyk J, Witman GB: Proteomic analysis of a eukaryotic cilium. J Cell Biol 2005;170:103–113.
79 Bartz PJ, Driscoll DJ, Dearani JA, et al: Early and late results of the modified Fontan operation for heterotaxy syndrome: 30 years of experience in 142 patients. J Am Coll Cardiol 2006;48:2301–2305.
80 Yildirim SV, Tokel K, Varan B, et al: Clinical investigations over 13 years to establish the nature of the cardiac defects in patients having abnormalities of lateralization. Cardiol Young 2007;17:275–282.
81 Takeuchi K, McGowan FX Jr, Bacha EA, et al: Analysis of surgical outcome in complex double-outlet right ventricle with heterotaxy syndrome or complete atrioventricular canal defect. Ann Thorac Surg 2006;82:146–152.
82 Kim SJ, Kim WH, Lim HG, et al: Outcome of 200 patients after an extracardiac Fontan procedure. J Thorac Cardiovasc Surg 2008; 136:108–116.
83 Swisher M, Jonas R, Tian X, et al: Increased postoperative and respiratory complications in patients with congenital heart disease associated with heterotaxy. J Thorac Cardiovasc Surg 2011;141:637–644.e3
84 Harden B, Tian X, Giese R, et al: Increased postoperative respiratory complications in heterotaxy congenital heart disease patients with respiratory ciliary dysfunction. J Thorac Cardiovasc Surg 2014;147:1291–1298.e2.

Dr. Cecilia Lo
Department of Developmental Biology
University of Pittsburgh School of Medicine, 8120 Rangos Research Center
530 45th Street
Pittsburgh, PA 15201 (USA)
E-Mail cel36@pitt.edu

Muenke M, Kruszka PS, Sable CA, Belmont JW (eds): Congenital Heart Disease: Molecular Genetics, Principles of Diagnosis and Treatment. Basel, Karger, 2015, pp 178–185
DOI: 10.1159/000375215

Molecular Genetics of Isolated Cardiovascular Malformations

Teresa M. Lee · Wendy K. Chung

Department of Pediatrics, Columbia University Medical Center, New York, N.Y., USA

Abstract

Most cardiac lesions occur as isolated birth defects. Yet the genetic basis of nonsyndromic congenital heart disease (CHD) has been difficult to elucidate due to genetic heterogeneity, incomplete penetrance, polygenics, and other nongenetic contributions. Families with Mendelian, nonsyndromic CHD have provided insight into some of the genes causing CHD, such as *NKX2.5* and *GATA4*. Common types of genes have begun to emerge, including transcription factors, chromatin modifiers, and signaling receptors and ligands. This chapter discusses a few highly penetrant cardiac lesions caused by mutations in genes that act in an autosomal dominant manner due to haploinsufficiency. Recent advances in genomic technology have also identified copy number variants and de novo mutations as common causes of CHD. Finally, strategies for genetic counseling and genetic testing are discussed.

As seen in prior chapters, single-gene disorders and copy number variants (CNVs) associated with syndromic congenital heart disease (CHD) are relatively well characterized. However, most heart lesions occur as isolated birth defects [1], and the genetics of nonsyndromic CHD has been much more difficult to elucidate compared to syndromic CHD due to genetic heterogeneity, genetic complexity, and the contribution of nongenetic factors.

Multiple epidemiological studies suggest there is a genetic contribution to CHD. Even as early as 1953, families with multiple affected family members with CHD were noted [2]. Twin studies support a genetic contribution; monozygotic twins have a concordance rate of 25% for CHD (although the exact lesion may differ between the twins) as compared to 4.9% in dizygotic twins [3]. Moreover, having a first-degree relative with CHD is associated with a relative risk of 3.2 to have CHD [4]. Overall, the estimated heritability for

CHD is 35 as compared to 85 for schizophrenia [5]. Risk differs by lesion, and some lesions like atrial septal defect (ASD), ventricular septal defect (VSD), tetralogy of Fallot, and hypoplastic left-heart syndrome (HLHS) have a 3% recurrence risk when 1 child is affected and the parents are unaffected, while other lesions like Ebstein's anomaly have a lower (1%) recurrence risk [6]. Known environmental factors, such as maternal diabetes, rubella, phenylketonuria, and certain medications such as thalidomide and indomethacin are thought to account for 2% of isolated CHD cases [7].

Families with Mendelian, nonsyndromic CHD have provided insight into the genes important for cardiac development, including *NKX2.5* and *GATA4*. Common mechanisms causing CHD have begun to emerge, such as the developmental importance of transcription factors, chromatin modifiers, and signaling receptors and ligands [8]. These monogenic conditions are highly penetrant and act in an autosomal dominant manner due to haploinsufficiency with sensitivity to gene dosage. Some of these genes will be discussed in relationship to the specific cardiac lesion with which they are commonly associated (table 1). Fewer X-linked and autosomal recessive genes have also been identified. For the most part, familial CHD has been associated with milder lesions that do not greatly impact survival or reproductive fitness since previous generations of individuals with severe CHD lesions often did not live long enough in order to transmit these genes.

There is significant heterogeneity in CHD with many different genes causing the same type of cardiac lesion and with a single gene causing many different types of CHD. For example, mutations in *NOTCH1* can cause a relatively benign lesion such as a bicuspid aortic valve (BAV) or a severe lesion such as HLHS [9]. Some genes like *JAG1* are commonly associated with a genetic syndrome such as the Alagille syndrome, which includes CHD, but may also cause nonsyndromic CHD [10, 11].

In addition to monogenic causes of isolated CHD, CNVs account for about 10% of CHDs (fig. 1). Furthermore, genome-wide association studies suggest that common variants may also play a role in CHD along with other epigenetic and environmental factors.

Finally, strategies for genetic counseling and testing are important for families concerned about recurrence or who seek to understand the underlying cause of the CHD and desire additional prognostic information.

Monogenic Cardiovascular Malformations

Atrial Septal Defects

ASD is a common cardiac lesion with an incidence of 1 in 1,500 live births [12]. In 1998, Schott et al. [13] identified the first gene associated with isolated CHD by studying 4 large families with autosomal dominant secundum ASD. Genome-wide linkage analysis demonstrated linkage to 5q35 that included *NKX2.5,* which had already been implicated in cardiac morphogenesis in other species [14]. Sequencing *NKX2.5* identified two premature stop mutations and a highly conserved missense mutation that segregated with ASD. These 4 families also had atrioventricular conduction defects, suggesting that *NKX2.5* mutations may alter conduction. Subsequently, additional groups have also reported other cases of ASD with and without conduction defects caused by *NKX2.5* mutations [15, 16]. Many mutations cluster in the homeodomain and significantly reduce transcriptional activation, but mutations also occur outside this region [13, 17]. *NKX2.5* mutations explain about 1–4% of sporadic, isolated ASD [18] and up to 12.5% of familial cases [18].

Additional studies have also identified *NKX2.5* mutations in other cardiac lesions, such as conotruncal anomalies, left-sided lesions, Ebstein's anomaly, and pulmonary atresia [19, 20]. Furthermore, even in the absence of CHD, *NKX2.5* can cause atrioventricular conduction defects, and these conduction defects can progress to complete heart block and even cause sudden cardiac death [17].

GATA4 encodes a zinc finger transcription factor with activity modulated by interaction with other proteins, such as those in the NKX2 family. Missense and frameshift mutations throughout

Table 1. Well-established single-gene causes of isolated CHD

Gene	Mode of inheritance	Cardiac defects (% of cases accounted for by gene)	Type of mutations	CNVs	Clinical testing available	Reference No.
NKX2.5	AD	ASD with/without conduction defects (1–4% sporadic; 12.5% familial) VSD CoA DORV Ebstein's anomaly Heterotaxy HLHS IAA TGA ToF	Missense Nonsense Frameshift Insertion Deletion Splice site		Yes	8, 16, 18
GATA4	AD	ASD without conduction delay (12.5% familial) VSD PS AVSD HRV PAPVR ToF	Missense Frameshift Insertion Deletion	8p23.1	Yes	8
TBX20	AD	ASD VSD MS, HLHS PDA	Missense Nonsense		Yes	8
NOTCH1	AD	BAV (4% sporadic) AS CoA HLHS (6.6%)	Missense Nonsense Deletion		Yes	8, 34
ELN	AD	SVAS AS PS	Missense Frameshift Splice site		Yes	8, 35
CRELD1	AD	AVSD (6%) ASD	Missense		Yes	8, 37

AD = Autosomal dominant; AS = aortic stenosis; CoA = coarctation of the aorta; DORV = double-outlet right ventricle; HRV = hypoplastic right ventricle; IAA = interruption of the aortic arch; MS = mitral stenosis; PAPVR = partial anomalous pulmonary venous return; PDA = patent ductus arteriosus; PS = pulmonary valve stenosis; SVAS = supravalvar AS; TGA = transposition of the great arteries; ToF = tetralogy of Fallot.

the *GATA4* gene have been identified in secundum ASD without conduction defects [21–24]. In one study of 16 families, *GATA4* mutations were identified in 2 of the families [15]. *GATA4* mutations are also frequently associated with VSD and pulmonary stenosis among other outflow tract lesions [25, 26].

T-box transcription factors are expressed in the developing heart and contribute to CHD [27]. *TBX5* interacts with *NKX2.5* and *GATA4* and causes syn-

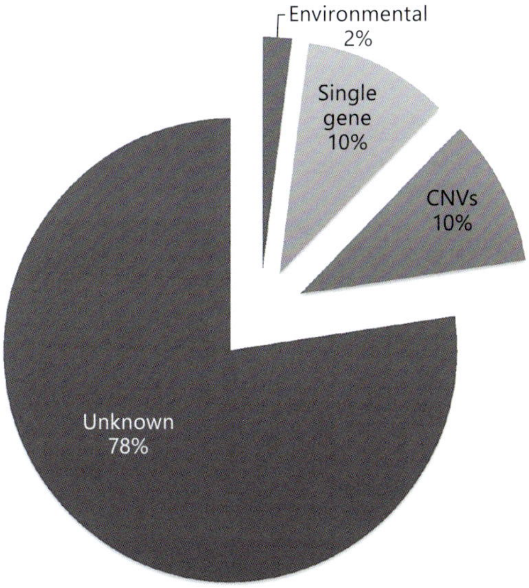

Fig. 1. Causes of isolated CHD. Only 20% of isolated CHD is currently accounted for by known single-gene disorders and CNVs. A small fraction is caused by known environmental teratogens. The vast majority of causes (78%) remain unknown.

dromic CHD associated with the Holt-Oram syndrome [see also the chapter by Borlak and Ciribilli, p. 131]. Missense and nonsense mutations in a related gene, *TBX20*, are associated with ASD [28]. One large family with secundum ASD was found to have a gain-of-function mutation in *TBX20* that enhanced transcriptional activity (opposite to the loss-of-function mechanism of the majority of *TBX20* mutations) demonstrating sensitivity to gene dosage in either direction [29]. When the *TBX20* gain-of-function mutation was coexpressed with *NKX2.5* and *GATA4/5*, the transcriptional activity of *TBX20* was synergistically increased demonstrating the common molecular pathway through which these mutations act.

Ventricular Septal Defects

VSD is the most frequent type of CHD, comprising over 20% of all CHD, with an incidence of 6 in 1,000 live births [30]. It is frequently associated with many of the syndromes discussed in the other chapters, but also frequently occurs in isolation. *NKX2.5*, *GATA4*, and *TBX20* mutations are all associated with VSD [25, 28]. Multiple studies have identified missense mutations throughout *GATA4* in VSD [25], and in one study this gene accounted for approximately 12.5% of isolated VSD cases [15]. Another zinc finger transcription factor, *GATA6*, has also been shown to segregate with autosomal dominantly inherited VSD [31].

Bicuspid Aortic Valves

In addition to the association with Turner syndrome [see also the chapter by Bondy, p. 91], BAV is a common anomaly that is often familial [32]. Although likely an underestimate, almost 2% of the population has BAV [33]. *NOTCH1* mutations have been associated with BAV in 4% of sporadic cases [34]. *NOTCH1* mutations have also been associated with aortic calcification even with an anatomically normal tricuspid aortic valve [34]. Many other studies have also implicated *NOTCH1* variants in other left-sided obstructive lesions, including HLHS [9].

Supravalvar Aortic Stenoses

Supravalvar aortic stenosis can be associated with the Williams-Beuren syndrome (see chapter by Lalani p. 115) or can occur in isolation in a familial form that is autosomal dominantly inherited. Missense, nonsense, frameshift, translation initiation, and splice site mutations have been identified in the elastin gene, *ELN* [35, 36], in individuals who lack the other phenotypic characteristics associated with the Williams-Beuren syndrome (a contiguous gene deletion syndrome that encompasses *ELN*).

Additional Lesions

The genes previously discussed are also implicated in multiple other lesions, such as atrioventricular septal defects (AVSDs), conotruncal lesions, and D-transposition of the great arteries. Although most AVSDs are observed in patients with Down syndrome [see also the chapter by Kruszka, p. 82], 6% of isolated, nonsyndromic AVSD can be caused by

4

missense mutations in *CRELD1*, a cell adhesion molecule [37]. Conotruncal lesions are commonly associated with the 22q11 deletion [see also the chapter by Goldmuntz, p. 100], and isolated conotruncal lesions can be caused by mutations in *NKX2.5*, *GATA4*, and *NOTCH1*. *TBX1* is located within the 22q11 microdeletion interval, and rare variants in *TBX1* are associated with nonsyndromic interrupted aortic arch and VSD [38].

Recent Advances

Copy Number Variants

CNVs are segmental aneuploidies, usually of several contiguous genes. CNVs have been implicated in CHD, especially syndromic forms such as the 22q11 deletion syndrome [see also the chapter by Goldmuntz, p. 100]. There are also multiple recurrent CNVs associated with nonsyndromic CHD [8]. Up to 10% of nonsyndromic CHD may be due to rare CNVs [8]. Some CNVs encompass genes related to CHD such as 8p23.1, which includes *GATA4* [39, 40], or 9q34.3, which includes *NOTCH1* [41]. The overall frequency of rare CNVs is higher in CHD cases compared to controls [42].

As in monogenic disorders, there is significant phenotypic variability in the type of CHD associated with most CNVs. CNVs explain ~10% of CHD cases with 5% of those CNVs being de novo [43]. On average, CNVs associated with isolated CHD have fewer genes and are smaller than CNVs associated with syndromic CHD [44]. Identifying the minimal critical interval within a series of overlapping CNVs allows for the identification of candidate genes for isolated CHD.

De novo Variants

Given that CHD often impairs survival and reproductive fitness, de novo variants are a likely mechanism of disease for either single-nucleotide variants or CNVs. The Pediatric Cardiac Genomics Consortium performed whole exome sequencing on 362 parent-child trios in which the child was affected with a severe type of CHD (left-ventricular outflow obstruction, conotruncal lesions, or heterotaxy) and found that de novo single-nucleotide variants explain ~10% of CHD cases [45]. Specifically, there was an excess of de novo mutations in histone-modifying genes *KDM5A*, *KDM5B*, *MLL2*, *RNF20*, *SMAD2*, *UBE2B*, *USP44*, and *WDR5*. These genes are involved in the production, removal, or reading of histone 3 lysine 4 methylation. These findings highlight the importance of histone methylation in cardiac development.

Genome-Wide Association Studies

Even with extensive genomic characterization, we are only able to explain the etiology in about 20% of isolated CHD cases [46]. The remaining fraction may be harder to elucidate as some of the CHD types are likely to be part of complex genetic diseases with multiple genetic, epigenetic, and environmental factors. Large genome-wide association studies have identified possible common single-nucleotide polymorphisms contributing to CHD. One study of 945 ASD or VSD cases and 1,246 controls identified significant associations with 1p12 near *TBX15* [47].

Clinical Genetic Evaluation and Testing

Many parents want to know why their child is affected with CHD, and what the chance is to have another affected child. Empirically, after having one affected child with CHD, the risk to the parents to have another child with CHD is 3–6% with variability in the type of lesion [48]. If one of the parents has CHD, they have on average a 4% risk of having an affected child although that risk can be as high as 20% if the affected parent is the mother as opposed to the father [6].

Genetic testing can clarify etiology and refine the recurrence risk. Genetic evaluation includes an evaluation of any syndromic feature by a clinical geneticist. Chromosome microarray testing may be recommended to evaluate CNVs and should be used rather than karyotyping because of the increased resolution. Testing for a single gene or a panel of genes may be performed, but has a low yield and is rarely clinically useful. Whole exome sequencing is a new diagnostic option for sequencing the coding region (exons) throughout the genome comprehensively. Analysis of the data is most efficient if it includes all affected individuals in the family as well as both parents of the proband. Insurance coverage for the testing is variable, so there are practical limitations to its utilization in some cases.

If a pathogenic variant is identified, predictive testing can be performed on other members of the family to determine who is personally at increased risk for CHD and to facilitate cascade genetic testing throughout the family and provide information about the recurrence risk. Mutation carriers have multiple reproductive options, including prenatal testing via chorionic villus sampling or amniocentesis. Preimplantation genetic diagnosis is performed on embryos created through in vitro fertilization prior to implantation and has the advantage of avoiding the concerns of pregnancy termination.

Conclusion

Our understanding of the genetics of isolated CHD is rapidly advancing. Linkage studies of monogenic forms of CHD identified transcription factors such as NKX2.5, GATA-binding proteins, and T-box proteins, which are important in cardiac development. Newer technology, like whole exome sequencing, has identified novel genes, including histone modifiers. However, all of these genes still only account for a small portion of isolated CHD cases. A more complete understanding of the complex genetic underpinnings of CHD will require continued large, collaborative efforts.

References

1 Garg V: Insights into the genetic basis of congenital heart disease. Cell Mol Life Sci 2006;63:1141–1148.
2 McKeown T, Macmahon B, Parsons CG: The familial incidence of congenital malformation of the heart. Br Heart J 1953;15:273–277.
3 Nora JJ, Gilliland JC, Sommerville RJ, McNamara DG: Congenital heart disease in twins. N Engl J Med 1967;277:568–571.
4 Oyen N, Poulsen G, Boyd HA, Wohlfahrt J, Jensen PK, Melbye M: Recurrence of congenital heart defects in families. Circulation 2009;120:295–301.
5 Turnpenny PD, Ellard S: Emery's Elements of Medical Genetics. Philadelphia, Elsevier/Churchill Livingstone, 2012.
6 van der Bom T, Zomer AC, Zwinderman AH, Meijboom FJ, Bouma BJ, Mulder BJ: The changing epidemiology of congenital heart disease. Nat Rev Cardiol 2011;8:50–60.
7 Kuciene R, Dulskiene V: Selected environmental risk factors and congenital heart defects. Medicina (Kaunas) 2008;44:827–832.
8 Fahed AC, Gelb BD, Seidman JG, Seidman CE: Genetics of congenital heart disease: the glass half empty. Circ Res 2013;112:707–720.
9 McBride KL, Riley MF, Zender GA, Fitzgerald-Butt SM, Towbin JA, Belmont JW, Cole SE: NOTCH1 mutations in individuals with left ventricular outflow tract malformations reduce ligand-induced signaling. Hum Mol Genet 2008;17:2886–2893.
10 Krantz ID, Smith R, Colliton RP, Tinkel H, Zackai EH, Piccoli DA, Goldmuntz E, Spinner NB: Jagged1 mutations in patients ascertained with isolated congenital heart defects. Am J Med Genet 1999;84:56–60.
11 Eldadah ZA, Hamosh A, Biery NJ, Montgomery RA, Duke M, Elkins R, Dietz HC: Familial tetralogy of Fallot caused by mutation in the jagged1 gene. Hum Mol Genet 2001;10:163–169.
12 Hoffman JI: Congenital heart disease: incidence and inheritance. Pediatr Clin North Am 1990;37:25–43.
13 Schott JJ, Benson DW, Basson CT, Pease W, Silberbach GM, Moak JP, Maron BJ, Seidman CE, Seidman JG: Congenital heart disease caused by mutations in the transcription factor NKX2-5. Science 1998;281:108–111.
14 Lyons I, Parsons LM, Hartley L, Li R, Andrews JE, Robb L, Harvey RP: Myogenic and morphogenetic defects in the heart tubes of murine embryos lacking the homeo box gene Nkx2-5. Genes Dev 1995;9:1654–1666.
15 Hirayama-Yamada K, Kamisago M, Akimoto K, Aotsuka H, Nakamura Y, Tomita H, Furutani M, Imamura S, Takao A, Nakazawa M, Matsuoka R: Phenotypes with GATA4 or NKX2.5 mutations in familial atrial septal defect. Am J Med Genet A 2005;135:47–52.
16 Sarkozy A, Conti E, Neri C, D'Agostino R, Digilio MC, Esposito G, Toscano A, Marino B, Pizzuti A, Dallapiccola B: Spectrum of atrial septal defects associated with mutations of NKX2.5 and GATA4 transcription factors. J Med Genet 2005;42:e19.
17 Benson DW, Silberbach GM, Kavanaugh-McHugh A, Cottrill C, Zhang Y, Riggs S, Smalls O, Johnson MC, Watson MS, Seidman JG, Seidman CE, Plowden J, Kugler JD: Mutations in the cardiac transcription factor NKX2.5 affect diverse cardiac developmental pathways. J Clin Invest 1999;104:1567–1573.
18 Ikeda Y, Hiroi Y, Hosoda T, Utsunomiya T, Matsuo S, Ito T, Inoue J, Sumiyoshi T, Takano H, Nagai R, Komuro I: Novel point mutation in the cardiac transcription factor CSX/NKX2.5 associated with congenital heart disease. Circ J 2002;66:561–563.

19 Elliott DA, Kirk EP, Yeoh T, Chandar S, McKenzie F, Taylor P, Grossfeld P, Fatkin D, Jones O, Hayes P, Feneley M, Harvey RP: Cardiac homeobox gene NKX2-5 mutations and congenital heart disease: associations with atrial septal defect and hypoplastic left heart syndrome. J Am Coll Cardiol 2003;41:2072–2076.
20 McElhinney DB, Geiger E, Blinder J, Benson DW, Goldmuntz E: NKX2.5 mutations in patients with congenital heart disease. J Am Coll Cardiol 2003; 42:1650–1655.
21 Garg V, Kathiriya IS, Barnes R, Schluterman MK, King IN, Butler CA, Rothrock CR, Eapen RS, Hirayama-Yamada K, Joo K, Matsuoka R, Cohen JC, Srivastava D: GATA4 mutations cause human congenital heart defects and reveal an interaction with TBX5. Nature 2003; 424:443–447.
22 Okubo A, Miyoshi O, Baba K, Takagi M, Tsukamoto K, Kinoshita A, Yoshiura K, Kishino T, Ohta T, Niikawa N, Matsumoto N: A novel GATA4 mutation completely segregated with atrial septal defect in a large Japanese family. J Med Genet 2004;41:e97.
23 Rajagopal SK, Ma Q, Obler D, Shen J, Manichaikul A, Tomita-Mitchell A, Boardman K, Briggs C, Garg V, Srivastava D, Goldmuntz E, Broman KW, Benson DW, Smoot LB, Pu WT: Spectrum of heart disease associated with murine and human GATA4 mutation. J Mol Cell Cardiol 2007;43: 677–685.
24 Chen Y, Han ZQ, Yan WD, Tang CZ, Xie JY, Chen H, Hu DY: A novel mutation in GATA4 gene associated with dominant inherited familial atrial septal defect. J Thorac Cardiovasc Surg 2010; 140:684–687.
25 Yang YQ, Li L, Wang J, Liu XY, Chen XZ, Zhang W, Wang XZ, Jiang JQ, Liu X, Fang WY: A novel GATA4 loss-of-function mutation associated with congenital ventricular septal defect. Pediatr Cardiol 2012;33:539–546.
26 Xiang R, Fan LL, Huang H, Cao BB, Li XP, Peng DQ, Xia K: A novel mutation of GATA4 (K319E) is responsible for familial atrial septal defect and pulmonary valve stenosis. Gene 2013, Epub ahead of print.
27 Wang H, Chen D, Ma L, Meng H, Liu Y, Xie W, Pang S, Yan B: Genetic analysis of the TBX1 gene promoter in ventricular septal defects. Mol Cell Biochem 2012;370:53–58.
28 Kirk EP, Sunde M, Costa MW, Rankin SA, Wolstein O, Castro ML, Butler TL, Hyun C, Guo G, Otway R, Mackay JP, Waddell LB, Cole AD, Hayward C, Keogh A, Macdonald P, Griffiths L, Fatkin D, Sholler GF, Zorn AM, Feneley MP, Winlaw DS, Harvey RP: Mutations in cardiac T-box factor gene TBX20 are associated with diverse cardiac pathologies, including defects of septation and valvulogenesis and cardiomyopathy. Am J Hum Genet 2007;81:280–291.
29 Posch MG, Gramlich M, Sunde M, Schmitt KR, Lee SH, Richter S, Kersten A, Perrot A, Panek AN, Al Khatib IH, Nemer G, Megarbane A, Dietz R, Stiller B, Berger F, Harvey RP, Ozcelik C: A gain-of-function TBX20 mutation causes congenital atrial septal defects, patent foramen ovale and cardiac valve defects. J Med Genet 2010;47:230–235.
30 Moller JH, Moodie DS, Blees M, Norton JB, Nouri S: Symptomatic heart disease in infants: comparison of three studies performed during 1969–1987. Pediatr Cardiol 1995;16:216–222.
31 Zheng GF, Wei D, Zhao H, Zhou N, Yang YQ, Liu XY: A novel GATA6 mutation associated with congenital ventricular septal defect. Int J Mol Med 2012;29:1065–1071.
32 Huntington K, Hunter AG, Chan KL: A prospective study to assess the frequency of familial clustering of congenital bicuspid aortic valve. J Am Coll Cardiol 1997;30:1809–1812.
33 Pierpont ME, Basson CT, Benson DW Jr, Gelb BD, Giglia TM, Goldmuntz E, McGee G, Sable CA, Srivastava D, Webb CL, American Heart Association Congenital Cardiac Defects Committee, Council on Cardiovascular Disease in the Young: Genetic basis for congenital heart defects: current knowledge: a scientific statement from the American Heart Association Congenital Cardiac Defects Committee, Council on Cardiovascular Disease in the Young: endorsed by the American Academy of Pediatrics. Circulation 2007;115:3015–3038.
34 Garg V, Muth AN, Ransom JF, Schluterman MK, Barnes R, King IN, Grossfeld PD, Srivastava D: Mutations in NOTCH1 cause aortic valve disease. Nature 2005;437:270–274.
35 Metcalfe K, Rucka AK, Smoot L, Hofstadler G, Tuzler G, McKeown P, Siu V, Rauch A, Dean J, Dennis N, Ellis I, Reardon W, Cytrynbaum C, Osborne L, Yates JR, Read AP, Donnai D, Tassabehji M: Elastin: mutational spectrum in supravalvular aortic stenosis. Eur J Hum Genet 2000;8:955–963.
36 Micale L, Turturo MG, Fusco C, Augello B, Jurado LA, Izzi C, Digilio MC, Milani D, Lapi E, Zelante L, Merla G: Identification and characterization of seven novel mutations of elastin gene in a cohort of patients affected by supravalvular aortic stenosis. Eur J Hum Genet 2010;18:317–323.
37 Robinson SW, Morris CD, Goldmuntz E, Reller MD, Jones MA, Steiner RD, Maslen CL: Missense mutations in CRELD1 are associated with cardiac atrioventricular septal defects. Am J Hum Genet 2003;72:1047–1052.
38 Rauch A, Devriendt K, Koch A, Rauch R, Gewillig M, Kraus C, Weyand M, Singer H, Reis A, Hofbeck M: Assessment of association between variants and haplotypes of the remaining TBX1 gene and manifestations of congenital heart defects in 22q11.2 deletion patients. J Med Genet 2004;41:e40.
39 Pehlivan T, Pober BR, Brueckner M, Garrett S, Slaugh R, Van Rheeden R, Wilson DB, Watson MS, Hing AV: GATA4 haploinsufficiency in patients with interstitial deletion of chromosome region 8p23.1 and congenital heart disease. Am J Med Genet 1999;83: 201–206.
40 Soemedi R, Wilson IJ, Bentham J, Darlay R, Topf A, Zelenika D, Cosgrove C, Setchfield K, Thornborough C, Granados-Riveron J, Blue GM, Breckpot J, Hellens S, Zwolinkski S, Glen E, Mamasoula C, Rahman TJ, Hall D, Rauch A, Devriendt K, Gewillig M, O'Sullivan J, Winlaw DS, Bu'Lock F, Brook JD, Bhattacharya S, Lathrop M, Santibanez-Koref M, Cordell HJ, Goodship JA, Keavney BD: Contribution of global rare copy-number variants to the risk of sporadic congenital heart disease. Am J Hum Genet 2012;91:489–501.
41 Greenway SC, Pereira AC, Lin JC, DePalma SR, Israel SJ, Mesquita SM, Ergul E, Conta JH, Korn JM, McCarroll SA, Gorham JM, Gabriel S, Altshuler DM, Quintanilla-Dieck Mde L, Artunduaga MA, Eavey RD, Plenge RM, Shadick NA, Weinblatt ME, De Jager PL, Hafler DA, Breitbart RE, Seidman JG, Seidman CE: De novo copy number variants identify new genes and loci in isolated sporadic tetralogy of Fallot. Nat Genet 2009;41: 931–935.
42 Goldmuntz E, Paluru P, Glessner J, Hakonarson H, Biegel JA, White PS, Gai X, Shaikh TH: Microdeletions and microduplications in patients with congenital heart disease and multiple congenital anomalies. Congenit Heart Dis 2011;6: 592–602.
43 Yuan S, Zaidi S, Brueckner M: Congenital heart disease: emerging themes linking genetics and development. Curr Opin Genet Dev 2013;23:352–359.

44 Silversides CK, Lionel AC, Costain G, Merico D, Migita O, Liu B, Yuen T, Rickaby J, Thiruvahindrapuram B, Marshall CR, Scherer SW, Bassett AS: Rare copy number variations in adults with tetralogy of Fallot implicate novel risk gene pathways. PLoS Genet 2012;8:e1002843.

45 Zaidi S, Choi M, Wakimoto H, Ma L, Jiang J, Overton JD, Romano-Adesman A, Bjornson RD, Breitbart RE, Brown KK, Carriero NJ, Cheung YH, Deanfield J, DePalma S, Fakhro KA, Glessner J, Hakonarson H, Italia MJ, Kaltman JR, Kaski J, Kim R, Kline JK, Lee T, Leipzig J, Lopez A, Mane SM, Mitchell LE, Newburger JW, Parfenov M, Pe'er I, Porter G, Roberts AE, Sachidanandam R, Sanders SJ, Seiden HS, State MW, Subramanian S, Tikhonova IR, Wang W, Warburton D, White PS, Williams IA, Zhao H, Seidman JG, Brueckner M, Chung WK, Gelb BD, Goldmuntz E, Seidman CE, Lifton RP: De novo mutations in histone-modifying genes in congenital heart disease. Nature 2013;498:220–223.

46 Erdogan F, Larsen LA, Zhang L, Tumer Z, Tommerup N, Chen W, Jacobsen JR, Schubert M, Jurkatis J, Tzschach A, Ropers HH, Ullmann R: High frequency of submicroscopic genomic aberrations detected by tiling path array comparative genome hybridisation in patients with isolated congenital heart disease. J Med Genet 2008;45:704–709.

47 Hu Z, Shi Y, Mo X, Xu J, Zhao B, Lin Y, Yang S, Xu Z, Dai J, Pan S, Da M, Wang X, Qian B, Wen Y, Wen J, Xing J, Guo X, Xia Y, Ma H, Jin G, Yu S, Liu J, Zhou Z, Wang X, Chen Y, Sha J, Shen H: A genome-wide association study identifies two risk loci for congenital heart malformations in Han Chinese populations. Nat Genet 2013;45:818–821.

48 Hoess K, Goldmuntz E, Pyeritz RE: Genetic counseling for congenital heart disease: new approaches for a new decade. Curr Cardiol Rep 2002;4:68–75.

Dr. Wendy K. Chung
Department of Pediatrics, Columbia University Medical Center
1150 St. Nicholas Avenue
New York, NY 10032 (USA)
E-Mail wkc15@columbia.edu

4

Muenke M, Kruszka PS, Sable CA, Belmont JW (eds): Congenital Heart Disease: Molecular Genetics, Principles of Diagnosis and Treatment. Basel, Karger, 2015, pp 186–195
DOI: 10.1159/000375216

Other Single-Gene Disorders Causing Congenital Heart Disease

Mark W. Russell · Mark Hannibal

Departments of Pediatrics and Human Genetics, University of Michigan, Ann Arbor, Mich., USA

Abstract

This chapter describes single-gene syndromes that include congenital heart malformations as part of their phenotype. With the exception of Goldenhar syndrome (craniofacial microsomia syndrome), at least one known causative gene has been identified in the described syndromes. Even though a genetic etiology has yet to be discovered for Goldenhar syndrome, we felt that this syndrome was important to describe due to its association with congenital heart diseases. There are many more single-gene syndromes that have been discovered, or are yet to be discovered, that have a congenital heart malformation as part of their phenotype, but the syndromes reviewed in this chapter are amongst the most commonly found in clinical practice. They span multiple disciplines and require the care of pediatricians, internists, cardiologists, and geneticists.

Developmental processes are commonly shared by multiple tissues and organs during development. While, in some instances, the genes responsible for each process are restricted to a single tissue, it is not uncommon for a gene critical for cardiac development to have also an important developmental role in another organ or tissue. Therefore, cardiac defects can occur as part of syndromes that have significant extracardiac developmental abnormalities. In this chapter, we will review developmental syndromes that are commonly associated with congenital heart diseases. These syndromes, not unlike the Marfan, DiGeorge (22q11.2 deletion or velocardiofacial syndrome; see Goldmuntz chapter p. 100) Williams (see Lalani chapter p. 115), and CHARGE (see Corsten-Janssen and van Ravenswaaij-Arts p. 145) syndromes, which are covered elsewhere in this book, have important extracardiac manifestations that influence the care of patients with these conditions.

VACTERL Association

The VACTERL association is a developmental disorder characterized by congenital malformations involving at least three of the following conditions: vertebral anomalies, anal atresia, cardiac defects, tracheoesophageal fistula, renal anomalies, and limb defects. Since the spectrum of defects is variable and there is no definitive test, it is difficult to determine the true incidence of the association, but it is estimated to occur in approximately 1 in 10,000–40,000 live births [1, 2]. The differential diagnosis is extensive and includes many of the disorders covered elsewhere in this book. Establishing the diagnosis of the VACTERL association requires a multidisciplinary evaluation coordinated by a geneticist. Only rarely is a genetic cause of the association identified, with some X-linked cases attributed to mutations/deletions of *ZIC3* (a gene which has also been implicated in X-linked heterotaxy) or *FANCB* (a gene responsible for one type of Fanconi anemia) [3, 4]. In approximately 90% of the cases, the condition appears to be sporadic without a prior family history of congenital malformations; in the remainder (10% of the cases), one or more defects characteristic of the VACTERL association can be identified in at least one relative, but rarely is there full manifestation of the VACTERL association [5].

Cardiac defects are reported to occur in 67% of the patients meeting the criteria for the VACTERL association [6]. The most common heart defects noted were ventricular septal defects, which occurred in just over half of the patients. For those patients with tracheoesophageal fistulas, determination of arch sidedness (whether there is a right- or left-sided aortic arch) is important for the planning of the tracheoesophageal repair.

Diagnosis/Evaluation

The diagnosis is often considered based on the finding of anal atresia or tracheoesophageal fistula, especially when they occur in a patient with limb anomalies which may include extra digits (polydactyly) or a proximally placed thumb. Once the diagnosis is considered, subsequent evaluation usually includes a chest and abdominal radiograph to detect vertebral anomalies, a renal ultrasound, and an echocardiogram. Some X-linked cases with hydrocephalus have been reported [7], and a cranial ultrasound should be considered particularly if the subject is male. Genetic testing to identify a mutation or deletion of *ZIC3* can be considered if the patient is male and may be helpful in estimating the recurrence risk within a given family. Fanconi anemia screening by laboratory testing for chromosome breakage should be considered in cases with hydrocephalus, microcephaly, and radial ray defects.

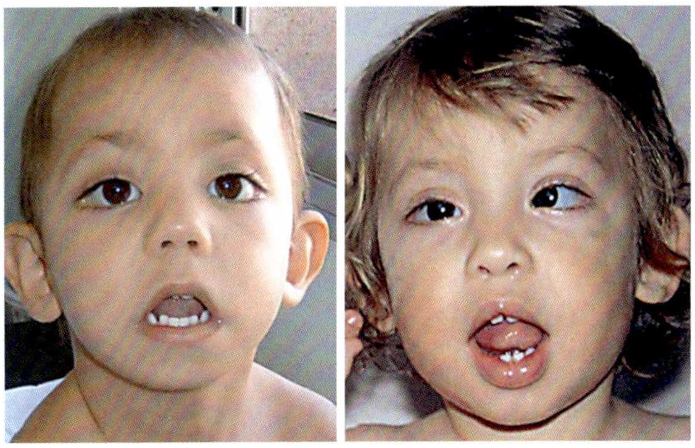

Fig. 1. The images show many of the facial features of the Kabuki syndrome, including eversion of the lateral one third of the lower eyelids, arched eyebrows, a broad and flat tip of the nose, and enlarged ears (http://creativecommons.org/licenses/by/2.0). http://en.wikipedia.org/wiki/File:Kabuki_syndrome.jpg. http://commons.wikimedia.org/wiki/File:KabukiSyndrome2.jpg

4

The Kabuki Syndrome

The Kabuki syndrome is a multisystem disorder characterized by intellectual disability, dwarfism, and unusual facies (fig. 1) [8]; its prevalence ranges from 1 in 32,000 in Japan [9] to 1 in 86,000 in Australia and New Zealand [10]. The eversion of the lateral one third of the lower eyelids was felt to be reminiscent of the makeup worn by actors of a traditional Japanese theater form known as Kabuki. Other characteristic features include arched eyebrows, ptosis, a broad and flat tip of the nose, persistence of fetal fingertip pads, enlarged ears, a cleft or high-arched palate, and skeletal abnormalities such as scoliosis and shortened fifth digit. In one study, cardiac defects were noted in 35 of 60 patients [11] evaluated with an echocardiogram. The most frequent heart defects included coarctation of the aorta, and atrial and ventricular septal defects in 14, 12, and 10 of the 60 patients, respectively. Another left outflow tract lesion in addition to coarctation of the aorta and hypoplastic left-heart syndrome was reported in a series of 3 patients with the Kabuki syndrome [12].

The Kabuki syndrome has been attributed to mutations in the *KMT2D* (formerly *MLL2*) and *KMD6A* genes, which encode for lysine-specific methyltransferase 2D and demethylase 6A, respectively [13, 14]. Both regulate histone H3 methylation during cellular differentiation and organ development [15], and interact with other transcriptional regulators and chromatin modulators to direct gene expression. Mutations of *KMT2D* can be identified in 60–70% of cases and are usually predicted to result in protein truncation and haploinsufficiency of the KMT2D protein [16]. Most cases are due to de novo mutations, but few are inherited in an autosomal dominant fashion. *KMD6A* mutations occur less commonly (in approximately 6% of cases) and are due to de novo mutations although X-linked transmission could occur. There are important phenotypic differences between patients with *KMT2D* and *KMD6A* mutations as patients with *KMT2D* mutations were more likely to have the characteristic facial features and patients with *KMD6A* mutations were more likely to have postnatal growth compromise [17].

Diagnosis/Evaluation

The diagnosis of the Kabuki syndrome may be difficult or delayed, since young infants may not be recognized with the characteristic facies. The Kabuki syndrome should be considered in any patient with facial features characteristic of the disorder and neonatal hypotonia and/or developmental delay. A clinical scoring system was developed by Makrythanasis et al. [18] and can be used to direct genetic testing. Genetic testing for sequence variants and/or deletions/duplications involving *KMT2D* and *KMD6A* is available to confirm the diagnosis. In addition to a cardiac evaluation, there should be an assessment for feeding difficulties, vision/hearing deficits, and possible genitourinary anomalies, and a high index of suspicion for immunologic abnormalities and seizures.

The Ellis-van Creveld Syndrome

The Ellis-van Creveld syndrome (EVC) is an autosomal recessive disorder characterized by skeletal abnormalities and cardiac defects. Skeletal abnormalities include short limbs, short ribs, and postaxial polydactyly. Other characteristic physical features include dysplastic/dystrophic nails and dental abnormalities, including natal teeth and conical teeth with wide spacing. Although typically characterized as an autosomal recessive disorder, heterozygous individuals do occasionally demonstrate some features of EVC, including postaxial polydactyly, teeth abnormalities, and cardiac defects [19]. Studies of consanguineous families affected by EVC have identified two genes that, when mutated or deleted, can cause EVC. The genes are adjacent to each other on human chromosome 4p16.2 and the clinical findings are indistinguishable regardless of which gene is responsible. The two genes identified to date are *EVC* and *EVC2* (encodes the protein limbin) [19, 20]. Their functions are unknown but they are coexpressed during development in a spatiotemporally restricted manner. During mouse development, both genes were expressed in (i) the vertebrae, ribs, and limbs (more prominent in distal than proximal limbs), (ii) the epithelium of the lung and the kidney, and (iii) the secondary heart field and the structures to which it contributes, including the atrial septum and the atrioventricular cushion [20, 21]. The expression pattern of both genes corresponded to the tissues affected by EVC and their overlap in expression suggests coordinate roles in development. They have both been localized to the basal bodies of primary cilia, and a mouse model of EVC (which lacks EVC expression) demonstrates abnormalities in hedgehog signaling [22]. Based on these findings, it was proposed that the proteins EVC and limbin might have tissue-specific functions in the hedgehog signaling pathway.

Based on the expression patterns and proposed function, it is not surprising that, of the approximately 60% of patients with EVC that demonstrate some form of structural congenital heart disease, most exhibit defects in atrioventricular septation. A review of the Pediatric Cardiac Care Consortium database identified 32 patients with the diagnosis of EVC, 28 (88%) of the 32 patients had an atrioventricular septal defect, and 15 of the 28 had primary failure of atrial septation leading to a common atrium [23]. Other frequently associated cardiac anomalies included persistence of the left superior vena cava and abnormalities of pulmonary venous drainage. The constellation of cardiac defects was similar to defects seen in heterotaxy syndromes, leading the authors to propose that the cardiac manifestations of EVC were within the heterotaxy spectrum and lending further support to the assertion that the genes responsible for EVC might have a role in ciliary function, a central determinant of left-right sidedness.

Diagnosis/Evaluation

The diagnosis of EVC should be suspected in any patient with cardiac and skeletal features characteristic of the disorder, especially if there is a history of consanguinity within the family. Genetic testing for sequence variants and/or deletions/duplications involving *EVC* or *EVC2* is available to confirm the diagnosis of EVC. Surgical repair of the cardiac defect is often required and may be complicated in the postoperative period by respiratory insufficiency. Thoracic dystrophy is not an uncommon finding in patients with EVC and, when present, can lead to restrictive lung disease that may prolong the need for mechanical ventilatory support. Difficulties achieving adequate ventilation even with mechanical support can increase the length of the intensive care unit stay and secondarily increase the morbidity and mortality associated with the operative repair.

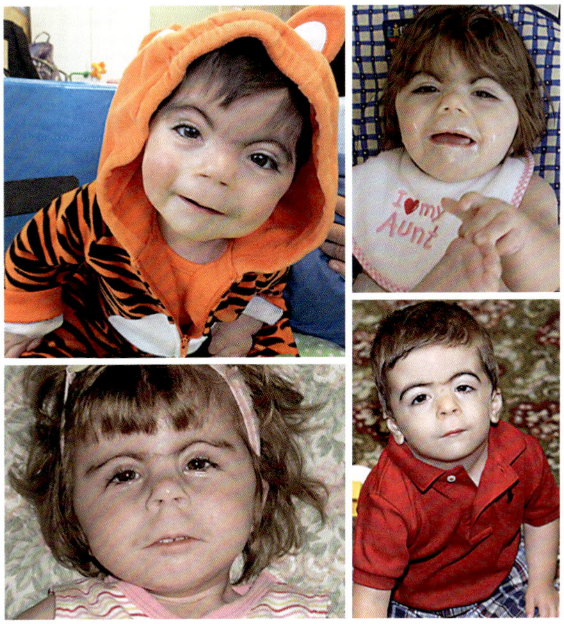

Fig. 2. The images show many of the common facial features in patients with CdLS, including a low anterior hairline, arched eyebrows, synophrys (meeting of the eyebrows), and characteristic mouth and nose (images were provided by families through the Cornelia de Lange Syndrome Foundation).

The Cornelia de Lange Syndrome

The Cornelia de Lange syndrome (CdLS) is characterized by growth restriction, microcephaly, intellectual disability, and facial dysmorphism, which includes a low anterior hairline, arched eyebrows, synophrys, long, thick eyelashes, a long, smooth philtrum, a thin upper lip, and micrognathia (fig. 2). Clinical manifestations can range from mild to severe, and patients may have palatal, dental, skeletal, renal, gastrointestinal, endocrine, neurologic, and cardiac abnormalities. Skeletal abnormalities can include upper limb anomalies, oligodactyly and proximally placed thumbs; syndactyly of the 2nd and 3rd toes is common. Structural abnormalities of the kidney and/or urinary tract were identified in 25 of 61 (41%) patients evaluated, and reduced renal function was noted in 9 patients (15%) [24]. Gastroesophageal reflux is quite common, with pathological reflux occurring in 28 of 43 (65%) patients evaluated [24]. Hearing loss was also quite common, occurring in 40 of 50 patients examined. Most commonly, hearing loss was due to middle ear effusions resulting in conductive hearing loss, with a minority, 10 of the 50 (20%) patients, having sensorineural deficits [25].

Heart defects occurred in 33% of the patients evaluated by echocardiogram [26]. The most common lesion was isolated valvar pulmonary stenosis, which occurred in 11 of 87 (13%) patients evaluated. Other common abnormalities included atrial and ventricular septal defects, and isolated, late-onset, atrioventricular (mitral or tricuspid) valve regurgitation.

Mutations in several members of the cohesin complex proteins, which regulate the separation of sister chromatids during mitosis and meiosis, have been implicated in causing CdLS. Approximately 50–60% of the cases are due to a mutation in the nipped-B-like 1 *(NIPBL)* gene [27, 28], which encodes for a cohesin-loading factor that is broadly expressed during vertebrate development. The second most common genetic abnormality identified, which occurs in ~5% of cases, involves mutations in the *SMC1A* gene on the X chromosome [29]. Other genes that have been implicated in causing CdLS include the *SMC3* and *RAD21* genes. *NIPBL*, SMC1A, *SMC,* and *RAD21* all encode for elements of the cohesion complex. A fifth CdLS gene encodes for *HDAC8*, a histone deacetylase for SMC3. Usually, CdLS occurs as the result of a de novo mutation, but cases of autosomal dominant and X-linked (*SMC1A*- and *HDAC8*-type) transmission have also been identified [30].

Diagnosis/Evaluation

Genetic testing can help confirm the diagnosis of CdLS and determine the risk of recurrence. An evaluation by a pediatric geneticist is indicated and will help guide the comprehensive evaluation that needs to be performed in a patient with known or suspected CdLS. Imaging of the heart and renal/urinary tract is indicated, as is referral for endocrine, hearing/otolaryngology, and gastroenterology evaluations.

The Mowat-Wilson Syndrome

The Mowat-Wilson syndrome is a multisystem disorder characterized by developmental delay and abnormal facial features, including microcephaly, hypertelorism, uplifted ear lobes with a central depression, and a prominent, pointed chin. Certain facial features become more prominent with time, including a convex nasal profile, pointed chin, and wedge-shaped eyebrows with a broad medial flare. Frequently associated abnormalities include epilepsy, hypoplasia or agenesis of the corpus callosum, cardiac defects, Hirschsprung's disease, and hypospadias. Cardiac defects occur in approximately 47% [31]. The cardiac defects range from mild to severe, and include pulmonary artery and valve abnormalities, patent ductus arteriosus (PDA), ventricular septal defects, and coarctation of the aorta. The Mowat-Wilson syndrome has been attributed to mutations or deletions of *ZEB2* [32], a zinc finger protein that binds to E-cadherin. The majority of *ZEB2* mutations described to date are large gene deletions or truncating mutations [33].

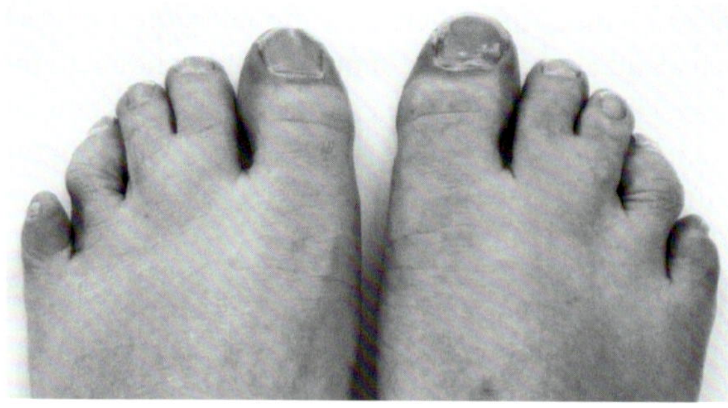

Fig. 3. Syndactyly in a patient with SLOS. Syndactyly of the 2nd and 3rd digits of the feet are a common finding in patients with SLOS [image by courtesy of Wikimedia Commons (http://en.wikipedia.org/wiki/File:Feets_with_partial_simple_syndactyly.jpg) (Creative Commons Attribution-Share Alike 3.0)].

Diagnosis/Evaluation

Genetic testing for deletions and/or sequence variants involving *ZEB2* is available to confirm the diagnosis of the Mowat-Wilson syndrome. Testing should be considered in patients with developmental delay and characteristic facial features especially if there is also a history of seizures or Hirschsprung's disease.

The Smith-Lemli-Opitz Syndrome

The Smith-Lemli-Opitz syndrome (SLOS) is an autosomal recessive disorder characterized by intellectual disability and multiple congenital anomalies. The association of microcephaly, intellectual disability, ambiguous genitalia, and short nose with anteverted nares was first described by Smith, Lemli and Opitz [34] in 1964. As additional patients were identified, other common features were noted, including syndactyly of the 2nd and 3rd toes (fig. 3), postaxial polydactyly, cleft palate, and a high frequency of cardiac and renal abnormalities as well as intestinal disorders (such as Hirschsprung's disease) and irregularities of the liver, pancreas, and lungs. Characteristic facial features include a narrow forehead, epicanthal folds, eyelid ptosis, a short, upturned nose, and palatal anomalies. This pervasive developmental disorder was determined to be secondary to a defect in sterol metabolism due to mutations in the gene encoding for the enzyme 7-dehydrocholesterol (DHC) reductase. [35, 36]. In some populations, including those of northern and central European ancestry, SLOS can be quite common, occurring in approximately 1 in 20,000–30,000 births [37]. As an autosomal recessive disorder, this would suggest a carrier frequency of *DHCR7* mutations of 1–2% in those populations [38]. This would make SLOS second only to cystic fibrosis in terms of disease incidence for a recessive condition.

Cardiac defects occur in approximately 44% of patients with SLOS [39, 40]. As might be expected, cardiac defects are more common in those patients with more severe extracardiac manifestations, occurring in approximately 80% of patients with severe SLOS [41]. From a spectrum of cardiac defects, atrioventricular septal defect and anomalous pulmonary venous return are most common. Other septal defects, including atrial and ventricular septal defects, were also noted. Given the nature of cardiac defects and the constellation of extracardiac abnormalities, in particular postaxial polydactyly, it was proposed that SLOS may be similar to a heterotaxy-like syndrome due to a defect in SHH (sonic hedgehog) signaling; the SHH pathway participates in the development of midline structures (such as the palate) and left right patterning [42].

Diagnosis/Evaluation

The diagnosis of SLOS should be suspected in any patient with multiple congenital anomalies, postaxial polydactyly, ambiguous genitalia, including 46,XY disorder of sex development with female phenotype (sex reversal), hypospadias and cryptorchidism, and microcephaly. The diagnosis is made by elevated serum levels of 7-DHC. Individuals with SLOS usually have low cholesterol levels, but they may also have cholesterol values in the normal range. *DHCR7* gene analysis is available as secondary confirmation and familial recurrence risk testing.

Treatment

The abnormality of steroid processing in patients with SLOS leads to growth and developmental delay, and life-long behavioral and cognitive deficits. While the anatomic defects of the heart and other organs are due to developmental abnormalities that are present at birth, therapy to compensate for the biochemical defect in sterol metabolism can potentially improve cognition and learning, reduce behavioral abnormalities (such as irritability, hyperactivity, sleep disturbance, and self-injury), and improve growth. Since patients with SLOS are unable to synthesize sufficient levels of cholesterol for necessary cellular processes, dietary supplementation of cholesterol has been used as a therapeutic intervention with success. The benefits of cholesterol supplementation appear to be twofold in that, in addition to supplying the cholesterol needed, the increase in cholesterol levels serves to inhibit HMG CoA reductase activity and secondarily prevent the accumulation of toxic cholesterol precursors such as 7-DHC and 8-DHC. It should be noted that cholesterol supplementation has not been tested in randomized controlled trials. In addition, HMG CoA reductase inhibitors (i.e. statins) have been used to directly inhibit the accumulation of the toxic precursors but alone may not be sufficient to raise serum cholesterol levels [43, 44]. Early intervention with occupational therapy, physical therapy, and nutritional services is helpful. Severely affected patients may require stress-related dose adjustment of steroids during illness. Finally, airway management during anesthesia may be difficult in patients with SLOS.

The Rubinstein-Taybi Syndrome

The Rubinstein-Taybi syndrome (RTS) is characterized by multiple congenital anomalies including intellectual disability, microcephaly, postnatal growth deficiency (weight and height), high-arched palate, broad and angulated thumbs and toes, and dysmorphic facies (including a beaked nose, downslanting

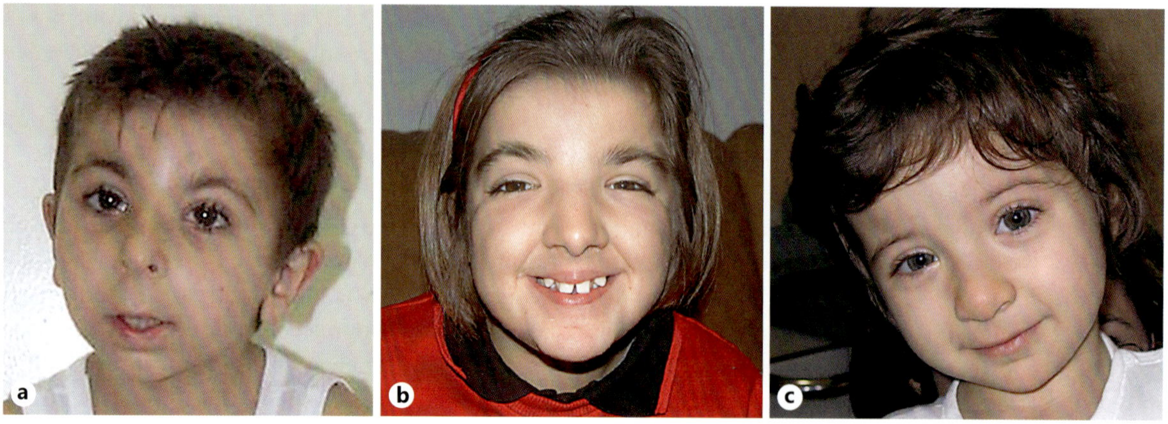

Fig. 4. Characteristic findings in patients with RTS. **a–c** Facial features include beaked nose, downslanting palpebral fissures, micrognathia, and arched eyebrows with long eyelashes. Patients also commonly have short and broad first digits of the hand and feet (not shown; http://creativecommons.org/licenses/by/2.0). http://sv.wikipedia.org/wiki/Fil:Rubinstein-Taybi_Syndrome2.jpg.

palpebral fissures, mild micrognathia, and arched eyebrows with long eyelashes; fig. 4). Multiorgan involvement includes eye anomalies, laryngomalacia, cardiac defects, intestinal dysmotility (megacolon or constipation), renal anomalies, and joint hypermobility. Patients with RTS also appear to be susceptible to frequent respiratory infections and tumors, which can be malignant or benign, most often involving the central nervous system. Cardiac defects occur in approximately 30% of patients, with atrial and ventricular septal defects or PDA being the most common [45].

Mutations in two genes, *CREBBP* and *EP300*, have been identified in patients with RTS and account for 50–70% and ~3% of the cases, respectively. Both genes encode for transcription regulators that interact to promote histone acetyltransferase activity and thereby affect chromatin remodeling at specific gene targets. Both genes are broadly expressed and are critical to development of the multiple tissues affected. Virtually all cases are caused by autosomal dominant de novo mutations (which can range from single amino acid changes to chromosomal rearrangements), and familial occurrences are exceptionally rare. It is an uncommon disorder occurring in approximately 1 in 100,000–125,000 newborns.

Diagnosis/Evaluation

Genetic testing for deletions/duplications and/or sequence variants involving *CREBBP* or *EP300* is available to confirm the diagnosis of RTS in approximately 55% of the identified cases. For the other 45%, the diagnosis is based on clinical features. If RTS is suspected, then cardiac and extracardiac (genetic, ophthalmologic, neurodevelopmental, and renal) evaluations are warranted. Perhaps, the most important early interventions include an evaluation for glaucoma, surgical correction of undescended testes (if present), and prompt management or feeding difficulties. A concise but thorough review of the management of RTS was presented by Hennekam [46]. Surgical correction of cardiac abnormalities can be complicated by airway issues, including tracheal collapse after exposure to muscle relaxants.

The Char Syndrome

The co-occurrence of PDA and unusual facial features was first noted by Char [47] in 1978. It was further characterized by Davidson [48], who described a large multigenerational family with multiple members with PDA and facial abnormalities (elongated nose, flattened nasal bridge, everted 'duck-bill' lips, mild ptosis, hypertelorism, and low-set ears), and by Slavotinek et al. [49], who first noted the association with hand abnormalities, including clinodactyly, syndactyly, and other defects involving the fifth digit. The syndrome exhibits autosomal dominant inheritance, and linkage studies in large families ultimately led to the identification of mutations in the *TFAP2B* gene [50], which encodes for a transcription factor expressed in the neural crest that has an important role in retinoic acid-induced differentiation [51]. There is significant variability in the Char syndrome phenotype, with some families (depending on the exact nature of their mutation) exhibiting more prominent facial and skeletal abnormalities than others [52]. In some instances, *TFAP2B* mutations have been identified in patients and families with PDA only and no detectable skeletal or facial abnormalities [53, 54]. While other cardiac defects have been noted in patients with *TFAP2B* mutations [55], their significance is unknown, and certainly the most consistent cardiac manifestation of the Char syndrome is PDA.

Diagnosis/Evaluation

Genetic testing for *TFAP2B* mutations can be performed to confirm the diagnosis; approximately half of the individuals with the Char syndrome will be found to have a mutation in *TFAP2B*. The co-occurrence of characteristic facial features and digit abnormalities would support the need for a cardiac evaluation with an echocardiogram.

The Goldenhar Syndrome

The Goldenhar syndrome, which is also called hemifacial or craniofacial microsomia syndrome and oculo-auriculo-vertebral dysplasia, is characterized by unilateral hypoplasia of the external ear and face. It is a relatively common disorder, occurring in approximately 1 in 3,000–5,000 live births. The defects can involve all of the derivatives of the first and second branchial arches, including the vertebrae and central nervous system. Most cases are sporadic, but, occasionally, it can recur in families where it demonstrates an autosomal dominant or autosomal recessive mode of transmission. Congenital heart defects occur in approximately 30% of patients [56]. Common types of defects include tetralogy of Fallot and ventricular septal defects (~21% of those with congenital heart defects, respectively). Atrial septal defects and other conotruncal defects are also frequently noted. The causes of Goldenhar syndrome are not yet known and may involve multiple genes and/or an interaction between genetic predisposing factors and environmental (e.g. the in utero environment) conditions. It has been proposed that the observed defects, at least in some cases, are due to an in utero vascular accident that affects tissues within the distribution of the affected vessel [57].

Diagnosis/Evaluation

Since there is no known cause of Goldenhar syndrome, there is no specific test to aid in the diagnosis, so it is usually based on clinical findings. Treatment may include craniofacial reconstruction, speech and language therapy, and hearing aids. Surgical repair of an associated cardiac defect is often required, and endotracheal intubation may be more difficult due to craniofacial and oropharyngeal abnormalities.

Conclusion

Congenital cardiac defects can occur in isolation or as part of a syndrome that affects multiple tissues and organs. It is important to recognize when a patient with a cardiac condition has an associated syndrome, as other features of the syndrome may significantly affect the patient's care, including the approach to the treatment of the cardiac abnormality. Close collaboration between pediatric cardiologists, geneticists, and other health care providers can help identify patients with these conditions, and direct appropriate diagnostic procedures and therapeutic approaches.

Acknowledgments

This work was supported in part by the Braylon Gift of Hope Fund and the Aaron Stern Professorship (M.W.R.). We would like to thank the families from the Cornelia de Lange Syndrome Foundation and the other patients and families who provided images for this chapter.

References

1 Botto LD, Khoury MJ, Mastroiacovo P, Castilla EE, Moore CA, Skjaerven R, et al: The spectrum of congenital anomalies of the VATER association: an international study. Am J Med Genet 1997;71:8–15.

2 Khoury MJ, Cordero JF, Greenberg F, James LM, Erickson JD: A population study of the VACTERL association: evidence for its etiologic heterogeneity. Pediatrics 1983;71: 815–820.

3 Wessels MW, Kuchinka B, Heydanus R, Smit BJ, Dooijes D, de Krijger RR, et al: Polyalanine expansion in the ZIC3 gene leading to X-linked heterotaxy with VACTERL association: a new polyalanine disorder? J Med Genet 2010;47:351–355.

4 McCauley J, Masand N, McGowan R, Rajagopalan S, Hunter A, Michaud JL, et al: X-linked VACTERL with hydrocephalus syndrome: further delineation of the phenotype caused by FANCB mutations. Am J Med Genet A 2011;155A:2370–2380.

5 Solomon BD, Pineda-Alvarez DE, Raam MS, Cummings DA: Evidence for inheritance in patients with VACTERL association. Hum Genet 2010;127:731–733.

6 Cunningham BK, Hadley DW, Hannoush H, Meltzer AC, Niforatos N, Pineda-Alvarez D, et al: Analysis of cardiac anomalies in VACTERL association. Birth Defects Res A Clin Mol Teratol 2013;97:792–797.

7 Lomas FE, Dahlstrom JE, Ford JH: VACTERL with hydrocephalus: family with X-linked VACTERL-H. Am J Med Genet 1998;76:74–78.

8 Cuscó I, del Campo M, Vilardell M, González E, Gener B, Galán E, Toledo L, Pérez-Jurado LA: Array-CGH in patients with Kabuki-like phenotype: identification of two patients with complex rearrangements including 2q37 deletions and no other recurrent aberration. BMC Med Genet 2008;9:27.

9 Niikawa N, Kuroki Y, Kajii T, Matsuura N, Ishikiriyama S, Tonoki H, Yamada Y, Fujita M, Umemoto H, Fukushima Y, Nako Y, Matsui I, Urakami T, Aritaki S, Hara M, Suzuki Y, Chyo H, Sugio Y, Hasegawa T, Yamanaka T, Tsukino R, Yoshida A, Nomoto N, Kawahito S, Aihara R, Toyota S, Ieshima A, Funaki H, Ishitobi K, Ogura S, Furumae T, Yoshino M, Tsuji Y, Kondoh T, Matsumoto T, Abe K, Harada N, Miike T, Ohdo S, Naritomi K, Abushwereb AK, Braun OH, Schmid E: Kabuki make-up (Niikawa-Kuroki) syndrome: a study of 62 patients. Am J Med Genet 1988;31:565–589.

10 White SM, Thompson EM, Kidd A, Savarirayan R, Turner A, Amor D, Delatycki MB, Fahey M, Baxendale A, White S, Haan E, Gibson K, Halliday JL, Bankier A: Growth, behavior, and clinical findings in 27 patients with Kabuki (Niikawa-Kuroki) syndrome. Am J Med Genet A 2004;127A:118–127.

11 Digilio MC, Marino B, Toscano A, Giannotti A, Dallapiccola B: Congenital heart defects in Kabuki syndrome. Am J Med Genet 2001;100:269–274.

12 Kung GC, Chang PM, Sklansky MS, Randolph LM: Hypoplastic left heart syndrome in patients with Kabuki syndrome. Pediatr Cardiol 2010;31:138–141.

13 Ng SB, Bigham AW, Buckingham KJ, Hannibal MC, McMillin MJ, Gildersleeve HI, Beck AE, Tabor HK, Cooper GM, Mefford HC, Lee C, Turner EH, Smith JD, Rieder MJ, Yoshiura K, Matsumoto N, Ohta T, Niikawa N, Nickerson DA, Bamshad MJ, Shendure J: Exome sequencing identifies MLL2 mutations as a cause of Kabuki syndrome. Nat Genet 2010;42:790–793.

14 Lederer D, Grisart B, Digilio MC, Benoit V, Crespin M, Ghariani SC, Maystadt I, Dallapiccola B, Verellen-Dumoulin C: Deletion of KDM6A, a histone demethylase interacting with MLL2, in three patients with Kabuki syndrome. Am J Hum Genet 2012;90:119–124.

15 Lan F, Bayliss PE, Rinn JL, Whetstine JR, Wang JK, Chen S, Iwase S, Alpatov R, Issaeva I, Canaani E, Roberts TM, Chang HY, Shi Y: A histone H3 lysine 27 demethylase regulates animal posterior development. Nature 2007;449:689–694.

16 Hannibal MC, Buckingham KJ, Ng SB, Ming JE, Beck AE, McMillin MJ, Gildersleeve HI, Bigham AW, Tabor HK, Mefford HC, Cook J, Yoshiura K, Matsumoto T, Matsumoto N, Miyake N, Tonoki H, Naritomi K, Kaname T, Nagai T, Ohashi H, Kurosawa K, Hou JW, Ohta T, Liang D, Sudo A, Morris CA, Banka S, Black GC, Clayton-Smith J, Nickerson DA, Zackai EH, Shaikh TH, Donnai D, Niikawa N, Shendure J, Bamshad MJ: Spectrum of MLL2 (ALR) mutations in 110 cases of Kabuki syndrome. Am J Med Genet A 2011;155A:1511–1516.

17 Miyake N, Koshimizu E, Okamoto N, Mizuno S, Ogata T, Nagai T, Kosho T, Ohashi H, Kato M, Sasaki G, Mabe H, Watanabe Y, Yoshino M, Matsuishi T, Takanashi J, Shotelersuk V, Tekin M, Ochi N, Kubota M, Ito N, Ihara K, Hara T, Tonoki H, Ohta T, Saito K, Matsuo M, Urano M, Enokizono T, Sato A, Tanaka H, Ogawa A, Fujita T, Hiraki Y, Kitanaka S, Matsubara Y, Makita T, Taguri M, Nakashima M, Tsurusaki Y, Saitsu H, Yoshiura K, Matsumoto N, Niikawa N: MLL2 and KDM6A mutations in patients with Kabuki syndrome. Am J Med Genet A 2013; 161:2234–2243.

18 Makrythanasis P, van Bon BW, Steehouwer M, Rodríguez-Santiago B, Simpson M, Dias P, Anderlid BM, Arts P, Bhat M, Augello B, Biamino E, Bongers EM, Del Campo M, Cordeiro I, Cueto-González AM, Cuscó I, Deshpande C, Frysira E, Izatt L, Flores R, Galán E, Gener B, Gilissen C, Granneman SM, Hoyer J, Yntema HG, Kets CM, Koolen DA, Marcelis Cl, Medeira A, Micale L, Mohammed S, de Munnik SA, Nordgren A, Psoni S, Reardon W, Revencu N, Roscioli T, Ruiterkamp-Versteeg M, Santos HG, Schoumans J, Schuurs-Hoeijmakers JH, Silengo MC, Toledo L, Vendrell T, van der Burgt I, van Lier B, Zweier C, Reymond A, Trembath RC, Perez-Jurado L, Dupont J, de Vries BB, Brunner HG, Veltman JA, Merla G, Antonarakis SE, Hoischen A: MLL2 mutation detection in 86 patients with Kabuki syndrome: a genotype-phenotype study. Clin Genet 2013;84:539–545.

19 Ruiz-Perez VL, Ide SE, Strom TM, Lorenz B, Wilson D, Woods K, et al: Mutations in a new gene in Ellis-van Creveld syndrome and Weyers acrodental dysostosis. Nat Genet 2000;24:283–286.

20 Ruiz-Perez VL, Tompson SW, Blair HJ, Espinoza-Valdez C, Lapunzina P, Silva EO, et al: Mutations in two nonhomologous genes in a head-to-head configuration cause Ellis-van Creveld syndrome. Am J Hum Genet 2003;72:728–732.

21 Sund KL, Roelker S, Ramachandran V, Durbin L, Benson DW: Analysis of Ellis van Creveld syndrome gene products: implications for cardiovascular development and disease. Hum Mol Genet 2009;18:1813–1824.

22 Ruiz-Perez VL, Goodship JA: Ellis-van Creveld syndrome and Weyers acrodental dysostosis are caused by cilia-mediated diminished response to hedgehog ligands. Am J Med Genet C Semin Med Genet 2009; 151C:341–351.

23 Hills CB, Kochilas L, Schimmenti LA, Moller JH: Ellis-van Creveld syndrome and congenital heart defects: presentation of an additional 32 cases. Pediatr Cardiol 2011; 32:977–982.

24 Selicorni A, Sforzini C, Milani D, Cagnoli G, Fossali E, Bianchetti MG: Anomalies of the kidney and urinary tract are common in de Lange syndrome. Am J Med Genet A 2005; 132A:395–397.

25 Marchisio P, Selicorni A, Pignataro L, Milani D, Baggi E, Lambertini L, Dusi E, Villa L, Capaccio P, Cerutti M, Esposito S, Principi N: Otitis media with effusion and hearing loss in children with Cornelia de Lange syndrome. Am J Med Genet A 2008;146A:426–432.

26 Selicorni A, Colli AM, Passarini A, Milani D, Cereda A, Cerutti M, Maitz S, Alloni V, Salvini L, Galli MA, Ghiglia S, Salice P, Danzi GB: Analysis of congenital heart defects in 87 consecutive patients with Brachmann-de Lange syndrome. Am J Med Genet A 2009; 149A:1268–1272.

27 Krantz ID, McCallum J, DeScipio C, Kaur M, Gillis LA, Yaeger D, Jukofsky L, Wasserman N, Bottani A, Morris CA, Nowaczyk MJ, Toriello H, Bamshad MJ, Carey JC, Rappaport E, Kawauchi S, Lander AD, Calof AL, Li HH, Devoto M, Jackson LG: Cornelia de Lange syndrome is caused by mutations in NIPBL, the human homolog of Drosophila melanogaster Nipped-B. Nat Genet 2004; 36:631–635.
28 Tonkin ET, Wang TJ, Lisgo S, Bamshad MJ, Strachan T: NIPBL, encoding a homolog of fungal Scc2-type sister chromatid cohesion proteins and fly Nipped-B, is mutated in Cornelia de Lange syndrome. Nat Genet 2004;36:636–641.
29 Musio A, Selicorni A, Focarelli ML, Gervasini C, Milani D, Russo S, Vezzoni P, Larizza L: X-linked Cornelia de Lange syndrome owing to SMC1L1 mutations. Nat Genet 2006;38:528–530.
30 Rohatgi S, Clark D, Kline AD, Jackson LG, Pie J, Siu V, Ramos FJ, Krantz ID, Deardorff MA: Facial diagnosis of mild and variant CdLS: insights from a dysmorphologist survey. Am J Med Genet A 2010;152A:1641–1653.
31 Zweier C, Temple IK, Beemer F, Zackai E, Lerman-Sagie T, Weschke B, Anderson CE, Rauch A: Characterisation of deletions of the ZFHX1B region and genotype-phenotype analysis in Mowat-Wilson syndrome. J Med Genet 2003;40:601–605.
32 Wakamatsu N, Yamada Y, Yamada K, Ono T, Nomura N, Taniguchi H, Kitoh H, Mutoh N, Yamanaka T, Mushiake K, Kato K, Sonta S, Nagaya M: Mutations in SIP1, encoding Smad interacting protein-1, cause a form of Hirschsprung disease. Nat Genet 2001;27: 369–370.
33 Dastot-Le Moal F, Wilson M, Mowat D, Collot N, Niel F, Goossens M: ZFHX1B mutations in patients with Mowat-Wilson syndrome. Hum Mutat 2007;28:313–321.
34 Smith DW, Lemli L, Opitz JM: A newly recognized syndrome of multiple congenital anomalies. J Pediatr 1964;64:210–217.
35 Wassif CA, Maslen C, Kachilele-Linjewile S, Lin D, Linck LM, Connor WE, et al: Mutations in the human sterol delta7-reductase gene at 11q12-13 cause Smith-Lemli-Opitz syndrome. Am J Hum Genet 1998;63:55–62.
36 Fitzky BU, Witsch-Baumgartner M, Erdel M, Lee JN, Paik YK, Glossmann H, et al: Mutations in the delta7-sterol reductase gene in patients with the Smith-Lemli-Opitz syndrome. Proc Natl Acad Sci U S A 1998;95: 8181–8186.
37 Ryan AK, Bartlett K, Clayton P, Eaton S, Mills L, Donnai D, et al: Smith-Lemli-Opitz syndrome: a variable clinical and biochemical phenotype. J Med Genet 1998;35:558–565.
38 Chasalow FI, Blethen SL, Taysi K: Possible abnormalities of steroid secretion in children with Smith-Lemli-Opitz syndrome and their parents. Steroids 1985;46:827–843.
39 Robinson CD, Perry LW, Barlee A, Mella GW: Smith-Lemli-Opitz syndrome with cardiovascular abnormality. Pediatrics 1971;47:844–847.
40 Lin AE, Ardinger HH, Ardinger RH Jr, Cunniff C, Kelley RI: Cardiovascular malformations in Smith-Lemli-Opitz syndrome. Am J Med Genet 1997;68:270–278.
41 Curry CJ, Carey JC, Holland JS, Chopra D, Fineman R, Golabi M, et al: Smith-Lemli-Opitz syndrome-type II: multiple congenital anomalies with male pseudohermaphroditism and frequent early lethality. Am J Med Genet 1987;26:45–57.
42 Digilio MC, Marino B, Giannotti A, Dallapiccola B, Opitz JM: Specific congenital heart defects in RSH/Smith-Lemli-Opitz syndrome: postulated involvement of the sonic hedgehog pathway in syndromes with postaxial polydactyly or heterotaxia. Birth Defects Res A Clin Mol Teratol 2003;67: 149–153.
43 Elias ER, Irons MB, Hurley AD, Tint GS, Salen G: Clinical effects of cholesterol supplementation in six patients with the Smith-Lemli-Opitz syndrome (SLOS). Am J Med Genet 1997;68:305–310.
44 Linck LM, Lin DS, Flavell D, Connor WE, Steiner RD: Cholesterol supplementation with egg yolk increases plasma cholesterol and decreases plasma 7-dehydrocholesterol in Smith-Lemli-Opitz syndrome. Am J Med Genet 2000;93:360–365.
45 Stevens CA, Bhakta MG: Cardiac abnormalities in the Rubinstein-Taybi syndrome. Am J Med Genet 1995;59:346–348.
46 Hennekam RC: Rubinstein-Taybi syndrome. Eur J Hum Genet 2006;14:981–985.
47 Char F: Peculiar facies with short philtrum, duck-bill lips, ptosis and low-set ears – a new syndrome? Birth Defects Orig Artic Ser 1978;14:303–305.
48 Davidson HR: A large family with patent ductus arteriosus and unusual face. J Med Genet 1993;30:503–505.
49 Slavotinek A, Clayton-Smith J, Super M: Familial patent ductus arteriosus: a further case of CHAR syndrome. Am J Med Genet 1997;71:229–232.
50 Satoda M, Zhao F, Diaz GA, Burn J, Goodship J, Davidson HR, Pierpont ME, Gelb BD: Mutations in TFAP2B cause Char syndrome, a familial form of patent ductus arteriosus. Nat Genet 2000;25:42–46.
51 Knight RD, Javidan Y, Zhang T, Nelson S, Schilling TF: AP2-dependent signals from the ectoderm regulate craniofacial development in the zebrafish embryo. Development 2005;132:3127–3138.
52 Zhao F, Weismann CG, Satoda M, Pierpont ME, Sweeney E, Thompson EM, et al: Novel TFAP2B mutations that cause Char syndrome provide a genotype-phenotype correlation. Am J Hum Genet 2001;69:695–703.
53 Chen YW, Zhao W, Zhang ZF, Fu Q, Shen J, Zhang Z, et al: Familial nonsyndromic patent ductus arteriosus caused by mutations in TFAP2B. Pediatr Cardiol 2011;32:958–965.
54 Khetyar M, Syrris P, Tinworth L, Abushaban L, Carter N: Novel TFAP2B mutation in nonsyndromic patent ductus arteriosus. Genet Test 2008;12:457–459.
55 Xiong F, Li Q, Zhang C, Chen Y, Li P, Wei X, et al: Analyses of GATA4, NKX2.5, and TFAP2B genes in subjects from southern China with sporadic congenital heart disease. Cardiovasc Pathol 2013;22:141–145.
56 Digilio MC, Calzolari F, Capolino R, Toscano A, Sarkozy A, de Zorzi A, et al: Congenital heart defects in patients with oculo-auriculo-vertebral spectrum (Goldenhar syndrome). Am J Med Genet A 2008; 146A:1815–1819.
57 Soltan HC, Holmes LB: Familial occurrence of malformations possibly attributable to vascular abnormalities. J Pediatr 1986;108: 112–114.

4

Dr. Mark W. Russell
Departments of Pediatrics and Human Genetics, University of Michigan
1500 East Medical Center Drive
Ann Arbor, MI 48109 (USA)
E-Mail mruss@med.umich.edu

5 Arrhythmias, Cardiomyopathies, and Connective Tissue Disorders

Muenke M, Kruszka PS, Sable CA, Belmont JW (eds): Congenital Heart Disease: Molecular Genetics, Principles of Diagnosis and Treatment. Basel, Karger, 2015, pp 198–209
DOI: 10.1159/000375217

Genetic Arrhythmias (Channelopathies)

Andrea Mazzanti[a] · Kevin Ng[a] · Silvia G. Priori[a–c]

[a]Molecular Cardiology, IRCCS Salvatore Maugeri Foundation, and [b]Department of Molecular Medicine, University of Pavia, Pavia, Italy; [c]Cardiovascular Genetics Program, Leon H. Charney Division of Cardiology, New York University School of Medicine, New York, N.Y., USA

Abstract

'Genetic arrhythmias' or 'channelopathies' (long QT syndrome, short QT syndrome, Brugada syndrome and catecholaminergic polymorphic ventricular tachycardia) are inheritable disorders caused by mutations in genes coding for channel proteins that regulate the electrical function of the heart. These mutations favor the onset of life-threatening ventricular arrhythmias either by altering the balance of ionic currents in the cardiac action potential or by impairing the process of electromechanical coupling in cardiomyocytes. Channelopathies are lethal disorders, accounting for about one quarter of sudden cardiac deaths in young individuals with a morphologically 'normal' autopsy. Every time a channelopathy is identified in a patient, other individuals in his/her family might be at risk of cardiac events. If a timely diagnosis is made, however, simple and efficacious preventative measures may be applied. Genetic studies play a pivotal role in the diagnosis of channelopathies and may help in the management of patients and their relatives.

'Genetic arrhythmias' or 'channelopathies' are a group of inheritable disorders caused by mutations in genes coding for channel proteins that regulate the electrical function of the heart. In the absence of overt structural heart defects, these mutations favor the onset of ventricular tachycardia (VT) either by altering the balance of ionic currents in the cardiac action potential or by impairing the process of electromechanical coupling in cardiomyocytes. The clinical relevance of channelopathies is demonstrated by the observation that they account for 15–25% of sudden cardiac deaths (SCD) in young individuals with a morphologically 'normal' autopsy.

In the following sections, we will outline the key features of the most prevalent channelopathies, making reference to two consensus documents released by the major international heart rhythm societies for the diagnosis and management of 'inherited primary arrhythmia syndromes' [1] and for the appropriate use of genetic testing in these heritable conditions [2].

Long QT Syndrome

The long QT syndrome (LQTS) is the archetype of channelopathies, having been described half a century ago by independent observations of Norwegian, Italian and Irish physicians. Nowadays, the term LQTS indicates a family of diseases characterized by the following traits: (1) prolonged ventricular repolarization, reflected by the QT interval on surface electrocardiograms (ECG); (2) morphological abnormalities in T waves, and (3) the propensity to develop polymorphic VT, especially during phases of adrenergic stimulation.

Epidemiology

Patients with LQTS have been described in all ethnic groups. The prevalence of the autosomal dominant LQTS in Caucasians is estimated at 1: 2,000 [1], whereas the autosomal recessive form is rarer (1:200,000).

Genetic Variants

Thirteen variants of congenital LQTS are known; they are caused by mutations in genes encoding for subunits of potassium, sodium or calcium voltage-dependent ion channels (table 1).

The first three subtypes, LQT1–LQT3, account for 75% of LQTS cases: 70% of all LQTS are secondary to loss-of-function mutations involving either the Kv7.1 potassium channel (LQT1, gene *KCNQ1*) or the Kv11.1 potassium channel (LQT2, gene *KCNH2*), while about 5% are secondary to gain-of-function mutations in the Nav1.5 sodium channel (LQT3, gene *SCN5A*). The other 'minor' LQTS genes are responsible for 5% of cases, while for 20% of patients the genetic background remains elusive [2].

From a practical standpoint, the subtypes of LQTS may be grouped in the following three categories:

(1) Autosomal dominant LQTS (also called Romano-Ward syndrome), which includes LQT1–LQT6 and LQT9–LQT13, and is characterized by an isolated prolongation of the QT interval.

(2) Autosomal dominant LQTS with extracardiac manifestation, which is comprised of:

- the Andersen-Tawil syndrome (ATS), characterized by prolonged QT intervals, prominent U waves, facial dysmorphisms and hyper-/hypokalemic periodic paralysis; half of the ATS cases are caused by mutations in the *KCNJ2*-encoded Kir2.1 potassium channel (LQT7);
- the Timothy syndrome (TS; LQT8), which shows a prolonged QT interval, syndactyly, cardiac malformations, autism spectrum disorders and facial dysmorphisms. LQT8 results from gain-of-function mutations in the *CACNA1C*-encoded L-type calcium channel α-subunit.

(3) Autosomal recessive LQTS (Jervell and Lange-Nielsen syndrome, JLNS), which combines an extremely prolonged QT interval and congenital deafness. It is caused by the same (homozygous) or different (compound heterozygous) *KCNQ1* or *KCNE1* mutations, received from both parents.

Diagnosis

The diagnosis of LQTS relies primarily on the measurement of the QT interval corrected for heart rate (QTc) using Bazett's formula. According to the current definition [1], LQTS is diagnosed in patients with a cardiac arrest (CA) or syncope and a QTc >480 ms. In asymptomatic individuals without a pathogenic mutation or a family history of LQTS, a QTc >500 ms is required to establish the diagnosis [1]. Secondary causes of QT prolongation (drugs or electrolyte imbalance) need to be excluded when assessing the ECG.

In cases showing less evident QT prolongation, a quantitative score, which combines the patient's age, clinical and family history, and QTc duration, assists in the diagnosis of LQTS [3].

Although a prolonged ventricular repolarization is the hallmark of LQTS, up to one third of the carriers of a pathogenic mutation exhibit normal QTc values (incomplete penetrance). Due to their higher risk of arrhythmia compared with the general population (10% from birth to 40 years [4]), these 'silent' mutation carriers are considered as 'affected' and consequently need treatment [1].

Aside from the prolonged ventricular repolarization, patients with LQTS present with peculiar electromorphological alterations, which tend to be gene specific (fig. 1) and may help in raising suspicion for

Table 1. Clinical forms of LQTS and related genes

Type	Gene symbol	Locus	Protein	Functional effect
Autosomal dominant LQTS without extracardiac manifestations (Romano-Ward syndrome)				
LQT1	*KCNQ1*	11p15.5-p15.4	Potassium channel, voltage-gated, KQT-like subfamily, member 1	Loss of function; reduction in IKs current
LQT2	*KCNH2*	7q36.1	Potassium channel, voltage-gated, subfamily H, member 2	Loss of function; reduction in IKr current
LQT3	*SCN5A*	3p22.2	Sodium channel, voltage-gated, type V, α-subunit	Gain of function; increase in sodium current
LQT4	*ANK2*	4q25-q26	Ankyrin 2	Loss of function (several target proteins)
LQT5	*KCNE1*	21q22.11-q22.12	Potassium channel, voltage-gated, ISK-related subfamily, member 1	Loss of function; reduction in IKs current
LQT6	*KCNE2*	21q22.11	Potassium channel, voltage-gated, ISK-related subfamily, member 2	Loss of function; reduction in IKr current
LQT9	*CAV3*	3p25.3	Caveolin 3	Secondary gain of function in sodium channel
LQT10	*SCN4B*	11q23.3	Sodium channel, voltage-gated, type IV, β-subunit	Secondary gain of function in sodium channel
LQT11	*AKAP9*	7q21.2	A-kinase anchor protein 9	Loss of function; reduction in IKs current
LQT12	*SNTA1*	20q11.21	Syntrophin, α-1	Secondary gain of function in sodium channel
LQT13	*KCNJ5*	11q24.3	Potassium channel, inwardly rectifying, subfamily J, member 5	Loss of function; reduction in IK-Ach current
Autosomal dominant LQTS with extracardiac manifestations				
LQT7 (ATS)	*KCNJ2*	17q24.3	Potassium channel, inwardly rectifying, subfamily J, member 2	Loss of function; reduction in IK1 current
LQT8 (TS)	*CACNA1C*	12p13.33	Calcium channel, voltage-dependent, L-type, α-1C-subunit	Gain of function; increase in calcium current
Autosomal recessive LQTS with congenital deafness (JNLS)				
JLN1	*KCNQ1*	11p15.5-p15.4	Potassium channel, voltage-gated, KQT-like subfamily, member 1	Loss of function; reduction in IKs current
JLN2	*KCNE1*	21q22.11	Potassium channel, voltage-gated, ISK-related subfamily, member 1	Loss of function; reduction in IKs current

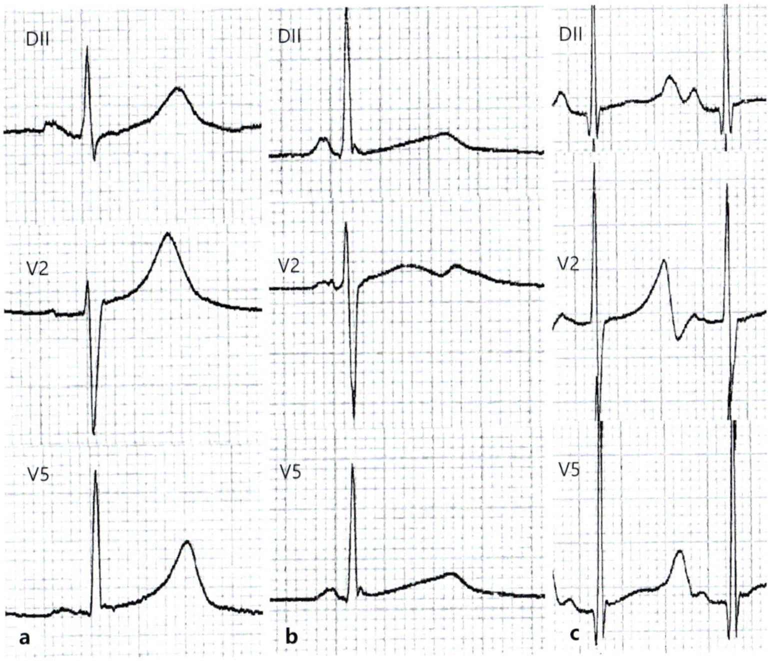

Fig. 1. Different electrocardiographic phenotypes of LQTS. ECG patterns of different LQTS genotypes. **a** LQT1: the T wave is broad based, smooth, with an accentuated ascending limb. **b** LQT2: the T wave is bifid (particularly in V2) and of low amplitude. **c** LQT3: the late-onset T wave is peaked, with a steep upstroke (evident in DII and V5).

an arrhythmia syndrome. Notches on the T wave are typical for LQT2 and indicate a higher risk for arrhythmic events. Long sinus pauses are common among LQT3 patients.

Clinical Manifestations

The clinical manifestations of LQTS are related to a unique form of VT, termed *torsade de pointes*, characterized by fast bursts of ventricular complexes that twist by 180° around the isoelectric line and lead to syncopal events. The precipitants for arrhythmias are often gene specific, with most events occurring during physical or emotional stress in LQT1, startling noises in LQT2 and during sleep in LQT3 patients [1].

The mean age at symptom onset is 14 years [5]; earlier manifestations forecast a severe prognosis. Among untreated patients, the natural history is represented by the occurrence of several syncopal episodes, eventually leading to SCD (annual incidence of SCD between 0.3 and 0.6% from birth to 40 years [4]). In a proportion of patients, SCD is the first manifestation of the syndrome and hence the rationale for treating asymptomatic patients.

Risk Stratification

A stepwise approach incorporating clinical, electrocardiographic, genetic and demographic parameters should be employed in the risk stratification of LQTS patients.

Symptomatic patients present a higher risk of SCD compared with asymptomatic ones, especially if arrhythmias occur during the 1st year of life. CA survivors have a high risk of recurrence, even while receiving β-blockers (14% within 5 years [6]) and, in general, should also receive an implantable cardioverter defibrillator (ICD) as secondary prevention. Similarly, the occurrence of syncope during therapy with adequate dosage of β-blockers is an ominous sign calling for aggressive treatment.

In asymptomatic individuals, the QT interval itself is the principal indicator of risk [4], whereby patients presenting with QTc >500 ms (and especially >550 ms) are at high risk for SCD. Additional ECG markers to consider are the presence of T-wave alternans and long sinus pauses followed by T-wave abnormalities as signs of high cardiac electrical instability [1].

It is also possible to delineate a gene-specific profile for the risk of SCD: LQT1 patients are in the lowest risk category, while LQT2 and LQT3 show a higher risk of CA. Recent advances have correlated mutations in specific regions of a protein to clinical severity. Mutations in the cytoplasmic loops of LQT1 [7] and mutations in the pore region of LQT2 [8] are associated with a higher risk.

Among genotyped patients, LQT1 males remaining asymptomatic up to puberty are at low risk of becoming symptomatic later on in life. Conversely, females (especially LQT2 females) show a high risk after adolescence and throughout adult life, peaking 9 months postpartum.

Finally, syndromic forms of LQTS, such as JLNS and TS, are malignant and manifest with major arrhythmias early in life, with poor response to therapy.

Management

Lifestyle modifications to limit the exposure to arrhythmic triggers should be routine care for LQTS patients. These include: avoidance of drugs prolonging QT intervals (for a comprehensive list, see www.qtdrugs.org), abstention from strenuous exercise (especially swimming) in LQT1 patients and reduction in exposure to abrupt loud noises in LQT2 patients.

β-Blockers are the mainstay in managing LQTS [1]. They are indicated in all LQTS patients, including those with a genetic diagnosis and normal QTc, unless there is a contraindication. Long-acting non-selective β-blockers (e.g. nadolol or sustained-release propranolol) should be preferred to improve compliance. Selective β-blockers (e.g. metoprolol) may have a role in asthmatic patients [1].

In LQT3 patients refractory to β-blockers, sodium channel blockers (mexiletine or flecainide [9]) have shown promising preliminary results in terms of QT-interval shortening.

In high-risk patients who are intolerant or refractory to β-blockers, especially infants and children in whom ICD therapy may be relatively dangerous, left cardiac sympathetic denervation is indicated to reduce the probability of arrhythmia [1].

ICD therapy is indicated in the few patients with a high arrhythmic risk despite therapy, such as CA survivors or patients who experienced syncope while on β-blockers [1]. On the contrary, the use of an ICD in asymptomatic individuals who have never tried β-blockers is generally not indicated [1]. Prophylactic ICD therapy might be considered, on a case-by-case basis, in high-risk patients, such as: (1) women with LQT2 and QTc ≥550 ms; (2) patients with QTc ≥550 ms and signs of electrical instability, and (3) patients with high-risk genetic profiles (carriers of two mutations, e.g. JLNS, or TS).

Short QT Syndrome

The short QT syndrome (SQTS) is the antithesis of LQTS, since it results in an abbreviated duration of cardiac repolarization, constituting both the diagnostic sign and the substrate for the development of dangerous arrhythmias. Back in the 1990s, an association between a shorter than normal QT interval with an increased risk of dying suddenly was postulated, and in 2003 SQTS was linked to familial SCD [10].

Epidemiology

Less than 200 SQTS patients have been reported in the literature [11, 12], demonstrating the rarity of the disease (estimated prevalence <1:10,000).

Genetic Variants

SQTS is an autosomal dominant disease and has been associated with five genes encoding for potassium (*KCNH2*, *KCNQ1* and *KCNJ2*) and calcium (*CACNA1C* and *CACNB2*) conducting channels. The yield of genetic screening is low (20% overall [12]); each gene accounts for <5% of index cases [2, 12].

Interestingly, three of these genes are also associated with variants in LQTS (LQT2, LQT1 and LQT7). This peculiarity, wherein mutations in the same genes may result in both abnormally prolonged and abnormally shortened repolarization, has a straightforward biophysical explanation. Mutations responsible for LQTS cause a decrease (loss of function) in the potassium current conducted by the ion channels encoded by the *KCNQ1*, *KCNH2* and *KCNJ2* genes. Conversely, mutations responsible for SQTS cause an increase (gain of function) in the cur-

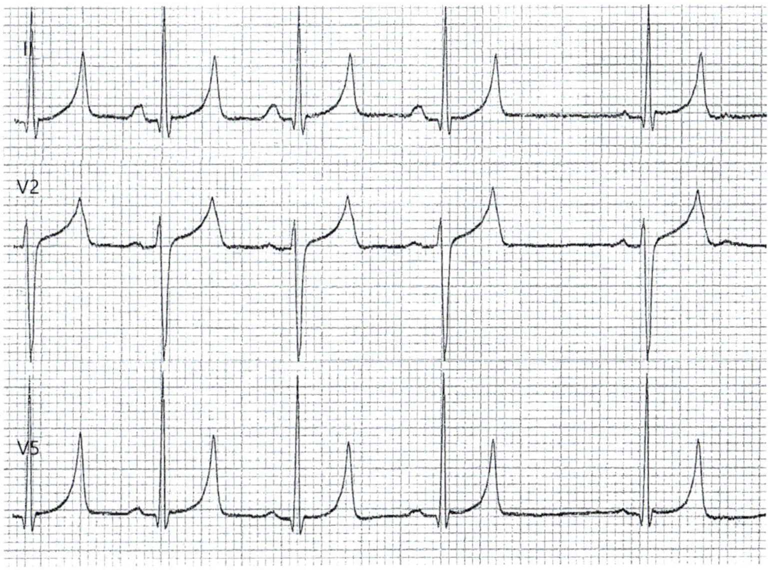

Fig. 2. SQTS: ECG from a 16-year-old girl with palpitations. Genetic screening revealed a missense mutation in the *KCNJ2* gene [24]. RR interval 1,000 ms, QT/QTc interval 330 ms. The T wave is narrow, peaked and asymmetrical with a relatively normal ascending limb but a remarkably rapid terminal phase.

rent conducted by the same potassium channels, thus shortening repolarization. On the contrary, loss of function mutations in the genes encoding α- and β-subunits of the L-type cardiac calcium channel *(CACNA1C* and *CACNB2)* have been associated with a mixed phenotype of SQTS and the Brugada syndrome (BrS).

Despite the reduced number of families with a positive genotype reported in the literature, some genotype-phenotype correlations have been attempted [11]. Patients with SQT1 constitute a subgroup with shorter QT intervals, higher prevalence of atrial fibrillation (AF) at a young age and a more relevant and constant response to quinidine in comparison to those lacking SQT1.

Diagnosis

Diagnostic thresholds for SQTS are debated. In general, QTc values <360 ms combined with SCD symptoms or a familial history of SCD at a young age are suggestive of the disease [1]. Individuals with QTc <330/340 ms should also be considered affected, even if asymptomatic [1, 12]. As for the LQTS, it is important that the QT interval is measured when the heart rate is close to 60 beats/min, to avoid over- or undercorrection using Bazett's formula (fig. 2).

Clinical Manifestations

SQTS is highly lethal and the probability of CA by the age of 40 years is >40% [12]; unfortunately, CA is the first manifestation of the disease in 40% of probands [12]. Symptoms may begin extremely early, even in the neonatal period [10, 12]. In some patients, SQTS manifests as early-onset 'lone' AF [10].

Risk Stratifications and Management

The clinical manifestations of SQTS are variable, even within the same family, but a risk stratification scheme for these patients is not yet available [1]. At variance with LQTS, a relation between QT-interval shortening and increased susceptibility to arrhythmias has not been demonstrated [12], nor have there been any data in support of the use of genotype determination to assess cardiac risk [12]. Furthermore, no clinical risk factors have been identified in asymptomatic individuals [12].

SQTS patients at high risk of SCD (e.g. CA survivors) should receive an ICD as secondary prevention, because the rate of recurrence reaches 10% per year [1, 12]. In a similar way, an ICD is recommended in patients who have documented spontaneous VT, with or without syncope [1]. On the contrary, there are no data to support the implantation of an ICD in asymptomatic SQTS patients.

Among the pharmacological options available to reduce the occurrence of life-threatening arrhythmias, quinidine (a class Ia antiarrhythmic drug) seems particularly promising, because it may normalize the duration of the QT interval (especially in patients with *KCNH2* mutations) and it may also reduce ventricular vulnerability during programmed electrical stimulation, irrespective of the genotype [11, 13]. According to current recommendations, quinidine may be considered in asymptomatic patients with a diagnosis of SQTS and a family history of SCD [1].

Brugada Syndrome

BrS is characterized by a typical electrocardiographic pattern of 'right bundle branch block and ST segment elevation in (right) precordial leads'.

Epidemiology

The prevalence of BrS is estimated at 1:1,000 worldwide, with a higher frequency in Southeast Asia than in Western countries [1]. A possible explanation for the higher frequency of BrS in Southeast Asia might be the existence of an Asian-specific variant in the promoter region of the *SCN5A* gene that reduces the sodium current, thus creating a predisposition to manifest the Brugada phenotype [14].

Besides ethnicity, age and gender play a role in the penetrance of BrS. Despite its congenital nature, clinical manifestations of the disease begin after adolescence. Additionally, notwithstanding the disease being inherited as an autosomal dominant condition in both genders, clinical manifestations are 8-fold higher in men than in women [1]. The presence of a more prominent transient outward potassium repolarizing current in cardiac action potentials in men and the higher levels of testosterone could contribute to this skewed distribution.

Genetic Variants

At least 12 genes have been associated with BrS, but genetic abnormalities are found in only one third of the patients. In all the variants described, either a decrease in the inward (depolarizing) sodium or calcium current, or an increase in one of the outward (repolarizing) potassium currents has been shown to be associated with the BrS phenotype. Only two genes (*SCN5A* and *CACN1Ac*) account for >5% of positively genotyped patients individually: the former, encoding the Nav1.5 sodium channel, explains the vast majority (75%) of genotype-positive cases [2].

Diagnosis

BrS is diagnosed when its hallmark ECG pattern, a coved ST-segment elevation ≥2 mm (termed type 1 ECG) is observed in ≥1 right precordial leads (V1–V2), which are placed in a standard or a superior position (up to the 2nd intercostal space) [1]. Since the type 1 ECG pattern appears intermittently, with a trend to become more evident during sleep or after a meal, multiple ECG recordings are required to establish the diagnosis.

When the phenotype is not completely evident during basal conditions, a provocative test may be performed to unmask otherwise concealed cases, by intravenous infusion of sodium channel-blocking agents (ajmaline, flecainide and pilsicainde) or by oral administration of procainamide (fig. 3) [1].

Besides the altered ventricular repolarization, ECG features frequently found in patients with BrS include: AF; atrioventricular conduction delays; fragmented QRS; late potentials on signal-averaged ECG, and spontaneous ventricular premature beats from the right ventricle.

Though BrS is considered a primary 'electrical' disorder, without clear structural heart abnormalities, several clinical studies have reported mild ventricular anomalies.

Clinical Manifestations

BrS typically manifests during adulthood (mean age at SCD 41 ± 15 years [15]). Symptoms often manifest as syncopal spells after meals or episodes of nocturnal agonal respiration reported by bed partners. Fever, excessive alcohol intake, large meals and all vagotonic triggers may unmask the type 1 ECG pattern, predisposing to SCD. Up to one third of BrS patients present with atrial arrhythmias, of which AF is the most common (10% of cases [16]).

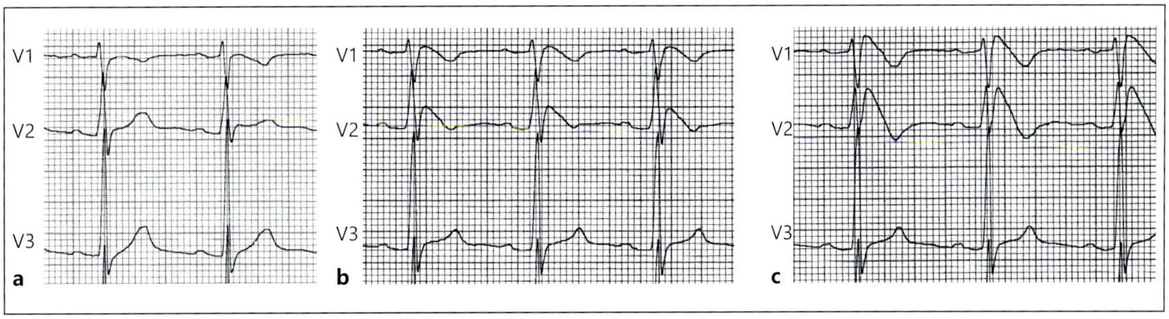

Fig. 3. BrS: right precordial leads (V1–V3) from the ECG of a 35-year-old asymptomatic man with BrS. **a** Basal ECG showing negative T waves in lead V1 but no significant ST segment elevation in the right precordial leads. **b** ECG showing occurrence of coved ST segments in leads V1 and V2 (type 1 Brugada pattern after infusion of 1 mg/kg ajmaline). **c** ECG with altered right precordial lead position (leads V1 and V2 at the 2nd intercostal space) showing more evident type 1 Brugada pattern.

Risk Stratification

Risk stratification in BrS is based on clinical parameters and is still debated. CA survivors are at high risk of recurrence (13.5%/year [17]). The presence of syncope in patients with a spontaneous type 1 ECG (i.e. without conditions unmasking the signature pattern, like drugs or fever) involves a high risk of CA (~3%/year) [17].

In asymptomatic individuals, several indicators of risk have been proposed, including the presence of fragmented QRS [18], an effective ventricular refractory period <200 ms [18] or the occurrence of AF [1]. Male gender has also been associated with increased arrhythmic events [1].

Data coupling genetic status to prognosis are scarce. Different outcomes related to the underlying gene defect have not been reported and, from a meta-analysis, there appears to be no difference even when *SCN5A* is involved [19]. However, in a subset analysis of patients with *SCN5A*-mediated BrS, there may be a better prognosis in case of a *SCN5A* missense mutation compared with a truncated protein [20].

The prognostic value of programmed electrical stimulation has been much debated; recent clinical studies have not confirmed its positive or negative predictive value for the occurrence of CA at follow-up [18].

Management

Lifestyle adjustments should be applied to all patients with clinically diagnosed BrS and may also be useful for asymptomatic *SCN5A* mutation-positive subjects [1]. Precautions include the reduction in body temperature during febrile illnesses and the avoidance of drugs that decrease sodium channel availability/functionality, therefore increasing arrhythmic risk (see www.brugadadrugs.org).

The only treatment able to reduce SCD in BrS is the ICD; therefore, the device is indicated in patients with CA [1], documented VT [1] or in those presenting with a spontaneous type 1 ECG and a history of syncope [1].

Asymptomatic BrS patients do not qualify for an ICD as their risk for CA is low [1]. In this group of patients, individual assessment of associated risk factors (e.g. gender and baseline ECG) should be performed.

Quinidine has been proposed as preventive therapy in BrS patients based on data showing that it could reduce ventricular vulnerability and ICD shocks in symptomatic patients [1]. A clinical trial (NCT00789165) with quinidine in asymptomatic BrS patients is ongoing.

BrS patients who experience arrhythmic storms may be treated with isoproterenol infusion [1]. Recent findings suggest that catheter ablation of fragmented potentials over the anterior right ventricular outflow tract epicardium may prevent arrhythmic storms in BrS patients with recurrent episodes [21]. However, randomized data on the efficacy of catheter ablation of spontaneous arrhythmias are lacking.

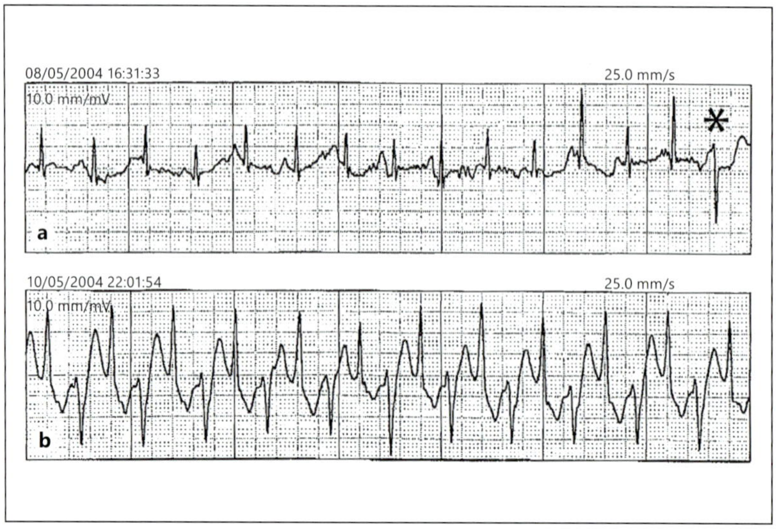

Fig. 4. CPVT with RyR2 mutation: Holter recordings from a 16-year-old girl with a history of recurrent syncope during exercise since the age of 10 years. **a** Continuous strips showing sinus tachycardia interrupted by a ventricular extrasystolic beat (*). **b** Trace showing a typical bidirectional VT characterized by beat-to-beat alternations in the frontal QRS axis.

Catecholaminergic Polymorphic Ventricular Tachycardia

Catecholaminergic polymorphic VT (CPVT) is a malignant arrhythmogenic syndrome characterized by adrenergic-induced bidirectional and polymorphic VT.

Epidemiology

The prevalence of the disease is unknown, with the most commonly quoted figure being 1:10,000. This is a rough estimate, because CPVT patients have a normal resting ECG: it is impossible to distinguish between low frequency of the disease and diagnostic underestimation.

Genetic Variants

Two CPVT genetic variants are known: an autosomal dominant one, related to mutations in the *RyR2* gene encoding for the cardiac ryanodine receptor, and an autosomal recessive form, resulting from mutations in the *CASQ2* gene, which encodes for cardiac calsequestrin. Genetic defects in both proteins alter calcium homeostasis in cardiac myocytes, facilitating diastolic calcium release, which leads to the development of delayed afterdepolarizations and subsequent triggered activity, which may precipitate supraventricular and ventricular arrhythmias.

Approximately 55% of CPVT index cases carry a mutation in the *RyR2* gene, while the prevalence of *CASQ2* mutations is estimated at 5% [2]. As for LQTS, the recessive form is more malignant than the dominant variant. Because it is unclear whether *CASQ2* mutations may also cause autosomal dominant transmission of the phenotype, it is rational to screen *CASQ2* in sporadic *RyR2*-negative index cases.

A partial phenotypic overlap exists between LQTS and CPVT: some carriers of LQT4 (gene *Ank2*) or LQT7 (ATS) variants may exhibit bidirectional VT in their ECG. It is currently unknown whether these cases should be regarded as variants of LQTS that mimic CPVT or whether *KCNJ2* and *Ank2* should be considered as new CPVT genes.

Diagnosis

CPVT patients show normal resting ECGs. Lower than normal heart rates and prominent U waves have been reported in some patients, but neither finding is sufficiently specific for a diagnosis. Typically, exercise stress testing or strong emotions elicit the appearance of ventricular escape beats that increase in complexity in parallel with the heart rate and culminate with the pathognomonic bidirectional or polymorphic VT. The term bidirectional refers to the 180° rotation on the frontal plane of the QRS complexes of the ectopic beats (fig. 4) [1]. Adrenergically mediated supraventricular arrhythmias (premature atrial contractions, runs of supraventricular tachycardia and bursts of AF) are also common in CPVT.

Clinical Manifestations

Clinical manifestations of CPVT are stress-induced syncope and CA. The mean age at symptom onset is 8 years [22], but first symptoms may also occur in adulthood. The clinical course is severe, as 30% of patients experience symptoms before age 10 years and nearly 60% of affected individuals have at least one syncopal episode before age 40 years [22].

Sudden CA can be the first clinical presentation in up to 30% of cases [22]. Therefore, *RyR2* mutations may be regarded as a cause of adrenergically mediated idiopathic ventricular fibrillation, which may justify genetic testing in such instances [2].

Risk Stratifications

There are few risk factors indicating an adverse outcome in CPVT. The occurrence of CA before diagnosis, but not of syncope, is associated with a higher risk of arrhythmic episodes at follow-up. Similarly, diagnosis in childhood is a predictor of severe prognosis. After diagnosis, the lack of β-blocker therapy is an independent predictor for arrhythmic events [1]. Furthermore, the persistence of complex ventricular arrhythmias during exercise testing is a marker for a worse outcome [1].

Genetic information has not yet been able to contribute to risk stratification in CPVT patients, but genotype-phenotype correlations are beginning to develop. Current data have shown that patients with a *RyR2* mutation in the C-terminal channel-forming domain showed an increased risk of nonsustained VT compared with those with N-terminal domain mutations [1].

Management

The first-line therapy for patients with CPVT are β-blockers combined with exercise restriction. High-dose nadolol (1–2 mg/kg per day) is our preferred prophylactic therapy and requires a faultless compliance [1].

Holter recordings and exercise tests should be repeated periodically to ensure that the rate response to effort is adequately suppressed. Asymptomatic ventricular escape beats usually persist with an unmodified threshold of appearance, but their complete suppression does not seem to be mandatory. Despite the appropriate use of β-blockers, up to one third of CPVT patients experience recurrence of arrhythmic events and additional treatments are indicated.

As in LQTS, left cardiac sympathetic denervation may have a role, especially in the first few years of life, when implantation of an ICD is associated with a high rate of complications [1].

Flecainide has been demonstrated as a useful addition to β-blockers to reduce the burden of ventricular arrhythmias. One clinical trial (NCT01117454) is ongoing to investigate the efficacy of flecainide in addition to standard therapy in patients with an ICD. Until results of the trial become available, ICD implantation should be considered the preferred therapy for CA survivors who continue to experience syncopal episodes despite β-blocker treatment and those who have sustained VT at exercise stress testing [1].

Careful programming of the ICD (long delays before shock delivery and high cutoff rates) is important in CPVT patients to avoid inappropriate and painful shocks that may have a proarrhythmic effect.

Considering the early age at CPVT manifestation, it is reasonable that in families with a known CPVT-associated mutation, confirmatory genetic testing should be performed at birth to allow prompt initiation of β-blocker therapy in mutation-positive subjects, even after a negative exercise test [1].

The next therapeutic target for channelopathies is the search for a cure aimed at restoring normal gene function. Promising experimental approaches to gene therapy are currently underway in CPVT, with encouraging results from animal models. Such studies achieved favorable results in the autosomal recessive form of CPVT (related to the *CASQ2* gene). Our group demonstrated that infection of a viral vector carrying wild-type calsequestrin induces long-term expression of a properly functioning gene in a knockout murine model [23].

Conclusions

The seminal discovery of LQTS about 50 years ago sealed the concept that the predisposition to SCD may be an inheritable trait, paving the way to the characterization of a set of primary electrical cardiac disorders with a genetic basis, the so-called channelopathies.

From the collaborative efforts of cardiologists, geneticists and basic scientists, genetic information has entered into the arena of clinical practice, giving origin to a vital and specialized branch of medicine: the so-called 'molecular cardiology'.

Genetic studies now play a key role in the diagnosis of channelopathies and may assist in the early detection of apparently unaffected individuals. The emergence of gene-based risk stratification algorithms and gene-specific treatments has led to the possibility of the implementation of preventive measures with the intention of defusing the potential lethality associated with these diseases.

The next step in the evolution of genetic studies is the search for the elusive cure which is aimed at restoring the normal function of a gene. The future, fortunately, is not as far away as it seems with several promising experimental approaches to gene therapy currently underway.

References

1 Priori SG, Wilde AA, Horie M, Cho Y, Behr ER, Berul C, Blom N, Brugada J, Chiang CE, Huikuri H, Kannankeril P, Krahn A, Leenhardt A, Moss A, Schwartz PJ, Shimizu W, Tomaselli G, Tracy C: HRS/EHRA/APHRS expert consensus statement on the diagnosis and management of patients with inherited primary arrhythmia syndromes. Heart Rhythm 2013;10:1932–1963.

2 Ackerman MJ, Priori SG, Willems S, Berul C, Brugada R, Calkins H, Camm AJ, Ellinor PT, Gollob M, Hamilton R, Hershberger RE, Judge DP, Le Marec H, McKenna WJ, Schulze-Bahr E, Semsarian C, Towbin JA, Watkins H, Wilde A, Wolpert C, Zipes DP: HRS/EHRA expert consensus statement on the state of genetic testing for the channelopathies and cardiomyopathies: this document was developed as a partnership between the Heart Rhythm Society (HRS) and the European Heart Rhythm Association (EHRA). Europace 2011;13:1077–1109.

3 Schwartz PJ, Crotti L: QTc behavior during exercise and genetic testing for the long-QT syndrome. Circulation 2011;124:2181–2184.

4 Priori SG, Schwartz PJ, Napolitano C, Bloise R, Ronchetti E, Grillo M, Vicentini A, Spazzolini C, Nastoli J, Bottelli G, Folli R, Cappelletti D: Risk stratification in the long-QT syndrome. N Engl J Med 2003;348:1866–1874.

5 Moss AJ, Schwartz PJ, Crampton RS, Tzivoni D, Locati EH, MacCluer J, Hall WJ, Weitkamp L, Vincent GM, Garson A Jr, et al: The long QT syndrome. Prospective longitudinal study of 328 families. Circulation 1991;84:1136–1144.

6 Moss AJ, Zareba W, Hall WJ, Schwartz PJ, Crampton RS, Benhorin J, Vincent GM, Locati EH, Priori SG, Napolitano C, Medina A, Zhang L, Robinson JL, Timothy K, Towbin JA, Andrews ML: Effectiveness and limitations of beta-blocker therapy in congenital long-QT syndrome. Circulation 2000;101:616–623.

7 Barsheshet A, Goldenberg I, O-Uchi J, Moss AJ, Jons C, Shimizu W, Wilde AA, McNitt S, Peterson DR, Zareba W, Robinson JL, Ackerman MJ, Cypress M, Gray DA, Hofman N, Kanters JK, Kaufman ES, Platonov PG, Qi M, Towbin JA, Vincent GM, Lopes CM: Mutations in cytoplasmic loops of the KCNQ1 channel and the risk of life-threatening events: implications for mutation-specific response to β-blocker therapy in type 1 long-QT syndrome. Circulation 2012;125:1988–1996.

8 Moss AJ, Zareba W, Kaufman ES, Gartman E, Peterson DR, Benhorin J, Towbin JA, Keating MT, Priori SG, Schwartz PJ, Vincent GM, Robinson JL, Andrews ML, Feng C, Hall WJ, Medina A, Zhang L, Wang Z: Increased risk of arrhythmic events in long-QT syndrome with mutations in the pore region of the human ether-a-go-go-related gene potassium channel. Circulation 2002;105:794–799.

9 Moss AJ, Windle JR, Hall WJ, Zareba W, Robinson JL, McNitt S, Severski P, Rosero S, Daubert JP, Qi M, Cieciorka M, Manalan AS: Safety and efficacy of flecainide in subjects with long QT-3 syndrome (deltaKPQ mutation): a randomized, double-blind, placebo-controlled clinical trial. Ann Noninvasive Electrocardiol 2005;10:59–66.

10 Gaita F, Giustetto C, Bianchi F, Wolpert C, Schimpf R, Riccardi R, Grossi S, Richiardi E, Borggrefe M: Short QT syndrome: a familial cause of sudden death. Circulation 2003;108:965–970.

11 Giustetto C, Schimpf R, Mazzanti A, Scrocco C, Maury P, Anttonen O, Probst V, Blanc JJ, Sbragia P, Dalmasso P, Borggrefe M, Gaita F: Long-term follow-up of patients with short QT syndrome. J Am Coll Cardiol 2011;58:587–595.

12 Mazzanti A, Kanthan A, Monteforte N, Memmi M, Bloise R, Novelli V, Miceli C, O'Rourke S, Borio G, Zienciuk-Krajka A, Curcio A, Surducan AE, Colombo M, Napolitano C, Priori SG: Novel insight into the natural history of short QT syndrome. J Am Coll Cardiol 2014;63:1300–1308.

13 Gaita F, Giustetto C, Bianchi F, Schimpf R, Haissaguerre M, Calo L, Brugada R, Antzelevitch C, Borggrefe M, Wolpert C: Short QT syndrome: pharmacological treatment. J Am Coll Cardiol 2004; 43:1494–1499.

14 Bezzina CR, Shimizu W, Yang P, Koopmann TT, Tanck MW, Miyamoto Y, Kamakura S, Roden DM, Wilde AA: Common sodium channel promoter haplotype in Asian subjects underlies variability in cardiac conduction. Circulation 2006;113:338–344.

15 Priori SG, Napolitano C, Gasparini M, Pappone C, Della Bella P, Giordano U, Bloise R, Giustetto C, De Nardis R, Grillo M, Ronchetti E, Faggiano G, Nastoli J: Natural history of Brugada syndrome: insights for risk stratification and management. Circulation 2002;105:1342–1347.

16 Giustetto C, Cerrato N, Gribaudo E, Scrocco C, Castagno D, Richiardi E, Giachino D, Bianchi F, Barbonaglia L, Ferraro A: Atrial fibrillation in a large population with Brugada electrocardiographic pattern: prevalence, management, and correlation with prognosis. Heart Rhythm 2014;11:259–265.
17 Fauchier L, Isorni MA, Clementy N, Pierre B, Simeon E, Babuty D: Prognostic value of programmed ventricular stimulation in Brugada syndrome according to clinical presentation: an updated meta-analysis of worldwide published data. Int J Cardiol 2013;168:3027–3029.
18 Priori SG, Gasparini M, Napolitano C, Della Bella P, Ottonelli AG, Sassone B, Giordano U, Pappone C, Mascioli G, Rossetti G, De Nardis R, Colombo M: Risk stratification in Brugada syndrome: results of the PRELUDE (PRogrammed ELectrical stimUlation preDictive valuE) registry. J Am Coll Cardiol 2012;59:37–45.
19 Gehi AK, Duong TD, Metz LD, Gomes JA, Mehta D: Risk stratification of individuals with the Brugada electrocardiogram: a meta-analysis. J Cardiovasc Electrophysiol 2006;17:577–583.
20 Meregalli PG, Tan HL, Probst V, Koopmann TT, Tanck MW, Bhuiyan ZA, Sacher F, Kyndt F, Schott JJ, Albuisson J, Mabo P, Bezzina CR, Le Marec H, Wilde AA: Type of SCN5A mutation determines clinical severity and degree of conduction slowing in loss-of-function sodium channelopathies. Heart Rhythm 2009;6:341–348.
21 Nademanee K, Veerakul G, Chandanamattha P, Chaothawee L, Ariyachaipanich A, Jirasirirojanakorn K, Likittanasombat K, Bhuripanyo K, Ngarmukos T: Prevention of ventricular fibrillation episodes in Brugada syndrome by catheter ablation over the anterior right ventricular outflow tract epicardium. Circulation 2011;123:1270–1279.
22 Priori SG, Napolitano C, Memmi M, Colombi B, Drago F, Gasparini M, DeSimone L, Coltorti F, Bloise R, Keegan R, Cruz Filho FE, Vignati G, Benatar A, DeLogu A: Clinical and molecular characterization of patients with catecholaminergic polymorphic ventricular tachycardia. Circulation 2002;106:69–74.
23 Denegri M, Bongianino R, Lodola F, Boncompagni S, De Giusti VC, Avelino-Cruz JE, Liu N, Persampieri S, Curcio A, Esposito F, Pietrangelo L, Marty I, Villani L, Moyaho A, Baiardi P, Auricchio A, Protasi F, Napolitano C, Priori SG: Single delivery of an adeno-associated viral construct to transfer the CASQ2 gene to knock-in mice affected by catecholaminergic polymorphic ventricular tachycardia is able to cure the disease from birth to advanced age. Circulation 2014;129:2673–2681.
24 Priori SG, Pandit SV, Rivolta I, Berenfeld O, Ronchetti E, Dhamoon A, Napolitano C, Anumonwo J, di Barletta MR, Gudapakkam S, Bosi G, Stramba-Badiale M, Jalife J: A novel form of short QT syndrome (SQT3) is caused by a mutation in the KCNJ2 gene. Circ Res 2005;96:800–807.

Dr. Silvia G. Priori
Molecular Cardiology
IRCCS Salvatore Maugeri Foundation
Via Maugeri 10, IT–27100 Pavia (Italy)
E-Mail silvia.priori@fsm.it

Muenke M, Kruszka PS, Sable CA, Belmont JW (eds): Congenital Heart Disease: Molecular Genetics, Principles of Diagnosis and Treatment. Basel, Karger, 2015, pp 210–225
DOI: 10.1159/000375218

Genetic Cardiomyopathies

Jeffrey A. Towbin

University of Tennessee Health Science Center, St. Jude Children's Research Hospital and Le Bonheur Children's Hospital, Memphis, Tenn., USA

Abstract

Cardiomyopathies (diseases of the heart muscle) are major causes of morbidity and mortality. A significant percentage of patients with cardiomyopathies have genetic-based, inheritable disease and, over the past 2 decades, the genetic causes of these disorders have been increasingly discovered. The causes of these disorders are mutations of gene(s) that appear to encode proteins that frame a 'final common pathway' for a specific disorder, but the specifics of the phenotype, including age at onset, severity, and outcome, are variable for reasons not yet understood. The 'final common pathways' for the classified forms of cardiomyopathy include the sarcomere in the primarily diastolic dysfunction disorders (hypertrophic and restrictive cardiomyopathy), the linkage of the sarcomere and sarcolemma in systolic dysfunction (dilated cardiomyopathy), and the desmosome in arrhythmogenic ventricular cardiomyopathy. Left-ventricular noncompaction cardiomyopathy (LVNC) is an overlap disorder and it appears that any of these 'final common pathways' can be involved depending on the specific form of LVNC. The genetics and mechanisms responsible for these clinical phenotypes will be described.

Cardiomyopathies are major causes of morbidity and mortality and, over the past 25 years, limited improvements in outcome have been reported [1, 2]. However, the understanding of the major forms of cardiomyopathy has improved over that time, in large part due to advances in imaging, genetics, and genomics [3, 4]. A new classification scheme was recently developed for the cardiomyopathies, in which five forms of disease were formally classified as distinct forms of cardiomyopathy: dilated cardiomyopathy (DCM), hypertrophic cardiomyopathy (HCM), restrictive cardiomyopathy (RCM), arrhythmogenic ventricular cardiomyopathy (AVC), and left-ventricular (LV) noncompaction cardiomyopathy (LVNC) [5]. These were further classified into genetic/inherited forms and acquired/noninherited forms. All forms occur at all ages except for AVC, which is almost always identified in teenagers and young adults.

Our understanding of the genetic causes of cardiomyopathy has expanded significantly over the last decade. In many cases, the genetic and mechanistic causes of these disorders follow a disturbance in a particular, disease-specific 'final common pathway' [6]. For instance, HCM is now viewed as predominantly an inherited abnormality of contractile protein function ('disease of the sarcomere'). Progress in understanding the genetics of familial DCM has been complicated by its heterogeneous etiologies, but a genetic cause is thought to occur in approximately 50% of subjects, with higher rates in children [3–5]. The genes identified to date as causative appear to disturb most commonly the func-

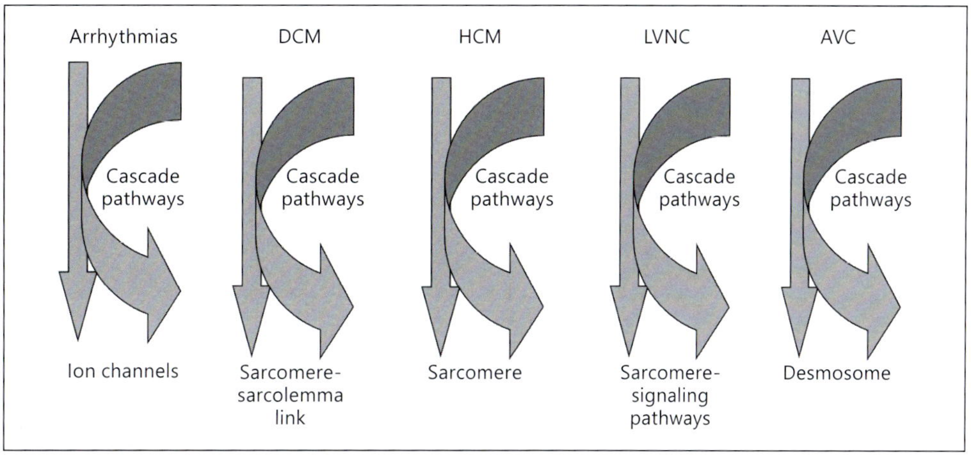

Fig. 1. Final common pathway hypothesis: illustration outlining the proposed 'final common pathways' for arrhythmia disorders DCM, HCM or RCM, LVNC, and AVC.

tional link between the cytoskeleton and sarcomere [4]. Multiple genes have been identified for AVC, most resulting in disturbed desmosome/intercalated disk function [4, 7]. Although understanding the genetic basis for the development of RCM and LVNC has been more elusive, genes for both have been identified and appear to include sarcomere dysfunction as critical factors [8].

In this chapter, we will review the current genetic knowledge of each cardiomyopathy phenotype and will describe how disruption of these 'final common pathways' leads to DCM (sarcolemma-sarcomere link), HCM (sarcomere), RCM (sarcomere), AVC (desmosome), and LVNC (sarcolemma and sarcomere).

Final Common Pathways

Over the past 2 decades, many of the genes responsible for the development of the different cardiomyopathies have been identified. In an initial attempt to target genes for genetic study, we developed the 'final common pathway hypothesis', which stated that genes encoding proteins with similar functions or involved in the same pathway are responsible for a particular disease or syndrome phenotype [6]. As a result, others and we identified structure-function similarities of proteins encoded by genes that, when disrupted, led to a somewhat predictable gross clinical phenotype. For instance, the genes identified as causative for inherited arrhythmia disorders tend to encode for ion channels, those for HCM encode for sarcomeric proteins, and those for AVC cell-cell junction proteins, for example (fig. 1). In addition, it appears that the proteins disturbed by the mutated gene directly disrupt the normal function of the structures in which it is integrated (such as the sarcomere in HCM when the mutated gene encodes a sarcomeric protein) most commonly, but, in some instances, they disrupt a binding partner protein that causes a downstream disturbance of the 'final common pathway' (such as a Z-disk protein disrupting the cell-cell junction via a maladaptive binding to desmin, which negatively interacts with a desmosomal protein causing AVC; fig. 1).

Dilated Cardiomyopathy

DCM is the most common cardiomyopathy, accounting for approximately 55% of cardiomyopathies [5]. The annual incidence is 2–8 in 100,000 per year (0.57 in 100,000/year in children) with an estimated prevalence of 1 in 2,500 [5, 9]. The percentage

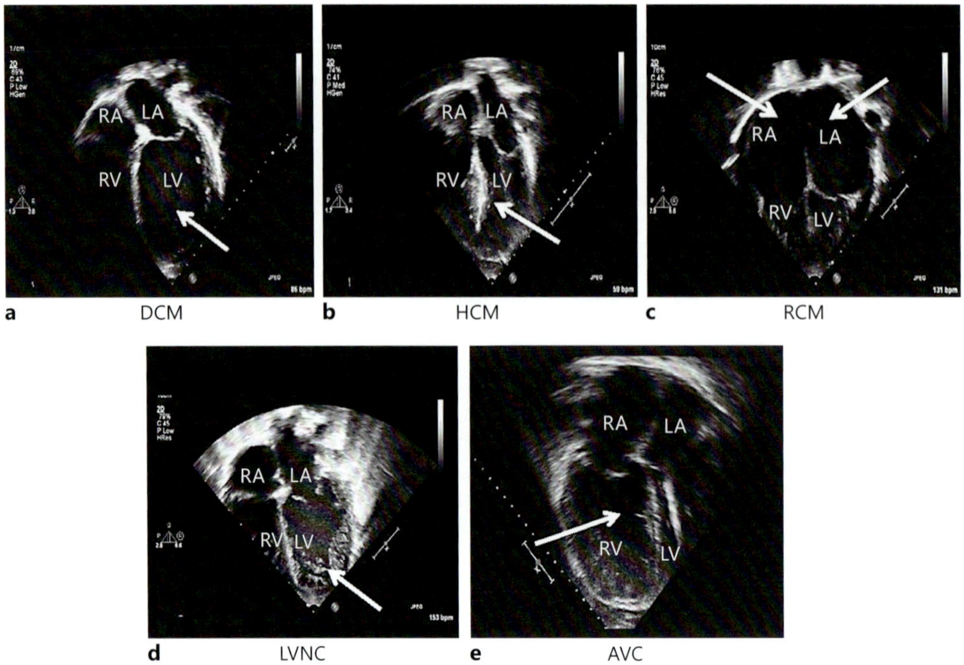

Fig. 2. Echocardiographic features of cardiomyopathies. **a–e** Four-chamber echocardiographic views show DCM (**a**), HCM (**b**), RCM (**c**), LVNC (**d**), and AVC (**e**). LA = Left atrium; RA = right atrium. Note the dilated LV (arrow; **a**); the thickened mid-portion of the interventricular septum (arrow; **b**); the dilated atria (arrows; **c**); the hypertrabeculation in the LV (arrow; **d**), and the dilated, trabeculated RV (arrow; **e**); commonly, an aneurysm of the RV or RV outflow tract can be seen, particularly by MRI.

of cases with a genetic etiology is approximately 30–50% based on the presence of a family history [10–12]. DCM is characterized by LV dilation and systolic dysfunction (a reduction in myocardial force generation) and is the most common indication for cardiac transplantation (fig. 2) [5, 9–12]. Clinical manifestations include heart failure (HF), thromboembolism, and sudden cardiac death (SCD). The age at onset ranges from newborn through late adulthood, although most patients are diagnosed between 20 and 50 years of age [12].

The genetic forms of DCM usually result from mutated genes encoding two major subgroups of proteins: cytoskeletal and sarcomeric proteins [3, 4, 6, 13]. DCM can also present with muscular involvement and may be the presenting or primary clinical feature of several multisystem conditions, including the Emery-Dreifuss muscular dystrophy, Barth syndrome, myofibrillar myopathy, limb-girdle muscular dystrophy, and the Duchenne (DMD) or Becker muscular dystrophy (BMD) [14].

Genetics of Dilated Cardiomyopathy

Inherited, familial DCM has been shown to occur in 30–50% of cases of DCM, and autosomal dominant inheritance is the predominant pattern of transmission; X-linked, autosomal recessive, and mitochondrial inheritance is less common [10–12, 15, 16]. Over the past 20+ years, substantial progress has been made in the understanding of the genetic etiology of familial DCM (table 1). Initial progress was made in the early 1990s studying families with X-linked forms of DCM, with the autosomal dominant forms unraveling shortly thereafter.

X-linked DCM, occurring in males in the teen years and early twenties with rapid progression from HF to death due to arrhythmias or transplantation, is distinguished by elevated serum creatine kinase muscle isoforms [16, 17]. Female carriers develop milder, slowly progressive DCM (5th decade). Towbin et al. [17] identified dystrophin as the disease-causing gene and demonstrated significant reduction or absence of

Table 1. DCM genetics

Gene	Gene name
ABCC9	ATP-binding cassette, subfamily C, member 9
ACTC	α-Cardiac actin
ACTN2	α-Actinin-2
ANKRD1	Cardiac ankyrin repeat, domain 1
BAG3	BCL2-associated athanogene 3
CSRP3	Cysteine- and glycine-rich protein 3
CTF1	Cardiotrophin-1
DES	Desmin
DYS	Dystrophin
DNAJC19	DnaJ (Hsp40) homolog, subfamily C, member 19
DSC2	Desmocollin-2
DSG2	Desmoglein-2
DSP	Desmoplakin
EMD	Emerin
EYA4	Eyes absent homolog 4
FHL2	Four and a half LIM domains 2
FKTN	Fukutin
FOXD4	Forkhead box D4
LAMA4	α_4-Laminin
LAMP2	Lysosomal-associated membrane protein 2
LDB3	LIM-domain binding 3
LMNA	Lamin A/C
MYBPC3	Myosin binding protein C
MYH6	β-Myosin heavy chain 6
MYH7	β-Myosin heavy chain 7
MYPN	Myopalladin
NEBL	Nebulette
NEXN	Nexilin (F actin binding protein)
PLN	Phospholamban
PSEN1	Presenilin 1
PSEN2	Presenilin 2
RBM20	RNA binding motif protein 20
SCN5A	Voltage-gated sodium channel, α subunit
SDHA	Succinate dehydrogenase complex, subunit A, flavoprotein
SGCD	δ-Sarcoglycan
SYNE1	Spectrin repeat containing nuclear protein 1
SYNE2	Spectrin repeat containing nuclear protein 2
TAZ	Tafazzin
TCAP	Titin-cap (telethonin)
TMPO	Thymopoeitin
TNNC1	Cardiac troponin C, type 1
TNNI3	Cardiac troponin I, type 3
TNNT2	Cardiac troponin T, type 2
TPM1	α-Tropomyosin 1
TTN	Titin
TTR	Transthyretin
VCL	Vinculin

dystrophin protein in the heart. These findings were later confirmed by Muntoni et al. [18] and others [19], with mutations generally occurring in the 5′-end of the gene. Dystrophin, a cytoskeletal protein which provides structural support to myocytes by creating a lattice-like network to the sarcolemma, links the contractile apparatus (sarcomere) to the sarcolemma and extracellular matrix (ECM; fig. 3) [16]. When mutated, dystrophin causes DMD/BMD, skeletal myopathies that present in males early in life with elevated creatine kinase MM isoforms and lead to the early need for wheelchairs (before 12 years of age in DMD and ≥16 years in BMD) [20–22] with DCM usually occurring between 10 and 25 years [16–22].

In addition to dystrophin protein dysfunction, mutations in the dystrophin gene secondarily affect proteins which interact with dystrophin. At the amino terminus, dystrophin binds to the sarcomeric thin-filament protein actin. At the carboxy terminus, dystrophin interacts with the dystrophin-associated membrane-bound proteins α-dystroglycan, syntrophins, and dystrobrevins [23, 24], which, in turn, interact with α_2-laminin and ECM (fig. 3). Mutations in these genes also lead to muscular dystrophies with or without DCM, information which led us to hypothesize that DCM is a disease of cytoskeleton/sarcolemma-sarcomere linkage, the 'final common pathway' of DCM (fig. 1) [6, 16].

The most common form of inheritance of DCM is autosomal dominant [6, 13, 15], presenting either as classic 'pure' DCM or DCM associated with early-onset conduction system disease (CDDC). Genetic heterogeneity exists for autosomal dominant DCM with more than 40 genes identified for DCM and CDDC [3, 4, 13, 24, 25], with most genes encoding either cytoskeletal, sarcomeric, or Z-disk proteins, although mutations in a small number of ion channel- and desmosome-encoding genes have also been identified (table 1). These include genes primarily encoding cytoskeletal proteins [δ-sarcoglycan *(SGCD)*, β-sarcoglycan *(SGCB)*, desmin *(DES)*, lamin A/C *(LMNA)*, and vinculin *(VCL)*], sarcomeric/myofibrillar proteins [α-cardiac actin *(ACTC)*, troponin T *(TNNT2)*, troponin I *(TNNI3)*, β-myosin heavy chain *(MYH7)*, myosin binding protein C *(MBPC3)*, and α-tropomyosin *(TPM1)*], and Z-disk proteins [muscle LIM protein (MLP)/cysteine- and

5

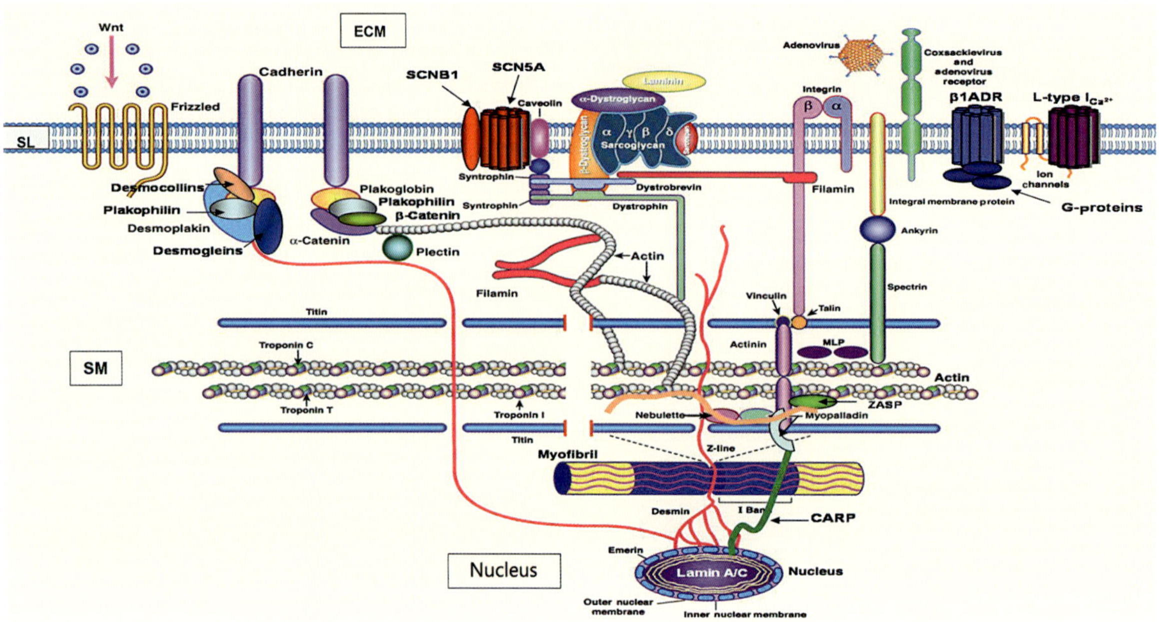

Fig. 3. Cardiac myocyte cytoarchitecture. Schematic illustration of key proteins of the ECM, sarcolemma (SL), sarcomere (SM), and nucleus, and some of their protein-protein interactions. Note: the sarcolemmal proteins include ion channels such as SCN5A and L-type calcium channels, for example, as well as the dystrophin-associated binding proteins that interact with dystrophin and other cytoplasmic cytoskeletal proteins (dystroglycans, sarcoglycans, syntrophins, dystrobrevin, sarcospan, and caveolin), and cadherins that bind with desmosomal proteins (desmocollin, plakophillin, desmoplakin, and plakoglobin). The integral sarcolemmal membrane proteins interact with the ECM via α-dystroglycan-laminin α_2 connections. The sarcomere includes thick- and thin-filament contractile proteins and Z-disk proteins. The amino terminus of dystrophin binds actin and connects dystrophin with the sarcomere intracellularly, the sarcolemma and ECM. The nucleus includes important membrane proteins: lamin A/C and emerin. The intermediate-filament protein desmin is another important and prominent linker protein. MLP = Muscle LIM protein.

glycine-rich protein 3 *(CSRP3)*, titin *(TTN)*, telethonin/TCAP, α-actinin-2 *(ACTN2)*, nebulette *(NEBL)*, myopalladin *(MYPN)*, ANKRD1/CARP, and ZASP/LIM-domain binding 3 *(LBD3)*] (table 1; fig. 3). Ion channel-encoding genes identified to date include the cardiac sodium channel gene *SCN5A* and the calcium homeostasis regulator phospholamban *(PLN)* [24, 25] while associated desmosome-encoding genes include desmoplakin *(DSP)*, desmoglein-2 *(DSG2)*, and desmocollin-2 *(DSC2)*, which have also been shown to result in a DCM phenotype (table 1; fig. 3) [26]. In the case of CDDC, LMNA is the most common cause, but other causes include DES and SCN5A (table 1; fig. 3) [27, 28]. Mechanistically, cytoskeletal proteins are thought to cause defects in force transmission resulting in the DCM phenotype, while defects in force generation have been speculated to be associated with sarcomere protein-induced DCM [29, 30]. The altered desmosomal proteins appear to disrupt the links between the intercalated disk, Z-disk, and sarcomere [31, 32]. Purevjav et al. [33, 34] recently showed that a gene mutation may disrupt protein binding partners, and, depending on this interaction, differential phenotypes and severity may occur.

Mutations in the sarcomere may produce variable forms of cardiomyopathy (tables 1–4; fig. 3). As previously noted, abnormalities in force generation or transmission are thought to contribute to the development of DCM [29, 30, 35, 36]. α-Cardiac actin, a sarcomeric thin-filament protein that interacts with tropomyosin and the troponin complex, links the sarcomere to the sarcolemma via its binding to the N terminus of dystrophin. DCM-causing actin mutations disturb dystrophin-actin binding [37, 38] and thus cause force transmission abnormalities and DCM. Furthermore, actin interacts in the sarcomere with troponin T and β-myosin heavy chain; muta-

Table 2. HCM genetics

Gene	Gene name
ACTC	α-Cardiac actin
ACTN2	α-Actinin-2
ANKRD1	Cardiac ankyrin repeat, domain 1
CAV3	Caveolin 3
COX15	COX 15 homolog, cytochrome C oxidase assembly protein
CRYAB	Crystallin αB
CSRP3	Cysteine- and glycine-rich protein 3
GLA	α-Galactosidase
LAMP2	Lysomal-associated membrane protein 2
MYBPC3	Myosin binding protein C
MYH6	β-Myosin heavy chain 6
MYH7	β-Myosin heavy chain 7
MYL2	Myosin regulatory light chain 2, slow
MYL3	Myosin light chain 3, slow
MYLK2	Myosin light chain kinase 2
MYO6	Unconventional myosin VI
MYOZ2	Myozenin 2
NEXN	Nexilin (F actin binding protein)
PLN	Phospholamban
PRKAG2	AMP-activated protein kinase, γ_2, noncatalytic subunit
TNNC1	Cardiac troponin C, type 1
TAZ	Tafazzin
TCAP	Titin-cap (telethonin)
TNNI3	Cardiac troponin I, type 3
TNNT2	Cardiac troponin T, type 2
TPM1	α-Tropomyosin 1
TTN	Titin
TTR	Transthyretin
VCL	Vinculin

Table 3. RCM genetics

Gene	Gene name
ACTC1	α-Cardiac actin1
BAG3	BCL2-associated athanogene 3
DES	Desmin
GLA	α-Galactosidase
MYH7	β-Myosin heavy chain 7
MYL2	Myosin regulatory light chain 2, slow
MYL3	Myosin light chain 3, slow
MYPN	Myopalladin
TNNI3	Cardiac troponin I, type 3
TNNT2	Cardiac troponin T, type 2
TPM1	α-Tropomyosin 1
TTN	Titin
TTR	Transthyretin

Table 4. LVNC genetics

Gene	Gene name
ACTC1	α-Cardiac actin1
CASQ2	Cardiac calsequestrin 2
DTNA	α-Dystrobrevin
DYS	Dystrophin
GLA	α-Galactosidase
LDB3	LIM-domain binding 3
LMNA	Lamin A/C
MYBPC3	Myosin binding protein C
MYH7	β-Myosin heavy chain 7
TAZ	Tafazzin
TNNT2	Cardiac troponin T, type 2

tions in these genes cause DCM or HCM, depending on the position of the mutation [38], via development of force generation abnormalities. For MYH7, this probably occurs by perturbing the actin-myosin interaction or altering cross-bridge movement during contraction [35–38]. TNNT2 mutations disrupt calcium-sensitive troponin C binding [35–38]. Mutations in PLN have also been identified, which further support calcium handling as a potentially important mechanism in DCM development [35–38]. *TPM1* mutations alter its surface charge, causing impaired interaction with actin and potentially changing its secondary structure, its binding to actin and position on the thin filament, and alternating actin-myosin interactions and myofilament Ca^{2+} sensitivity.

Another molecular level target for DCM is the Z-disk [39–41]. Knoll et al. [40] identified mutations in *MLP/CSPR3* which disturb their interaction with TCAP and its stretch sensor activity. Mutations in CSPR3 cause abnormalities in the T-tubule system and Z-disk architecture as well [42]. Mutations in ACTN2, which binds CSPR3, are involved in cross-linking actin filaments and share a common actin-binding domain with dystrophin, and disrupt CSPR3 binding and stretch sensing [39–42]. Mutations in *ZASP/LBD3* cause DCM and LVNC, as well as myofibrillar myopathy [39–41, 43]. This protein, which interacts with ACTN2, the FATZ/calsarcin/myozenin protein family, the myotilin (myotilin, myopalladin, and palladin) family and

TCAP, forms a complex with the cardiac sodium channel, NEBL, and phosphoglucomutase 1, and disrupts the actin cytoskeleton when mutated [44]. *TTN*, which encodes a giant sarcomeric cytoskeletal protein, contributes to the maintenance of sarcomere organization and myofibrillar elasticity, and interacts with these proteins at the Z-disk/I-band transition zone and causes DCM or AVC when mutated [45].

Due to significant locus and allelic heterogeneity, genetic testing for DCM has been of limited utility, with pathogenic variants identified in 17–40% of cases using the current 40-gene panels, with most genes contributing only to a small percentage of the pathogenic variants [4, 13, 24, 25]. Clear genotype-phenotype correlations are rare. Exceptions include variants in *LMNA* and *SCN5A*, which usually cause DCM and conduction/rhythm abnormalities [24, 25, 27]. Desmosomal genes, traditionally known to cause AVC, also cause arrhythmia-prone DCM (table 1) [26]. *TTN* reportedly contributes to up to 25% of familial and 18% of sporadic DCM cases, making it the most commonly mutated gene in DCM [45].

Muscle Is Muscle: Cardiomyopathy and Skeletal Myopathy Genes Overlap

Interestingly, nearly all of the genes identified for inherited DCM are also known to cause skeletal myopathy in humans and/or mouse models: dystrophin mutations cause DMD/BMD, SGCD causes limb-girdle muscular dystrophy type 2F, LMNA causes autosomal dominant Emery-Dreifuss muscular dystrophy and limb-girdle muscular dystrophy type 1B, and ACTC and DES cause nemaline myopathy. In addition, tafazzin (TAZ), α-dystrobrevin, LBD3, CSRP3, ACTN2, TTN, and SGCB mutations also cause skeletal myopathy, suggesting that cardiac and skeletal muscle function is interrelated; skeletal muscle fatigue seen in patients with DCM with and without HF may be due to primary skeletal muscle disease and not only related to cardiac dysfunction. It also suggests that striated muscle dysfunction results from disturbed 'final common pathways', and both sets of muscles should be evaluated in DCM.

Hypertrophic Cardiomyopathy

HCM is characterized by asymmetric or concentric wall thickening (fig. 2) in the absence of an underlying systemic condition or other cardiac disease [5, 6, 13, 16, 46]. The major impact of this disorder on human health is its predilection to be inherited, its reputation as the most common cause of SCD in young, healthy individuals, and its potential to result in HF due to diastolic factors or development of systolic dysfunction [5, 47].

Gene Identification in Familial Hypertrophic Cardiomyopathy

HCM is among the most common inherited cardiac disorders, with a prevalence of 1 in 500 in young adults [5]. During the last 20+ years, molecular genetic studies have given important insights into the pathogenesis of HCM and provided new perspectives for the diagnosis and management of affected patients. Genetic causes for HCM have been described and over 20 genes have been discovered to date, with most affecting the sarcomere; however, mutations in genes encoding proteins of the Z-disk or intracellular calcium modulators have also been identified (table 2). Eight causative genes encode sarcomere proteins, with most (~80%) mutations being found in the *MYH7* and *MYBPC3* genes (fig. 3) [4, 5, 13, 46]. Mutations identified in sarcomeric genes are typically single-nucleotide substitutions, and in most instances the mutant protein is thought to incorporate into the sarcomere, exerting a poison peptide effect (dominant negative mutations), with the only exception being MYBPC3, where deletions or insertions leading to a frameshift, a truncated protein with no function, result in haploinsufficiency [48]. In addition to defects in the sarcomere-encoding genes, HCM patients have been identified hosting mutations in Z-disk and other non-sarcomere-encoding genes [4, 13, 33, 49]. The giant protein titin and its interactive Z-disk proteins, including MLP, ZASP, telethonin, nexilin, myopalladin, myozenin-2, α-actinin-2, CARP, and vinculin, have been identified as causes of HCM when their gene is mutated (table 2; fig. 3) [49]. For Z-disk and calcium modulator genes, the specific mechanism has not been clearly elucidated.

Recent clinical guidelines for HCM recommend comprehensive testing for five HCM genes (*MYBPC3, MYH7, TNNI3, TNNT2*, and *TPM1*) although current next-generation sequencing approaches have facilitated much broader testing panels to be widely available from commercial laboratories [19] (http://www.genetests.org and http://www.ncbi.nlm.nih.gov/gtr). Currently, genetic testing for HCM is primarily used to identify families with a detectable genetic cause of disease and to screen at-risk family members. In our clinic, mutations are seen in approximately 65–70% of all subjects. The use of genetic test results in guiding clinical management is limited due to limited genotype-phenotype correlations. Although almost 1,000 variants for HCM have been identified to date [4, 13, 33, 49, 50], most are private and can, therefore, be detected only through comprehensive genetic testing.

Genotype-Phenotype Correlation in Hypertrophic Cardiomyopathy

Sarcomere variants are identified in up to 60–70% of patients with HCM who also have a family history and in 40–60% of patients with sporadic HCM [13, 50]. Genotype-phenotype correlations for HCM are incompletely defined, in part due to the private nature of the mutations. Those that have been established are broad correlations at the gene level, but extensive heterogeneity exists and reported correlations are somewhat controversial. For example, it was originally reported that some, but not all, *TNNT2* mutations are associated with only minor hypertrophy but an appreciable risk of arrhythmia [51]. However, there is clearly a subgroup of patients with significant hypertrophy. MYH7 variants generally seem to lead to significant LV hypertrophy by the 2nd decade of life and are thought to be associated with an increased risk of HF and SCD [50]. However, there are young children who present with *MYH7* mutations in infancy and childhood [52]. Similarly, although pathogenic variants in *MYBPC3* were initially reported to be associated with a later age at onset, there are young children with disease-causing *MYBPC3* mutations [52]. Most *MYBPC3* variants in pediatric patients reportedly have missense changes, contrasting the high prevalence of loss-of-function variants in adult HCM, suggesting missense variants have more severe functional consequences [52].

The pattern and extent of LV hypertrophy in patients with HCM, as well as outcomes, are heterogeneous even in first-degree relatives. This heterogeneity has made it difficult to correlate genotype and phenotype, including outcome. A systematic review and meta-analysis of genotype-phenotype correlations in 2,459 patients and 53 families with sarcomeric gene mutations reported in 18 publications showed that the presence of any sarcomere gene mutation was associated with younger age at presentation (38.4 vs. 46.0 years), a family history of HCM (50.6 vs. 23.1%), a family history of SCD (27.0 vs. 14.9%), and greater LV wall thickness (21.0 vs. 19.3 mm) [53]. Regarding outcome, the prognosis for patients with different MYH7 mutations has been shown to vary: the R403Q mutation was initially reported to be associated with markedly reduced survival, whereas others, such as V606M, appeared more benign [54]; *TNNT2* mutations were associated with a 20% incidence of nonpenetrance, relatively mild and sometimes subclinical hypertrophy, but a high incidence of sudden death occurring even in the absence of significant clinical LV hypertrophy [55]; mutations in *MYBPC3*, on the other hand, were initially characterized by specific clinical features with a mild phenotype in young subjects, delayed age at symptom onset, and favorable prognosis before 40 years of age [56]. However, despite these assertions, the notion of mutation-specific clinical outcomes was challenged by Van Driest et al. [57], who demonstrated that 'benign' mutations were uncommon (5/253) and that the mutations studied all reflected severe clinical disease.

The relationship between cardiac morphology, mutated genes, and outcome has also been evaluated [58–60]. Bos et al. [58, 59] studied 359 patients, and 34% were genotype positive for a putative HCM-associated mutation in one or more genes. Echocardiographic reverse curve morphological subtype (fig. 4), age at diagnosis younger than 45 years, maximum LV wall thickness of ≥20 mm, a family history of HCM, and a family history of SCD were identified as positive predictors of mutation identification; hypertension was a negative predictor. A score, based on the number of predictors of a positive genetic test result, predicted

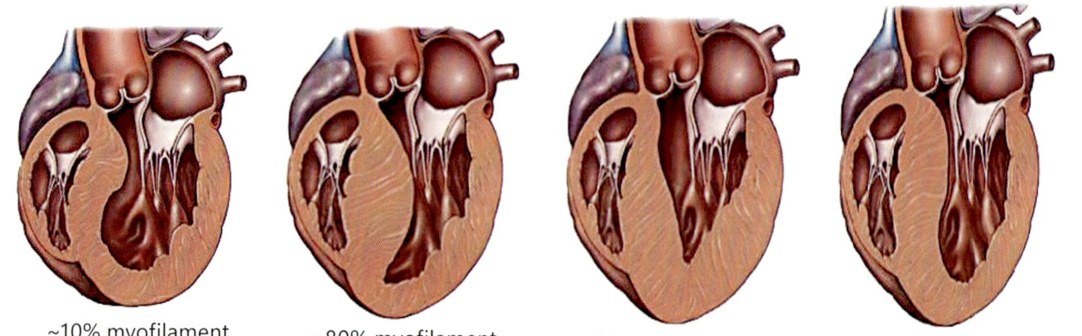

Fig. 4. Septal morphologies in HCM and the relationship to sarcomeric myofilament-encoding gene mutations. The four subgroups of septal morphology in HCM (sigmoidal, reverse curve, apical, and neutral) are shown, along with the percentage of HCM cases represented by each morphology and the likelihood of identifying a mutation in a myofilament-encoding gene (with permission from Bos et al. [59]).

mutation identification in 6% when only hypertension was present compared to 80% when all five positive predictive markers were present. Geske et al. [61] studied 131 patients (age 55 ± 15 years) with clinically diagnosed HCM by echocardiography with LV strain imaging to evaluate LV dimensions and ejection fraction, septal contour and thickness, and obstructive physiology, and found correlations as well. Multiple mutations in causative genes (i.e. compound or digenic heterozygotes) are detected in 3–5% of genotype-positive patients, with a more severe phenotype and increased incidence of SCD notable, suggesting a gene-dosage effect contributes to disease severity. One of the mutations usually involves *MYBPC3* [62, 63].

Restrictive Cardiomyopathy

RCM is the rarest form of cardiomyopathy; it is characterized by dilated atria, and increased ventricular stiffness with normal ventricular wall thickness and systolic function (fig. 2) [5, 8]. SCD or a life-threatening cardiac event due to ventricular arrhythmias or heart block is common, as is HF; death occurs within a few years of diagnosis [5, 8]. Some reports suggest clinical overlap between RCM and HCM [64, 65].

Genetics

RCM usually has autosomal dominant inheritance, but autosomal recessive, X-linked, and mitochondrial-transmitted disease also occurs. Most genes identified encode sarcomere or Z-disk proteins, such as *TNNI3, TNNT2, MYH7, ACTC1, TPM1, MYL3,* and *MYL2* (table 3) [8, 66]. Z-disk protein-encoding genes, including *MYPN, TTN,* and *BAG3,* have also been noted [4, 5, 8, 13, 33]. Missense variants in DES have been identified in several families with desmin-related myopathy, which can present with RCM, with or without skeletal myopathy and/or atrioventricular block [8]. Transthyretin is associated with amyloid-related RCM [8].

Left-Ventricular Noncompaction Cardiomyopathy

LVNC is a heterogeneous myocardial disorder characterized by prominent trabeculae most evident in the LV apex, intratrabecular recesses, and LV myocardium having two distinct layers: compacted and noncompacted myocardium (fig. 2) [5, 13, 16, 67]. Although LVNC primarily affects the LV, isolated right ventricle (RV) and biventricular noncompaction also occurs [67]. Multiple forms of

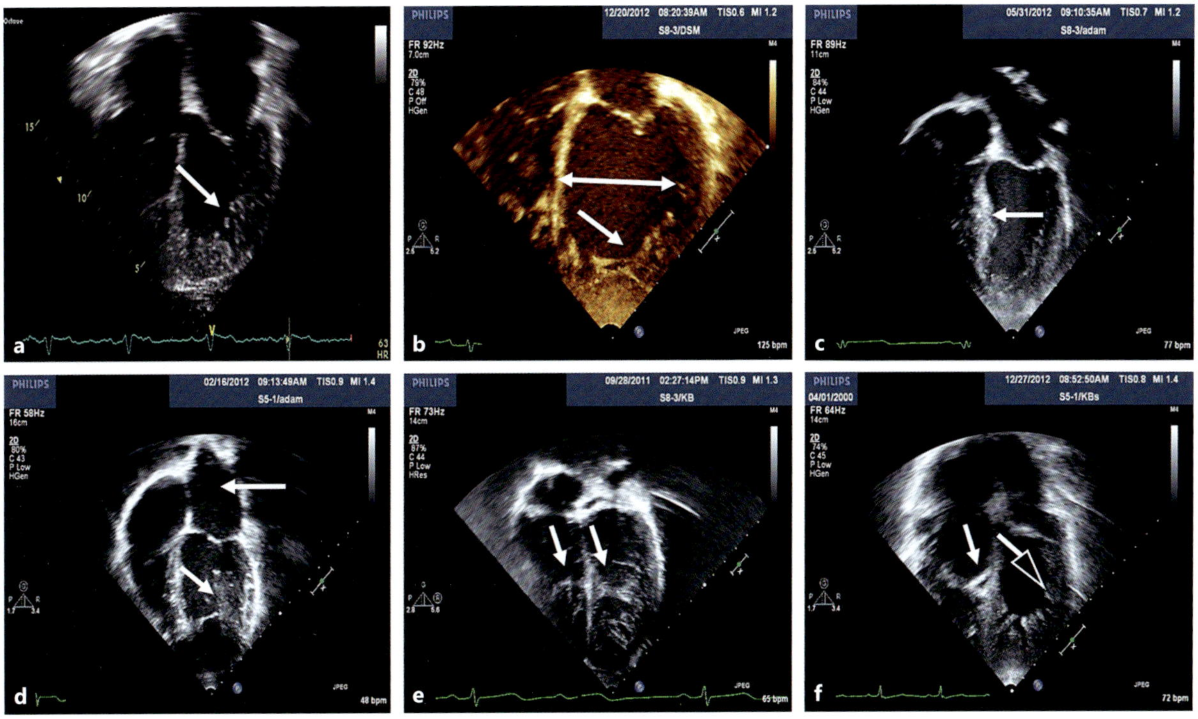

Fig. 5. Echocardiographic heterogeneous features of the LV noncompaction phenotype. Four-chamber views demonstrate normal atrial and ventricular sizes and thickness with a hypertrabeculated LV wall and apex (arrow; **a**); normal atrial sizes with a dilated and hypertrabeculated LV wall and apex (arrow; **b**); hypertrophic and hypertrabeculated ventricular walls and apex with a hypertrophic septum (arrow; **c**); normal to small ventricular sizes with dilated atria bilaterally (arrows) and a hypertrabeculated LV (**d**); normal atrial sizes with severely hypertrabeculated LV and RV wall and apices (arrows; **e**); and Ebstein's anomaly with LVNC, which demonstrates a normal left atrial size with a large right atrium, displaced tricuspid valve towards the RV (closed arrowhead), and a severely hypertrabeculated LV wall and apex (open arrowhead; **f**).

LVNC occur and these include primary myocardial forms, a form associated with arrhythmia, and LVNC associated with congenital heart disease (CHD), including atrial and ventricular septal defects, hypoplastic left-heart syndrome, and right-heart obstructive abnormalities, including pulmonic stenosis and Ebstein's anomaly (fig. 5), for example [67]. Outcomes appear to differ based on the specifics of the phenotype.

Genetics

LVNC most commonly has X-linked recessive or autosomal dominant inheritance, with reports suggesting 70% having autosomal dominant and 30% X-linked inheritance, at least in childhood [67–69]. Autosomal recessive and mitochondrial inheritance also occurs [67]. When LVNC is associated with CHD, the congenital cardiac defect may be heterogeneous in families, but this form of LVNC is transmitted as an autosomal dominant trait along with the CHD; affected members may have no CHD at initial evaluation because the cardiac defects include 'minor' forms of CHD (small ventricular and atrial septal defects, and patent ductus arteriosus), which have spontaneously normalized or penetrance may be reduced, while others may have severe forms of CHD (e.g. hypoplastic left-heart syndrome or Ebstein's anomaly) [67, 70]. Ichida et al. [68] reported that 44% of their patients had inherited LVNC, with 70% having autosomal dominant and 30% X-linked inheritance. In addition, patients with chromosomal abnormalities are associated with LVNC.

The first genetic cause of isolated LVNC was initially described by Bleyl et al. [71]; they identified mutations in the X-linked *TAZ* gene, the gene also responsible for the Barth syndrome, in patients and carrier females (table 3). Multiple genes causing autosomal dominant LVNC have now been identified, including mutations in genes causing CHD with LVNC. In patients with hypoplastic left-heart syndrome and LVNC, the cytoskeletal gene α-dystrobrevin was identified while mutations in *NKX2.5* in children with LVNC and atrial septal defects and *MYH7* in patients with LVNC and Ebstein's anomaly have also been reported (table 3) [67, 72–75]. In LVNC without CHD, mutations in the Z-line protein-encoding ZASP/LDB3 gene and the sarcomere-encoding genes *(MYH7, ACTC, TNNT2, MYBPC3, TMP1*, and *TNNI3)* appear to account for 20% or more of LVNC [67, 76, 77]. Hoedemaekers et al. [77] additionally demonstrated an association of LVNC with genetic variants in two calcium-handling genes, as well as *TAZ* and *LMNA*, while Probst et al. [76] further showed that sarcomere gene mutations are important in LVNC, showing a prevalence of 29%, with *MYH7* and *MYBPC3* being most frequently mutated (13 and 8%, respectively). Dellefave et al. [78] also identified sarcomere mutations in LVNC, including those presenting with HF in infancy with and without compound heterozygosity.

In addition to genes encoding the sarcomere and cytoskeleton, mutations in the sodium channel gene, *SCN5A*, are associated with LVNC and rhythm disturbance [72]. Dystrophin mutations have also been seen in boys with LVNC and DMD/BMD [14], while a homozygous 2-bp deletion (5208_5209delAG) in an alternatively spliced region of the desmosomal protein-encoding gene DSP, which is known to cause AVC and DCM, has also been identified in LVNC patients [79]. Mitochondrial genome mutations have also been found to be associated with LVNC [80] and, as noted, chromosomal abnormalities and syndromic patients also have been associated with LVNC [81], including the 1p36 deletion, 7p14.3-7p14.1 deletion, 18p subtelomeric deletion, 22q11.2 deletion, distal 22q11.2 deletion, trisomies 18 and 13, 8p23.1 deletion, tetrasomy 5q35.2–5q35, the Coffin-Lowry syndrome (*RPS6KA3* mutation), the Sotos syndrome (*NSD1* mutation), and Charcot-Marie-Tooth disease type 1A (*PMP22* duplication). Diagnostic testing in patients with LVNC appears to have a detection rate of clinically significant variants in 35–40% of individuals, and sarcomere-encoding genes are most commonly found to be mutated [4, 82].

Arrhythmogenic Cardiomyopathies

AVC, previously referred to as arrhythmogenic *right*-ventricular dysplasia or cardiomyopathy, and recently renamed in a consensus statement [5], constitutes a hereditary cardiomyopathy usually with an autosomal dominant inheritance pattern, although a recessive cardiocutaneous disorder also occurs [83]. The RV was initially thought to be solely affected in AVC, and therefore any associated disease of the LV was considered exclusionary for the diagnosis in the original 'Task Force criteria' for diagnosis but, more recently, it has been recognized that the LV can also be involved and actually is often associated with severe disease and a worse prognosis [84]. Classically, however, the RV is dilated with fibrofatty infiltration with no or only minimal LV involvement [5, 7]. Clinically, progressive disease is characterized by systolic impairment and biventricular dilation (with or without a ventricular aneurysm) with clinical features of HF (fig. 2). In most parts of the world, phenotypic expression is more common in men than in women (2–3:1) [85]. AVC commonly manifests during late childhood or adolescence but can also emerge in the elderly and has a prevalence of 1 in 2,000, which can be higher in certain geographical regions such as the Veneto region or the Greek island Naxos [86]. AVC is recognized as a leading cause of SCD in young adults ≤35 years of age and may account for up to 10% of cardiovascular deaths in the <65-year age group [5, 7].

Genetics

Analyses of first- and second-degree relatives of patients with AVC suggest that up to 50% of AVC cases are familial [5, 7, 87]. AVC is most commonly inherited as an autosomal dominant trait with incomplete penetrance [5, 7, 87], although two autosomal recessive forms have been described [83]. To date, 15 genes have been reported to cause AVC (ta-

Table 5. AVC genetics

Gene	Gene name
CTNNA3	αT-catenin
DES	Desmin
DNAJC19	DnaJ (Hsp40) homolog, subfamily C, member 19
DSC2	Desmocollin-2
DSG2	Desmoglein-2
DSP	Desmoplakin
JUP	Junctional plakoglobin
LMNA	Lamin A/C
PKP2	Plakophilin 2
PKP4	Plakophilin 4
RYR2	Ryanodine receptor 2
STRN	Striatin
TGFβ3	Transforming growth factor-β_3
TMEM43	Transmembrane 43
TTN	Titin

ble 5) [4, 5, 7, 13, 88]. We and others demonstrated that compound and digenic heterozygosity is involved in AVC pathogenesis in up to 20% of cases and leads to a more severe disease [89, 90]. As penetrance is incomplete, genetically affected relatives often demonstrate a variable and mild (or no) phenotype, and the prevalence of familial disease is often underestimated in clinical practice [13, 85]. In addition, patients with fully penetrant arrhythmogenic RV cardiomyopathy and dermatologic abnormalities of the palms, plantar fascia, and hair were found clustered in families on the Greek island Naxos, now called Naxos disease, and they were shown to have autosomal recessive inheritance. In addition, a similar autosomal recessive cardiocutaneous disorder with an LV dominant cardiomyopathy was also reported in Ecuador (Carvajal syndrome) [83].

The first gene to be identified in AVC was junctional plakoglobin *(JUP)* when a homozygous 2-nucleotide deletion in *JUP* was reported in patients with Naxos disease [7, 83, 85]. This gene encodes the plakoglobin protein, a key protein of the desmosome in the intercalated disk. In autosomal dominant AVC, the desmosomal protein-encoding DSP gene was identified as disease causing [7, 83, 85]. Since myocytes and epidermal cells share similar intercalated disks (desmosomes and fascia adherens) and both are exposed to high shear stress, particularly during strenuous physical activity and increased cardiac workload, it makes sense that this (impaired intercalated-disk integrity) could be the 'final common pathway' of AVC (fig. 1) [91].

Three groups of desmosomal proteins are known: (1) transmembrane desmosomal cadherins, including DSC2 and DSG2; (2) DSP, a plakin family protein that attaches directly to intermediate filaments (desmin in the myocardium), and (3) linker proteins such as armadillo family proteins, including JUP and plakophilin 2 (PKP2) that mediate interactions between the desmosomal cadherin tails and DSP [92]. In about 80% of cases with confirmed pathogenic mutations, PKP2, DSP, and DSG2 are altered [86]. Besides desmosomal gene mutations, mutations in genes encoding proteins that interact with desmosomal proteins were also found. These include: (1) the transforming growth factor β_3 that conveys cytokine-stimulating fibrosis and modulates cell adhesion and growth; (2) the transmembrane protein 43 (TMEM43), which functions as a PPAR-γ response element, (3) an adipogenic transcription factor; (4) DES, which binds desmoplakin, and (5) TTN, which bridges the sarcomere along its longitudinal axis and forms a continuous filament along the myofibril (table 5) [4, 7, 13, 85, 91, 92].

Genetically determined disruption of intercalated-disk integrity is a key factor promoting the development of AVC and SCD. Recent data indicate that loss of desmosomal integrity can substantially affect gap junctions, sodium channel function, and electrical propagation, thereby promoting ventricular arrhythmias in the absence of overt structural damage [93, 94]. Accordingly, lethal ventricular arrhythmias often occur. Delmar and McKenna [93] postulated that mutations in desmosomal genes may affect the integrity of other molecular complexes adjacent to desmosomes, such as connexins and voltage-gated sodium channels, and are crucial for electrical synchrony, thus providing an overlapping phenotype (cardiomyopathy plus arrhythmias) due to disruption of two 'final common pathways' (desmosomes and ion channels) [91, 95].

Conclusions

The cardiomyopathies appear to occur due to disruption of 'final common pathways'. These disruptions may be due to purely genetic causes, such as mutations in a single gene that results in a dysfunctional protein, which leads to a domino effect of downstream protein interaction abnormalities and ultimately in the phenotype. In other situations, multiple mutations in the same gene (compound heterozygosity) or in different genes (digenic heterozygosity) may lead to a phenotype that may be classic, more severe, or even overlapping with other disease forms. In some cases, different intersecting pathways may become disturbed, resulting in complex phenotypes. Furthermore, acquired causes may play a role by causing disruption of these functional pathways. For instance, DCM results from disruption of the 'final common pathway' linking the sarcomere and sarcolemma, and mutations in the affected genes are responsible for cardiac and skeletal muscle dysfunction. The mechanisms of disease, which include disruption of the linkage due to protein-protein interaction abnormalities occurring from dysfunctional proteins, as well as the interplay of other factors, such as mechanical stress and stretch, are being elucidated in detail with the development of animal models of the corresponding human disease. Many of the genes identified are now clinically available in fee-for-service laboratories. Novel therapies have resulted from the improved understanding of this clinical phenotype, as noted above. Similarly, the genetic basis and mechanistic understanding of HCM as a disturbance of sarcomere function has occurred over the past 2 decades, and genetic tests are clinically available. The development of novel targeted therapies has been somewhat slow in coming but expected in the near future. In the case of LVNC, the 'new kid on the block', genetic understanding is in the early phases. The future of cardiomyopathy care is poised to shift in the next decade due to these new developments, as well as the growing science of stem cell therapy. Since children have 'pure' disease states, unfettered by comorbidities, the dream of 'cures' of (cardiac/skeletal) muscle disease will likely be realized more fully in this population. We must move toward that goal.

References

1 Lee CS, Chien CV, Bidwell JT, Gelow JM, Denfeld QE, Creber RM, Buck HG, Mudd JO: Comorbidity profiles and inpatient outcomes during hospitalization for heart failure: an analysis of the U.S. Nationwide inpatient sample. BMC Cardiovasc Disord 2014;14:73.

2 Shamszad P, Hall M, Rossano JW, Denfield SW, Knudson JD, Penny DJ, Towbin JA, Cabrera AG: Characteristics and outcomes of heart failure-related intensive care unit admissions in children with cardiomyopathy. J Card Fail 2013; 19:672–677.

3 Cahill TJ, Ashrafian H, Watkins H: Genetic cardiomyopathies causing heart failure. Circ Res 2013;113:660–675.

4 Teekakirikul P, Kelly MA, Rehm HL, Lakdawala NK, Funke BH: Inherited cardiomyopathies: molecular genetics and clinical genetic testing in the postgenomic era. J Mol Diagn 2013;15:158–170.

5 Maron BJ, Towbin JA, Thiene G, Antzelevitch C, Corrado D, Arnett D, Moss AJ, Seidman CE, Young JB; American Heart Association; Council on Clinical Cardiology, Heart Failure and Transplantation Committee; Quality of Care and Outcomes Research and Functional Genomics and Translational Biology Interdisciplinary Working Groups; Council on Epidemiology and Prevention: Contemporary definitions and classification of the cardiomyopathies: an American Heart Association Scientific Statement from the Council on Clinical Cardiology, Heart Failure and Transplantation Committee; Quality of Care and Outcomes Research and Functional Genomics and Translational Biology Interdisciplinary Working Groups; and Council on Epidemiology and Prevention. Circulation 2006;113:1807–1816.

6 Bowles NE, Bowles KR, Towbin JA: The 'final common pathway' hypothesis and inherited cardiovascular disease. The role of cytoskeletal proteins in dilated cardiomyopathy. Herz 2000;25:168–175.

7 Ellinor PT, MacRae CA, Thierfelder L: Arrhythmogenic right ventricular cardiomyopathy. Heart Fail Clin 2010;6: 161–177.

8 Sen-Chowdhry S, Syrris P, McKenna WJ: Genetics of restrictive cardiomyopathy. Heart Fail Clin 2010;6:179–186.

9 Towbin JA, Lowe AM, Colan SD, Sleeper LA, Orav EJ, Clunie S, Messere J, Cox GF, Lurie P, Hsu D, Canter C, Wilkinson JD, Lipshultz SE: Incidence, causes and outcomes of dilated cardiomyopathy in children. JAMA 2006;296:1867–1876.

10 Fatkin D; members of the CSANZ Cardiac Genetic Diseases Council Writing Group: Guidelines for the diagnosis and management of familial dilated cardiomyopathy. Heart Lung Circ 2011;20: 691–693.

11 Givertz MM, Mann DL: Epidemiology and natural history of recovery of left ventricular function in recent onset dilated cardiomyopathies. Curr Heart Fail Rep 2013;10:321–330.

12 Dec GW, Fuster V: Idiopathic dilated cardiomyopathy. N Engl J Med 1994; 331:1564–1575.
13 Ackerman MJ, Priori SG, Willems S, Berul C, Brugada R, Calkins H, Camm AJ, Ellinor PT, Gollob M, Hamilton R, Hershberger RE, Judge DP, Le Marec H, McKenna WJ, Schulze-Bahr E, Semsarian C, Towbin JA, Watkins H, Wilde A, Wolpert C, et al: HRS/EHRA expert consensus statement on the state of genetic testing for the channelopathies and cardiomyopathies: this document was developed as a partnership between the Heart Rhythm Society (HRS) and the European Heart Rhythm Association (EHRA). Heart Rhythm 2011;8:1308–1339.
14 Finsterer J, Stöllberger C, Wahbi K: Cardiomyopathy in neurological disorders. Cardiovasc Pathol 2013;22:389–400.
15 Hershberger RE, Lindenfeld J, Mestroni L, Seidman CE, Taylor MR, Towbin JA; Heart Failure Society of America: Genetic evaluation of cardiomyopathy – a Heart Failure Society of America practice guideline. J Card Fail 2009;15:83–97.
16 Towbin JA, Bowles NE: The failing heart. Nature 2002;415:227–233.
17 Towbin JA, Hejtmancik JF, Brink P, et al: X-linked dilated cardiomyopathy. Molecular genetic evidence of linkage to the Duchenne muscular dystrophy gene at the Xp21 locus. Circulation 1993;87:1854–1865.
18 Muntoni F, Cau M, Ganau A, et al: Brief report: deletion of the dystrophin muscle-specific promoter region associated with X-linked dilated cardiomyopathy. N Engl J Med 1993;329:921–925.
19 Diegoli M, Grasso M, Favalli V, Serio A, Gambarin FI, Klersy C, Pasotti M, Agozzino E, Scelsi L, Ferlini A, Febo O, Piccolo G, Tavazzi L, Narula J, Arbustini E: Diagnostic work-up and risk stratification in X-linked dilated cardiomyopathies caused by dystrophin defects. J Am Coll Cardiol 2011;58:925–934.
20 Rahimov F, Kunkel LM: The cell biology of disease: cellular and molecular mechanisms underlying muscular dystrophy. J Cell Biol 2013;201:499–510.
21 Constantin B: Dystrophin complex functions as a scaffold for signalling proteins. Biochim Biophys Acta 2014;1838:635–642.
22 Chelly J, Desguerre I: Progressive muscular dystrophies. Handb Clin Neurol 2013;113:1343–1366.
23 Gumerson JD, Michele DE: The dystrophin-glycoprotein complex in the prevention of muscle damage. J Biomed Biotechnol 2011;2011:210797.
24 Morales A, Hershberger RE: Genetic evaluation of dilated cardiomyopathy. Curr Cardiol Rep 2013;15:375.
25 Mestroni L, Taylor MR: Genetics and genetic testing of dilated cardiomyopathy: a new perspective. Discov Med 2013;15:43–49.
26 Garcia-Pavia P, Syrris P, Salas C, Evans A, Mirelis JG, Cobo-Marcos M, Vilches C, Bornstein B, Segovia J, Alonso-Pulpon L, Elliott PM: Desmosomal protein gene mutations in patients with idiopathic dilated cardiomyopathy undergoing cardiac transplantation: a clinicopathological study. Heart 2011;97:1744–1752.
27 Wolf CM, Wang L, Alcalai R, Pizard A, Burgon PG, Ahmad F, Sherwood M, Branco DM, Wakimoto H, Fishman GI, See V, Stewart CL, Conner DA, Berul CI, Seidman CE, Seidman JG: Lamin A/C haploinsufficiency causes dilated cardiomyopathy and apoptosis-triggered cardiac conduction system disease. J Mol Cell Cardiol 2008;44:293–303.
28 Taylor MR, Slavov D, Ku L, Di Lenarda A, Sinagra G, Carniel E, Haubold K, Boucek MM, Ferguson D, Graw SL, Zhu X, Cavanaugh J, Sucharov CC, Long CS, Bristow MR, Lavori P, Mestroni L; Familial Cardiomyopathy Registry; BEST (Beta-Blocker Evaluation of Survival Trial) DNA Bank: Prevalence of desmin mutations in dilated cardiomyopathy. Circulation 2007;115:1244–1251.
29 Debold EP, Schmitt JP, Patlak JB, Beck SE, Moore JR, Seidman JG, Seidman C, Warshaw DM: Hypertrophic and dilated cardiomyopathy mutations differentially affect the molecular force generation of mouse alpha-cardiac myosin in the laser trap assay. Am J Physiol Heart Circ Physiol 2007;293:H284–H291.
30 Ehler E, Perriard JC: Cardiomyocyte cytoskeleton and myofibrillogenesis in healthy and diseased heart. Heart Fail Rev 2000;5:259–269.
31 Basso C, Czarnowska E, Della Barbera M, Bauce B, Beffagna G, Wlodarska EK, Pilichou K, Ramondo A, Lorenzon A, Wozniek O, Corrado D, Daliento L, Danieli GA, Valente M, Nava A, Thiene G, Rampazzo A: Ultrastructural evidence of intercalated disc remodelling in arrhythmogenic right ventricular cardiomyopathy: an electron microscopy investigation on endomyocardial biopsies. Eur Heart J 2006;27:1847–1854.
32 Yang Z, Bowles NE, Scherer SE, Taylor MD, Kearney DL, Ge S, Nadvoretskiy VV, DeFreitas G, Carabello B, Brandon LI, Godsel LM, Green KJ, Saffitz JE, Li H, Danieli GA, Calkins H, Marcus F, Towbin JA: Desmosomal dysfunction due to mutations in desmoplakin causes arrhythmogenic right ventricular dysplasia/cardiomyopathy. Circ Res 2006; 99:646–655.
33 Purevjav E, Arimura T, Augustin S, Huby AC, Takagi K, Nunoda S, Kearney DL, Taylor MD, Terasaki F, Bos JM, Ommen SR, Shibata H, Takahashi M, Itoh-Satoh M, McKenna WJ, Murphy RT, Labeit S, Yamanaka Y, Machida N, Park JE, Alexander PM, Weintraub RG, Kitaura Y, Ackerman MJ, Kimura A, Towbin JA: Molecular basis for clinical heterogeneity in inherited cardiomyopathies due to myopalladin mutations. Hum Mol Genet 2012;21:2039–2053.
34 Purevjav E, Varela J, Morgado M, Kearney DL, Li H, Taylor MD, Arimura T, Moncman CL, McKenna W, Murphy RT, Labeit S, Vatta M, Bowles NE, Kimura A, Boriek AM, Towbin JA: Nebulette mutations are associated with dilated cardiomyopathy and endocardial fibroelastosis. J Am Coll Cardiol 2010; 56:1493–1502.
35 Fatkin D, Graham RM: Molecular mechanisms of inherited cardiomyopathies. Physiol Rev 2002;82:945–980.
36 McNally EM, Golbus JR, Puckelwartz MJ: Genetic mutations and mechanisms in dilated cardiomyopathy. J Clin Invest 2013;123:19–26.
37 Olson TM, Michels VV, Thibodeau SN, Tai YS, Keating MT: Actin mutations in dilated cardiomyopathy, a heritable form of heart failure. Science 1998;280:750–752.
38 Kamisago M, Sharma SD, DePalma SR, et al: Mutations in sarcomere protein genes as a cause of dilated cardiomyopathy. N Engl J Med 2000;343:1688–1696.
39 Pyle WG, Solaro RJ: At the crossroads of myocardial signaling: the role of Z-discs in intracellular signaling and cardiac function. Circ Res 2004;94:296–305.
40 Knoll R, Hoshijima M, Hoffman HM, et al: The cardiac mechanical stretch sensor machinery involves a Z disc complex that is defective in a subset of human dilated cardiomyopathy. Cell 2002;11:943–955.
41 Vatta M, Sinagra G, Brunelli L, Faulkner G: Remodeling of dystrophin and sarcomeric Z-band occurs in pediatric cardiomyopathies: a unifying mechanism for force transmission defect. J Cardiovasc Med (Hagerstown) 2009;10:149–156.

42 Mohapatra B, Jimenez S, Lin JH, Bowles KR, Coveler KJ, Marx JG, Chrisco MA, Murphy RT, Lurie PR, Schwartz RJ, Elliott PM, Vatta M, McKenna W, Towbin JA, Bowles NE: Mutations in the muscle LIM protein and alpha-actinin-2 genes in dilated cardiomyopathy and endocardial fibroelastosis. Mol Genet Metab 2003;80:207–215.
43 Lin X, Ruiz J, Bajraktari I, Ohman R, Banerjee S, Gribble K, Kaufman JD, Wingfield PT, Griggs RC, Fischbeck KH, Mankodi A: Z-disc-associated, alternatively spliced, PDZ motif-containing protein (ZASP) mutations in the actin-binding domain cause disruption of skeletal muscle actin filaments in myofibrillar myopathy. J Biol Chem 2014;289: 13615–13626.
44 Martinelli VC, Kyle WB, Kojic S, Vitulo N, Li Z, Belgrano A, Maiuri P, Banks L, Vatta M, Valle G, Faulkner G: ZASP interacts with the mechanosensing protein Ankrd2 and p53 in the signalling network of striated muscle. PLoS One 2014;9:e92259.
45 LeWinter MM, Granzier HL: Cardiac titin and heart disease. J Cardiovasc Pharmacol 2014;63:207–212.
46 Maron BJ, Maron MS: Hypertrophic cardiomyopathy. Lancet 2013;381:242–255.
47 O'Mahony C, Elliott PM: Prevention of sudden cardiac death in hypertrophic cardiomyopathy. Heart 2014;100:254–260.
48 Marston S, Copeland O, Jacques A, Livesey K, Tsang V, McKenna WJ, Jalilzadeh S, Carballo S, Redwood C, Watkins H: Evidence from human myectomy samples that MYBPC3 mutations cause hypertrophic cardiomyopathy through haploinsufficiency. Circ Res 2009;105: 219–222.
49 Lopes LR, Zekavati A, Syrris P, Hubank M, Giambartolomei C, Dalageorgou C, Jenkins S, McKenna W; Uk10k Consortium, Plagnol V, Elliott PM: Genetic complexity in hypertrophic cardiomyopathy revealed by high-throughput sequencing. J Med Genet 2013;50:228–239.
50 Ho CY: Genetics and clinical destiny: improving care in hypertrophic cardiomyopathy. Circulation 2010;122:2430–2440.
51 Watkins H, McKenna WJ, Thierfelder L, Suk HJ, Anan R, O'Donoghue A, et al: Mutations in the genes for cardiac troponin T and α-tropomyosin in hypertrophic cardiomyopathy. N Engl J Med 1995;332:1058–1064.
52 Morita H, Rehm HL, Menesses A, McDonough B, Roberts AE, Kucherlapati R, et al: Shared genetic causes of cardiac hypertrophy in children and adults. N Engl J Med 2008;358:1899–1908.
53 Lopes LR, Rahman MS, Elliott PM: A systematic review and meta-analysis of genotype-phenotype associations in patients with hypertrophic cardiomyopathy caused by sarcomeric protein mutations. Heart 2013;99:1800–1811.
54 Watkins H, Rosenzweig T, Hwang DS, Levi T, McKenna W, Seidman CE, Seidman JG: Characteristics and prognostic implications of myosin missense mutations in familial hypertrophic cardiomyopathy. N Engl J Med 1992;326:1108–1114.
55 Moolman JC, Corfield VA, Posen B, Ngumbela K, Seidman C, Brink PA, Watkins H: Sudden death due to troponin T mutations. J Am Coll Cardiol 1997;29: 549–555.
56 Charron P, Dubourg O, Desnos M, Bennaceur M, Carrier L, Camproux AC, Isnard R, Hagege A, Langlard JM, Bonne G, Richard P, Hainque B, Bouhour JB, Schwartz K, Komajda M: Clinical features and prognostic implications of familial hypertrophic cardiomyopathy related to cardiac myosin-binding protein C gene. Circulation 1998;97:2230–2236.
57 Van Driest SL, Ackerman MJ, Ommen SR, Shakur R, Will ML, Nishimura RA, Tajik AJ, Gersh BJ: Prevalence and severity of 'benign' mutations in the β-myosin heavy chain, cardiac troponin T, and α-tropomyosin genes in hypertrophic cardiomyopathy. Circulation 2002;106:3085–3090.
58 Bos JM, Will ML, Gersh BJ, Kruisselbrink TM, Ommen SR, Ackerman MJ: Characterization of a phenotype-based genetic test prediction score for unrelated patients with hypertrophic cardiomyopathy. Mayo Clin Proc 2014;89: 727–737.
59 Bos JM, Towbin JA, Ackerman MJ: Diagnostic, prognostic, and therapeutic implications of genetic testing for hypertrophic cardiomyopathy. J Am Coll Cardiol 2009;54:201–211.
60 Theis JL, Bos JM, Bartleson VB, et al: Echocardiographic-determined septal morphology in Z-disc hypertrophic cardiomyopathy. Biochem Biophys Res Commun 2006;351:896–902.
61 Geske JB, Bos JM, Gersh BJ, Ommen SR, Eidem BW, Ackerman MJ: Deformation patterns in genotyped patients with hypertrophic cardiomyopathy. Eur Heart J Cardiovasc Imaging 2014;15:456–465.
62 Van Driest SL, Vasile VC, Ommen SR, et al: Myosin binding protein C mutations and compound heterozygosity in hypertrophic cardiomyopathy. J Am Coll Cardiol 2004;44:1903–1910.
63 Olivotto I, Girolami F, Ackerman MJ, et al: Myofilament protein gene mutation screening and outcome of patients with hypertrophic cardiomyopathy. Mayo Clin Proc 2008;83:630–638.
64 Rivenes SM, Kearney DL, Smith EO, Towbin JA, Denfield SW: Sudden death and cardiovascular collapse in children with restrictive cardiomyopathy. Circulation 2000;102:876–882.
65 Walsh MA, Grenier MA, Jefferies JL, Towbin JA, Lorts A, Czosek RJ: Conduction abnormalities in pediatric patients with restrictive cardiomyopathy. Circ Heart Fail 2012;5:267–273.
66 Caleshu C, Sakhuja R, Nussbaum RL, Schiller NB, Ursell PC, Eng C, De Marco T, McGlothlin D, Burchard EG, Rame JE: Furthering the link between the sarcomere and primary cardiomyopathies: restrictive cardiomyopathy associated with multiple mutations in genes previously associated with hypertrophic or dilated cardiomyopathy. Am J Med Genet A 2011;155A:2229–2235.
67 Towbin JA: Left ventricular noncompaction: a new form of heart failure. Heart Fail Clin 2010;6:453–469.
68 Ichida F, Hamamichi Y, Miyawaki T, et al: Clinical features of isolated noncompaction of the ventricular myocardium: long-term clinical course, hemodynamic properties, and genetic background. J Am Coll Cardiol 1999;34:233–240.
69 Sasse-Klaassen S, Gerull B, Oechslin E, Jenni R, Thierfelder L: Isolated noncompaction of the left ventricular myocardium in the adult is an autosomal dominant disorder in the majority of patients. Am J Med Genet Part A 2003;119A:162–167.
70 Stahli BE, Gebhard C, Biaggi P, et al: Left ventricular non-compaction: prevalence in congenital heart disease. Int J Cardiol 2013;167:2477–2481.
71 Bleyl SB, Mumford BR, Brown-Harrison MC, et al: Xq28-linked noncompaction of the left ventricular myocardium: prenatal diagnosis and pathologic analysis of affected individuals. Am J Med Genet 1997;72:257–265.
72 Udeoji DU, Philip KJ, Morrissey RP, Phan A, Schwarz ER: Left ventricular noncompaction cardiomyopathy: updated review. Ther Adv Cardiovasc Dis 2013;7:260–273.
73 Ouyang P, Saarel E, Bai Y, et al: A de novo mutation in NKX2.5 associated with atrial septal defects, ventricular noncompaction, syncope and sudden death. Clin Chim Acta 2011;412:170–175.
74 Postma AV, van Engelen K, van de Meerakker J, et al: Mutations in the sarcomere gene MYH7 in Ebstein anomaly. Circ Cardiovasc Genet 2011;4:43–50.

75 Vermeer AM, van Engelen K, Postma AV, Baars MJ, Christiaans I, De Haij S, Klaassen S, Mulder BJ, Keavney B: Ebstein anomaly associated with left ventricular noncompaction: an autosomal dominant condition that can be caused by mutations in MYH7. Am J Med Genet C Semin Med Genet 2013;163C:178–184.
76 Probst S, Oechslin E, Schuler P, et al: Sarcomere gene mutations in isolated left ventricular noncompaction cardiomyopathy do not predict clinical phenotype. Circ Cardiovasc Genet 2011;4:367–374.
77 Hoedemaekers YM, Caliskan K, Michels M, et al: The importance of genetic counseling, DNA diagnostics, and cardiologic family screening in left ventricular noncompaction cardiomyopathy. Circ Cardiovasc Genet 2010;3:232–239.
78 Dellefave LM, Pytel P, Mewborn S, et al: Sarcomere mutations in cardiomyopathy with left ventricular hypertrabeculation. Circ Cardiovasc Genet 2009;2:442–449.
79 Williams T, Machann W, Kühler L, Hamm H, Müller-Höcker J, Zimmer M, Ertl G, Ritter O, Beer M, Schönberger J: Novel desmoplakin mutation: juvenile biventricular cardiomyopathy with left ventricular non-compaction and acantholytic palmoplantar keratoderma. Clin Res Cardiol 2011;100:1087–1093.
80 Tang S, Batra A, Zhang Y, Ebenroth ES, Huang T: Left ventricular noncompaction is associated with mutations in the mitochondrial genome. Mitochondrion 2010;10:350–357.
81 Digilio M, Bernardini L, Gagliardi M, et al: Syndromic non-compaction of the left ventricle: associated chromosomal anomalies. Clin Genet 2013;84:362–367.
82 Shieh JT: Implications of genetic testing in noncompaction/hypertrabeculation. Am J Med Genet C Semin Med Genet 2013;163C:206–211.
83 Protonotarios N, Tsatsopoulou A: Naxos disease and Carvajal syndrome: cardiocutaneous disorders that highlight the pathogenesis and broaden the spectrum of arrhythmogenic right ventricular cardiomyopathy. Cardiovasc Pathol 2004;13:185–194.
84 Marcus FI, McKenna WJ, Sherrill D, et al: Diagnosis of arrhythmogenic right ventricular cardiomyopathy/dysplasia: proposed modification of the task force criteria. Circulation 2010;121:1533–1541.
85 Azaouagh A, Churzidse S, Konorza T, Erbel R: Arrhythmogenic right ventricular cardiomyopathy/dysplasia: a review and update. Clin Res Cardiol 2011;100:383–394.
86 Herren T, Gerber PA, Duru F: Arrhythmogenic right ventricular cardiomyopathy/dysplasia: a not so rare 'disease of the desmosome' with multiple clinical presentations. Clin Res Cardiol 2009;98:141–158.
87 Hamid MS, Norman M, Quraishi A, Firoozi S, Thaman R, Gimeno JR, Sachdev B, Rowland E, Elliott PM, McKenna WJ: Prospective evaluation of relatives for familial arrhythmogenic right ventricular cardiomyopathy/dysplasia reveals a need to broaden diagnostic criteria. J Am Coll Cardiol 2002;40:1445–1450.
88 Te Rijdt WP, Jongbloed JD, de Boer RA, Thiene G, Basso C, van den Berg MP, van Tintelen JP: Clinical utility gene card for: arrhythmogenic right ventricular cardiomyopathy (ARVC). Eur J Hum Genet 2014;22.
89 Xu T, Yang Z, Vatta M, Rampazzo A, Beffagna G, Pilichou K, Scherer SE, Saffitz J, Kravitz J, Zareba W, et al: Compound and digenic heterozygosity contributes to arrhythmogenic right ventricular cardiomyopathy. J Am Coll Cardiol 2010;55:587–597.
90 Bauce B, Nava A, Beffagna G, Basso C, Lorenzon A, Smaniotto G, De Bortoli M, Rigato I, Mazzotti E, Steriotis A, Marra MP, Towbin JA, Thiene G, Danieli GA, Rampazzo A: Multiple mutations in desmosomal proteins encoding genes in arrhythmogenic right ventricular cardiomyopathy/dysplasia. Heart Rhythm 2010;7:22–29.
91 Vatta M, Marcus F, Towbin JA: Arrhythmogenic right ventricular cardiomyopathy: a 'final common pathway' that defines clinical phenotype. Eur Heart J 2007;28:529–530.
92 Patel DM, Green KJ: Desmosomes in the heart: a review of clinical and mechanistic analyses. Cell Commun Adhes 2014;21:109–128.
93 Delmar M, McKenna WJ: The cardiac desmosome and arrhythmogenic cardiomyopathies: from gene to disease. Circ Res 2010;107:700–714.
94 Noorman M, Hakim S, Kessler E, Groeneweg JA, Cox MG, Asimaki A, van Rijen HV, van Stuijvenberg L, Chkourko H, van der Heyden MA, et al: Remodeling of the cardiac sodium channel, connexin43, and plakoglobin at the intercalated disk in patients with arrhythmogenic cardiomyopathy. Heart Rhythm 2013;10:412–419.
95 Towbin JA, Lorts A: Arrhythmias and dilated cardiomyopathy: common pathogenetic pathways? J Am Coll Cardiol 2011;57:2169–2171.

Prof. Jeffrey A. Towbin
University of Tennessee Health Science Center
St. Jude Children's Research Hospital, and Le Bonheur Children's Hospital
50 N. Dunlap Street, 3rd Floor
Memphis, TN 38103 (USA)
E-Mail jtowbin1@uthsc.edu

Muenke M, Kruszka PS, Sable CA, Belmont JW (eds): Congenital Heart Disease: Molecular Genetics, Principles of Diagnosis and Treatment. Basel, Karger, 2015, pp 226–235
DOI: 10.1159/000375219

Congenital Thoracic Aortic Aneurysm

Mark E. Lindsay[a] · Harry C. Dietz[b, c]

[a]Departments of Medicine and Pediatrics, Thoracic Aortic Center, Massachusetts General Hospital, Harvard Medical School, Boston, Mass., and [b]McKusick-Nathans Institute of Genetic Medicine, Departments of Pediatrics, Medicine, and Molecular Biology and Genetics, Johns Hopkins University School of Medicine, and [c]Howard Hughes Medical Institute, Baltimore, Md., USA

Abstract

Inherited forms of thoracic aortic aneurysm (TAA) can generally be grouped into those with extra-aortic manifestations (syndromic) and those without (nonsyndromic). Syndromic conditions generally include many disorders historically classified as 'connective tissue disorders' such as the Marfan syndrome and Loeys-Dietz syndrome. Nonsyndromic familial TAA demonstrates similar patterns of inheritance and cardiovascular manifestations, but patients lack external findings on physical examination that can alert the clinician to underlying aortic enlargement. Diagnostic algorithms incorporate anthropomorphic phenotyping, cardiovascular imaging, and molecular genetic testing. Proper treatment requires accurate genetic evaluation, as medical and surgical decision-making is increasingly genotype driven. Optimal medical care requires a team of physicians and surgeons familiar with this unique group of individuals.

Aortic aneurysm is a common cardiovascular condition defined by dilation of the lumen of the aorta (fig. 1). Aortic dilation produces a risk of tear or 'dissection' commensurate with the degree of enlargement. Aortic aneurysm is generally asymptomatic and therefore its true incidence is unknown, but the incidence of the clinically evident aortic dissection has been estimated to be 1 in 100,000 patient years [1]. Aortic dissection is life threatening primarily through arterial obstruction that accompanies the tear. Depending on the anatomic segment affected, this can result in compromise of blood flow to the heart, brain, limbs, or mesentery. Less commonly, an aortic tear can span from the lumen to the extravascular space and result in internal hemorrhage within the thorax or abdomen. Abdominal aortic aneurysm (AAA), the most common aortic disease in humans, is associated with both genetic and environmental risk factors closely correlated with those causing myocardial infarction, such as hypertension, atherosclerosis, and diabetes [1, 2]. In contrast, thoracic aortic aneurysm (TAA) is more commonly related to dysfunction of a single gene demonstrating Mendelian inheritance, sometimes as an aspect of a named syndrome.

Thoracic aortic dissection typically presents in adulthood with an average age in the mid-7th decade

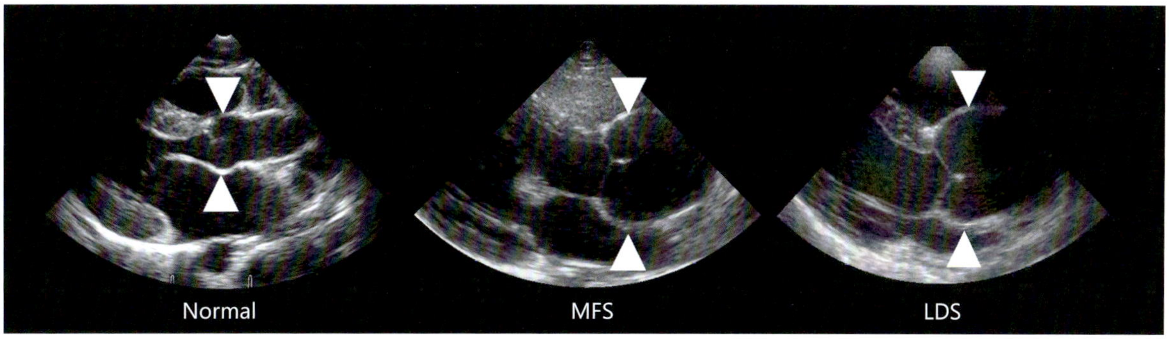

Fig. 1. Parasternal long-axis echocardiographic stills of a normal aorta, a patient with MFS, and a patient with LDS. Arrowheads indicate the aortic sinuses of valsalva.

[3]. Most of these cases are sporadic in nature (80–90%), without known family history of aortic disease. However, a sizable fraction of thoracic aortic dissection cases represents complications of familial TAA syndromes. In the International Registry of Aortic Dissection, up to 15% of patients cite a family history of aortic disease, with clear syndromic association in up to 5% [4]. As more patients with TAA have been prospectively identified at younger ages, it has become increasingly clear that TAA is a phenotype that begins in childhood with continued progression into adulthood and, when unrecognized, results in catastrophic consequences. Aortic dissection is only very rarely a clinical concern during childhood or young adulthood, and then only in severe cases of genetically triggered disease [5]. In light of these observations, many presentations of TAA should be considered a congenital cardiovascular predisposition and understood in the same context as other, more easily identifiable structural cardiovascular lesions.

Gene Discovery

Genetic investigation over the last several decades has uncovered the basis of multiple TAA syndromes. In 1991, mutations in the gene *FBN1* were described as the cause of the most commonly recognized genetic syndrome associated with TAA, the Marfan syndrome (MFS) [6]. *FBN1* encodes the protein fibrillin-1, the major component of extracellular microfibrils. Subsequent experiments in animal models of MFS, with now confirmatory findings in humans, have elucidated the importance of the TGF-β signaling pathway in the multisystem pathogenesis of MFS [7–10]. Unexpectedly for an extracellular polymeric protein, fibrillin-1 was discovered to physically interact with and play an active role in modulating TGF-β bioavailability and signaling. The central role of this pathway in TAA pathogenesis was confirmed with the implication of mutations in the genes encoding the receptor subunits for TGF-β (*TGFBR1* and *TGFBR2*) in the Marfan-related disorder, Loeys-Dietz syndrome (LDS). Since the initial description of this condition, two other genes have been implicated as causal in LDS. Mutations in the *SMAD3* gene, encoding the intracellular effector of TGF-β signaling, were demonstrated to cause aneurysms in the proximal aorta and other vascular segments in association with typical craniofacial, skeletal, and cutaneous manifestations of LDS, with the added feature of strong predisposition for osteoarthritis [11], an entity referred to as aneurysm-osteoarthritis syndrome or LDS type 3 [12]. More recently, loss of function mutations in the *TGFB2* gene, encoding one of the three TGF-β isoforms (TGF-β_2), were shown to cause a syndromic presentation of aneurysm with substantial overlap with typical LDS, referred to as LDS type 4 [13, 14]. An additional disorder with significant phenotypic overlap with LDS is a rare condition, the Shprintzen-Goldberg syndrome (SGS). SGS phenocopies virtually all of the craniofacial, skeletal cutaneous, and

5

Table 1. Human aneurysm genes

Gene (protein)	Human syndrome
Extracellular matrix proteins	
COL3A1 (collagen 3 α_1) [24]	vEDS
EFEMP2 (fibulin-4) [25]	Cutis laxa with aneurysm
TGF-β pathway	
FBN1 (fibrillin-1) [6]	MFS
TGFBR1 (tgfbr1) [33, 45]	LDS type 1; iFTAAD
TGFBR2 (tgfbr2) [33, 45, 46]	LDS type 2; iFTAAD
TGFB2 (tgfb2) [13, 14]	LDS type 4; iFTAAD
SMAD3 (SMAD family member 3) [47, 48]	Aneurysm-osteoarthritis syndrome; LDS type 3; iFTAAD
SKI (v-SKI sarcoma oncogene homolog) [15]	SGS
Cytoskeletal/smooth muscle Contraction apparatus proteins	
ACTA2 (α-SMA) [19]	iFTAAD with livedo reticularis and iris flocculi
MYH11 (smooth muscle myosin) [17, 18]	iFTAAD with patent ductus arteriosus
FLNA (filamin A) [49]	Periventricular nodular heterotopia with Ehlers-Danlos features
MYLK (myosin light chain kinase) [20]	iFTAAD
PRKG1 (protein kinase, cGMP dependent, type I) [21]	iFTAAD
RAS-related disorder	
NF1 (neurofibromin 1) [28]	Neurofibromatosis
PTPN11 (SH2 domain-containing protein tyrosine phosphatase-2) [26, 50]	Noonan syndrome and the LEOPARD syndrome
Miscellaneous	
SLC2A10 (glucose transporter 10) [29]	Arterial tortuosity syndrome
NOTCH1 (notch1) [22]	BAV-AscAA
45,X0 [30]	Turner syndrome

cardiovascular manifestations of LDS and MFS, with the added feature of highly penetrant cognitive disability. Vascular disease in SGS tends to be restricted to the aortic root, and is both less penetrant and less severe than in either LDS or MFS. Mutations in the *SKI* gene, encoding a repressor of TGF-β signaling, were recently shown to account for a majority of cases (table 1) [15, 16].

A second group of genes with a related functional theme has been described as causal in in isolated familial TAA and thoracic aortic dissection (iFTAAD). Mutations in several genes that encode components of the smooth muscle contractile apparatus have now been shown to cause iFTAAD. Patients do not show external connective tissue phenotypes and patients are not typically recognized as syndromic, although manifestations of systemic smooth muscle dysfunction such as livedo reticularis or mydriasis with iris flocculi can be observed. Extra-aortic manifestations, when they exist, are often subtle or nonspecific for aortic disease. Some presentations of iFTAAD can be associated with a more widespread vasculopathy, rarely including a predisposition for coronary artery disease and obstructive lesions of the cerebral vasculature (Moyamoya disease) in some families. The first gene described within this group was *MYH11* [17, 18]. *MYH11* encodes smooth muscle-specific myosin heavy chain (also known as myosin heavy chain 11) that is expressed at high levels in definitive vascular, urinary, and enteric smooth muscle cells. Patients with mutations in *MHY11* demonstrate iFTAAD and a high penetrance of patent ductus arteriosus. Investigation of a large family with iFTAAD and livedo reticularis next implicated the *ACTA2* gene encoding the binding partner of smooth muscle-specific myosin heavy chain [19]. *ACTA2* encodes α-smooth muscle actin (SMA). In smooth muscle cells, actin-myosin interaction is regulated by phosphorylation of the regulatory myosin subunit by myosin light chain kinase. Based on findings of mutations in *ACTA2* and *MYH11* in familial TAA, this positive regulator of actin-myosin interaction, encoded by the gene *MYLK*, was investigated by candidate analysis and found to be a rare cause of iFTAAD [20]. Analysis of identified mutations confirmed a decrement in kinase activity consistent with a loss-of-function mechanism. Most recently, using exome sequencing of probands, a recurrent mutation (p.Arg^{177}Gln) in the gene *PRKG1* was identified in four autosomal dominant families presenting with iFTAAD [21]. This mutation appears to induce constitutive activity of the type I cGMP-dependent protein kinase (PKG-1), a described negative regulator of myosin light chain kinase activity. Therefore, loss-of-function mutations in *MYLK* and the gain-of-function mutation in *PRKG1* are mechanistically consistent with the findings of *ACTA2* and *MYH11* alterations and clearly implicate decreased vascular smooth muscle cell actin-myosin interaction as a predisposing biochemical activity for iFTAAD.

TAA has been reported as an aspect of many additional genetic conditions. Bicuspid aortic valve (BAV) is the most common congenital heart defect, occurring in 1–2% of the general population with strong male predominance. A sizeable percentage of people with BAV show the predisposition for TAA, most typically with predominant involvement of the ascending aortic segment just distal to the aortic root. Importantly, BAV with ascending aortic aneurysm (AscAA) can segregate in families as an autosomal dominant trait with incomplete penetrance and variable expressivity. Family members of individuals with BAV-AscAA often show AscAA without the accompanying BAV, mandating follow-up of family members irrespective of the status of their aortic valve. While a tiny fraction of people with BAV and/or BAV-AscAA have mutations in *NOTCH1*, the gene encoding the receptor for Jagged ligands, this most often occurs in association with early and aggressive calcification of the aortic valve and/or other congenital heart lesions [22, 23]. The connective tissue disorder, vascular Ehlers-Danlos syndrome (vEDS), has some phenotypic overlap with LDS, particularly in the skin, but is caused by mutations in *COL3A1* encoding type III collagen [24]. TAA is actually uncommon in vEDS, and dissection of any large- to medium-sized arteries typically occurs in this condition without precedent aneurysmal dilation. Impaired collagen and elastin homeostasis is an important component of autosomal recessive cutis laxa, a disorder of the skin and vascular tissue caused by mutations in *EFEMP2* [25]. TAA has been reported in Noonan syndrome [26], in patients with 22q11 contiguous gene deletion [27], and neurofibromatosis type 1 *(NF1)* [28], albeit infrequently. TAA can be seen in the autosomal recessive arterial tortuosity syndrome caused by loss-of-function mutations in *SLC2A10*, although segmental tortuosity and stenoses are more common manifestations [29]. Finally, TAA is a notable aspect of the Turner syndrome, often accompanied by BAV [30].

Inheritance and Genetic Counseling

TAA is a highly heritable medical condition. Pedigree analyses in families with aneurysm and/or dissections have noted a 20% chance of having an affected first-degree relative [31]. This may represent an underestimate, as the identification of a familial aneurysm condition often occurs after the first aortic dissection within an affected family. Taken in this light, the presence of ascending TAA should be considered a result of an inherited condition, especially in young individuals without identified risk factors for atherosclerosis-induced acquired aneurysms, such as hypertension, smoking, diabetes, and hypercholesterolemia. Diagnosis should prompt radiologic screening in all first-degree relatives at the time of diagnosis and thorough genetic evaluation of all at-risk family members. Appreciation of the strong genetic contribution to TAA is now reflected in the official recommendations for the management of TAA, which mandates screening of first-degree relatives [32].

5

In general, genetic conditions causing thoracic aortic disease have been discovered to represent autosomal dominant conditions with varying degrees of expressivity [33, 34]. When inherited, penetrance of TAA is variable between conditions, from near 100% in MFS [35], to approximately 90% in LDS [33], to 50% or less in iFTAAD or BAV-AscAA. In conditions such as MFS or LDS, the identification of causal mutations by molecular genetic testing is common, allowing straightforward genetic counseling. Molecular testing is less effective in iFTAAD, with identification of causal mutations occurring in less than 10% of cases. Reproductive counseling in these conditions often involves both the risk of transmission to the offspring as well as the cardiovascular risk of pregnancy to an affected mother, a risk that can be significant. For patients with identified genetic mutations, prenatal or preimplantation genetic diagnosis can be applied to prevent recurrence. For these reasons, preconception planning and pregnancy in TAA families should optimally involve a team consisting of maternal cardiology and medical genetic specialists, and a high-risk obstetrician.

Clinical Findings and Diagnoses

Connective tissue disorders were initially organized into a coherent group through the recognition of repetitive external phenotypes [36]. These phenotypes were generally explained as representations of structural failure of the connective tissue in a regional manner dictated by the expression pattern and functional importance of the specific connective tissue protein under consideration. Commonly involved tissues include the skeleton, eye, skin, integument, and vasculature. MFS, the archetype of connective tissue disorders associated with ascending aortic enlargement, offers an instructive example. Over time, delineation of the full phenotype has discovered dysfunction in almost every tissue examined. In the ocular system, multiple levels of dysfunction are noted, including eye lens dislocation, myopia caused by increased globe length, early cataract formation, glaucoma, and retinal disease with a high risk of detachment or tear. In the musculoskeletal system, bone overgrowth causes the characteristic dolichostenomelia, arachnodactyly of fingers and toes, and rib overgrowth resulting in sternal deformity such as pectus carinatum or excavatum. Joint laxity is a common finding. Scoliosis is common, representing a combined dysfunction of muscle, bone, and sinew. Skeletal muscle hypoplasia and myopathy has emerged as a source of morbidity, particularly in severely affected young children and in more typical presentations with advancing age. Clinical manifestations of musculoskeletal dysfunction often include pain from both primary joint dysfunction as well as early osteoarthritis due to enhanced wear and tear of unstable joints. Hip pain can result from improper articulation due to a deep hip socket (protrusio acetabulae), and peripheral neuromuscular impairment can result from expansion of the dural sac (dural ectasia) with consequent nerve impingement. Cardiovascular manifestations include the highly penetrant finding of aortic root aneurysm and dissection, but also valvular and consequent myocardial dysfunction as a result of myxomatous degeneration of the mitral valve and/or progressive aortic valve regurgitation due to stretching of the annulus by an expanding root aneurysm. Aneurysms and primary dissections can less commonly occur in other aortic segments, prominently including the proximal descending thoracic aorta and the abdominal aorta. More widespread vascular risk has become clinically apparent as proximal aortic surgery has extended the lifespan of MFS patients.

Early diagnostic algorithms for MFS emphasized external clinical features with the requirement for involvement in disparate body systems. Recently, the criteria for the diagnosis of MFS have been revised to emphasize the central role of the aorta in clinical care and patient outcomes as well as to accommodate the role of molecular testing in routine diagnosis. The revised Ghent criteria published in 2010 (table 2) recognize aortic enlargement as the defining clinical feature of the MFS phenotype. As a result, it is now necessary to demonstrate either a personal or family history of aortic disease to MFS diagnosis. Mutations in *FBN1* can contribute strongly to the diagnosis, particularly when a specific mutation has previously been associated with MFS, in-

Table 2. Revised Ghent criteria for the diagnosis of MFS

In the absence of a family history	
Aortic root (Z score ≥2) and ectopia lentis	
Aortic root (Z score ≥2) and qualifying mutation in *FBN1* gene	
Aortic root (Z score ≥2) and systemic score (≥7 points)	
Ectopia lentis and qualifying mutation in *FBN1* gene previously described to cause aortic disease	
In the presence of a family history	
Ectopia lentis and family history of MFS	
Systemic score (≥7 points) and family history of MFS	
Aortic root (Z score ≥2 above 20 years and ≥3 below 20 years) and family history of MFS	
Systemic score	
phenotypic features	points
Wrist and thumb sign	3
Wrist or thumb sign	1
Pectus carinatum	2
Pectus excavatum or chest asymmetry	1
Hindfoot deformity	2
Plain flat foot (pes planus)	1
Pneumothorax	2
Dural ectasia	2
Protrusio acetabulae	2
Reduced upper segment/lower segment and increased arm span/height ratios	1
Scoliosis or thoracolumbar kyphosis	1
Reduced elbow extension	1
3/5 facial features	1
Skin striae	1
Myopia	1
Mitral valve prolapse	1

To be used only without distinguishing features of SGS, LDS, or vEDS [adapted directly from Loeys et al. [35]].

cluding the predisposition for aortic root aneurysm, but are neither necessary nor sufficient to make the diagnosis.

An important clinical challenge is to differentiate MFS from the closely related condition LDS. Discriminating features of LDS can be overt or subtle, but commonly include findings in the craniofacial (e.g. craniosynostosis, hypertelorism, cleft palate and/or bifid uvula), skeletal (e.g. cervical spine malformation and/or instability, or clubfoot), ocular (e.g. exotropia and lack of ectopia lentis), cutaneous (e.g. translucent skin or easy bruising, dystrophic scars), and immunologic systems (allergy, e.g. food allergy, eczema, eosinophilic esophagitis, or inflammatory bowel disease). Most importantly, all etiologies of LDS (mutations in *TGFBR1*, *TGFBR2*, *SMAD3*, and *TGFB2*) have been associated with a strong predisposition for widespread and aggressive vascular disease, including arterial tortuosity (most prominently of the head and neck vessels) and aneurysms throughout the entire arterial tree, commonly including the aortic root, the more distal ascending aorta, the descending thoracic and abdominal aorta, the proximal subclavian, carotid, vertebral, and iliac arteries, and the base of the superior mesenteric and celiac arteries. Aortic root aneurysms tend to tear or rupture at smaller dimensions and younger ages when compared to all other etiologies. Taken together, these findings highlight the importance of diagnostic accuracy in the development of an individualized management plan. Discrimination between MFS and LDS is typically accomplished using a combination of careful clinical assessment and molecular testing (table 3).

The clinical presentation of smooth muscle contraction vasculopathies is distinguishable from the more commonly appreciated connective tissue disorders. Described patients primarily exhibit isolated aortic disease without skeletal or ocular involvement prompting the classification as 'iFTAAD'. Mutations in the gene encoding α-SMA *(ACTA2)* are the most common cause of iFTAAD yet described and thought to occur in 15–20% of classic pedigrees [19]. In addition to TAA, patients with *ACTA2* mutations exhibit an increased rate of nonaortic vascular disease, including stroke, myocardial infarction, and a variant of the Moyamoya neurovascular malformation [37]. Deletions or premature termination codons causing nonsense-mediated mRNA decay have yet to be described within the *ACTA2* spectrum, perhaps indicating that protein expression and a trans-dominant mechanism of action is required for disease expression. This type of mechanism has been invoked in one particularly severe presentation of *ACTA2*-associated disease, the p.Arg^{179}His mutation. This recurrent mutation in heterozygosity has been reported to cause a severe syndrome of multi-

5

Table 3. Discriminating between MFS and LDS

Phenotypic features	MFS	LDS		
	FBN1	*TGFBR1/2*	*SMAD3*	*TGFB2*
Discriminating features of MFS				
Ectopia lentis	+++	–	–	–
Discriminating features of LDS				
Cleft palate/bifid uvula	–	++	+	+
Hypertelorism	–	++	+	+
Clubfoot	–	+	+	++
Arterial tortuosity	–	++	++	++
BAV	–	+	+	+
Shared features				
Tall stature	+++	+	+	+
Chest wall deformity	++	++	++	++
Osteoarthritis	++	+	+++	+
Aortic root aneurysm	+	+	+	+
Other aneurysm	+	++	++	+
Skin striae	++	+	+	+
Hernia	+	+	+	++
Dural ectasia	+	+	+	+

– = Absent or at population frequency; + = observed; ++ = common; +++ = typical. Adapted from Lindsay et al. [13].

system smooth muscle dysfunction, in essence a smooth muscle dystrophy [38]. Characteristics include vascular disease, including aortic aneurysm and patent ductus arteriosus, pulmonary hypertension, and cerebrovascular disease within the Moyamoya spectrum, including tapering of the terminal internal carotid arteries and cerebrovascular vessel malformation. Visceral and renal involvement includes impaired gastrointestinal motility, hydronephrosis, and hypotonic bladder. Short-bowel syndrome and intestinal malrotation were also observed. In the ocular system, congenital mydriasis is completely penetrant.

In contrast to *ACTA2* patients, mutations in *MYH11* have not been described to cause features outside of the cardiovascular system. Instead, the disease is entirely cardiovascular with a combination of TAA and an increased rate of patent ductus arteriosus [18]. Similarly, external features of connective tissue disease were not reported in patients with mutations in *MYLK* [20] and *PRKG1* [21], making the prospective identification of affected patients, prior to an aortic dissection, an important clinical challenge.

Management and Molecular Pathogenesis

The primary goal of clinical management of patients with aortic enlargement is to prevent aortic dissection. Except in rare instances, simple aortic enlargement is neither painful nor harmful to the patient, but is useful as a proxy to estimate the risk of aortic dissection. Management strategies in general use a two-tiered approach with initial medical management as the first-line therapy for ascending aortic enlargement.

Antihypertensive agents have been recommended therapy in aortic aneurysm from diverse etiologies based largely on a hemodynamic rationale. As the aorta enlarges, radial wall stress increases causing a vicious cycle of dilation leading to increased stress and increased dilation. Additionally, the aorta undergoes both lateral and radial strain during the cardiac cycle, with the diseased aorta inducing a loss of distensibility and further hemodynamic derangement. Therefore, strategies have been focused on decreasing arterial pressure as a means to decrease hemodynamic stress on the aortic wall. According to this rationale, any intervention that effectively decreases blood pressure should be equally efficacious in controlling aneurysm growth. β-Blockade has been the 'standard of care' in the treatment of MFS aortic disease since the first – and still largest – randomized, open-label trial of any medication in 1994 [39]. The rationale for the use of β-blockers in this trial was to decrease the rate of increase in the aortic pressure wave or 'dP/dt'. Retrospective analyses also supported the use of β-blockers in children with MFS [40]. More recent experimentation has provided the rationale to treat intrinsic dysfunction of the Marfan aortic wall [9].

A dramatic change in our understanding of the pathogenesis of MFS has come with the implication of the TGF-β signaling pathway in aneurysmal disease progression. Experiments performed in an animal model of MFS initially uncovered the involvement of TGF-β signaling in the pathogenesis of pulmonary disease in MFS [8] and observed improvement of phenotypes through antagonism of TGF-β signaling. It was, therefore, reasoned that type-1 angiotensin receptor blockers (ARBs) could have clinical utility in MFS due to their well-described TGF-β signaling antagonism properties. In animals, these observations were eventually extended to myxomatous mitral valve disease [7] and finally to MFS aortic aneurysm [9]. Initial experience in humans was gathered treating a small group of children with severe MFS with the ARB losartan [41]. These promising initial results lead to the initiation of multiple randomized trials around the world to compare the activity of ARBs versus β-blockade in MFS. The results of many of these trials have not been reported, but initial experience with losartan in two trials has been positive [42, 43].

If medical management is ineffective at controlling growth of the aorta, surgical replacement of the affected portion of the aorta with synthetic graft material is effective at preventing aortic tear [44]. Surgical recommendations for prophylactic aortic surgery have been established for clinical practice and, importantly, are genotypically based due to divergent clinical behavior (see Costello chapter on Surgical Management of Marfan syndrome on p. 285). For instance, untreated patients with MFS most commonly experience a first dissection during the 4th decade [4], while patients with LDS often dissect in the 3rd decade and even earlier in childhood [33]. For MFS, most centers recommend replacement of the aortic root and ascending aorta for slowly growing aneurysms at an aortic diameter approaching 5.0 cm, while for LDS a smaller diameter (4.0 cm) has been proposed due to the aggressive nature of the vascular disease [12]. In both conditions, these thresholds should be individualized through consideration of factors such as family history and knowledge about the specific gene and mutation involved. Rapid growth of TAA in either condition is an indication for surgical treatment of the ascending aorta [32]. Genotype-specific surgical recommendations have increased the importance of proper genetic diagnosis in the care of TAA patients.

As described above, genetic conditions associated with TAA show marked discrepancy in the risk of vascular aneurysms and dissections in arterial beds outside of the aorta. Therefore, in addition to surgical recommendations, risk predictions and therefore follow-up imaging regimens are based upon proper genetic diagnosis [12]. For these reasons, genetic evaluation and identification is now a necessary and integrated component for the proper care of TAA patients.

Conclusions

The last decade has provided a wealth of information about the genetic underpinnings of thoracic aortic disease. Novel gene loci have been elucidated at an increasing pace and the study of these conditions in the laboratory has provided an intellectual basis for rationale medical therapy. Despite the excitement regarding new medical therapeutic approaches in genetically triggered TAA, prophylactic aortic surgery remains the most effective method of preventing cardiovascular death due to aortic dissection. Proper genetic diagnosis in TAA syndromes is a critical component of a team approach to identify at risk family members as well as for medical and surgical management of the individual TAA patient.

References

1 Tsai TT, Nienaber CA, Eagle KA: Acute aortic syndromes. Circulation 2005;112:3802–3813.
2 Helgadottir A, Thorleifsson G, Magnusson KP, et al: The same sequence variant on 9p21 associates with myocardial infarction, abdominal aortic aneurysm and intracranial aneurysm. Nat Genet 2008;40:217–224.
3 Hagan PG, Nienaber CA, Isselbacher EM, et al: The International Registry of Acute Aortic Dissection (IRAD): new insights into an old disease. JAMA 2000;283:897–903.
4 Januzzi JL, Marayati F, Mehta RH, et al: Comparison of aortic dissection in patients with and without Marfan's syndrome (results from the International Registry of Aortic Dissection). Am J Cardiol 2004;94:400–402.
5 Januzzi JL, Isselbacher EM, Fattori R, et al: Characterizing the young patient with aortic dissection: results from the International Registry of Aortic Dissection (IRAD). J Am Coll Cardiol 2004;43:665–669.
6 Dietz HC, Cutting GR, Pyeritz RE, et al: Marfan syndrome caused by a recurrent de novo missense mutation in the fibrillin gene. Nature 1991;352:337–339.
7 Ng CM, Cheng A, Myers LA, et al: TGF-beta-dependent pathogenesis of mitral valve prolapse in a mouse model of Marfan syndrome. J Clin Invest 2004;114:1586–1592.
8 Neptune ER, Frischmeyer PA, Arking DE, et al: Dysregulation of TGF-beta activation contributes to pathogenesis in Marfan syndrome. Nat Genet 2003;33:407–411.
9 Habashi JP, Judge DP, Holm TM, et al: Losartan, an AT1 antagonist, prevents aortic aneurysm in a mouse model of Marfan syndrome. Science 2006;312:117–121.
10 Matt P, Schoenhoff F, Habashi J, et al: Circulating transforming growth factor-beta in Marfan syndrome. Circulation 2009;120:526–532.
11 van de Laar IM, Oldenburg RA, Pals G, et al: Mutations in SMAD3 cause a syndromic form of aortic aneurysms and dissections with early-onset osteoarthritis. Nat Genet 2011;43:121–126.
12 MacCarrick G, Black JH 3rd, Bowdin S, et al: Loeys-Dietz syndrome: a primer for diagnosis and management. Genet Med 2014;16:576–587.
13 Lindsay ME, Schepers D, Bolar NA, et al: Loss-of-function mutations in TGFB2 cause a syndromic presentation of thoracic aortic aneurysm. Nat Genet 2012;44:922–927.
14 Boileau C, Guo DC, Hanna N, et al: TGFB2 mutations cause familial thoracic aortic aneurysms and dissections associated with mild systemic features of Marfan syndrome. Nat Genet 2012;44:916–921.
15 Doyle AJ, Doyle JJ, Bessling SL, et al: Mutations in the TGF-β repressor SKI cause Shprintzen-Goldberg syndrome with aortic aneurysm. Nat Genet 2012;44:1249–1254.
16 Carmignac V, Thevenon J, Adès L, et al: In-frame mutations in exon 1 of SKI cause dominant Shprintzen-Goldberg syndrome. Am J Hum Genet 2012;91:950–957.
17 Zhu L, Vranckx R, Khau Van Kien P, et al: Mutations in myosin heavy chain 11 cause a syndrome associating thoracic aortic aneurysm/aortic dissection and patent ductus arteriosus. Nat Genet 2006;38:343–349.
18 Pannu H, Tran-Fadulu V, Papke CL, et al: MYH11 mutations result in a distinct vascular pathology driven by insulin-like growth factor 1 and angiotensin II. Hum Mol Genet 2007;16:2453–2462.
19 Guo DC, Pannu H, Tran-Fadulu V, et al: Mutations in smooth muscle alpha-actin (ACTA2) lead to thoracic aortic aneurysms and dissections. Nat Genet 2007;39:1488–1493.
20 Wang L, Guo DC, Cao J, et al: Mutations in myosin light chain kinase cause familial aortic dissections. Am J Hum Genet 2011;87:701–707.
21 Guo DC, Regalado E, Casteel DE, et al: Recurrent gain-of-function mutation in PRKG1 causes thoracic aortic aneurysms and acute aortic dissections. Am J Hum Genet 2013;93:398–404.
22 Garg V, Muth AN, Ransom JF, et al: Mutations in NOTCH1 cause aortic valve disease. Nature 2005;437:270–274.
23 Kent KC, Crenshaw ML, Goh DL, Dietz HC: Genotype-phenotype correlation in patients with bicuspid aortic valve and aneurysm. J Thorac Cardiovasc Surg 2013;146:158–165.e1.
24 Superti-Furga A, Gugler E, Gitzelmann R, Steinmann B: Ehlers-Danlos syndrome type IV: a multi-exon deletion in one of the two COL3A1 alleles affecting structure, stability, and processing of type III procollagen. J Biol Chem 1988;263:6226–6232.
25 Dasouki M, Markova D, Garola R, et al: Compound heterozygous mutations in fibulin-4 causing neonatal lethal pulmonary artery occlusion, aortic aneurysm, arachnodactyly, and mild cutis laxa. Am J Med Genet A 2007;143A:2635–2641.
26 Purnell R, Williams I, Von Oppell U, Wood A: Giant aneurysms of the sinuses of Valsalva and aortic regurgitation in a patient with Noonan's syndrome. Eur J Cardiothorac Surg 2005;28:346–348.
27 John AS, McDonald-McGinn DM, Zackai EH, Goldmuntz E: Aortic root dilation in patients with 22q11.2 deletion syndrome. Am J Med Genet A 2009;149A:939–942.
28 Friedman JM, Arbiser J, Epstein JA, et al: Cardiovascular disease in neurofibromatosis 1: report of the NF1 Cardiovascular Task Force. Genet Med 2002;4:105–111.
29 Coucke PJ, Willaert A, Wessels MW, et al: Mutations in the facilitative glucose transporter GLUT10 alter angiogenesis and cause arterial tortuosity syndrome. Nat Genet 2006;38:452–457.
30 Lopez L, Arheart KL, Colan SD, et al: Turner syndrome is an independent risk factor for aortic dilation in the young. Pediatrics 2008;121:e1622–e1627.
31 Albornoz G, Coady MA, Roberts M, et al: Familial thoracic aortic aneurysms and dissections – incidence, modes of inheritance, and phenotypic patterns. Ann Thorac Surg 2006;82:1400–1405.
32 Hiratzka LF, Bakris GL, Beckman JA, et al: 2010 ACCF/AHA/AATS/ACR/ASA/SCA/SCAI/SIR/STS/SVM Guidelines for the diagnosis and management of patients with thoracic aortic disease. A Report of the American College of Cardiology Foundation/American Heart Association Task Force on Practice Guidelines, American Association for Thoracic Surgery, American College of Radiology, American Stroke Association, Society of Cardiovascular Anesthesiologists, Society for Cardiovascular Angiography and Interventions, Society of Interventional Radiology, Society of Thoracic Surgeons, and Society for Vascular Medicine. J Am Coll Cardiol 2010;55:e27–e129.
33 Loeys BL, Schwarze U, Holm T, et al: Aneurysm syndromes caused by mutations in the TGF-beta receptor. N Engl J Med 2006;355:788–798.
34 Lindsay ME, Dietz HC: Lessons on the pathogenesis of aneurysm from heritable conditions. Nature 2011;473:308–316.
35 Loeys BL, Dietz HC, Braverman AC, et al: The revised Ghent nosology for the Marfan syndrome. J Med Genet 2010;47:476–485.

36 McKusick V: Heritable Disorders of Connective Tissue. St. Louis, Mosby, 1973.
37 Guo DC, Papke CL, Tran-Fadulu V, et al: Mutations in smooth muscle alpha-actin (ACTA2) cause coronary artery disease, stroke, and Moyamoya disease, along with thoracic aortic disease. Am J Hum Genet 2009;84:617–627.
38 Milewicz DM, Østergaard JR, Ala-Kokko LM, et al: De novo ACTA2 mutation causes a novel syndrome of multisystemic smooth muscle dysfunction. Am J Med Genet A 2010; 152A:2437–2443.
39 Shores J, Berger KR, Murphy EA, Pyeritz RE: Progression of aortic dilatation and the benefit of long-term beta-adrenergic blockade in Marfan's syndrome. N Engl J Med 1994;330:1335–1341.
40 Ladouceur M, Fermanian C, Lupoglazoff JM, et al: Effect of beta-blockade on ascending aortic dilatation in children with the Marfan syndrome. Am J Cardiol 2007;99:406–409.
41 Brooke BS, Habashi JP, Judge DP, et al: Angiotensin II blockade and aortic-root dilation in Marfan's syndrome. N Engl J Med 2008;358:2787–2795.
42 Chiu HH, Wu MH, Wang JK, et al: Losartan added to beta-blockade therapy for aortic root dilation in Marfan syndrome: a randomized, open-label pilot study. Mayo Clin Proc 2013;88:271–276.
43 Groenink M, den Hartog AW, Franken R, et al: Losartan reduces aortic dilatation rate in adults with Marfan syndrome: a randomized controlled trial. Eur Heart J 2013;34:3491–3500.
44 Gott VL, Cameron DE, Alejo DE, et al: Aortic root replacement in 271 Marfan patients: a 24-year experience. Ann Thorac Surg 2002;73:438–443.
45 Loeys BL, Chen J, Neptune ER, et al: A syndrome of altered cardiovascular, craniofacial, neurocognitive and skeletal development caused by mutations in TGFBR1 or TGFBR2. Nat Genet 2005; 37:275–281.
46 Mizuguchi T, Collod-Beroud G, Akiyama T, et al: Heterozygous TGFBR2 mutations in Marfan syndrome. Nat Genet 2004;36:855–860.
47 van de Laar IM, Oldenburg RA, Pals G, et al: Mutations in SMAD3 cause a syndromic form of aortic aneurysms and dissections with early-onset osteoarthritis. Nat Genet 2010;43:121–126.
48 Regalado ES, Guo DC, Villamizar C, et al: Exome sequencing identifies SMAD3 mutations as a cause of familial thoracic aortic aneurysm and dissection with intracranial and other arterial aneurysms. Circ Res 2011;109:680–686.
49 Sheen VL, Jansen A, Chen MH, et al: Filamin A mutations cause periventricular heterotopia with Ehlers-Danlos syndrome. Neurology 2005;64:254–262.
50 Iwasaki Y, Horigome H, Takahashi-Igari M, et al: Coronary artery dilatation in LEOPARD syndrome. A child case and literature review. Congenit Heart Dis 2009;4:38–41.

Dr. Mark E. Lindsay
Massachusetts General Hospital, Harvard Medical School
Richard B. Simches Research Building, Room 3224
185 Cambridge Street, Boston, MA 02114 (USA)
E-Mail Lindsay.Mark@mgh.harvard.edu

6 Evaluation

Muenke M, Kruszka PS, Sable CA, Belmont JW (eds): Congenital Heart Disease: Molecular Genetics, Principles of Diagnosis and Treatment. Basel, Karger, 2015, pp 238–256
DOI: 10.1159/000375221

The Genetic Workup for Congenital Structural Heart Disease: From Clinical to Genetic Evaluation

Paul S. Kruszka[a] · Craig A. Sable[b] · John W. Belmont[c] · Maximilian Muenke[a]

[a]National Human Genome Research Institutes, National Institutes of Health, Bethesda, Md., [b]Division of Cardiology, Children's National Health System, Washington, D.C., and [c]Department of Molecular and Human Genetics, Children's Nutrition Research Center, Houston, Tex., USA

Abstract

Genetic testing is an important consideration in all congenital heart conditions. Given that congenital heart diseases (CHDs) are disorders of abnormal heart development, it is probable that pathogenic variants in genes that affect early embryonic differentiation and cardiac organogenesis play a large role in CHD. Over the last 50 years, evidence for genetic contributions to the etiologies of CHD has been reinforced by the discovery of CHD associations with specific chromosomal abnormalities, genomic disorders, and rare single-gene disorders. In these patients, genetic evaluation has clinical utility. Precision genetic diagnosis can guide cardiovascular monitoring protocols, allow for evaluation of developmental anomalies of other organ systems, promote early interventions such as speech and developmental therapies, and direct medical and surgical interventions. Additionally, genetic diagnosis allows cascade testing of at-risk relatives, recurrence risk information determination, and preimplantation and prenatal diagnosis if patient-specific mutations are known. Next-generation sequencing has radically changed genetic testing and has already begun to accelerate the pace of discovery of new single-gene mutations in CHD. This chapter will review an algorithm for the evaluation of CHD, the genetic testing options available to clinicians, appropriate genetic counseling of patients when giving results to the patient, and nongenetic causes of CHD to consider.

Multiple etiologies influence congenital heart disease (CHD), which will be defined as structural heart malformations present at birth, including altered gene function or dosage, and the effects of environmental or stochastic factors [1–3]. Given that CHDs are disorders of abnormal heart development, it is probable that pathogenic variants in genes that affect early embryonic differentiation and cardiac organogenesis play a large role in CHD [4]. Over the last 50 years, evidence for genetic contributions to the etiologies of CHD has been reinforced by the discovery of CHD associations with specific chromosomal abnormalities, genomic disorders, and rare single-gene disorders. In addition, epidemiological data suggest additional undiscovered genetic components based on the increased recurrence risk of CHD for couples with an affected child [5], the increased risk of CHD in the offspring of individuals with CHD [6, 7], the rare families with multigenerational occurrence of CHD, parental consanguinity associated with a 2- to 3-fold increased offspring risk of CHD [8, 9], and differences in the frequency of specific CHD among populations [10, 11]. In Scandinavia, where congenital malformations have been registered for decades and linked to population-based data sets with pedigree information, inferences about the genetic components of CHD can be made. A large Danish study evaluated 1.8 million people from 1977 to 2005, of whom 18,708 had CHD [12]. After excluding chromosomal abnormalities, 4.2% of heart defects in the population were attributed to a CHD family history. Relative risks ratios (ratio of the prevalence of the disease in relatives to the prevalence of the disease in the general population) for 1st-degree relatives varied depending on specific heart lesions, ranging from 79.1 for heterotaxy to 3.4 for ventricular septal defect. These results strongly support the role for genetic factors in CHD and provide motivation for CHD gene discovery research. It is important to note, though, that familial occurrence of CHD could be confounded with unmeasured and unknown shared environmental factors. The reduction in CHD recurrence after moving to a new city [13, 14] suggests that environmental factors do contribute to the CHD risk. With the ability to interrogate the entire genome, researchers are now able to answer some of the causes of nonsyndromic complex CHD. Complex genetic effects, in which a few or many genes contribute in aggregate, may increase the risk of CHD. Gene-environment interactions are also implied by the increased 1st-degree relative risk and risk caused by known teratogens.

It has been known for many years that chromosome abnormalities, like trisomy 21, are often accompanied by heart defects. It was very difficult, and remains so, to determine which genes were most influential in causing CHD in chromosome disorders. A new era of genetics began with the 2001 draft sequence of the human genome by the Human Genome Project (HGP) and thrust genetics and the genetic basis of CHD into the genomic era [15]. HGP created a reference map of human genes, and parallel projects have identified their orthologues in model organisms like mice and zebrafish. The comparison of human genes with model organisms has been an invaluable tool in identifying genes that influence normal cardiac development. HGP also allowed refinement of physical gene mapping techniques. Physical mapping technology evolved in the last decade supporting the development of efficient and inexpensive microarray assays for DNA copy number variants (CNVs). Subsequent studies have shown that recurrent copy number abnormalities, especially deletions, e.g. the 22q11 deletion, are a major cause of CHD. HGP has also powered such projects as HapMap, which cataloged common single nucleotide polymorphisms (SNPs) in several human populations and enabled genome-wide association studies (GWAS) for hundreds of human diseases and medical phenotypes [16]. GWAS focuses on common SNPs (present in 1–5% of the population) addressing the genetic components of common diseases contributed by multiple common variants. GWAS has had a limited impact on our understanding of CHD so far [17] and can be expected to explain only a small fraction of the heritability [18]. Using information from the HGP, linkage and positional cloning techniques have been used successfully to identify some important genes that cause CHD [19–22]. Positional cloning is ideal for the discovery of rare family-specific mutations that are seen in conditions like familial atrial septal defect, Holt-Oram syndrome and Noonan syndrome. But there are two major factors that have made it difficult to use these methods for CHD: (a) it is difficult to find large families affected with CHD (possibly because of reduced survival and reproductive fitness of affected individuals) and (b) there are a large number of genes that can cause CHD, and, therefore, it is not feasible to analyze small families together for linkage and gene identification. Genetic syndromes and familial cases only explain roughly 20% of CHD causes [12]. Over the past few years, the introduction of next-generation sequencing (NGS) technology has resulted in less expensive and faster interrogation of the human genome in the form of massive parallel sequencing, giving researchers and clinicians a new and powerful research and diagnostic tool. NGS has made an immediate impact on identifying the potential contribution of de novo mutations in CHD [23]. These new technologies are now allowing us to explore complex CHD etiologies that may be attributed to genes with decreased penetrance, mutations in noncoding regions, gene-environment interactions, and multigenic etiologies (modifier genes). Beyond the euphoria of new genomic technology, these new tools available for the workup of CHD present an enormous challenge to the researcher considering the vast amount of data generated.

Genetic evaluation has clinical utility in patients with CHD. Precision genetic diagnosis can guide cardiovascular monitoring protocols, for example echocardiography for hypertrophic cardiomyopathy in Noonan syndrome. CHD patients often have developmental anomalies of other organs and knowledge of that risk can direct clinically indicated imaging and other laboratory studies [24]. Knowledge of specific complications associated with a genetic diagnosis can govern early interventions, such as speech and developmental therapies. Prognostic information may be used to guide medical and surgical interventions, and genetic conditions may sometimes offer an explanation for unexpected adverse surgical outcomes. A genetic diagnosis allows cascade testing of at-risk relatives, which can be particularly useful in case of age-related complications. Following identification of specific causal mutations, recurrence risk information can be provided to parents of CHD children and adults with CHD. Finally, the knowledge of patient-specific mutations can enable preimplantation and prenatal diagnosis. In cases of genetic syndromes with known associated cardiac malformations, such as tetralogy of Fallot in the 22q11 deletion syndrome or coarctation of the aorta in Turner syndrome, genetic testing is straightforward. However, most CHD is sporadic and thought to involve complex inheritance (not fully penetrant, not inherited in Mendelian fashion, contribution of more than one gene in a person, and gene-environment interactions) and there are not adequate methods to characterize those genetic factors in individual patients. Between these two extremes lie disorders in which genetic testing, albeit imperfectly, can significantly contribute to patient care.

This chapter will review an algorithm for the evaluation of CHD, the genetic testing available to clinicians, appropriate genetic counseling of patients when giving results to the patient, and nongenetic causes of CHD to consider.

Genetic Testing Algorithm

This section is an algorithm to help physicians determine appropriate genetic testing of CHD and is based on expert opinion and previous reviews [3, 4, 11, 24–26]. When a patient presents with CHD, the clinician deciding a genetic workup plan should consider several factors: the specific cardiac lesion, the presence of specific extracardiac malformations, whether there is any unexplained developmental or cognitive delay, the prenatal history including exposure to known teratogens, and the family history. A three-generation pedigree is important to identify known occurrences of CHD, pregnancy losses, and unexplained infant deaths [24]. The physical examination should include detailed growth measurements, including head circumference, specialized craniofacial anthropometrics, and thorough examination for visible developmental defects (e.g. chest, abdomen, and limbs). For newborns and children, we recommend that the examination be performed by individuals with specialized training, such as neonatologists, pediatric cardiologists, or medical geneticists. Adults with CHD should have a similar evaluation. Recognizing that many adult cardiologists have limited experience with developmental anomalies, evaluation by a specialist in medical genetics may be particularly helpful. Prior to any genetic testing, the clinical evaluation should include clinically indicated imaging, such as abdominal and renal ultrasound, skeletal X-rays, and brain MRI. For some lesions, particularly left-outflow-tract abnormalities, echocardiography is warranted for 1st-degree relatives [24, 27, 28]. Previous studies have shown that there is an increased occurrence of bicuspid aortic valve (BAV) and other anomalies in close relatives. The pedigree will help to construct clinical hypotheses about possible inheritance patterns, such

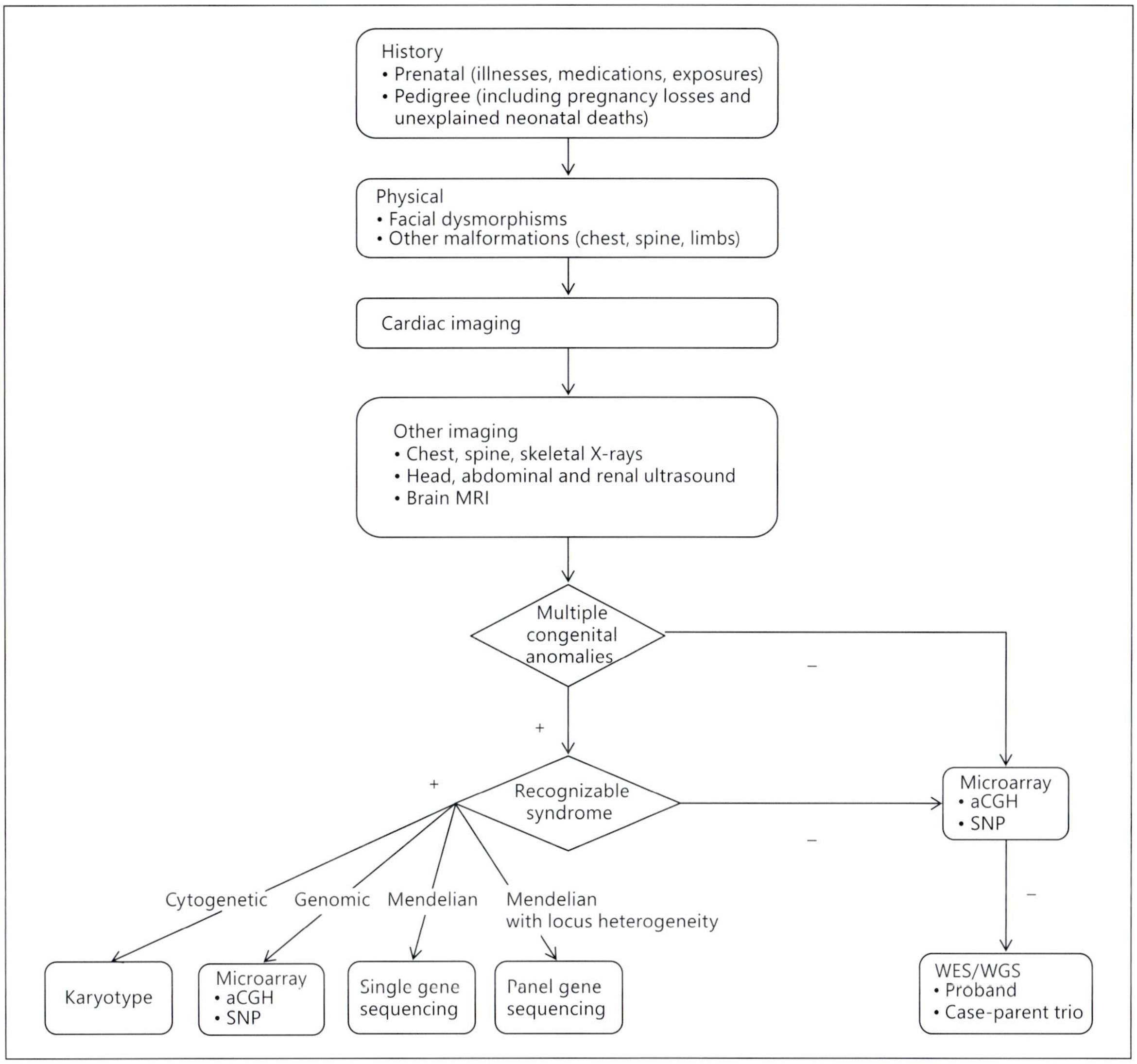

Fig. 1. Algorithm flow diagram for the genetic workup of CHD.

as autosomal dominant, autosomal recessive, X-linked, or de novo mutations. Most occurrences of CHD occur in the context of no previous family history, but this does not, by itself, preclude a genetic disorder.

Based on case-specific findings, appropriate genetic tests may be ordered. Figure 1 is an algorithm that outlines a strategy for genetic testing. This algorithm assumes that cardiac imaging will have been done (echocardiogram, cardiac MRI, or cardiac catheterization contrast study). Table 1 gives a comprehensive list of genetic diagnoses to consider organized by specific heart lesions and serves as a useful guide for developing a differential diagnosis.

In combination with the cardiac and extracardiac phenotype, the clinician will be able to divide the patient's CHD into large categories: syndromic CHD versus nonsyndromic CHD, and familial versus sporadic CHD. There is a higher yield in positive results of genetic testing for both syndromic CHD and familial CHD, adding increased attention to these groups; in a large study of over 2,000 participants with CHD, the positive yield on genetic testing in syndromic patients was 43%, in familial

Table 1. List of genetic disorders, associated genes and cardiovascular malformations (CVMs)

Syndrome	Gene	CVM
Absence of abdominal muscles with urinary tract abnormality	CHRM3	PDA
Acrocallosal syndrome	KIF7	ASD, VSD, PS
Acrofacial dysostosis, Nager type	SF3B4	TOF
Adams-Oliver syndrome	ARHGAP31, DOCK6, EOGT, RBPJ	ASD, VSD, PS, ToF
Alagille syndrome 1	JAG1	PS, ToF
α-Thalassemia/mental retardation syndrome	ATRX	VSD
Andersen cardiodysrhythmic periodic paralysis	KCNJ2	BAV, AS
Ankyloblepharon-ectodermal defects-cleft lip/palate	TP63	VSD, PDA
Antley-Bixler syndrome, Apert syndrome	FGFR2	VSD
Aortic valve disease	NOTCH1, SMAD6	AS, BAV
Aplasia cutis congenita, reticulolinear, with microcephaly	COX7B	ASD, VSD, ToF
Arterial tortuosity syndrome	SLC2A10	AS, PAS
Atrial septal defect	ACTC1, CITED2, GATA4, GATA6, NKX2-5, TBX20, TLL1	ASD, VSD
Atrioventricular septal defect AVSD2	CRELD1	AVSD
Axenfeld-Rieger syndrome	FOXC1	PDA, VSD
Baraitser-Winter syndrome	ACTB	BAV, AS, PDA
Bardet-Biedl syndrome	ARL6, BBS1, BBS2, BBS4, BBS5, BBS7, BBS9, BBS10, BBS12, CCDC28B, CEP290, LZTFL1, MKKS, MKS1, TMEM67, TRIM32, TTC21B, TTC8, WDPCP	Complex
Barth syndrome	TAZ	VSD
Basal cell nevus syndrome	PTCH1	Cardiac fibroma
Blepharophimosis-ptosis-intellectual disability syndrome	UBE3B	ASD, VSD, CoA
Bohring-Opitz syndrome	ASXL1	ASD, VSD
Brachydactyly-mental retardation syndrome	HDAC4	AS
Brittle cornea syndrome	ZNF469	MVP
C syndrome	CD96	VSD, PDA
Campomelic dysplasia	SOX9	ASD, VSD
Cantu syndrome	ABCC9	BAV
Cardiofaciocutaneous syndrome	BRAF	ASD, PS

Table 1. Continued

Syndrome	Gene	CVM
Carpenter syndrome with heterotaxy	MEGF8	Heterotaxy
Carpenter syndrome 1	RAB23	ASD, VSD, PS, ToF
Char syndrome	TFAP2B	PDA
CHARGE syndrome	CHD7	ToF, ASD, VSD, DORV, PDA, PS
Coffin-Lowry syndrome	RPS6KA3	MR
Cohen syndrome	VPS13B	MVP
Cornelia de Lange syndrome	NIPBL	ASD, VSD
Conotruncal heart malformations	CFC1, GDF1, GATA6, NKX2-5, NKX2-6, TBX1, ZFPM2	ToF, DORV, TA
Costello syndrome	HRAS	PS, MVP, VSD, ASD, hypertrophic cardiomyopathy, arrhythmias
Cranioectodermal dysplasia	IFT122, IFT43	BAV, PS
Cutis laxa, autosomal dominant	ELN	MR, AI, SVAS
Cutis laxa, autosomal recessive	FBLN5	SVAS, vascular tortuosity
Desmosterolosis	DHCR24	TAPVR
Diamond-Blackfan anemia	RPS19	VSD
DiGeorge syndrome	TBX1	VSD, ToF, DORV, IAA-B, TGA
Distal arthrogryposis, type 9	FBN2	ASD, VSD, BAV
Donnai-Barrow syndrome	LRP2	VSD
Duane-radial ray syndrome	SALL4	ASD, VSD
Ehlers-Danlos syndrome, cardiac valvular form	COL1A2	MVP, MR, AI
Ehlers-Danlos syndrome, vascular	COL3A1	MVP
Ellis-van Creveld syndrome	EVC, EVC2	Common atrium, ASD
Familial thoracic aortic aneurysm	MYH11	PDA
Fanconi anemia	FANCC, FANCA, FANCD2, RAD51C	ASD, VSD
Feingold syndrome	MYCN	PDA
Floating-Harbor syndrome	SRCAP	ASD, mesocardia, CoA, persistent left SVC
Frontonasal dysplasia	ALX3	ToF
Geleophysic dysplasia	ADAMTSL2, FBN1	AS, AI, MS, MR
Generalized arterial calcification of infancy	ABCC6, ENPP1	

Table 1. Continued

Syndrome	Gene	CVM
Genitopatellar syndrome, Ohdo syndrome	KAT6B	ASD, VSD
Hajdu-Cheney syndrome	NOTCH2	ASD, VSD, PDA
Hamamy syndrome	IRX5	AVSD, ASD, PDA
Heart-hand syndrome, Slovenian type	LMNA	Conduction
Hennekam lymphangiectasia-lymphedema syndrome	CCBE1	ASD, VSD, pericardial lymphangiectasia
Heterotaxy	ACVR2B, CCDC11, CFC1, CRELD1, FOXH1, GALNT11, GDF1, MED13L, MEGF8, NEK2, NKX2-5, NODAL, INVS, NPHP3, NPHP4, NUP188, PKD2, ROCK2, SHROOM3, TGFBR2, LZTFL1, BCL9L, ZIC3	Heterotaxy
Hirschsprung, cardiac defects and autonomic dysfunction	ECE1	PDA, VSD, ASD
Histiocytosis-lymphadenopathy plus syndrome	SLC29A3	ASD, VSD, MVP, BAV, cardiomyopathy
Holt-Oram syndrome	TBX5	ASD, VSD, HLHS, ToF, TAPVR
Hydrolethalus syndrome	HYLS1, KIF7	AVSD, VSD
Hypermethioninemia due to adenosine kinase deficiency	ADK	ASD, PS
Johanson-Blizzard syndrome	UBR1	ASD, VSD, heterotaxy
Joubert syndrome	TCTN3, TMEM237	VSD
Kabuki syndrome	KDM6A, KMT2D	ASD, VSD, CoA
Keutel syndrome	MGP	VSD
Kleefstra syndrome	EHMT1	VSD, ToF, DORV
Koolen-De Vries syndrome	KANSL1	ASD, VSD, PS, BAV, aortic dilatation
Larsen syndrome	FLNB	ASD, VSD
Left ventricular noncompaction	ACTC1, DTNA, LDB3, MIB1, MYBPC3, MYH7, PRDM16, TNNT2, TPM1	VSD, MR, HLHS, Ebstein's anomaly
Lethal restrictive dermopathy	ZMPSTE24	ASD, PDA
Loeys-Dietz syndrome	SMAD3, TGFB2, TGFBR1, TGFBR2	ASD
Lujan-Fryns syndrome	MED12	ASD, VSD, aortic aneurysm
Lymphedema-distichiasis syndrome	FOXC2	ToF

Table 1. Continued

Syndrome	Gene	CVM
Mandibulofacial dysostosis, Guion-Almeida type	EFTUD2	ASD, VSD
Marshall-Smith syndrome	NFIX	ASD, PDA
McKusick-Kaufman syndrome	MKKS	VSD
Megalencephaly-capillary malformation-polymicrogyria syndrome	PIK3CA	VSD
Megalencephaly-polymicrogyria-polydactyly-hydrocephalus syndrome	AKT3, PIK3R2	ASD, VSD, vascular ring
Microcephaly-capillary malformation syndrome	STAMBP	ASD, VSD
Microphthalmia with limb anomalies	SMOC1	Inferior vena cava interruption with azygous continuation
Microphthalmia, syndromic	BCOR, STRA6, HCCS	ASD, VSD, MVP, HLHS, SV, PS
Miller-Dieker lissencephaly syndrome	PAFAH1B1	VSD
Mosaic variegated aneuploidy syndrome	CEP57	ASD, VSD, AI, CoA, subaortic stenosis
Mowat-Wilson syndrome	ZEB2	VSD, ASD, PS, PDA, PAS, pulmonary artery sling
Mulibrey nanism	TRIM37	Myocardial fibrosis
Multiple congenital anomalies-hypotonia-seizures syndrome	PIGA, PIGN, PIGT	ASD, PDA
Multiple intestinal atresia	TTC7A	VSD
Multiple joint dislocations, short stature, craniofacial dysmorphism	B3GAT3	LVH, BAV, MVP, ASD, PFO
Multiple pterygium syndrome	CHRNA1, CHRND, CHRNG	Cardiac hypoplasia
Myhre syndrome	SMAD4	ASD, VSD, AS, PDA, CoA, pericardial effusion and fibrosis
Neonatal inflammatory skin and bowel disease	ADAM17	Left-ventricular dilation
Nephronophthisis	ANKS6, INVS, NPHP4	AS, PS, PDA, heterotaxy
Neurofibromatosis-Noonan syndrome	NF1	PS
Noonan syndrome	PTPN11, KRAS, SOS1, RAF1, NRAS, BRAF, MEK1, MEK2, SHOC2, CBL, SPRED1, RIT1	PS, ASD, CoA
Ogden syndrome	NAA10	VSD, ASD, conduction
Omodysplasia	GPC6	ASD, VSD
Opitz GBBB syndrome	MID1	VSD
Orofaciodigital syndrome	OFD1	VSD

Table 1. Continued

Syndrome	Gene	CVM
Osteopathia striata with cranial sclerosis	AMER1	ASD, VSD
Pallister-Hall syndrome	GLI3	VSD, CoA, PDA
Periventricular nodular heterotopia	FLNA	ToF, VSD
Perlman syndrome	DIS3L2	IAA
Peroxisome biogenesis disorder	PEX1	HLHS
Peters-plus syndrome	B3GALTL	ASD, VSD, PS
Polycystic kidney disease, autosomal dominant	PKD1	AS, MVP
Primary ciliary dyskinesia	AK7, CCDC103, CCDC114, CCDC39, CCDC40, DNAAF3, DNAH11, DNAH5, DNAI1, DNAI2, DNAL1, DYNC2H1, HEATR2, HYDIN, LRRC50, LRRC6, NME8, RSPH4A, RSPH6A, RSPH9	Heterotaxy
Psychomotor retardation, epilepsy, and craniofacial dysmorphism	SNIP1	AS, BAV
Renal-hepatic-pancreatic dysplasia	NPHP3	ASD, AS, PDA, heterotaxy
Renpenning syndrome 1	PQBP1	ASD, VSD, ToF, heterotaxy
Retinal arterial macroaneurysm with supravalvular pulmonic stenosis	IGFBP7	PS
Roberts syndrome	ESCO2	AS
Robinow syndrome, autosomal dominant	WNT5A	PS
Robinow syndrome, autosomal recessive	ROR2	PS, PAS
Rubinstein-Taybi syndrome	CREBBP	ASD, VSD, PDA
Saethre-Chotzen syndrome	TWIST1	ASD, VSD
Schinzel-Giedion syndrome	SETBP1	ASD
Severe congenital neutropenia	G6PC3	ASD
Short rib-polydactyly syndrome	NEK1	VSD, ASD
Sillence type I osteogenesis imperfecta	COL1A1	MR, AS
Simpson-Golabi-Behmel syndrome	GPC3	VSD, PS
Smith-Lemli-Opitz syndrome	DHCR7	ASD, VSD, CoA, PDA, HLHS
Smith-Magenis syndrome	RAI1	VSD
Sinoatrial node dysfunction and deafness	CACNA1D	Arrhythmia

Table 1. Continued

Syndrome	Gene	CVM
Sotos syndrome	NSD1	PAIVS, ASD, VSD, PDA
Spondylocostal dysostosis	DLL3, HES7, LFNG, MESP2, TBX6	VSD, PDA, dextrocardia, complex
Spondyloepimetaphyseal dysplasia with joint laxity	B3GALT6	ASD,VSD, MR, BAV
Spondyloepiphyseal dysplasia with congenital joint dislocations	CHST3	VSD, MS, MR, TS, AS, AI, PS
Stickler syndrome, type I	COL2A1	MVP
TARP syndrome	RBM10	ASD
Tetra-amelia, autosomal recessive	WNT3	Peripheral pulmonary vessel aplasia
Thiamine-responsive megaloblastic anemia	SLC19A2	ASD, VSD, conduction defects and arrhythmias, cardiomyopathy
Townes-Brocks syndrome	SALL1	ToF, VSD
Trichohepatoenteric syndrome	SKIV2L, TTC37	AI, PS, VSD, ToF, PS
Tuberous sclerosis	TSC1, TSC2	Cardiac rhabdomyoma
Ulnar-mammary syndrome	TBX3	VSD, WPW
VATER association	HOXD13	VSD, ToF, TGA
Warsaw breakage syndrome	DDX11	VSD, ToF
Weill-Marchesani syndrome	ADAMTS10	AS, PS, VSD, MR, PDA
Wolff-Parkinson-White syndrome		WPW
Yunis-Varon syndrome	FIG4	ToF, VSD

AI = Aortic insufficiency; AS = aortic valve stenosis; ASD = atrial septal defect; AVSD = atrioventricular septal defect; CoA = coarctation of the aorta; DORV = double-outlet right ventricle; HLHS = hypoplastic left-heart syndrome; IAA = interruption of the aortic arch; IAA-B = IAA type B; LVH = left-ventricular hypertrophy; MR = mitral regurgitation; MS = mitral stenosis; MVP = mitral valve prolapse; PAIVS = pulmonary artery stenosis with intact ventricular septum; PAS = pulmonary artery stenosis; PDA = patent ductus arteriosus; PFO = patent foramen ovale; PS = pulmonary valve stenosis; SV = single ventricle; SVC = superior vena cava; SVAS = supravalvar aortic stenosis; TA = truncus arteriosus; TAPVR = total anomalous pulmonary venous return; TGA = transposition of the great arteries; ToF = tetralogy of Fallot; TS = tricuspid stenosis; VSD = ventricular septal defect; WPW = Wolff-Parkinson-White conduction defect.

6

cases 32%, and in sporadic CHD just 8% [29]. When family history is present, consideration for cardiac evaluation and genetic testing of other family members is necessary as some cardiac lesions may be silent, such as BAV (see Genetic Counseling Section). There are broad trends of relationships between specific cardiac lesions and genetic disorders. Physicians should consider the strength of inferences about the embryological origin of the cardiac lesion and how that may relate to chromosomal, genomic, and single-gene disorders. For example, familial occurrence of heterotaxy in males could suggest mutations in the X-chromosome-encoded transcription factor ZIC3. ZIC3 is known to influence embryonic left-right patterning [30]. There are limits to this approach. Although pulmonary valve stenosis is the typical lesion seen in patients with Noonan syndrome, a variety of other CHDs may be seen in these patients. In the presence of other features of Noonan syndrome, physicians should consider the diagnosis even if a non-RVOTO lesion is present.

The following sections will review the modalities available to clinicians and will be divided into four categories: chromosome analysis for aneuploidies, microarray methods for abnormalities in DNA copy number, targeted single-gene and panel sequencing, and NGS of the whole genome or exome.

Aneuploidy

Cytogenetic analysis is the microscopic visualization of the chromosomes. Abnormalities in chromosomes can involve an extra or a missing chromosome such as trisomy 21 in Down syndrome (see Kruszka chapter on Down syndrome p. 82) or monosomy X in Turner syndrome (see Bondy chapter p. 91), respectively. Other chromosome anomalies may involve microscopically visible segmental monosomies or trisomies, unbalanced translocations, or inversions, for example. The cri-du-chat syndrome (5p–) is an example of a recurrent segmental chromosome abnormality with a high risk of CHD. Aneuploidy makes up the largest category of syndromic CHD; in one study, 51% of syndromic CHD cases were attributed to aneuploidy, with trisomy 21 being most common [29], and roughly 8–10% of total CHD to aneuploidy [31]. Aneuploidies are usually the easiest genetic conditions to diagnose based on their characteristic associated dysmorphic features. Additionally, cardiac defects associated with some aneuploidies assist in making a genetic diagnosis; for example, 50% of individuals with atrioventricular septal defects have trisomy 21 and over 50% of individuals with Turner syndrome have BAV, aortic coarctation, or anomalous pulmonary veins [32, see also chapter by Bondy, pp 91].

Karyotype with G-banding (Giemsa staining) gives a resolution of 5–10 Mb [33]. Fluorescence in situ hybridization (FISH) is another technique that can be used to detect aneuploidy. Fluorescent-labeled DNA probes that hybridize to sequences on chromosomes of interest can be used to rapidly screen for trisomy 18 or 13, for example. However, this method cannot distinguish between partial and complete trisomies and, therefore, should be used only as an intermediate diagnostic procedure. Before the advent of microarray technology, FISH was the standard method used to diagnose microdeletion syndromes like 22q11 deletion and Williams syndrome. FISH is still used to test parents of children with chromosomal and genomic disorders as part of the evaluation for de novo occurrence of these conditions.

There is an important continuing role for karyotype testing in the evaluation of individuals with CHD and other developmental disorders. If the patient has clinical features of Down syndrome, for example, more costly techniques like microarray (see below) are inappropriate. It is also important to note that microarrays and most types of FISH, unlike karyotyping, do not show balanced translocations and inversions. In the case of Robertsonian translocations, as an example, a parent with a balanced translocation involving chromosome 21 (fig. 2) is at risk for having recurrence of Down syndrome in future offspring, information that might be lost with other cytogenetic methods. We also note that the presence of a cytogenetic abnormality does not preclude a second genetic disorder. It is important for physicians to evaluate whether a detected chromosome abnormality fully explains the clinical presentation.

Copy Number and Structural Variants

CNVs are deletions or duplications of thousands to millions of base pairs. Most CNVs are rare variations that do not clearly cause any disease. However, an important subset, and especially de novo CNVs, are responsible for some well-known syndromes including many that involve CHD (see Lalani chapter p. 112). An important cause of recur-

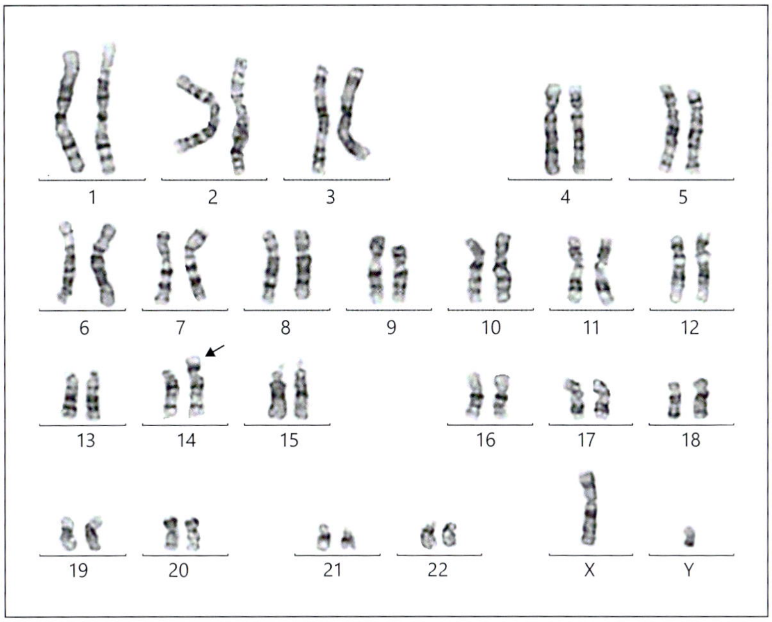

Fig. 2. Karyotype of a Robertsonian translocation. Arrow points to the fusion of chromosomes 14 and 21 at their centromeres, giving a third chromosome 21 [46,XY, rob(14;21)(q10;q10), +21] (courtesy of Dr. Jeanne Meck).

rent pathogenic CNVs is misalignment during replication and recombination of low copy repeat sequences (called nonallelic homologous recombination). These elements have rearrangement rates that are orders of magnitude greater than single-base mutations, explaining, in part, their frequent occurrence in the population. For example, the 22q11 deletion (see Goldmuntz chapter p. 100) occurs at a frequency of about 1 per 4,000 and is a leading contributor to congenital heart defects. The Database of Genomic Variants currently lists over 2 million CNVs in the human genome (http://dgv.tcag.ca/dgv/app/home) [34]. Structural variants are conventionally considered to be less than 1,000 bp in length. They have lower mutation rates than large CNVs and they contribute to the mutational 'spectrum' of most single-gene disorders. Structural variants which can include deletions, duplications, insertions, and inversions are particularly challenging to detect with current diagnostic methods. CNVs and structural variants result in more genetic variation in the human genome than SNPs [35].

Multiple techniques, including FISH, multiplex ligation-dependent probe amplification (MLPA), and chromosomal microarray, can be used to evaluate CNVs. MLPA relies on sequence-specific probe hybridization to DNA, and then PCR amplification of the probe, with subsequent semiquantitative analysis based on probe size; this technique is reviewed in detail by Sellner and Taylor [36]. Chromosomal microarrays utilize millions of probes that hybridize with sample DNA and can be used to efficiently scan the genome for copy number abnormalities. There are several competing microarray platforms and it is important for physicians to understand which platform has been used for their patients. There are two different types of chromosomal microarrays, array comparative genomic hybridization (aCGH) and SNP arrays, and both are commercially available as a combined aCGH-SNP array. Both of these different techniques are reviewed by Gijsbers and Ruivenkamp [37]. aCGH employs an internal control DNA and compares the relative signal produced by the patient and control to deduce the copy number. SNP arrays, which use only the patient's DNA, compare both the total fluorescent signal and the ratio of alleles at heterozygous positions to assess CNVs. An important advantage of SNP arrays is that they can be easily analyzed to detect runs of homozygosity, which may also be called absence of heterozygosity (AOH). Long AOH segments on a single chromosome are the hallmark of uniparental isodisomy. A high genome-wide fraction of AOH coming from some or all chromosomes signals the presence of consanguinity with its increased risk of recessive disorders. aCGH methods, on the other hand, are flexible in their design and have been used to detect small intragenic defects in developmentally important genes. Chromosomal microarrays have changed the discipline of cytogenetics allowing orders of magnitude better resolution than karyotyping. More than 200 clinical syndromes have been reported as caused by recurrent pathogenic CNVs. Rare de novo CNVs are also reported in many children with syndromic CHD [38]. Attribution of cause to these CNVs requires assessment of their length, whether they overlap with previously observed pathogenic CNVs and evaluation of their gene content. Lab-specific and public databases have been developed (ISCA/DECIPHER) to allow molecular and phenotypic comparisons to other overlapping but nonidentical CNV cases. As an example, the American College of Medical Genetics (ACMG) has recommended microarray testing for CNV as a first-line test in the postnatal evaluation of individuals with multiple anomalies not specific to a well-delineated genetic syndrome [39].

The most common pathogenic CNV is a 3-Mb deletion on chromosome 22q11.2 causing a syndrome with variable occurrence of conotruncal heart defects, craniofacial dysmorphisms, velopharyngeal insufficiency, cleft palate, developmental delay, immune deficiency secondary to hypoplastic thymus, renal anomalies, and endocrine abnormalities. Rarely patients may have eye and inner ear abnormalities that overlap with the CHARGE syndrome. When the classic triad of CHD (including aortic arch defects), hypocalcemia (parathyroid gland anomaly), and absent thymus occur together, the patient meets the diagnostic criteria for the DiGeorge syndrome. Approximately 90% of patients with the DiGeorge syndrome have 22q11 deletions. 22q11.2 deletions occur in 1 in 4,000–6,000 live births and make up a significant fraction of conotruncal abnormalities [40]; in one study, 50% of patients with interrupted aortic arch type B had 22q11.2 deletions [41]. The 22q11.2 deletion is the second most common genetic diagnosis in CHD after trisomy 21 [29]. The American Heart Association has suggested evaluating for 22q11.2 deletions in newborns with several specific heart lesions, including interrupted or anomalous aortic arch, truncus arteriosus, tetralogy of Fallot, and discontinuous branch pulmonary arteries [24].

Another consideration is the inheritance of CNVs. In the 22q11.2 deletion syndrome, the recurrence risk is significant with an estimation of up to 5% transmitted from a subtly affected parent and often only discovered after a proband is ascertained [42]. In a study of adults with tetralogy of Fallot and pulmonary atresia, 24 of 44 patients (54%) with 22q11.2 deletions were unknown before the study, emphasizing the need to examine family members of probands with CNVs [43].

When a clinician is confronted with a specific cardiac lesion and dysmorphic features, chromosomal microarray testing is now most often used to confirm a diagnosis, supplanting FISH and MLPA. CNV evaluation (fig. 3) should also be considered in nonsyndromic cases, as approximately 5–10% of sporadic nonsyndromic CHDs are due to rare CNVs [25]. Unlike syndromic cases where the CNV has a severe and broad effect and significantly reduces reproductive fitness (e.g. the Williams-Beuren syndrome), CNVs in nonsyndromic CHD may exhibit reduced penetrance and may be more difficult to decipher. Analysis of CNVs in CHD should focus on the gene content and the overlap of the CNV with known chromosomal syndromes. The analysis and challenges of CNVs in nonsyndromic CHD are reviewed by Breckpot et al. [38].

Targeted Gene Sequencing

The number of single genes responsible for CHD is rapidly increasing and can be tracked with various online resources. Locus heterogeneity, where mutations in more than one gene may cause a specific phenotype, and variable expressivity, where distinct cardiac phenotypes are caused by mutations in the same gene, are important features of the genetic architecture of CHD. Single-gene mutations account for approximately 3–5% of CHD and include syndromes such as Noonan syndrome, Alagille syndrome, and Holt-Oram syndrome [31]. There are

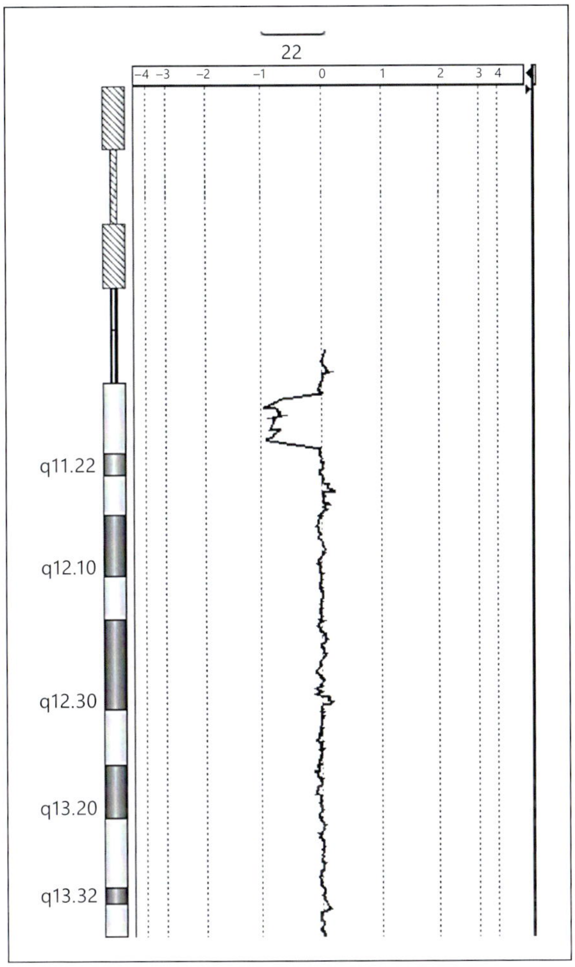

Fig. 3. CGH for a patient with the 22q11.2 deletion. The deletion is shown by the negative value on the $\log_2$ scale (courtesy of Dr. Jeanne Meck).

now at least 150 genes known to cause syndromic and nonsyndromic CHD. Some genes, for example *JAG1*, which can cause both Alagille syndrome (see chapter by Lin et al. p. 155) and isolated familial tetralogy of Fallot [44], may cause both syndromic and nonsyndromic cardiac defects. There are various free online resources such as CHD Wiki (http://homes.esat.kuleuven.be/~bioiuser/chdwiki/index.php/Main_Page) [45] and GeneReviews (http://www.ncbi.nlm.nih.gov/books/NBK1116/), which can be used to obtain updated lists of causative genes causing CHD. The Online Mendelian Inheritance in Man (OMIM, http://www.omim.org/) is a widely used professional resource with up-to-date information on thousands of rare disorders. The most frequent single-gene diseases associated with CHD are Noonan spectrum disorders, which are caused by mutations in at least 11 genes. Mutations in one of these genes, *PTPN11*, are responsible for 50% of cases [46]. These conditions are sometimes called RASopathies to indicate the unifying theme of disturbed regulation of the Ras/MAPK signaling pathway. One study found that 7% of all syndromes associated with CHD were attributed to the Noonan syndrome, and when compared to all syndromic CHD, Noonan syndrome was only behind Down syndrome (51%) and the 22q11.2 deletion syndrome (19%) [29].

Nonsyndromic single-gene causes of CHD, such as in the transcription factor *NKX2.5,* present a more challenging dilemma. Heterozygous mutations in *NKX2.5* were initially described in families with conduction abnormalities and septal defects affecting individuals in several generations [21]. Incomplete penetrance and variable expressivity have been described [47] in patients with rare mutations in *NKX2.5*. Rare variants with altered function are also observed in general population controls [48] suggesting caution in clinical interpretation unless there is additional supporting evidence for causation.

Sanger sequencing has been extensively used in clinical single-gene testing [49]. NGS has dramatically altered the cost structure for sequencing enabling large gene panel tests, whole exome sequencing (WES) and whole genome sequencing (WGS) to emerge as practical alternatives for individual patient diagnostic evaluation. The combination of NGS with Sanger confirmation allows highly accurate and reproducible results. Panel testing is cost effective when a substantial fraction of cases can be explained by a restricted group of genes. Again, this is nicely illustrated by Noonan spectrum disorders where >70% of patients can be given a gene-specific diagnosis using a panel of 11 genes. Physicians evaluating the results of single-gene and panel sequencing tests must assess the following: the prior probability that the patient has a mutation in the selected gene(s) based on the clinical phenotype; the putative pattern of inheritance of the suspected genetic disorder; the bioinformatic interpretation (functional prediction) of the mutation effect and the frequency of the putative mutation in the general population; the frequency of occurrence of similar functional mutations in the disease gene, and the occurrence of the mutation in any other affected family member. For some mutations, the bioinformatic interpretation is simple and clear, e.g. the occurrence of a stop codon in a gene known to be sensitive to haploinsufficiency. Many other mutations have less certain functional consequences. These are often reported as variants of unknown significance and the physicians must use other supporting information to support conclusions about pathogenicity. Recent experience has also demonstrated that some genes are more tolerant of amino acid substitutions (missense mutations) than other genes. This makes interpretation of missense variants particularly challenging with substantial caution in using the genetic test result in clinical decision making. The more specific the phenotype-genotype correlation, the more likely that a gene sequencing test will contribute to the diagnosis. We recommend single-gene sequencing when the clinical disease presentation is highly specific and a large fraction of cases are explained by one or a few genes. As an example, consider the Ellis-van Creveld syndrome where there are specific findings of a characteristic skeletal dysplasia, polydactyly, and CHD (most often common atrium). Mutations in *EVC* and *EVC2* account for all cases of the Ellis-van Creveld syndrome and, thus, targeted sequencing of those genes has high clinical validity. Panel testing is effective when the phenotype specificity is high even if there is substantial locus heterogeneity. Both single-gene and panel testing have technical limitations in the classes of alleles that can be detected. For example, a deletion mutation may not be detected by sequencing alone because the amplification procedure used to prepare the DNA for sequencing selectively misses the deleted DNA segments. Mutations that occur in noncoding elements, like deep intronic splice regulators, will not be detected in tests that target only the exons and their flanking sequences. No sequencing and mutation detection procedure, even those that incorporate methods to detect deletions and duplications, can be expected to have 100% sensitivity. It is always advisable to evaluate whether a putative mutation has been transmitted from a parent or has occurred de novo. In some families, it may be necessary to test siblings especially if they are also affected with CHD (test of cosegregation). Finally, we caution that panel testing, especially if not converted to NGS methodology, can be as costly as WES. In those clinical situations, WES may give a higher diagnostic success rate.

Whole Genome and Whole Exome Sequencing

NGS has radically changed genetic testing and has already begun to accelerate the pace of discovery of new single-gene mutations in CHD. In NGS, massively parallel sequencing of millions of small DNA fragments is carried out using highly optimized kit chemistry and dedicated instruments. The resulting short sequences are realigned to a reference sequence and variants from the reference called. The accuracy of the variant calling depends on the depth of the sequence data (how short sequences overlap with a particular base position), the ratio of variant to reference calls, and whether the variant is a single-nucleotide substitution or a short insertion/deletion-type variant. WGS evaluates the entire euchromatic human genome and, due to its costs and difficulty in interpretation, is not yet widely used on a clinical basis. There are 18,000–23,000 genes that code for proteins comprising approximately 1% of the genome (about 35–37 Mb). WES uses targeted capture techniques to sequence only the coding parts of the genome, and plummeting costs have made WES a widely used test at many clinical and academic centers, especially for undiagnosed clinical cases. WES has had relative success in highly penetrant Mendelian disorders, first demonstrated in a proof-of-concept paper when WES was shown to identify the gene for the Freeman-Sheldon syndrome in a small number of unrelated affected individuals [50].

In the first large-scale NGS study of CHD, Zaidi et al. [23] sequenced the exomes of 362 patients with CHD and their unaffected parents and compared the variants to 264 unaffected control trios. This study found that de novo mutations explained 10%

of the cardiac anomalies and implicated 28 genes as highly confident mutations. Interestingly, this group of de novo variants encoded an excess of proteins involved in histone modification, specifically trimethylation of histone H3, lysine 4 (H3K4me3). Epigenetic processes such as histone modification control gene expression during development. This concept of quantitative control of gene expression reinforces previous findings in CHD research associating heart anomalies with haploinsufficiency or heterozygous mutations in transcription factors (i.e. *NKX2.5*), which also regulate early development by controlling transcription [51]. The results of Zaidi et al. [23] provide early support for the use of WES in the diagnostic evaluation of CHD. WES can be an effective tool when the clinical presentation lacks key-specific clues to a single gene association. This is very typical in the early evaluation of infants with multiple congenital anomalies. It may not be possible to reliably recognize conditions like the Kleefstra, Mowat-Wilson and Kabuki syndromes in the neonatal period because of their low frequency and overlap with other similar disorders. In addition, some conditions like heterotaxy/primary ciliary dyskinesia, where there are now nearly 50 genes implicated, have such extensive locus heterogeneity that panel testing is currently unavailable or unfeasible.

NGS technology is now being used for complex inherited CHDs, which presents a bigger challenge than Mendelian disease. The BAV has been shown to be heritable with one study of 309 probands demonstrating the heritability (h2) of BAV to be 89% [52]. However, only two genes, *KCNJ2* and *NOTCH1*, have been identified, which account for <5% of all cases of known BAV [53–55]. In an attempt to further elucidate the genetic etiology of BAV using WES on a 17-person kindred with nonsyndromic BAV, Martin et al. [55] was unable to find a causative gene, highlighting the difficulty in analyzing CHD as a complex trait. Sporadic nonsyndromic CHD has been popularly attributed to the multifactorial model first suggested by Nora [56] in 1968. This model implies that multiple genes interact with the environment to cause a disease and has the following criteria: aggregates in families, recurrence rate in sibs of 1–5%, and evidence of environmental influences [56]. Although this hypothesis makes sense and is widely accepted, very few studies have provided examples of support [57–59]. If correct, the consequence of this model for clinical testing would be that single-gene mutations with large effect would explain only a minority of CHD cases. In such a scenario, clinical WES and even WGS would be ineffective. This hypothesis needs much more research before it can be concluded that only a small fraction of CHD cases are due to single-gene mutations. At the present time, clinical utility would be difficult or impossible to achieve if CHD causation is primarily polygenic and multifactorial.

NGS, especially WES, has limitations when addressing both syndromic and nonsyndromic CHD. WES only looks at protein-coding regions, and there may be changes outside these regions, i.e. in promoters, introns, and regulatory regions of the genome. As an example, familial amyotrophic lateral sclerosis in Finnish populations has hexanucleotide repeat mutations within the noncoding region of the *C9orf72* gene [60]. Additionally, some changes are not considered in the bioinformatic data filters, such as synonymous changes (missense changes that do not change the coded amino acid), which, in some cases, may cause disease due to cryptic splicing changes, as in the Hutchinson-Gilford progeria syndrome [61, 62]. There is also a chance to miss a mutation as WES does not have adequate coverage or reliable variant detection in approximately 5% of the genome.

There are a number of ethical and legal issues that have become apparent with widespread WGS testing. When doing genomic testing, whether that be SNP array or WGS, the technology looks at the entire genome, not just the areas of clinical interest, and may generate results unrelated to the clinical condition that prompted the test. For example, a whole exome test may be ordered to evaluate a child for a rare neurologic condition; however, the sequencing data provide information on *BRAC1* and *BRAC2* and other cancer susceptibility genes that may be important to that child later in life. The ACMG has recommended that laboratories report genetic variants for a minimum set of 56 genes that are medically actionable [63]. Given that 1–3% of patients will have incidental findings [64], this adds another layer of complexity to WGS and requires careful interpretation of these results by a clinical geneticist in the context of personal and family history, and examination of the patient. Additionally, the stance of the ACMG recommendations contradicts past policies on testing of minors, which has traditionally only recommended a genetic test if immediate benefit was possible from the results of the testing [65].

Genetic Counseling

Appropriate genetic counseling should accompany the return of all genetic results to provide the patient and family with a clear understanding of the results, education on a syndrome if diagnosed, and recurrence risks. All four layers of testing technology deserve genetic counseling, including karyotypes, chromosomal microarray, Sanger sequencing, and NGS. Given that more patients with CHD are surviving into adulthood and producing offspring, recurrence risks become even more relevant. A large British study of 727 individuals with major heart defects who had 393 live offspring found a recurrence risk of 4.1%. The sibling risk for this cohort was 2.1% [66]. Interestingly, more offspring of affected women had CHD than men in this study ($p = 0.021$). In unaffected parents, the risk of recurrence of CHD is found to be roughly 1–6% and increases to 10% if two siblings are affected [12, 67–68]. Given this information, genetic counseling for nonsyndromic, non-Mendelian CHD becomes complicated for both sides the counselor and the patient and family. The National Society of Genetic Counselors provides resources for genetic counseling (http://www.nsgc.org/).

Concluding Remarks

There is still much to be done in understanding and applying genetic technologies to CHD. We have become proficient at finding fully penetrant mutations that segregate in a Mendelian fashion; the next barrier to overcome will be understanding the functional and medical relevance of cardiac developmental genes and elucidating the underpinnings of genetically complex cardiac malformations. A key to this realization will be advances in technology and decreasing WGS costs, which will make WGS available to everyone in the near future.

References

1 Kurnit DM, Layton WM, Matthysse S: Genetics, chance, and morphogenesis. Am J Hum Genet 1987;41:979–995.
2 Jenkins KJ, Correa A, Feinstein JA, Botto L, Britt AE, Daniels SR, Elixson M, Warnes CA, Webb CL; American Heart Association Council on Cardiovascular Disease in the Young: Noninherited risk factors and congenital cardiovascular defects: current knowledge: a scientific statement from the American Heart Association Council on Cardiovascular Disease in the Young: endorsed by the American Academy of Pediatrics. Circulation 2007;115:2995–3014.
3 Bruneau BG: The developmental genetics of congenital heart disease. Nature 2008;451: 943–998.
4 Yuan S, Zaidi S, Brueckner M: Congenital heart disease: emerging themes linking genetics and development. Curr Opin Genet Dev 2013;23:352–359.
5 Mckeown T, Macmahon B, Parsons CG: The familial incidence of congenital malformation of the heart. Br Heart J 1953;15:273–277.
6 Drenthen W, Pieper PG, Roos-Hesselink JW, van Lottum WA, Voors AA, Mulder BJ, van Dijk AP, Vliegen HW, Yap SC, Moons P, Ebels T, van Veldhuisen DJ; ZAHARA Investigators: Outcome of pregnancy in women with congenital heart disease: a literature review. J Am Coll Cardiol 2007;49:2303–2311.
7 Chin-Yee NJ, Costain G, Swaby JA, Silversides CK, Bassett AS: Reproductive fitness and genetic transmission of tetralogy of Fallot in the molecular age. Circ Cardiovasc Genet 2014;7:102–109.
8 Nabulsi MM, Tamim H, Sabbagh M, Obeid MY, Yunis KA, Bitar FF: Parental consanguinity and congenital heart malformations in a developing country. Am J Med Genet A 2003;116A:342–347.
9 Yunis K, Mumtaz G, Bitar F, Chamseddine F, Kassar M, Rashkidi J, Makhoul G, Tamim H: Consanguineous marriage and congenital heart defects: a case-control study in the neonatal period. Am J Med Genet A 2006;140: 1524–1530.
10 Ferencz C, Rubin JD, Loffredo CA, Magee DA: Epidemiology of congenital heart disease: the Baltimore-Washington Infant Study 1981–1989; in Anderson RH (ed): Perspectives in Pediatric Cardiology. Mount Kisco, Futura Publishing, 1993.
11 Benson DW: Genetic origins of pediatric heart disease. Pediatr Cardiol 2010;31:422–429.
12 Øyen N, Poulsen G, Boyd HA, Wohlfahrt J, Jensen PK, Melbye M: Recurrence of congenital heart defects in families. Circulation 2009;120:295–301.
13 Kuehl KS, Loffredo CA: Population-based study of l-transposition of the great arteries: possible associations with environmental factors. Birth Defects Res A Clin Mol Teratol 2003;67:162–167.
14 Langlois PH, Brender JD, Suarez L, Zhan FB, Mistry JH, Scheuerle A, Moody K: Maternal residential proximity to waste sites and industrial facilities and conotruncal heart defects in offspring. Paediatr Perinat Epidemiol 2009;23:321–331.

15 Lander ES, Linton LM, Birren B, Nusbaum C, Zody MC, Baldwin J, Devon K, Dewar K, Doyle M, FitzHugh W, et al: International Human Genome Sequencing Consortium. Initial sequencing and analysis of the human genome. Nature 2001;409:860–921.
16 International HapMap Consortium, Frazer KA, Ballinger DG, Cox DR, Hinds DA, Stuve LL, Gibbs RA, et al: A second generation human haplotype map of over 3.1 million SNPs. Nature 2007;449:851–861.
17 Cordell HJ, Bentham J, Topf A, Zelenika D, Heath S, Mamasoula C, Cosgrove C, Blue G, Granados-Riveron J, Setchfield K, Thornborough C, Breckpot J, Soemedi R, Martin R, Rahman TJ, Hall D, van Engelen K, Moorman AF, Zwinderman AH, Barnett P, Koopmann TT, Adriaens ME, Varro A, George AL Jr, dos Remedios C, Bishopric NH, Bezzina CR, O'Sullivan J, Gewillig M, Bu'Lock FA, Winlaw D, Bhattacharya S, Devriendt K, Brook JD, Mulder BJ, Mital S, Postma AV, Lathrop GM, Farrall M, Goodship JA, Keavney BD: Genome-wide association study of multiple congenital heart disease phenotypes identifies a susceptibility locus for atrial septal defect at chromosome 4p16. Nat Genet 2013;45:822–824.
18 Manolio TA, Collins FS, Cox NJ, Goldstein DB, Hindorff LA, Hunter DJ, McCarthy MI, Ramos EM, Cardon LR, Chakravarti A, Cho JH, Guttmacher AE, Kong A, Kruglyak L, Mardis E, Rotimi CN, Slatkin M, Valle D, Whittemore AS, Boehnke M, Clark AG, Eichler EE, Gibson G, Haines JL, Mackay TF, McCarroll SA, Visscher PM: Finding the missing heritability of complex diseases. Nature 2009;461:747–753.
19 Basson CT, Bachinsky DR, Lin RC, et al: Mutations in human TBX5 cause limb and cardiac malformation in Holt-Oram syndrome. Nat Genet 1997;15:30–35.
20 Li QY, Newbury-Ecob RA, Terrett JA, et al: Holt-Oram syndrome is caused by mutations in TBX5, a member of the Brachyury (T) gene family. Nat Genet 1997;15:21–29.
21 Schott JJ, Benson DW, Basson CT, Pease W, Silberbach GM, Moak JP, Maron BJ, Seidman CE, Seidman JG: Congenital heart disease caused by mutations in the transcription factor NKX2-5. Science 1998;281:108–111.
22 Tartaglia M, Mehler EL, Goldberg R, Zampino G, Brunner HG, Kremer H, van der Borg I, Crosby AH, Ion A, Jeffery S, Kalidas K, Patton MA, Kucherlapati RS, Gelb BD: Mutations in PTPN11, encoding the protein tyrosine phosphatase SHP-2, cause Noonan syndrome. Nat Genet 2001;29:465–468.
23 Zaidi S, Choi M, Wakimoto H, Ma L, Jiang J, Overton JD, Romano-Adesman A, Bjornson RD, Breitbart RE, Brown KK, Carriero NJ, Cheung YH, Deanfield J, DePalma S, Fakhro KA, Glessner J, Hakonarson H, Italia MJ, Kaltman JR, Kaski J, Kim R, Kline JK, Lee T, Leipzig J, Lopez A, Mane SM, Mitchell LE, Newburger JW, Parfenov M, Pe'er I, Porter G, Roberts AE, Sachidanandam R, Sanders SJ, Seiden HS, State MW, Subramanian S, Tikhonova IR, Wang W, Warburton D, White PS, Williams IA, Zhao H, Seidman JG, Brueckner M, Chung WK, Gelb BD, Goldmuntz E, Seidman CE, Lifton RP: De novo mutations in histone-modifying genes in congenital heart disease. Nature 2013;498:220–223.
24 Pierpont ME, Basson CT, Benson DW Jr, Gelb BD, Giglia TM, Goldmuntz E, McGee G, Sable CA, Srivastava D, Webb CL; American Heart Association Congenital Cardiac Defects Committee, Council on Cardiovascular Disease in the Young: Genetic basis for congenital heart defects: current knowledge: a scientific statement from the American Heart Association Congenital Cardiac Defects Committee, Council on Cardiovascular Disease in the Young: endorsed by the American Academy of Pediatrics. Circulation 2007;115:3015–3038.
25 Fahed AC, Gelb BD, Seidman JG, Seidman CE: Genetics of congenital heart disease: the glass half empty. Circ Res 2013;112:707–720.
26 Marelli A, Beauchesne L, Mital S, Therrien J, Silversides CK: Canadian Cardiovascular Society 2009 Consensus Conference on the management of adults with congenital heart disease: introduction. Can J Cardiol 2010;26:e65–e69.
27 Hinton RB Jr, Martin LJ, Tabangin ME, Mazwi ML, Cripe LH, Benson DW: Hypoplastic left heart syndrome is heritable. J Am Coll Cardiol 2007;50:1590–1595.
28 Lewin MB, McBride KL, Pignatelli R, Fernbach S, Combes A, Menesses A, Lam W, Bezold LI, Kaplan N, Towbin JA, Belmont JW: Echocardiographic evaluation of asymptomatic parental and sibling cardiovascular anomalies associated with congenital left ventricular outflow tract lesions. Pediatrics 2004;114:691–696.
29 Fung A, Manlhiot C, Naik S, Rosenberg H, Smythe J, Lougheed J, Mondal T, Chitayat D, McCrindle BW, Mital S: Impact of prenatal risk factors on congenital heart disease in the current era. J Am Heart Assoc 2013;2:e000064.
30 Ware SM, Harutyunyan KG, Belmont JW: Heart defects in X-linked heterotaxy: evidence for a genetic interaction of Zic3 with the nodal signaling pathway. Dev Dyn 2006;235:1631–1637.
31 van der Bom T, Zomer AC, Zwinderman AH, Meijboom FJ, Bouma BJ, Mulder BJ: The changing epidemiology of congenital heart disease. Nat Rev Cardiol 2011;8:50–60.
32 Craig B: Atrioventricular septal defect: from fetus to adult. Heart 2006;92:1879–1885.
33 Smeets DF: Historical prospective of human cytogenetics: from microscope to microarray. Clin Biochem 2004;37:439–446.
34 MacDonald JR, Ziman R, Yuen RK, Feuk L, Scherer SW: The Database of Genomic Variants: a curated collection of structural variation in the human genome. Nucleic Acids Res 2014;42(database issue):D986–D992.
35 Redon R, Ishikawa S, Fitch KR, Feuk L, Perry GH, Andrews TD, Fiegler H, Shapero MH, Carson AR, Chen W, Cho EK, Dallaire S, Freeman JL, González JR, Gratacòs M, Huang J, Kalaitzopoulos D, Komura D, MacDonald JR, Marshall CR, Mei R, Montgomery L, Nishimura K, Okamura K, Shen F, Somerville MJ, Tchinda J, Valsesia A, Woodwark C, Yang F, Zhang J, Zerjal T, Zhang J, Armengol L, Conrad DF, Estivill X, Tyler-Smith C, Carter NP, Aburatani H, Lee C, Jones KW, Scherer SW, Hurles ME: Global variation in copy number in the human genome. Nature 2006;444:444–454.
36 Sellner LN, Taylor GR: MLPA and MAPH: new techniques for detection of gene deletions. Hum Mutat 2004;23:413–419.
37 Gijsbers AC, Ruivenkamp CA: Molecular karyotyping: from microscope to SNP arrays. Horm Res Paediatr 2011;76:208–213.
38 Breckpot J, Thienpont B, Arens Y, Tranchevent LC, Vermeesch JR, Moreau Y, Gewillig M, Devriendt K: Challenges of interpreting copy number variation in syndromic and non-syndromic congenital heart defects. Cytogenet Genome Res 2011;135:251–259.
39 Manning M, Hudgins L; Professional Practice and Guidelines Committee: Array-based technology and recommendations for utilization in medical genetics practice for detection of chromosomal abnormalities. Genet Med 2010;12:742–745.
40 Botto LD, May K, Fernhoff PM, Correa A, Coleman K, Rasmussen SA, Merritt RK, O'Leary LA, Wong LY, Elixson EM, Mahle WT, Campbell RM: A population-based study of the 22q11.2 deletion: phenotype, incidence, and contribution to major birth defects in the population. Pediatrics 2003;112(1 pt 1):101–107.
41 Lewin MB, Lindsay EA, Jurecic V, Goytia V, Towbin JA, Baldini A: A genetic etiology for interruption of the aortic arch type B. Am J Cardiol 1997;80:493–497.
42 Goldmuntz E: DiGeorge syndrome: new insights. Clin Perinatol 2005;32:963–978, ix–x.
43 van Engelen K, Topf A, Keavney BD, Goodship JA, van der Velde ET, Baars MJ, Snijder S, Moorman AF, Postma AV, Mulder BJ: 22q11.2 deletion syndrome is under-recognised in adult patients with tetralogy of Fallot and pulmonary atresia. Heart 2010;96:621–624.

44 Bauer RC, Laney AO, Smith R, Gerfen J, Morrissette JJ, Woyciechowski S, Garbarini J, Loomes KM, Krantz ID, Urban Z, Gelb BD, Goldmuntz E, Spinner NB: Jagged1 (JAG1) mutations in patients with tetralogy of Fallot or pulmonic stenosis. Hum Mutat 2010;31:594–601.
45 Barriot R, Breckpot J, Thienpont B, Brohée S, Van Vooren S, Coessens B, Tranchevent LC, Van Loo P, Gewillig M, Devriendt K, Moreau Y: Collaboratively charting the gene-to-phenotype network of human congenital heart defects. Genome Med 2010;2:16.
46 Allanson JE, Roberts AE: Noonan syndrome (2001; updated 2011); in Pagon RA, Adam MP, Ardinger HH, et al (eds): GeneReviews® [Internet]. Seattle, University of Washington, 1993–2015, http://www.ncbi.nlm.nih.gov/books/NBK1124/.
47 Benson DW, Silberbach GM, Kavanaugh-McHugh A, Cottrill C, Zhang Y, Riggs S, Smalls O, Johnson MC, Watson MS, Seidman JG, Seidman CE, Plowden J, Kugler JD: Mutations in the cardiac transcription factor NKX2.5 affect diverse cardiac developmental pathways. J Clin Invest 1999;104:1567–1573.
48 Akcaboy MI, Cengiz FB, Inceoglu B, Ucar T, Atalay S, Tutar E, Tekin M: The effect of p.Arg25Cys alteration in NKX2-5 on conotruncal heart anomalies: mutation or polymorphism? Pediatr Cardiol 2008;29:126–129.
49 Katsanis SH, Katsanis N: Molecular genetic testing and the future of clinical genomics. Nat Rev Genet 2013;14:415–426.
50 Ng SB, Turner EH, Robertson PD, Flygare SD, Bigham AW, Lee C, Shaffer T, Wong M, Bhattacharjee A, Eichler EE, Bamshad M, Nickerson DA, Shendure J: Targeted capture and massively parallel sequencing of 12 human exomes. Nature 2009;461:272–276.
51 Bruneau BG, Srivastava D: Congenital heart disease: entering a new era of human genetics. Circ Res 2014;114:598–599.
52 Cripe L, Andelfinger G, Martin LJ, Shooner K, Benson DW: Bicuspid aortic valve is heritable. J Am Coll Cardiol 2004;44:138–143.
53 Andelfinger G, Tapper AR, Welch RC, Vanoye CG, George AL Jr, Benson DW: KCNJ2 mutation results in Andersen syndrome with sex-specific cardiac and skeletal muscle phenotypes. Am J Hum Genet 2002;71:663–668.
54 Garg V, Muth AN, Ransom JF, Schluterman MK, Barnes R, King IN, Grossfeld PD, Srivastava D: Mutations in NOTCH1 cause aortic valve disease. Nature 2005;437:270–274.
55 Martin LJ, Pilipenko V, Kaufman KM, Cripe L, Kottyan LC, Keddache M, Dexheimer P, Weirauch MT, Benson DW: Whole exome sequencing for familial bicuspid aortic valve identifies putative variants. Circ Cardiovasc Genet 2014;7:677–683.
56 Nora JJ: Multifactorial inheritance hypothesis for the etiology of congenital heart diseases. The genetic-environmental interaction. Circulation 1968;38:604–617.
57 Garg V, Kathiriya IS, Barnes R, Schluterman MK, King IN, Butler CA, Rothrock CR, Eapen RS, Hirayama-Yamada K, Joo K, Matsuoka R, Cohen JC, Srivastava D: GATA4 mutations cause human congenital heart defects and reveal an interaction with TBX5. Nature 2003;424:443–447.
58 Roessler E, Pei W, Ouspenskaia MV, Karkera JD, Veléz JI, Banerjee-Basu S, Gibney G, Lupo PJ, Mitchell LE, Towbin JA, Bowers P, Belmont JW, Goldmuntz E, Baxevanis AD, Feldman B, Muenke M: Cumulative ligand activity of NODAL mutations and modifiers are linked to human heart defects and holoprosencephaly. Mol Genet Metab 2009;98:225–234.
59 van Beynum IM, Mooij C, Kapusta L, Heil S, den Heijer M, Blom HJ: Common 894G>T single nucleotide polymorphism in the gene coding for endothelial nitric oxide synthase (eNOS) and risk of congenital heart defects. Clin Chem Lab Med 2008;46:1369–1375.
60 Renton AE, Majounie E, Waite A, Simón-Sánchez J, Rollinson S, Gibbs JR, Schymick JC, Laaksovirta H, van Swieten JC, Myllykangas L, Kalimo H, Paetau A, Abramzon Y, Remes AM, Kaganovich A, Scholz SW, Duckworth J, Ding J, Harmer DW, Hernandez DG, Johnson JO, Mok K, Ryten M, Trabzuni D, Guerreiro RJ, Orrell RW, Neal J, Murray A, Pearson J, Jansen IE, Sondervan D, Seelaar H, Blake D, Young K, Halliwell N, Callister JB, Toulson G, Richardson A, Gerhard A, Snowden J, Mann D, Neary D, Nalls MA, Peuralinna T, Jansson L, Isoviita VM, Kaivorinne AL, Hölttä-Vuori M, Ikonen E, Sulkava R, Benatar M, Wuu J, Chiò A, Restagno G, Borghero G, Sabatelli M; ITALSGEN Consortium, Heckerman D, Rogaeva E, Zinman L, Rothstein JD, Sendtner M, Drepper C, Eichler EE, Alkan C, Abdullaev Z, Pack SD, Dutra A, Pak E, Hardy J, Singleton A, Williams NM, Heutink P, Pickering-Brown S, Morris HR, Tienari PJ, Traynor BJ: A hexanucleotide repeat expansion in C9ORF72 is the cause of chromosome 9p21-linked ALS-FTD. Neuron 2011;72:257–268.
61 De Sandre-Giovannoli A, Bernard R, Cau P, Navarro C, Amiel J, Boccaccio I, Lyonnet S, Stewart CL, Munnich A, Le Merrer M, Lévy N: Lamin a truncation in Hutchinson-Gilford progeria. Science 2003;300:2055.
62 Eriksson M, Brown WT, Gordon LB, Glynn MW, Singer J, Scott L, Erdos MR, Robbins CM, Moses TY, Berglund P, Dutra A, Pak E, Durkin S, Csoka AB, Boehnke M, Glover TW, Collins FS: Recurrent de novo point mutations in lamin A cause Hutchinson-Gilford progeria syndrome. Nature 2003;423:293–298.
63 Green RC, Berg JS, Grody WW, Kalia SS, Korf BR, Martin CL, McGuire AL, Nussbaum RL, O'Daniel JM, Ormond KE, Rehm HL, Watson MS, Williams MS, Biesecker LG; American College of Medical Genetics and Genomics: ACMG recommendations for reporting of incidental findings in clinical exome and genome sequencing. Genet Med 2013;15:565–574.
64 Dorschner MO, Amendola LM, Turner EH, et al: Actionable, pathogenic incidental findings in 1,000 participants' exomes. Am J Hum Genet 2013;93:631–640.
65 Ross LF, Saal HM, David KL, Anderson RR: Technical report: ethical and policy issues in genetic testing and screening of children. Genet Med 2013;15:234–245.
66 Burn J, Brennan P, Little J, Holloway S, Coffey R, Somerville J, Dennis NR, Allan L, Arnold R, Deanfield JE, Godman M, Houston A, Keeton B, Oakley C, Scott O, Silove E, Wilkinson J, Pembrey M, Hunter AS: Recurrence risks in offspring of adults with major heart defects: results from first cohort of British collaborative study. Lancet 1998;351:311–316.
67 Calcagni G, Digilio MC, Sarkozy A, Dallapiccola B, Marino B: Familial recurrence of congenital heart disease: an overview and review of the literature. Eur J Pediatr 2007;166:111–116.
68 Gill HK, Splitt M, Sharland GK, Simpson JM: Patterns of recurrence of congenital heart disease: an analysis of 6,640 consecutive pregnancies evaluated by detailed fetal echocardiography. J Am Coll Cardiol 2003;42:923–929.

Dr. Maximilian Muenke
National Human Genome Research Institutes, NIH
35 Convent Drive
Bethesda, MD 20892-3717 (USA)
E-Mail mamuenke@mail.nih.gov

Muenke M, Kruszka PS, Sable CA, Belmont JW (eds): Congenital Heart Disease: Molecular Genetics, Principles of Diagnosis and Treatment. Basel, Karger, 2015, pp 257–268
DOI: 10.1159/000375222

Imaging of Congenital Heart Defects for the Noncardiologist

Craig A. Sable

Division of Cardiology, Children's National Health System, Washington, D.C., USA

Abstract

Noninvasive imaging is used to make a definitive diagnosis of a congenital heart defect. The various modalities include echocardiography (ultrasound of the heart), cardiac magnetic resonance imaging (MRI), and cardiac computerized tomography (CT). Of these modalities, echocardiography is by far the most readily available and can almost always be used to make an initial diagnosis of the most common form of congenital heart defects. MRI and CT are often used for more detailed structural and functional assessments that fine-tune the diagnosis and help plan for surgical or catheter-based interventions. It is important for the pediatrician, neonatologist, geneticist, and anyone else who encounters patients with genetic conditions to have a basic understanding of the indications, timing, and limitations of echocardiography, the principles of ultrasound, and to have some familiarity with recognition of the most common lesions.

Types of Imaging

Noninvasive imaging can almost always be used to make a definitive diagnosis of a congenital heart defect. Modalities include echocardiography (ultrasound of the heart), cardiac magnetic resonance imaging (MRI), and cardiac computerized tomography (CT). Of these modalities, echocardiography is by far the most readily available and can almost always be used to make an initial diagnosis of the most common form of congenital heart defects. MRI and CT are often used for more detailed structural and functional assessment that fine-tune the diagnosis and help plan for surgical or catheter-based interventions. This chapter will primarily focus on the role of echocardiography in evaluating the patient with possible underlying genetic disorders. This includes a basic overview of ultrasound physics, the echocardiography examination, the setting in which echocardiography is performed, indications for echocardiography, timing of the echocardiographic examination, and echocardiographic features of the most common congenital cardiac lesions.

Ultrasound Physics

A detailed explanation of ultrasound physics is beyond the scope of this book, but there are some basic principles that are helpful for the clinician evaluating a child with a genetic disorder and suspected cardiac diagnosis. These principles are (1) penetra-

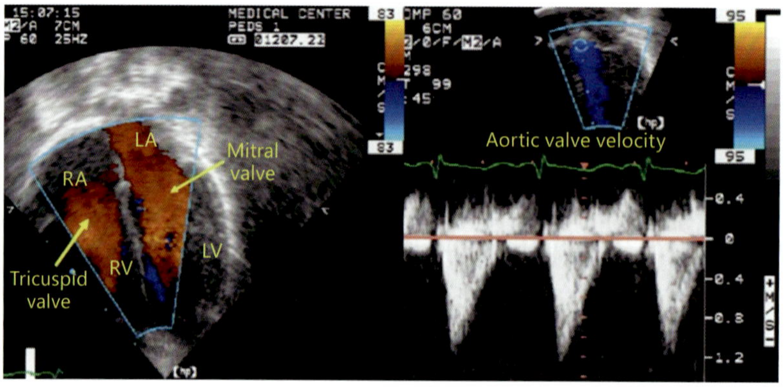

Fig. 1. Color (left) Doppler image of normal mitral valve inflow (red signifies flow coming towards the transducer) and spectral Doppler (right) of normal aortic outflow (below the line signifies flow going away from transducer). LA = Left atrium; LV = left ventricle; RA = right atrium; RV = right ventricle.

tion versus resolution, (2) spatial versus time resolution, and (3) Doppler.

Ultrasound images are created by sound waves at frequencies far above what the human ear can detect (2–12 MHz). Just as with a ship that sends ultrasound waves to the bottom of the ocean and waits for a signal to come back, an echocardiography transducer sends a high-frequency sound wave through the chest and it forms an image of the heart and sends it back to the transducers and machine to form an image. The first important principle arises from this frequency range: resolution versus penetration. Frequency is inversely proportional to wavelength: the higher the frequency, the shorter the wavelength. Shorter wavelengths allow for better resolution. However, there is a tradeoff; higher frequency signals are more readily absorbed by tissue and have limited ability to penetrate. The implication of this is that there are different size transducers used for different size patients and even within the same patient from different places on the body. As a result, image quality in newborns is far superior to adults because of the ability to use higher-frequency transducers. However, image quality can be adversely impacted by depth or size, air, obesity, and other factors that limit penetration. Thus, there is a tradeoff between penetration and resolution; higher-frequency transducers optimize resolution while lower-frequency transducers optimize penetration. Pediatric echocardiography laboratories must have at least three different size transducers while adult echocardiography laboratories only need the lowest frequency transducer. This may create challenges to imaging newborn babies born in hospitals that only have an adult echocardiography laboratory (the case for the vast majority of babies born in the United States).

Echocardiography and ultrasound machines look the same, but the key difference is based on the principle that the heart is moving, and the machine and transducers must be optimized to both spatial and time resolution. Frame rate is synonymous to time resolution; just like when watching a movie, if it were playing at a frame rate that is too low it would not blend together. This is even more important for infants with higher heart rates. The types of transducers and image processing required to account for time resolution are different than what is used for processing abdominal, brain or obstetrical imaging. Some machines can do both, but in general, provide suboptimal imaging. Therefore, in almost all hospitals and clinical practices, ultrasound and echocardiography departments use different equipment and are staffed by different personnel.

In addition to forming an image of the heart, echocardiography can evaluate hemodynamics by assessing the speed of blood using Doppler. The Doppler principle is based on the concept that a moving object will change the frequency of a sound wave. The echocardiography transducer sends out a pulse of sound that is altered by moving blood and has a different frequency when it returns to the transducer. The machine can determine the speed and direction of blood flow based on this frequency shift and display velocity as a color or spectral map (fig. 1).

Echocardiography Examination

A comprehensive pediatric echocardiographic examination involves obtaining images from multiple windows [1]. These include parasternal, apical, subcostal, and suprasternal notch positions. Two-dimensional and Doppler images are obtained from each window. Additionally, M-mode images are obtained from the parasternal window. M-mode displays a single dimension versus time and is used to measure chamber and wall thickness size as well as a measure of function known as shortening fraction. By obtaining orthogonal two-dimensional views from each position, the echocardiographer can put together a mental three-dimensional model of the heart and get a very good understanding of the anatomy. The examination is focused on exclusion of intracardiac communications, valvular abnormalities, abnormal venous or arterial connections, and major structural defects including situs abnormalities. The addition of Doppler helps localize shunts, blockages, and leakages, as well as quantitate severity of blockages and leakages.

Assessment of the size of cardiac chambers, walls, and valves is more complex in children than adults because of the wide range of ages and sizes of pediatric patients. Z scores are used to normalize values for body surface area. A Z score of 0 corresponds to the 50th percentile for body surface area, +2 to the 95th percentile and –2 to the 5th percentile. By convention, a structure (chamber or valve) is considered to be normal if the Z score is between 2 and –2. All pediatric reports should contain values and Z scores, which means that no pediatric echocardiogram is complete unless height and weight are recorded. There are several references for Z scores in pediatric echocardiography [2, 3] and the website www.parameterz.blogspot.com is an excellent resource.

Doppler echocardiography can be used to assess pressure gradients across valves and vessels using the simplified Bernoulli equation (pressure gradient = 4 × velocity^2). In general, a velocity <2 m/s corresponds to a normal gradient while a velocity >4 m/s (64 mm Hg) corresponds to a moderate-to-severe gradient. This varies based on the specific site of obstruction and clinical scenario.

Although the main focus in most pediatric patients with genetic disease is to exclude structural cardiac defects, quantitative assessment of cardiac function and hemodynamics is a routine part of any study [4]. The most common tool for measuring systolic function is ejection fraction. Ejection fraction is the difference between end-diastolic and end-systolic function divided by end-diastolic function. There are several different ways of obtaining ejection but all of these methods extrapolate data from one or two dimensions to come up with a volumetric assessment. A normal ejection fraction is between 55 and 70%, and an ejection fraction under 35% is considered severely depressed. It is important to keep in mind that although many noncardiologists who look at echocardiography reports consider cardiac function, contractility, and ejection fraction to be synonymous; this is far from the case. Preload, afterload, heart rate, wall motion, and image quality all impact ejection fraction, and it is critical to understand its limitations and not put too much weight on it. There are other more complex assessments of systolic and diastolic function that are beyond the scope of this chapter.

One of the most common questions asked of the pediatric cardiologist is to assess for pulmonary hypertension [4]. Pulmonary hypertension can be caused by a large-pressure unrestrictive communication at the ventricle or great vessel level, primary pulmonary vascular abnormalities, and/or elevation of pulmonary venous pressure (secondary to anatomy obstruction or left-ventricular diastolic dysfunction). Patients with pulmonary valve stenosis can have right-ventricular hypertension without pulmonary hypertension. Doppler of tricuspid regurgitation provides a measure of right-ventricular systolic pressure (and pulmonary artery pressure in the absence of pulmonary stenosis). When present (which is the case in 60–80% of normal patients), the Doppler velocity of tricuspid regurgitation can be converted to a pressure gradient using the modified Bernoulli equation. This gradient represents the difference between the right ventricle and the right atrium. In a patient with a tricuspid regurgitation velocity of 4 m/s, this would equate to a gradient of 64 mm Hg and a right-ventricular pressure of approximately 70 mm Hg (assuming a normal right-atrial pressure). In most cases, a tricuspid regurgitation velocity <2.5 m/s is normal and >3.0 m/s is high. Other tools to assess for pulmonary hypertension include Doppler velocity across a ventricular septal defect or patent ductus, pulmonary insufficiency Doppler and interventricular septal position. It is important to assess the pulmonary pressure in concert with the systemic pressure; the ratio may be more important than the actual number. Therefore, a cuff blood pressure is an essential part of any pediatric echocardiogram.

Echocardiography Logistics: Why, When, Where, Who

Indications

There are many indications for pediatric echocardiography; evaluation of a heart murmur, chest pain, and syncope are the most common. Concern for genetic abnormalities is also high on the list. As echocardiography has become more ubiquitous, it is expected that the majority of patients referred for evaluation of genetic disorders will get at least one echocardiogram. This is accepted as standard of care for many common genetic disorders with a high incidence of cardiovascular disease, such as trisomy 21, Turner syndrome, Noonan syndrome, Williams syndrome, and many others [5]. Is it really necessary to do echocardiograms or is clinical evaluation good enough? There are no data specifically related to genetic disease. Scholz and Kienzle [6] compared the diagnostic yield of echocardiograms ordered by pediatric cardiologists and community physicians as part of a telemedicine program in Iowa. They found no significant difference in the percentage of positive echocardiograms (85 vs. 73%) in patients under 1 year of age when ordered by a pediatric cardiologist or primary care provider. However, there was a large, statistically significant difference (75 vs. 17%) in the diagnostic yield in patients over 1 year old. This implies that in children over one year old, referral to a pediatric cardiologist for full evaluation may be more appropriate than simply ordering an echocardiogram.

Timing of Imaging

The timing of echocardiography will in part be dictated by when a genetic diagnosis is made. In some cases, pregnant mothers and children may be referred for echocardiography to help determine the likelihood of a genetic disorder (e.g. fetus with suspected trisomy 21 or older child with some features of Marfan syndrome). The transitional circulation in the newborn has important implications for the timing of echocardiography. Echocardiography will be much more informative on the 2nd or 3rd day of life than on day 1 of life in newborns who are stable but have a genetic diagnosis with a high probability of a congenital heart defect. The presence of patent ductus can mask some forms of congenital heart disease. Additionally, pulmonary-artery pressure falls precipitously over the first 24 h of life and then more gradually over the next 2–3 weeks. This normal elevation in pulmonary-artery pressure may lead to underestimation of the severity of pulmonary valve or branch stenosis or the amount of left-to-right shunting in a ventricular septal defect.

Many patients are sent for repair between 3 and 12 months of life. Imaging is usually ideal at this age, but cooperation may not be. Sedated echocardiography should strongly be considered for any child who is undergoing surgical repair in the 1st year of life (other than in the newborn period). A single normal echocardiogram is sufficient to exclude heart defects in some conditions (e.g. trisomy 21) while serial studies are needed to assess for later onset of cardiac complications in other conditions (e.g. Marfan syndrome).

Where/Who Does the Echocardiography

A complete echocardiogram is very different in children than in adults. Many babies are born in hospitals without direct access to pediatric cardiologist or certified pediatric sonographers. Many studies have shown that telemedicine can help to bridge this gap if an echocardiogram is required prior to hospital discharge [7–9]. For infants and children who are stable and referred for outpatient evaluation, it is always preferable to refer to a pediatric cardiologist than to an adult echocardiography laboratory. The pediatric cardiologist can help focus the echocardiography examination, insuring that all views are obtained during the visit. This may be especially important in uncooperative patients.

Table 1. The most common cardiac diagnoses and their associated genetic conditions that lead to echocardiography

	Most common genetic conditions/syndromes	Echocardiographic considerations
Atrial septal defect	Holt-Oram, Ellis van Creveld	Common atrium in Ellis van Creveld
Ventricular septal defect	30% of all congenital heart diseases, Holt-Oram, trisomy 21, 13, 18, Rubenstein-Taybi, VACTERL, Goldenhar	Assessment of hemodynamics is key in diagnosis and management
Atrioventricular septal defect	Trisomy 21	Assessment of atrioventricular valve position, balance and function is critical in surgical planning
Tetralogy of Fallot	22q11 deletion	Precise definition of pulmonary valve/ branches and coronary arteries most critical for surgical planning
Pulmonary stenosis	Noonan	Dysplastic pulmonary valve usually not responsive to catheterization/balloon valvuloplasty
Pulmonary artery branch stenosis	Alagille, Williams, Noonan	Diffuse pulmonary artery hypoplasia and stenoses in Alagille
Supravalvar aortic stenosis	Williams	Associated coronary artery ostial stenosis of some patients puts them at highest risk
Coarctation of the aorta	Turner	Associated bicuspid valve and ascending aorta dilatation

Common Lesions

Table 1 shows the most common cardiac diagnoses and their associated genetic conditions that lead to echocardiography.

Atrial Septal Defects

Transthoracic echocardiography is the mainstay of diagnosis of atrial septal defects. The presence of a patent foramen ovale or small atrial septal defect is almost universal in the newborn period and independent of other findings. An aneurysm of septum primum may also be present in the newborn period as a normal variant. The presence of right-ventricular volume overload is often apparent on initial parasternal long-axis images which reveal a large right ventricle even before the actual septal defect is seen. Parasternal short-axis imaging shows an enlarged right ventricle with diastolic interventricular septal flattening. The differential diagnosis of this finding includes atrial septal defects, anomalous pulmonary venous return, tricuspid regurgitation, and pulmonary insufficiency.

Although atrial septal defects may be seen from parasternal and apical windows, false positive and -negative findings may occur because the thin septum is parallel to the beam of sound. Subcostal windows provide the most specific diagnostic information about morphology, size, shape, location, and number of atrial septal defects since the transducer beam angle is perpendicular to the atrial septum. Secundum defects can be round or elliptical, central or eccentric, and single or multiple (including one or more fenestrations in septum primum). Color flow Doppler is very helpful to determine the direction and amount of shunting as well as venous abnormalities. Newer real-time transthoracic three-dimensional echocardiography transducers can provide additional information with biplane, surface-rendered, and 'en-face' views to aid in better delineating the borders of defects relative to surrounding structures (fig. 2). This information can be very important in

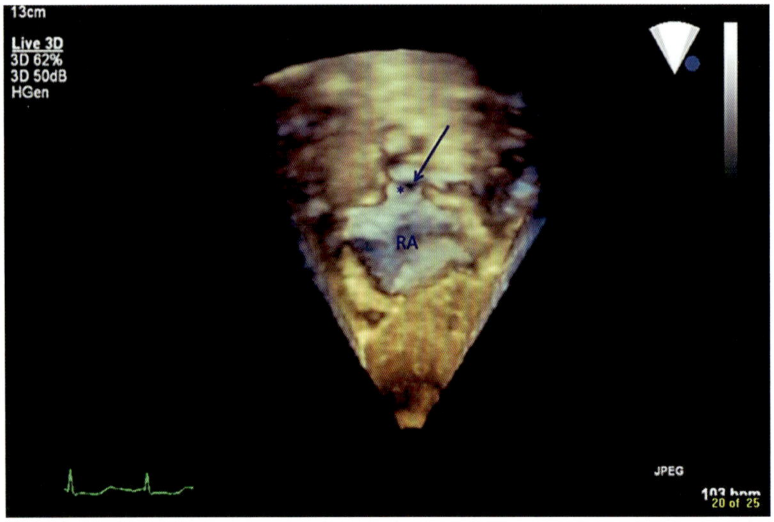

Fig. 2. Three-dimensional echocardiographic subcostal sagittal plane image as seen from the right atrium demonstrating superior sinus venosus septal defect and partial anomalous pulmonary venous return. Right upper pulmonary vein (arrow) and septal defect (asterisk) are shown. RA = Right atrium.

determining the suitability for transcatheter closure, especially in patients with large defects and concern for deficiency in the retroaortic rim.

Subcostal windows provide exquisite imaging in infants, but may be more challenging in older children. In older patients, asking the patient to inspire will significantly improve subcostal image quality. High right parasternal imaging with the transducer in near straight sagittal orientation and the patient lying on his or her right side can also provide detailed assessment of the atrial septum, including the relationship of the defect to right-pulmonary veins in sinus venosus defects.

The ratio of pulmonary to systemic blood flow can be estimated from spectral Doppler and two-dimensional assessment of the left- and right-ventricular outflow tracks. However, this estimation has some degree of error and should be interpreted in combination with other findings on echocardiography. In patients with a history of embolic stroke and suspected right-to-left atrial shunting, color-flow Doppler may not detect any shunting. Saline contrast injection through a peripheral vein may be helpful to detect a small right-to-left shunt but needs to be performed with enough volume and speed to completely opacify the right atrium. Mixing a small amount of blood or air with saline, 'agitating' the saline with two syringes and a stopcock, and having the patient Valsalva during the injection can increase the sensitivity of the test.

Transesophageal echocardiography is an excellent modality to image the atrial septum, but is rarely needed to make a primary diagnosis in children. In adults with poor transthoracic windows, it may be needed to define the anatomy of the atrial septum. Transesophageal echocardiography is more sensitive to rule out small defects and right-to-left shunts in patients with suspected cerebral embolic events. Transesophageal and intracardiac echocardiography are both used to help guide transcatheter device closure of atrial septal defects.

Cardiac MRI and CT scanning technology has dramatically improved and can provide useful information about atrial septal defects. Information about ventricular size and shunting can be obtained as well as the anatomic location of the defects. The most useful clinical scenario for cardiac MRI is in patients with abnormal pulmonary venous return.

Ventricular Septal Defects

Echocardiography is the mainstay of diagnosis of ventricular septal defects [10, 11]. Anatomy and physiology can be ascertained. Black and white and color-Doppler imaging from parasternal, apical, and subxiphoid windows is used to define the location, size, and number of defects as well as associated findings; such as tricuspid valve aneurysm tissue, aortic valve prolapse, and double-chamber right ventricle

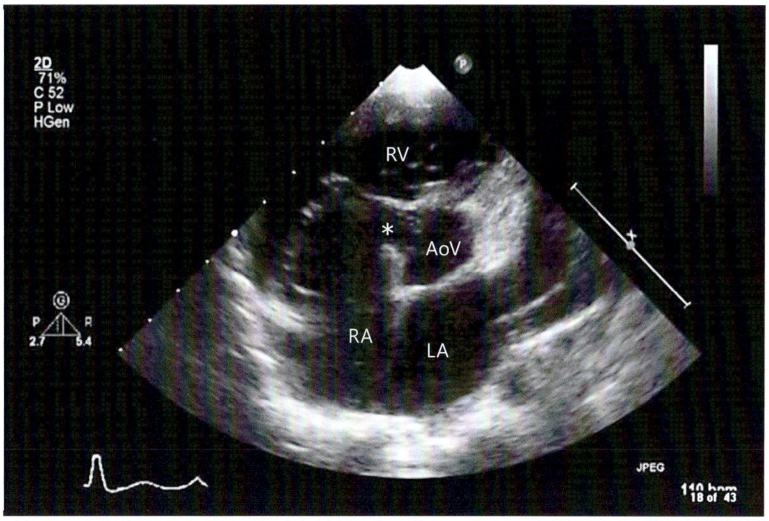

Fig. 3. Parasternal short-axis transthoracic image of a large membranous ventricular septal defect (asterisk). AoV = Aortic valve; LA = left atrium; RA = right atrium; RV = right ventricle.

[12]. The relative anterior/posterior position of each defect as well as its relation to all heart valves is very important, especially in patients who are referred for surgical repair. The morphology of multiple muscular defects may not be readily apparent until all views are assessed and a three-dimensional understanding of the defects is possible.

The distinction between perimembranous and conoseptal (supracristal or subpulmonary) defects is made by assessing the relation of the defect to the aortic, tricuspid; and pulmonary valves. On parasternal long axis and apical four-chamber views a perimembranous defect will be next to the tricuspid and aortic valves while a conoseptal defect will be closer to the pulmonary valve. On short-axis imaging, a perimembranous defect seen just inferior to the right aortic valve cusp near the tricuspid valve and right/nonaortic valve commissure (9–10 o'clock relative to the aortic valve from parasternal short axis; fig. 3). Tricuspid valve aneurysm tissue partially closing the defect is often present. A conoseptal defect is found adjacent to the pulmonary valve and right/left aortic valve commissure (12–1 o'clock relative to the aortic valve from parasternal short axis; fig. 4). There is often deficiency in or absence of conal septum in conoseptal defects, giving the appearance that the two valves are touching (instead of the normal appearance of them being separated by conal septum).

Color Doppler can be used to determine the direction of shunting, although a small amount of right-to-left shunting during isovolumic relaxation occurs in almost all defects. Spectral Doppler of flow across the ventricular septal defect, using the modified, Bernoulli equation, can be used to estimate the pressure drop across the defect when combined with a concurrent measure of systolic systemic blood pressure [13]. Tricuspid regurgitation velocity Doppler can also be used to estimate right-ventricular systolic pressure. Patients with high-velocity flow across the defect (>4 m/s) almost always have normal right-ventricular and pulmonary-artery systolic pressure.

There are pitfalls with using spectral Doppler to estimate right-ventricular and pulmonary pressure that need to be recognized. The angle of flow should be parallel to flow or the gradient may be underestimated. The amount of flow across a very small defect may not be adequate to obtain a clean envelope. Patients with large defects and low-velocity flow are likely to have near systemic or systemic pulmonary-artery systolic pressure. However, the pulmonary-artery diastolic and mean pressure may be subsystemic. Spectral Doppler represents the peak instantaneous pressure gradient across the defect. Left-ventricular pressure rises earlier in systole then the right-ventricular pressure; the peak instantaneous gradient may overestimate the true gradient and thus underesti-

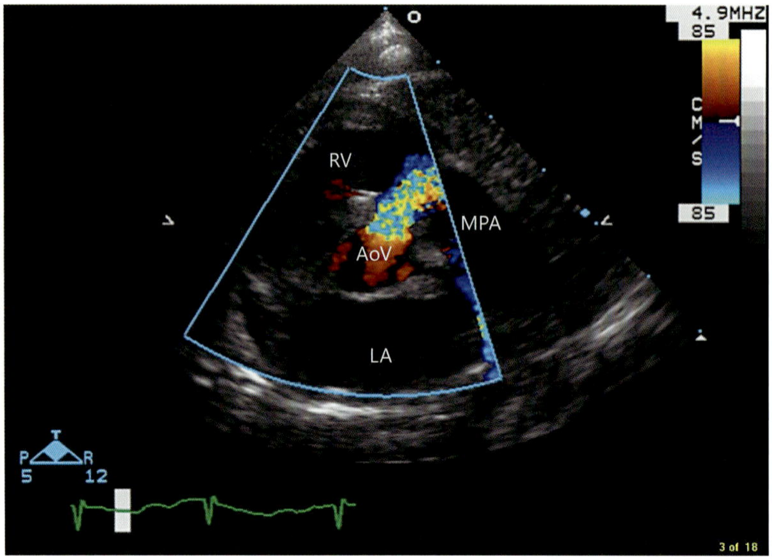

Fig. 4. Parasternal short-axis image of conoseptal ventricular septal defect showing color flow through the defect. AoV = Aortic valve; LA = left atrium; MPA = main pulmonary artery; RV = right ventricle.

mate the right-ventricular pressure. In patients with double-chambered right ventricle; a high-velocity signal may be interpreted as evidence of normal right-ventricular pressure but may actually represent mid cavity obstruction with normal pressure in the right-ventricular outflow but elevated pressure in the proximal right ventricle. Careful subxiphoid imaging of the right-ventricular outflow, especially from the sagittal short-axis plane and correlation with tricuspid-valve regurgitation velocity is important to exclude a double-chambered right ventricle. Assessment of right-ventricular outflow in postoperative patients and those with inlet ventricular septal defects may be complicated by the presence of a shunt from the left ventricle to right atrium. This may be interpreted as an elevated right-ventricular pressure when it is actually a measure of left-ventricular pressure.

Atrioventricular Septal Defects

Echocardiography is the primary mode of diagnosis for all types of atrioventricular septal defects [14–16]. The presence and size of atrial and ventricular septal defects, atrioventricular valve morphology and function, relative sizes [17] of the left and right atrium, ventricles, and atrioventricular valve components, and associated defects is clearly delineated by a combination of parasternal, apical, and subxiphoid windows. Apical four-chamber windows provide excellent details about the presence of defects and balance (fig. 5). It is important to sweep from posterior to anterior to gauge the extent of the ventricular septal defect. Color-flow Doppler helps define and quantify the degree of atrioventricular valve regurgitation. Spectral Doppler of tricuspid regurgitation may be used to estimate right-ventricular pressure, but many patients have left ventricular-to-right atrial shunts, which will cause falsely elevated estimation of right-ventricular pressure.

Subxiphoid coronal imaging at the plane of the atrioventricular valve provides a cross-sectional view of the valve leaflets and gives the best anatomic information about the valve morphology and relative distribution over each ventricle (fig. 6). The anterior leaflet can be assessed for being free floating or divided, as well as the presence or absence of attachments to the crest of the ventricular septum. Apical sweeping from this view can provide information about the number and spacing of left-ventricular papillary muscles.

Echocardiography is very important in the intra- and postoperative setting to assess for residual defects, including left ventricle-to-right atrial shunts, presence of left- and right-sided atrioventricular valve regurgitation, and subaortic obstruction. The presence of accessory atrioventricular valve tissue as well as superior displacement of the aorta can result in subaortic stenosis in a small but significant num-

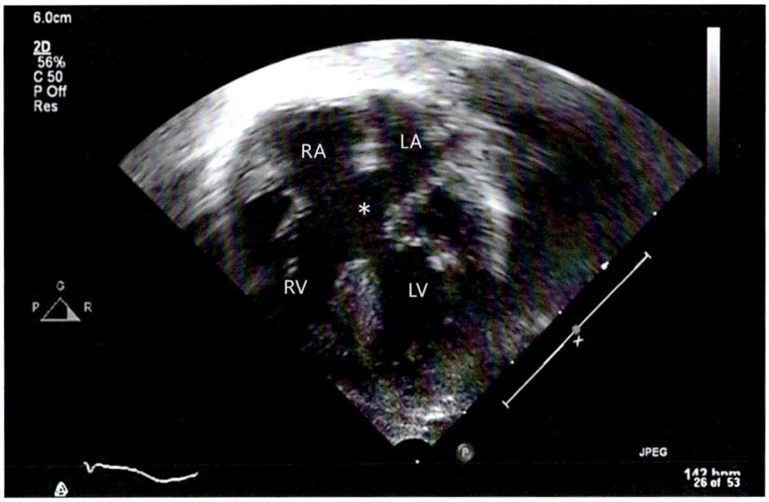

Fig. 5. Apical four-chamber transthoracic echocardiographic image of complete atrioventricular septal defect (asterisk) in diastole. LA = Left atrium; LV = left ventricle; RA = right atrium; RV = right ventricle.

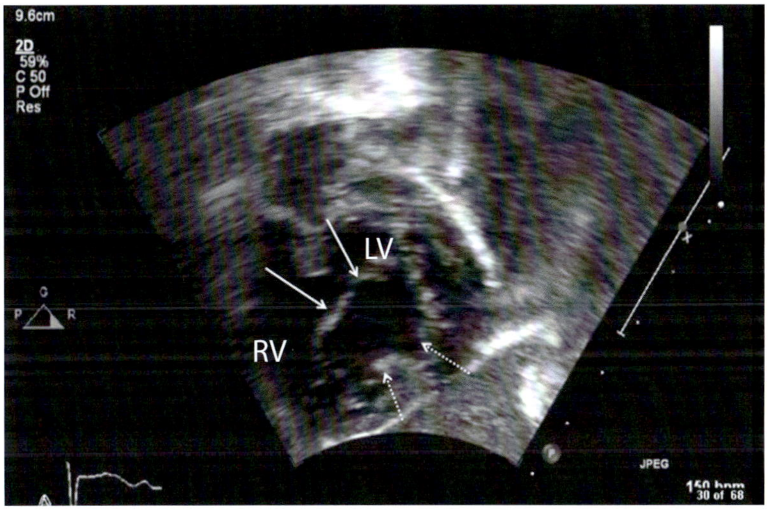

Fig. 6. Subcostal coronal plane transthoracic echocardiographic image of complete atrioventricular septal defect with undivided anterior bridging leaflet in diastole. Solid and dashed arrows show anterior and posterior atrioventricular valve leaflets, respectively. LV = Left ventricle; RV = right ventricle.

ber of patients after repair. In assessing residual left-sided atrioventricular valve regurgitation, it is important to try to assess if the leak is from a residual cleft or secondary to poor coaptation and leak through a commissure.

Patients with trisomy 21 and complete atrioventricular septal defects (see Kruszka chapter on Down syndrome p. 82) may have higher pulmonary vascular resistance than patients with similar heart defects without trisomy 21 [18]. This may be secondary to the presence of airway obstruction, central hypoventilation, and more frequent respiratory infections in patients with trisomy 21.

Tetralogy of Fallot

Tetralogy of Fallot is typically described as including the constellation of aortic override, right-ventricular outflow track obstruction, right-ventricular hypertrophy, and an anterior malalignment ventricular septal defect. Echocardiography is the primary mode of diagnosis and is usually sufficient for preoperative planning [19]. Anatomical definition of the ventricular septal defect and right-ventricular outflow is performed from all views (fig. 7). The degree of override distinguishes tetralogy of Fallot (<50%) from double-outlet right ventricle (>50%). In patients with trisomy 21, the ven-

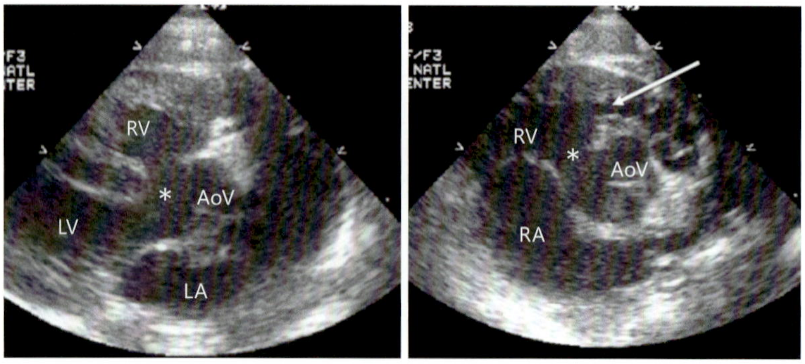

Fig. 7. Parasternal long (left)- and short (right)-axis images of tetralogy of Fallot showing anterior malaligned ventricular septal defect (asterisk) and very tight right-ventricular outflow track (arrow). AoV = Aortic valve; LA = left atrium; LV = left ventricle; RA = right atrium; RV = right ventricle.

tricular septal defect often extends to the inlet septum and can be associated with an atrioventricular septal defect, too.

There is a great degree of variability in the right-ventricular outflow obstruction. Some patients have a very discrete mid-cavity obstruction (or infundibular narrowing) while others have more diffuse tunnel-like obstruction (longer-segment infundibular narrowing). An oblique subcostal image of the right-ventricular outflow with the transducer pointing the left shoulder (between 12 and 3 o'clock), the so-called right anterior oblique or 'tet' view, is the best window to completely define the right-ventricular outflow. The pulmonary valve may be normal or stenotic, and the valve annulus itself can be hypoplastic or normal. The pulmonary branches may also be hypoplastic or have discrete stenosis. In many cases, they are in the lower range of normal. It is of critical importance to measure the pulmonary valve and branches and report as a Z score (see above). The surgeon uses these data in combination with interoperative measurements to determine whether a transannular patch or valve-sparing procedure can be performed. Spectral Doppler can define the pressure gradient across the right-ventricular outflow but this is not helpful in most cases as the definition of tetralogy of Fallot includes severe stenosis. Paradoxically, the lower the gradient the more severe the stenosis – limited pulmonary blood flow results in the inability to measure a gradient.

Other important features that are critical in preoperative planning include the presence of an atrial septal defect and coronary artery anatomy. A small atrial septal defect is often helpful in the early postoperative recovery. The thick noncompliant right ventricle can result in impaired cardiac output in the first hours and days after tetralogy of Fallot repair; the presence of a small right-to-left atrial shunt may allow a 'pop off'. This results in improved cardiac output at the expense of mild cyanosis and usually resolves as the right ventricle recovers. Approximately 5% of tetralogy of Fallot patients have an abnormal course of the left coronary artery that has a branch crossing over the right-ventricular outflow track. If this is not recognized, it may have devastating consequences at surgical repair, especially in patients who require an extensive right-ventricular outflow patch. Parasternal short-axis imaging can usually define the anatomy clearly.

Echocardiography is the mainstay of postoperative short- and intermediate-term follow-up with focus on residual ventricular septal defects, pulmonary valve and branch stenosis, and pulmonary insufficiency. MRI is the mainstay of long-term postoperative assessment of right-ventricular size and function in teenagers and adults, and MRI data are used to inform the need for pulmonary valve replacement in patients with pulmonary insufficiency [20, 21].

Pulmonary Valve Stenosis

The echocardiographic assessment of the anatomy in pulmonary valve stenosis likely has more direct impact on patient management than any other cardiac condition in individuals with genetic syndromes [22]. Patients with Noonan syndrome (see Gelb et al. chapter on Noonan syndrome p. 122) of-

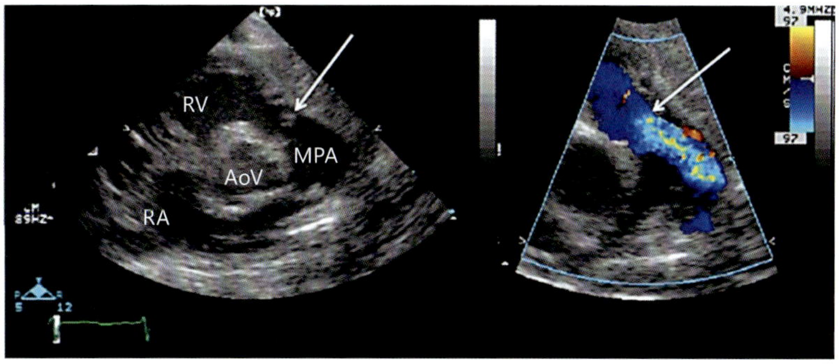

Fig. 8. Parasternal short-axis black and white (left) and color images of pulmonary valve stenosis showing doming leaflets (arrow), poststenotic main pulmonary artery dilatation, and an anteriorly directed color jet. AoV = Aortic valve; MPA = main pulmonary artery; RA = right atrium; RV = right ventricle.

Table 2. Features that should be assessed to determine likely successful catheter balloon dilation

	Good catheter candidate	Poor catheter candidate
Genetic syndrome	None	Noonan
Valve leaflets	Thin, doming, commissure fusion	Thickened, no doming
Supravalvar attachments	Absent	Present
Main pulmonary artery	Poststenotic dilatation	Normal or supravalvular narrowing
Color Doppler	Discrete color jet, often angled obliquely and anteriorly	Diffuse color Doppler jet

ten have dysplastic pulmonary valve stenosis that is unresponsive to catheter pulmonary balloon valvuloplasty and will need surgical repair [23]. Those without an underlying genetic syndrome more often have thin valve leaflets that are simply fused together and are usually treatable with balloon dilation in the catheterization laboratory (fig. 8). The pulmonary valve is best assessed from high parasternal short- and long-axis views, but it is also very well seen from the apical four-chamber window with anterior angulation. Table 2 lists the features that should be assessed to determine likely successful catheter balloon dilation.

The degree of pulmonary stenosis is assessed by the severity of the right-ventricular outflow gradient based on spectral Doppler. An estimated gradient of <30 mm Hg is usually mild and >60 mm Hg is usually severe. This may not be true in the first days of life when high pulmonary pressure can mask the severity of a gradient. In any newborn with suspected pulmonary valve stenosis, early follow-up is warranted. The presence and direction of shunting across an atrial septal defect is also an important consideration in patients with pulmonary valve stenosis and best assessed from subcostal imaging. Right-to-left shunting may indicate more severe stenosis.

Concluding Remarks

Echocardiography is almost always the first-line diagnostic test in any infant or young child with a suspected genetic diagnosis and congenital heart disease. The reader is referred to more detailed echocardiography textbooks for lesion-by-lesion descriptions of each congenital defect [24]. However, it is important for the pediatrician, neonatologist, geneticist, and anyone else who encounters these patients to have a basic understanding of the indications, timing, and limitations of echocardiography, the principles of ultrasound, and have some familiarity with recognition of the most common lesions.

References

1 Lai WW, Geva T, Shirali GS, Frommelt PC, Humes RA, Brook MM, Pignatelli RH, Rychik J: Guidelines and standards for performance of a pediatric echocardiogram: a report from the Task Force of the Pediatric Council of the American Society of Echocardiography. J Am Soc Echocardiogr 2006;19:1413–1430.

2 Olivieri L, Arling B, Friberg M, Sable C: Coronary artery Z score regression equations and calculators derived from a large heterogeneous population of children undergoing echocardiography. J Am Soc Echocardiogr 2009;22:159–164.

3 Pettersen MD, Du W, Skeens ME, Humes RA: Regression equations for calculation of z scores of cardiac structures in a large cohort of healthy infants, children, and adolescents: an echocardiographic study. J Am Soc Echocardiogr 2008;21:922–934.

4 Lopez L, Colan SD, Frommelt PC, Ensing GJ, Kendall K, Younoszai AK, Lai WW, Geva T: Recommendations for quantification methods during the performance of a pediatric echocardiogram: a report from the Pediatric Measurements Writing Group of the American Society of Echocardiography Pediatric and Congenital Heart Disease Council. J Am Soc Echocardiogr 2010;23:465–495.

5 Pierpont ME, Basson CT, Benson DW Jr, Gelb BD, Giglia TM, Goldmuntz E, McGee G, Sable CA, Srivastava D, Webb CL: Genetic basis for congenital heart defects: current knowledge: a scientific statement from the American Heart Association Congenital Cardiac Defects Committee, Council on Cardiovascular Disease in the Young: endorsed by the American Academy of Pediatrics. Circulation 2007;115:3015–3038.

6 Scholz TD, Kienzle MG: Optimizing utilization of pediatric echocardiography and implications for telemedicine. Am J Cardiol 1999;83:1645–1648.

7 Lewin M, Xu C, Jordan M, Borchers H, Ayton C, Wilbert D, Melzer S: Accuracy of paediatric echocardiographic transmission via telemedicine. J Telemed Telecare 2006;12:416–421.

8 Sable CA, Cummings SD, Pearson GD, Schratz LM, Cross RC, Quivers ES, Rudra H, Martin GR: Impact of telemedicine on the practice of pediatric cardiology in community hospitals. Pediatrics 2002;109:E3.

9 Webb CL, Waugh CL, Grigsby J, Busenbark D, Berdusis K, Sahn DJ, Sable CA: Impact of telemedicine on hospital transport, length of stay, and medical outcomes in infants with suspected heart disease: a multicenter study. J Am Soc Echocardiogr 2013;26:1090–1098.

10 Cheatham JP, Latson LA, Gutgesell HP: Ventricular septal defect in infancy: detection with two dimensional echocardiography. Am J Cardiol 1981;47:85–89.

11 Pieroni DR, Nishimura RA, Bierman FZ, Colan SD, Kaufman S, Sanders SP, Seward JB, Tajik AJ, Wiggins JW, Zahka KG: Second natural history study of congenital heart defects. Ventricular septal defect: echocardiography. Circulation 1993;87:I80–I88.

12 Hagler DJ, Edwards WD, Seward JB, Tajik AJ: Standardized nomenclature of the ventricular septum and ventricular septal defects, with applications for two-dimensional echocardiography. Mayo Clin Proc 1985;60:741–752.

13 Houston AB, Lim MK, Doig WB, Reid JM, Coleman EN: Doppler assessment of the interventricular pressure drop in patients with ventricular septal defects. Br Heart J 1988;60:50–56.

14 Minich LA, Snider AR, Bove EL, Lupinetti FM, Vermilion RP: Echocardiographic evaluation of atrioventricular orifice anatomy in children with atrioventricular septal defect. J Am Coll Cardiol 1992;19:149–153.

15 Smallhorn JF: Cross-sectional echocardiographic assessment of atrioventricular septal defect: basic morphology and preoperative risk factors. Echocardiography 2001;18:415–432.

16 Silverman NH, Zuberbuhler JR, Anderson RH: Atrioventricular septal defects: cross-sectional echocardiographic and morphologic comparisons. Int J Cardiol 1986;13:309–331.

17 Cohen MS, Jacobs ML, Weinberg PM, Rychik J: Morphometric analysis of unbalanced common atrioventricular canal using two-dimensional echocardiography. J Am Coll Cardiol 1996;28:1017–1023.

18 Hals J, Hagemo PS, Thaulow E, Sorland SJ: Pulmonary vascular resistance in complete atrioventricular septal defect. A comparison between children with and without Down's syndrome. Acta Paediatr 1993;82:595–598.

19 Silverman NH: The essential echocardiographic features of tetralogy of Fallot. Cardiol Young 2013;23:871–882.

20 Valente AM, Cook S, Festa P, Ko HH, Krishnamurthy R, Taylor AM, Warnes CA, Kreutzer J, Geva T: Multimodality imaging guidelines for patients with repaired tetralogy of Fallot: a report from the American Society of Echocardiography: developed in collaboration with the Society for Cardiovascular Magnetic Resonance and the Society for Pediatric Radiology. J Am Soc Echocardiogr 2014;27:111–141.

21 Geva T: Indications for pulmonary valve replacement in repaired tetralogy of Fallot: the quest continues. Circulation 2013;128:1855–1857.

22 Sullivan ID, Robinson PJ, Macartney FJ, Taylor JF, Rees PG, Bull C, Deanfield JE: Percutaneous balloon valvuloplasty for pulmonary valve stenosis in infants and children. Br Heart J 1985;54:435–441.

23 Burch M, Sharland M, Shinebourne E, Smith G, Patton M, McKenna W: Cardiologic abnormalities in Noonan syndrome: phenotypic diagnosis and echocardiographic assessment of 118 patients. J Am Coll Cardiol 1993;22:1189–1192.

24 Lai WW, Mertens L, Cohen MS, Geva T: Echocardiography in Pediatric and Congenital Heart Disease: From Fetus to Adult. Hoboken, Wiley-Blackwell, 2009.

Prof. Craig A. Sable
Division of Cardiology, Children's National Health System
111 Michigan Avenue, NW
Washington, DC 20010 (USA)
E-Mail csable@childrensnational.org

Muenke M, Kruszka PS, Sable CA, Belmont JW (eds): Congenital Heart Disease: Molecular Genetics, Principles of Diagnosis and Treatment. Basel, Karger, 2015, pp 269–278
DOI: 10.1159/000375223

Prenatal Evaluation of Congenital Heart Defects and Fetal Intervention

Jacqueline G. Weinberg · Anita Krishnan

Division of Cardiology, Children's National Health System, Washington, D.C., USA

Abstract

The majority of congenital heart defects (CHD) can be detected prenatally, although many patients still go undetected until after birth. The main goal of prenatal diagnosis is to improve the physical condition of the fetus and the outcome for the neonate. The ability to identify patients with cardiac lesions prenatally leads to the potential for identification of associated extracardiac abnormalities and underlying genetic etiologies. Similarly, the prenatal detection of extracardiac abnormalities or genetic derangements may provoke a fetal cardiac evaluation. The most common reason for fetal cardiac evaluation is the suspicion of a structural heart abnormality on obstetric ultrasound screening, with a rate of diagnosis of CHD as high as 70%. Fetal evaluation should also include an assessment of extracardiac abnormalities, which are seen in an estimated 37–45% of fetuses with CHD. The field of fetal intervention for CHD is still relatively young. Fetal therapies include maternal medication administration, ultrasound-guided and other minimally invasive techniques, and invasive open uterine fetal surgery.

The field of fetal cardiac diagnosis and intervention is rapidly evolving and becoming more sophisticated. The majority of congenital heart defects (CHD) can be detected prenatally, although many patients still go undetected until after birth. The ability to identify patients with cardiac lesions prenatally leads to the potential for identification of associated extracardiac abnormalities and underlying genetic etiologies. Similarly, the prenatal detection of extracardiac abnormalities or genetic derangements may provoke a fetal cardiac evaluation. Once a serious CHD is identified, it enables the health care team to better counsel the family, and, in certain cases, to improve fetal management and postnatal outcome, or prevent fetal demise. Fetal cardiac evaluation is described in this chapter, as well as the current status of fetal interventions.

Indications for Fetal Cardiac Evaluation

Indications for fetal cardiac evaluation include maternal factors, family history, or fetal factors which increase the risk for CHD above that of the

Table 1. Indications for fetal cardiac evaluation

Maternal factors
In vitro fertilization [45]
Maternal CHD [14, 46]
Cardiac teratogen [47]
Including retinoic acids, lithium, ethanol, anticonvulsants, and angiotensin-converting enzyme inhibitors
Maternal metabolic disorders
Diabetes mellitus (pregestational or diagnosed in the first trimester)
Phenylketonuria
Maternal first-trimester rubella infection or other infection with suspicion of fetal myocarditis
Maternal lupus erythematosus or Sjögren syndrome with positive SSA/SSB autoantibody [48]
Family history factors
First-degree relative with CHD [14, 46]
Previous sibling with CHD
Paternal CHD
First- or second-degree relatives with Mendelian syndrome associated with CHD [12]
Fetal factors
Extracardiac anomalies
Chromosomal [12]
Anatomic [49]
Increased nuchal fold thickness [3, 4]
Abnormality of umbilical cord, placenta or intra-abdominal venous anatomy
Fetal cardiac dysrhythmia
Persistent irregular rhythm [50]
Tachycardia (>180 b.p.m.) in the absence of amnionitis [51]
Fixed bradycardia [52]
Nonimmune hydrops fetalis or effusions (pericardial or pleural) [53]
Abnormal fetal situs
Suspected fetal heart malformation or lack of reassuring four-chamber view on screening ultrasound [54]

general population. Table 1 delineates common indications for referral.

The most common reason for fetal cardiac evaluation is the suspicion of a structural heart abnormality on obstetric ultrasound screening, with a rate of diagnosis of CHD as high as 70% [1, 2]. First-trimester nuchal translucency thickness, standardly assessed at approximately 11–13 weeks of gestation, has a high association with aneuploidy and other malformations, including CHD in chromosomally normal fetuses, and is an indication for fetal cardiac evaluation [3, 4]. The specificity can be increased with the addition of fetal echocardiographic evaluation of the ductus venosus blood flow pattern and tricuspid regurgitation [5].

Timing and Performance of Fetal Echocardiography

The timing of initial fetal echocardiography depends on the reason for referral and the gestational age at which any anomaly is detected by obstetric ultrasound screening. Generally, the initial echocardiogram is at 18–22 weeks of gestation, correlating with the timing of most routine mid-trimester obstetric ultrasound assessments. When CHD is identified, the timing of follow-up echocardiography is based on the nature and severity of the lesion and expected progression of the disease. For certain indications with the highest risks of CHD, such as a previous child with severe CHD, referral may be made earlier in gestation, including in the late first trimester and early second trimester [6].

A standard fetal echocardiogram includes M-mode, 2-dimensional and color flow imaging, and pulsed- and continuous-wave Doppler modalities (fig. 1). The components of a complete fetal echocardiogram are listed in table 2; they include evaluation of chamber size, relationships between cardiac structures, estimates of chamber pressures, assessment of cardiac rhythm, and ventricular and valvar function. Standardized Z-score measurements have been developed based on gestational age to assess the normal size of heart structures [7].

The Cardiovascular Profile Score proposed by Huhta [8] gives a measure of the overall cardiovascular health of the fetus and may predict the onset of cardiovascular decompensation.

Many new imaging technologies are now emerging to supplement fetal echocardiography, including three- and four-dimensional echocardiography, cardiovascular MRI, fetal electrocardiography, and magnetocardiography [9].

Fetal evaluation should also include an assessment of extracardiac abnormalities, which are seen

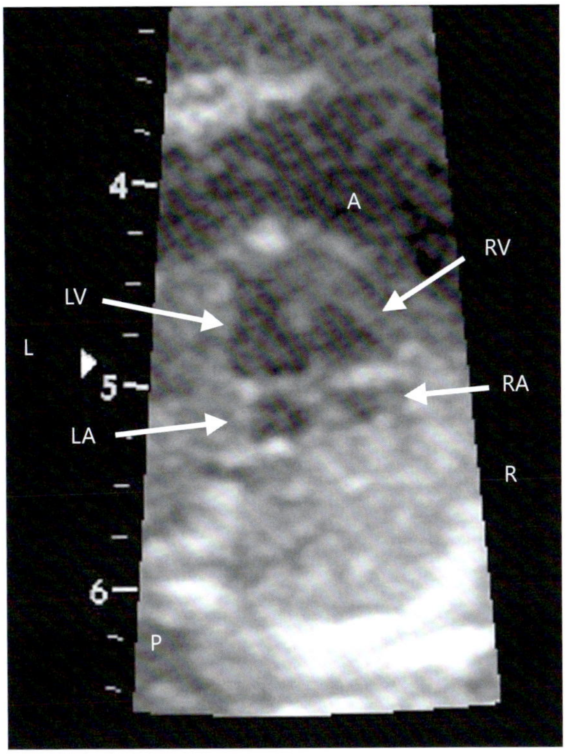

Fig. 1. First-trimester fetal cardiac evaluation. This image shows a standard four-chamber image from a fetus at 13 weeks of gestation. Four normal-sized chambers can be appreciated, with structurally normal mitral and tricuspid valves. The addition of color flow imaging allows for detection of atrioventricular valvar insufficiency or stenosis, and direction of foramen ovale flow. Abnormalities in the outflow tracts, such as transposition of the great arteries, cannot be seen on this four-chamber image. L = Left; R = right; A = anterior; P = posterior; LV = left ventricle; LA = left atrium; RV = right ventricle; RA = right atrium.

in an estimated 37–45% of fetuses with CHD [10, 11]. When CHD is identified, a thorough ultrasound examination or possibly fetal MRI should be performed [10].

Prenatal Diagnosis of Congenital Heart Defects Associated with Specific Genetic Defects

Congenital heart malformations have long been known to be associated with extracardiac anomalies, and there is an increasing body of knowledge of the genetic basis underlying these associations [11]. Based on the associations of chromosomal abnormalities in fetuses diagnosed with CHD [11], if major cardiac or visceral organ malformations are documented by prenatal ultrasound and/or fetal echocardiogram, cytogenetic testing should be considered [12, 13]. Table 3 lists chromosomal and genetic conditions associated with CHD.

Additionally, heterotaxy syndromes (see Lo et al. chapter on heterotaxy on p. 166) have been found to have a high rate of heritability, with a relative risk of recurrence 80 times higher than the population prevalence [14]. These clinical syndromes are characterized by abnormalities in laterality, with such findings on fetal echocardiography as abnormal visceral laterality, discordance in cardiac chamber laterality, and anomalous pulmonary or systemic venous drainage to the heart. If these findings are suggested by fetal cardiac evaluation, cytogenetic testing can be performed. Testable genes include *ZIC3*, *CFC1*, *ACVR2B*, *LEFTYA*, and *HTX3* [9].

Prenatal molecular testing options include amniocentesis, chorionic villus sampling, and noninvasive prenatal testing. The timing for the various testing modalities differs, which must be taken into consideration given the narrow window available for the option of termination.

Noninvasive prenatal testing modalities for common aneuploidies are now commercially available, and have emerged as a highly sensitive and specific method to detect the trisomies 21, 18 and 13, with sensitivity ranging from 59 to 100% and specificity ranging from 83 to 100% [15–17]. These tests sample maternal peripheral blood using massively parallel sequencing, which can evaluate DNA from circulating placental trophoblast tissue. Abnormalities found on these tests are an evolving indication for fetal echocardiography. These are promising for more widespread application when CHD and other major malformations are diagnosed prenatally.

Fetal Intervention

The field of fetal intervention for CHD is still relatively young. Fetal therapies include maternal medication administration, ultrasound-guided and other minimally invasive techniques, and invasive open uterine fetal surgery.

Table 2. Components of the fetal echocardiogram

2-dimensional imaging	
	Cardiac size (qualitative), axis, and position in the chest
	Right-left orientation of abdominal organs
	Systemic and pulmonary venous anatomy and connections to the heart
	Atrial size (qualitative), morphology, and location of atrial septal defect (if present)
	Relationship of atria, ventricles, and great arteries
	Tricuspid and mitral valve morphology, and quantitative and relative size
	Ventricular morphology, orientation, and quantitative and relative size
	Ventricular septal defect localization and morphology (if present)
	Pulmonary and aortic valve morphology, and quantitative and relative size
	Great artery relationship, and quantitative and relative size
	Aortic and ductal arch morphology, and position relative to trachea
	Proximal branch pulmonary arteries, and quantitative and relative size
	Assessment for pericardial effusions
Color flow map imaging	
	Tricuspid and mitral valves/ventricular inflows
	Pulmonary and aortic valves/ventricular outflows
	Aortic and ductal arches
	Ventricular and atrial septal flow
	Superior and inferior vena cavae
	Pulmonary veins
	Ductus venosus
	Proximal branch pulmonary arteries
	Umbilical artery and vein
Pulsed-wave Doppler	
	Tricuspid and mitral inflows
	Pulmonary and aortic outflows
	Ductus venosus
	Pulmonary veins
	Umbilical vein and artery
	Aortic and ductal arches
	Superior and inferior vena cavae
	Branch pulmonary arteries
	Middle cerebral Doppler
Continuous-wave Doppler	
	Valvar insufficiency (if present)
	Ventricular outflows (if abnormal pulsed-wave Doppler)
	Ductus arteriosus (if abnormal pulsed-wave Doppler)
Rhythm assessment	
	Heart rate
	Atrioventricular relationship and rhythm, mechanical atrioventricular interval
Ventricular function	
	Exclusion of hydrops and cardiomegaly
	Qualitative and quantitative assessment of ventricular function
	Examination of systemic and pulmonary venous flow pattern, and ventricular inflow pattern
	Right and left ventricular cardiac output
	Myocardial performance index
	Cardiovascular profile score

Table is based on guidelines in reference 9, Copyright Circulation 2014.

Table 3. CHD seen with common chromosomal and genetic abnormalities

Chromosomal or genetic syndrome	CHD rate, %	Common cardiac malformations	Other associated findings
Trisomy 21	40–50	AVSD, VSD, ASD common ToF, D-TGA less common	Increased nuchal thickness, macroglossia, hypoplastic fifth metacarpal, duodenal atresia, and sandal foot [55]
Trisomy 13	80	ASD, VSD, PDA, HLHS, laterality defects, and atrial isomerism	Holoprosencephaly, intrauterine growth restriction, and cleft lip and palate
Trisomy 18	90–100	ASD, VSD, PDA, ToF, DORV, D-TGA, coarctation of the aorta, bicuspid aortic valve, bicuspid pulmonary valve, and polyvalvular nodular dysplasia	Intrauterine growth restriction, clinodactyly, rocker-bottom feet, and esophageal atresia
Turner syndrome		Coarctation of the aorta and bicuspid aortic valve	Cervical cystic hygroma and pedal edema
22q11 deletion	75	IAA-B, truncus arteriosus, isolated Ao arch anomalies, ToF, VSD (perimembranous, conoseptal hypoplasia, or malalignment type)	
Noonan syndrome	60	Pulmonary valve stenosis with dysplastic leaflets, hypertrophic cardiomyopathy, and septal defects [56]	Prenatal testing can be done when the fetus is at risk for inheriting a defined *PTPN11* mutation from an affected parent [12]
Tuberous sclerosis		Intracardiac rhabdomyomas	CNS tubers may be detected by fetal brain MRI [57]
Heterotaxy		Systemic and pulmonary venous anomalies, congenitally corrected TGA, complex conotruncal defects, and septal defects	Ciliary dysfunction, abnormal abdominal organ laterality, gastrointestinal malrotation, and biliary atresia [12]

Ao = Aorta; ASD = atrial septal defect; AVSD = atrioventricular septal defect; DORV = double-outlet right ventricle; IAA-B = interruption of the aortic arch type B; PDA = patent ductus arteriosus; TGA = transposition of the great arteries; ToF = tetralogy of Fallot; VSD = ventricular septal defect.

Medical therapy can be used to manage fetal arrhythmias, such as atrial flutter or other supraventricular tachycardias. In certain cases, maternal administration of antiarrhythmic medication, with transplacental transfer to the fetus, can control the tachyarrhythmia. Other examples include maternal administration of steroids attempt to mitigate cardiovascular damage from anti-SSA or anti-SSA antibodies [18, 19].

Fetal cardiac catheter intervention was first described by Maxwell et al. [20] in 1991. Fetal cardiac intervention aims to improve the cardiac morphology and function to alter the natural history of a lesion such that it is either lifesaving to the fetus or results in an improved state at birth with reduction in short- or long-term morbidity or mortality.

The first and most well-described target for intervention is balloon dilatation of the aortic valve (fig. 2) in critical aortic stenosis (AS) in select patients thought to be evolving to hypoplastic left-heart syndrome (HLHS) [20–22]. Through relief of the AS, the procedure aims to halt or reverse ongoing myocardial damage, facilitating growth of left heart structures, and prevent the development of

6

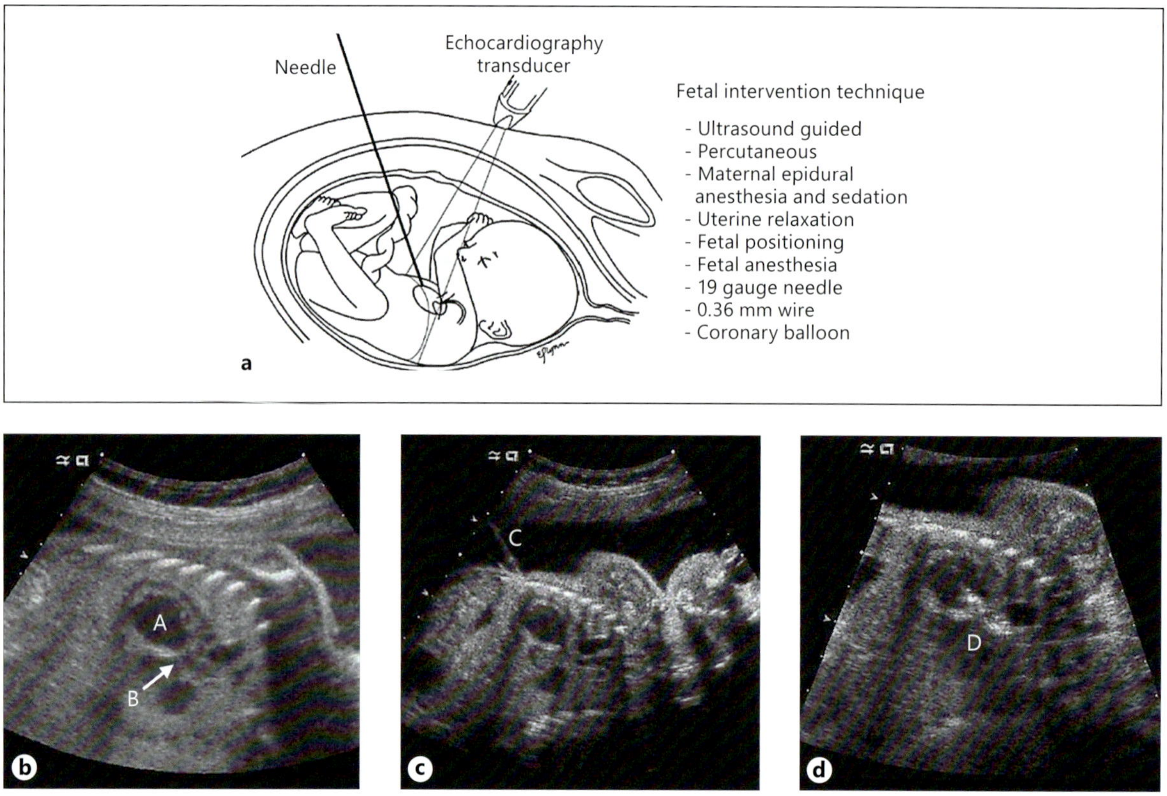

Fig. 2. Fetal cardiac intervention. This image shows the technique of fetal balloon aortic valvuloplasty, as well as images of the procedure. **a** Fetal intervention technique. **b** Echocardiographic images of a fetus at 26 weeks of gestation with critical AS with concern for evolving HLHS. The left ventricle appears dilated. The aortic valve is stenotic with thickened leaflets. A = Left ventricle; B = aortic valve. **c** The catheter is inserted through the uterus and fetal chest wall, directed through the dilated left ventricle towards the stenotic aortic valve. C = Needle. **d** A balloon is positioned over a wire through the fetal aortic valve and inflated. D = Balloon positioned across the aortic valve. Images used with permission from Wayne Tworetzky.

HLHS (fig. 3). Several groups have reported results, with the largest series reporting approximately one third of technically successful procedures leading to a biventricular outcome [23]. At present, it remains limited to a few centers and primarily a research protocol.

Other lesions have been targeted since that time, including balloon atrial septostomy in HLHS with intact atrial septum [24], critical AS with mitral regurgitation, giant left atrium and hydrops [25], and balloon pulmonary valvuloplasty in critical pulmonary stenosis or atresia with hypoplastic right-heart syndrome [26].

Fetal bradycardia and hemopericardium are common complications of fetal catheter interventions [21, 26, 27]. Although fetal cardiac interventions hold much promise, these procedures have not gained wide acceptance due to concerns about safety and efficacy [28, 29], and as standard postnatal palliative therapies are still an option in most situations. These procedures require substantial resources and interdisciplinary personnel to be safely and effectively performed.

Invasive fetal intervention, through hysterotomy and exposure of the fetus, or through laparoscopic techniques with a closed uterus, may be indicated for extracardiac anomalies, again if the procedure can save the life of the fetus or alter the natural history of a condition to improve postnatal outcome [30]. Examples of fetal surgical interventions currently offered include those for large congenital cystic adenomatoid malformations with signs of hydrops [31], giant sacrococcygeal teratomas [32], severe congenital diaphragmatic hernia [33], and meningomyeloceles [34].

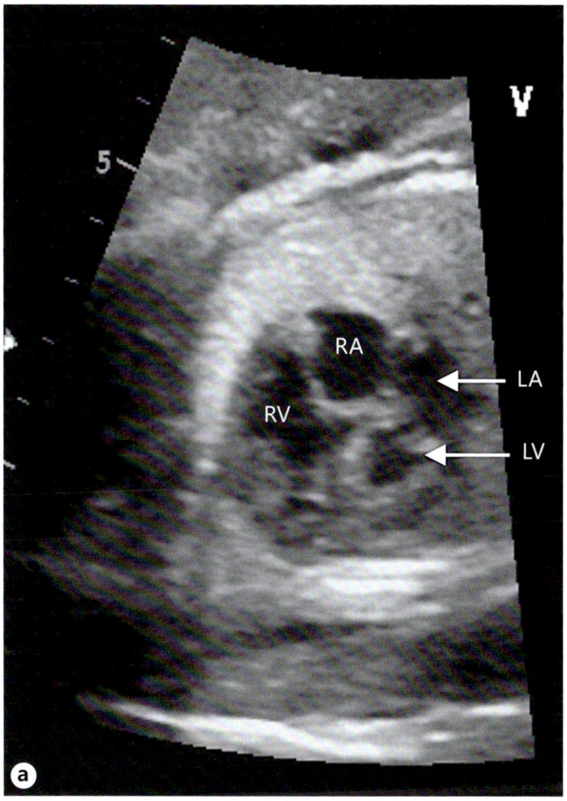

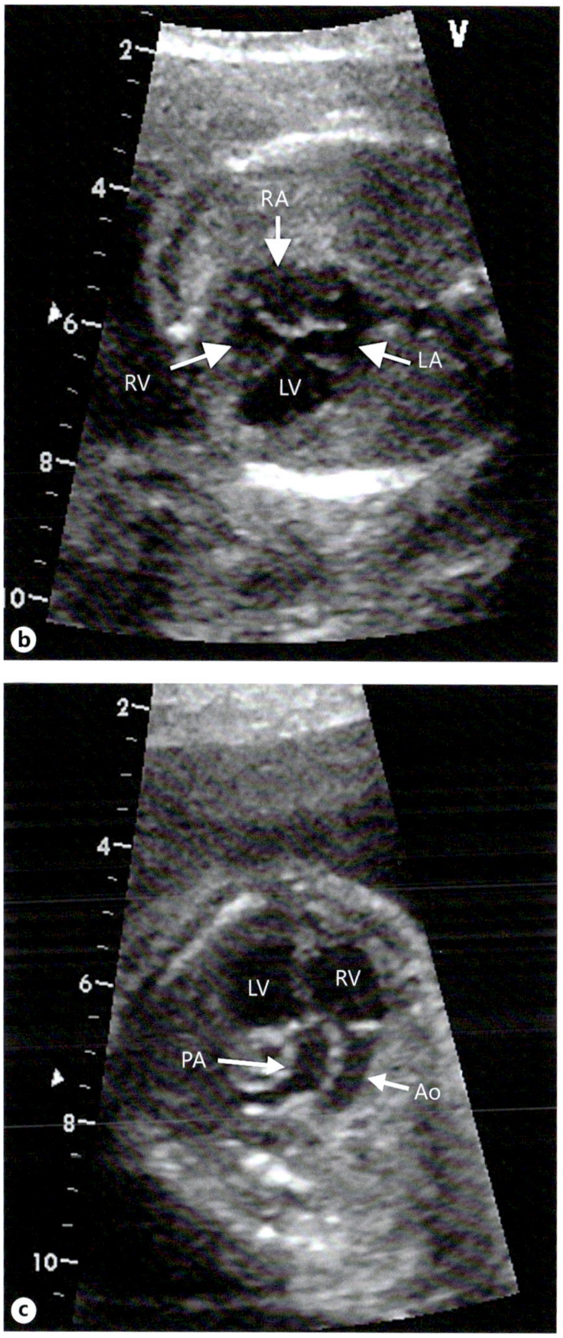

Fig. 3. Prenatal diagnosis of CHD. RA = Right atrium; RV = right ventricle; LA = left atrium; LV = left ventricle; Ao = aorta; PA = pulmonary artery. **a** HLHS: this fetus is at 33 weeks of gestation. The mitral valve is thick and severely stenotic with a hypoplastic left ventricle. **b** Hypoplastic right heart syndrome: this fetus is at 26 weeks of gestation. **c** Transposition of the great arteries: this fetus is at 22 weeks of gestation. The outflow tracts are seen coming from the right and left ventricles parallel to each other, instead of crossing as seen in a normal heart.

Importance of Fetal Diagnosis and Outcomes following Prenatal Detection of Congenital Heart Defects

The main goal of prenatal diagnosis is to improve the physical condition of the fetus and the outcome for the neonate. It also has important implications for the emotional well-being of the family, allowing additional time for counseling. Prenatal diagnosis can allow decisions to be made about the location of delivery, such as at or near a medical center with capabilities for specialized care and neonatal intervention, or specialized delivery room care [35]. Referral can also be made for possible fetal intervention when applicable.

Several studies have now shown an improvement in the preoperative status in neonates diagnosed prenatally, including less frequent and less severe acidosis [36–39], a lower incidence of ventricular dysfunction [38], a lower need for inotropic support [38] or intubation [40], and decreased preoperative neurologic insult [41]. A possible benefit in longer-term neurologic outcomes has also been described [36].

Despite these advances in preoperative status, data on mortality have been mixed. While some studies have shown an overall mortality benefit [37, 38, 42], others have shown no difference [39–41, 43], or even worse outcomes [44]. It is possible that the apparent lack of a benefit in outcome is due to the fact that prenatal diagnosis identifies those patients with more severe phenotypes and at higher risk for a poor outcome. Additionally, prior studies have not captured patients without a prenatal diagnosis who may die prior to arriving at the tertiary-care site.

It remains to be seen what effect the recent recommendation for universal newborn pulse oximetry screening will have on the outcome of those diagnosed with CHD. The implementation of this recommendation also aims to improve detection of those with CHD prior to clinical decompensation or irreversible damage. Despite the additional benefit that this will likely bring to overall outcomes and rates of CHD detection, we continue to strive for improved rates of prenatal detection through improved referral, improved echocardiographic techniques and equipment, as well as optimization of delivery planning.

References

1 Simpson LL: Indications for fetal echocardiography from a tertiary-care obstetric sonography practice. J Clin Ultrasound 2004;32:123–128.
2 Copel JA, Kleinman CS: The impact of fetal echocardiography on perinatal outcome. Ultrasound Med Biol 1986;12:327–335.
3 Nicolaides KH, Heath V, Cicero S: Increased fetal nuchal translucency at 11–14 weeks. Prenat Diagn 2002;22:308–315.
4 Makrydimas G, Sotiriadis A, Huggon IC, Simpson J, Sharland G, Carvalho JS, Daubeney PE, Ioannidis JP: Nuchal translucency and fetal cardiac defects: a pooled analysis of major fetal echocardiography centers. Am J Obstet Gynecol 2005;192:89–95.
5 Papatheodorou SI, Evangelou E, Makrydimas G, Ioannidis JP: First-trimester ductus venosus screening for cardiac defects: a meta-analysis. BJOG 2011;118:1438–1445.
6 Moon-Grady A, Shahanavaz S, Brook M, Rodriguez H, Hornberger LK: Can a complete fetal echocardiogram be performed at 12 to 16 weeks' gestation? J Am Soc Echocardiogr 2012;25:1342–1352.
7 Schneider C, McCrindle BW, Carvalho JS, Hornberger LK, McCarthy KP, Daubeney PE: Development of Z-scores for fetal cardiac dimensions from echocardiography. Ultrasound Obstet Gynecol 2005;26:599–605.
8 Huhta JC: Fetal congestive heart failure. Semin Fetal Neonatal Med 2005;10:542–552.
9 Donofrio MT, Moon-Grady AJ, Hornberger LK, Copel JA, Sklansky MS, Abuhamad A, Cuneo BF, Huhta JC, Jonas RA, Krishnan A, Lacey S, Lee W, Michelfelder EC Sr, Rempel GR, Silverman NH, Spray TL, Strasburger JF, Tworetzky W, Rychik J: Diagnosis and treatment of fetal cardiac disease: a scientific statement from the American Heart Association. Circulation 2014;129:2183–2242.
10 Song MS, Hu A, Dyamenahalli U, Chitayat D, Winsor EJ, Ryan G, Smallhorn J, Barrett J, Yoo SJ, Hornberger LK: Extracardiac lesions and chromosomal abnormalities associated with major fetal heart defects: comparison of intrauterine, postnatal and postmortem diagnoses. Ultrasound Obstet Gynecol 2009;33:552–559.
11 Paladini D, Calabro R, Palmieri S, D'Andrea T: Prenatal diagnosis of congenital heart disease and fetal karyotyping. Obstet Gynecol 1993;81:679–682.
12 Pierpont ME, Basson CT, Benson DW Jr, Gelb BD, Giglia TM, Goldmuntz E, McGee G, Sable CA, Srivastava D, Webb CL: Genetic basis for congenital heart defects: current knowledge: a scientific statement from the American Heart Association Congenital Cardiac Defects Committee, Council on Cardiovascular Disease in the Young: endorsed by the American Academy of Pediatrics. Circulation 2007;115:3015–3038.
13 Wimalasundera RC, Gardiner HM: Congenital heart disease and aneuploidy. Prenat Diagn 2004;24:1116–1122.
14 Oyen N, Poulsen G, Boyd HA, Wohlfahrt J, Jensen PK, Melbye M: Recurrence of congenital heart defects in families. Circulation 2009;120:295–301.
15 Lau TK, Cheung SW, Lo PS, Pursley AN, Chan MK, Jiang F, Zhang H, Wang W, Jong LF, Yuen OK, Chan HY, Chan WS, Choy KW: Non-invasive prenatal testing for fetal chromosomal abnormalities by low-coverage whole-genome sequencing of maternal plasma DNA: review of 1982 consecutive cases in a single center. Ultrasound Obstet Gynecol 2014;43:254–264.
16 Song Y, Liu C, Qi H, Zhang Y, Bian X, Liu J: Noninvasive prenatal testing of fetal aneuploidies by massively parallel sequencing in a prospective Chinese population. Prenat Diagn 2013;33:700–706.
17 Mersy E, Smits LJ, van Winden LA, de Die-Smulders CE, Paulussen AD, Macville MV, Coumans AB, Frints SG: Noninvasive detection of fetal trisomy 21: systematic review and report of quality and outcomes of diagnostic accuracy studies performed between 1997 and 2012. Hum Reprod Update 2013;19:318–329.
18 Trucco SM, Jaeggi E, Cuneo B, Moon-Grady AJ, Silverman E, Silverman N, Hornberger LK: Use of intravenous gamma globulin and corticosteroids in the treatment of maternal autoantibody-mediated cardiomyopathy. J Am Coll Cardiol 2011;57:715–723.

19 Friedman DM, Kim MY, Copel JA, Llanos C, Davis C, Buyon JP: Prospective evaluation of fetuses with autoimmune-associated congenital heart block followed in the PR interval and dexamethasone evaluation (PRIDE) study. Am J Cardiol 2009;103: 1102–1106.
20 Maxwell D, Allan L, Tynan MJ: Balloon dilatation of the aortic valve in the fetus: a report of two cases. Br Heart J 1991;65:256–258.
21 Tworetzky W, Wilkins-Haug L, Jennings RW, van der Velde ME, Marshall AC, Marx GR, Colan SD, Benson CB, Lock JE, Perry SB: Balloon dilation of severe aortic stenosis in the fetus: potential for prevention of hypoplastic left heart syndrome: candidate selection, technique, and results of successful intervention. Circulation 2004;110:2125–2131.
22 Arzt W, Wertaschnigg D, Veit I, Klement F, Gitter R, Tulzer G: Intrauterine aortic valvuloplasty in fetuses with critical aortic stenosis: experience and results of 24 procedures. Ultrasound Obstet Gynecol 2011;37: 689–695.
23 McElhinney DB, Marshall AC, Wilkins-Haug LE, Brown DW, Benson CB, Silva V, Marx GR, Mizrahi-Arnaud A, Lock JE, Tworetzky W: Predictors of technical success and postnatal biventricular outcome after in utero aortic valvuloplasty for aortic stenosis with evolving hypoplastic left heart syndrome. Circulation 2009;120:1482–1490.
24 Marshall AC, Levine J, Morash D, Silva V, Lock JE, Benson CB, Wilkins-Haug LE, McElhinney DB, Tworetzky W: Results of in utero atrial septoplasty in fetuses with hypoplastic left heart syndrome. Prenat Diagn 2008;28:1023–1028.
25 Rogers LS, Peterson AL, Gaynor JW, Rome JJ, Weinberg PM, Rychik J: Mitral valve dysplasia syndrome: a unique form of left-sided heart disease. J Thorac Cardiovasc Surg 2011;142:1381–1387.
26 Tworetzky W, McElhinney DB, Marx GR, Benson CB, Brusseau R, Morash D, Wilkins-Haug LE, Lock JE, Marshall AC: In utero valvuloplasty for pulmonary atresia with hypoplastic right ventricle: techniques and outcomes. Pediatrics 2009;124:e510–e518.
27 Mizrahi-Arnaud A, Tworetzky W, Bulich LA, Wilkins-Haug LE, Marshall AC, Benson CB, Lock JE, McElhinney DB: Pathophysiology, management, and outcomes of fetal hemodynamic instability during prenatal cardiac intervention. Pediatr Res 2007;62:325–330.
28 Kleinman CS: Fetal cardiac intervention: innovative therapy or a technique in search of an indication? Circulation 2006;113:1378–1381.
29 Latson LA: Aortic valvuloplasty in the fetus: technically possible but is it ready for prime time? J Pediatr 2005;147:424–426.
30 Adzick NS: Open fetal surgery for life-threatening fetal anomalies. Semin Fetal Neonatal Med 2010;15:1–8.
31 Szwast A, Tian Z, McCann M, Donaghue D, Bebbington M, Johnson M, Wilson RD, Rychik J: Impact of altered loading conditions on ventricular performance in fetuses with congenital cystic adenomatoid malformation and twin-twin transfusion syndrome. Ultrasound Obstet Gynecol 2007;30:40–46.
32 Hedrick HL, Flake AW, Crombleholme TM, Howell LJ, Johnson MP, Wilson RD, Adzick NS: Sacrococcygeal teratoma: prenatal assessment, fetal intervention, and outcome. J Pediatr Surg 2004;39:430–438; discussion 430–438.
33 Jani JC, Nicolaides KH, Gratacos E, Valencia CM, Done E, Martinez JM, Gucciardo L, Cruz R, Deprest JA: Severe diaphragmatic hernia treated by fetal endoscopic tracheal occlusion. Ultrasound Obstet Gynecol 2009;34:304–310.
34 Adzick NS, Thom EA, Spong CY, Brock JW 3rd, Burrows PK, Johnson MP, Howell LJ, Farrell JA, Dabrowiak ME, Sutton LN, Gupta N, Tulipan NB, D'Alton ME, Farmer DL: A randomized trial of prenatal versus postnatal repair of myelomeningocele. N Engl J Med 2011;364:993–1004.
35 Donofrio MT, Levy RJ, Schuette JJ, Skurow-Todd K, Sten MB, Stallings C, Pike JI, Krishnan A, Ratnayaka K, Sinha P, duPlessis AJ, Downing DS, Fries MI, Berger JT: Specialized delivery room planning for fetuses with critical congenital heart disease. Am J Cardiol 2013;111:737–747.
36 Calderon J, Angeard N, Moutier S, Plumet MH, Jambaque I, Bonnet D: Impact of prenatal diagnosis on neurocognitive outcomes in children with transposition of the great arteries. J Pediatr 2012;161:94.e1–98.e1.
37 Bonnet D, Coltri A, Butera G, Fermont L, Le Bidois J, Kachaner J, Sidi D: Detection of transposition of the great arteries in fetuses reduces neonatal morbidity and mortality. Circulation 1999;99:916–918.
38 Tworetzky W, McElhinney DB, Reddy VM, Brook MM, Hanley FL, Silverman NH: Improved surgical outcome after fetal diagnosis of hypoplastic left heart syndrome. Circulation 2001;103:1269–1273.
39 Sivarajan V, Penny DJ, Filan P, Brizard C, Shekerdemian LS: Impact of antenatal diagnosis of hypoplastic left heart syndrome on the clinical presentation and surgical outcomes: the Australian experience. J Paediatr Child Health 2009;45:112–117.
40 Levey A, Glickstein JS, Kleinman CS, Levasseur SM, Chen J, Gersony WM, Williams IA: The impact of prenatal diagnosis of complex congenital heart disease on neonatal outcomes. Pediatr Cardiol 2010;31:587–597.
41 Mahle WT, Clancy RR, McGaurn SP, Goin JE, Clark BJ: Impact of prenatal diagnosis on survival and early neurologic morbidity in neonates with the hypoplastic left heart syndrome. Pediatrics 2001;107:1277–1282.
42 Franklin O, Burch M, Manning N, Sleeman K, Gould S, Archer N: Prenatal diagnosis of coarctation of the aorta improves survival and reduces morbidity. Heart 2002;87:67–69.
43 Landis BJ, Levey A, Levasseur SM, Glickstein JS, Kleinman CS, Simpson LL, Williams IA: Prenatal diagnosis of congenital heart disease and birth outcomes. Pediatr Cardiol 2013;34:597–605.
44 Wright LK, Ehrlich A, Stauffer N, Samai C, Kogon B, Oster ME: Relation of prenatal diagnosis with one-year survival rate for infants with congenital heart disease. Am J Cardiol 2014;113:1041–1044.
45 Koivurova S, Hartikainen AL, Gissler M, Hemminki E, Sovio U, Jarvelin MR: Neonatal outcome and congenital malformations in children born after in-vitro fertilization. Hum Reprod 2002;17:1391–1398.
46 Burn J, Brennan P, Little J, Holloway S, Coffey R, Somerville J, Dennis NR, Allan L, Arnold R, Deanfield JE, Godman M, Houston A, Keeton B, Oakley C, Scott O, Silove E, Wilkinson J, Pembrey M, Hunter AS: Recurrence risks in offspring of adults with major heart defects: results from first cohort of British collaborative study. Lancet 1998;351:311–316.
47 Jenkins KJ, Correa A, Feinstein JA, Botto L, Britt AE, Daniels SR, Elixson M, Warnes CA, Webb CL: Noninherited risk factors and congenital cardiovascular defects: current knowledge: a scientific statement from the American Heart Association Council on Cardiovascular Disease in the Young: endorsed by the American Academy of Pediatrics. Circulation 2007;115: 2995–3014.
48 Buyon JP, Hiebert R, Copel J, Craft J, Friedman D, Katholi M, Lee LA, Provost TT, Reichlin M, Rider L, Rupel A, Saleeb S, Weston WL, Skovron ML: Autoimmune-associated congenital heart block: demographics, mortality, morbidity and recurrence rates obtained from a national neonatal lupus registry. J Am Coll Cardiol 1998; 31:1658–1666.
49 Tennstedt C, Chaoui R, Korner H, Dietel M: Spectrum of congenital heart defects and extracardiac malformations associated with chromosomal abnormalities: results of a seven year necropsy study. Heart 1999;82: 34–39.
50 Copel JA, Liang RI, Demasio K, Ozeren S, Kleinman CS: The clinical significance of the irregular fetal heart rhythm. Am J Obstet Gynecol 2000;182:813–817; discussion 817–819.

6

51 Fouron JC, Fournier A, Proulx F, Lamarche J, Bigras JL, Boutin C, Brassard M, Gamache S: Management of fetal tachyarrhythmia based on superior vena cava/aorta Doppler flow recordings. Heart 2003;89:1211–1216.
52 Schmidt KG, Ulmer HE, Silverman NH, Kleinman CS, Copel JA: Perinatal outcome of fetal complete atrioventricular block: a multicenter experience. J Am Coll Cardiol 1991;17:1360–1366.
53 Kleinman CS, Donnerstein RL, DeVore GR, Jaffe CC, Lynch DC, Berkowitz RL, Talner NS, Hobbins JC: Fetal echocardiography for evaluation of in utero congestive heart failure. N Engl J Med 1982;306:568–575.
54 Carvalho JS, Mavrides E, Shinebourne EA, Campbell S, Thilaganathan B: Improving the effectiveness of routine prenatal screening for major congenital heart defects. Heart 2002;88:387–391.
55 Allen HD, Driscoll DJ, Shaddy RE, et al: Moss and Adams' Heart Disease in Infants, Children, and Adolescents: Including the Fetus and Young Adult, ed 8. Philadelphia, Wolters Kluwer Health/Lippincott Williams & Wilkins, 2013.
56 Sharland M, Burch M, McKenna WM, Paton MA: A clinical study of Noonan syndrome. Arch Dis Child 1992;67:178–183.
57 Tworetzky W, McElhinney DB, Margossian R, Moon-Grady AJ, Sallee D, Goldmuntz E, van der Velde ME, Silverman NH, Allan LD: Association between cardiac tumors and tuberous sclerosis in the fetus and neonate. Am J Cardiol 2003;92:487–489.

Dr. Anita Krishnan
Division of Cardiology, Children's National Health System
111 Michigan Avenue NW, Suite WW 3-200
Washington, DC 20010 (USA)
E-Mail akrishna@childrensnational.org

7 Treatment

Muenke M, Kruszka PS, Sable CA, Belmont JW (eds): Congenital Heart Disease: Molecular Genetics, Principles of Diagnosis and Treatment. Basel, Karger, 2015, pp 280–288
DOI: 10.1159/000375224

Surgical Management

John P. Costello · Richard A. Jonas · Dilip S. Nath

Division of Cardiac Surgery, Children's National Medical Center, Washington, D.C., USA

Abstract

Congenital heart disease often requires surgical management for both cure and palliation of a large variety of cardiac abnormalities. The common association between genetic syndromes, including trisomy 21, DiGeorge syndrome, and Turner syndrome among others, and congenital heart defects makes an understanding of the general principles involved in operative repair an important topic for all clinicians focusing on the care of congenital heart disease. As atrioventricular canal defects, septal defects, and tetralogy of Fallot are frequently encountered in many of these patients, techniques and outcomes of operative repair for these lesions will be discussed. The use of mechanical circulatory support and heart transplantation in these unique patient populations will also be covered. Overall, surgical intervention for the treatment of congenital heart disease in the setting of comorbid genetic syndromes remains an integral component of the comprehensive management plan of these complex patients.

As congenital heart disease (CHD) is frequently associated with a wide range of genetic syndromes, it is imperative for CHD specialists to appreciate the variety of anomalies that exist and how these anomalies impact cardiac surgical care both inside and outside of the operating room. In addition, the great diversity that is present within this patient population poses unique surgical challenges that the congenital cardiac surgeon must grasp in breadth and depth. This discussion will focus on identifying key patient differences among these genetic syndromes from the operative and perioperative perspectives to help elucidate the key components of optimal surgical management.

Trisomy 21 – Down Syndrome

Trisomy 21 is the most frequent identifiable cause of mental retardation and has a high association with CHD (see Kruszka chapter on Down syndrome p. 82)[1]. The pediatric cardiologist and congenital cardiac surgeon encounter patients with Down syndrome on a regular basis. The most common cardiac abnormalities seen in Down syndrome are atrioventricular (AV) canal defects, atrial septal defects (ASD), ventricular septal defects (VSD), and tetralogy of Fallot. Tetralogy and AV canal defects can coexist and represent a particularly challenging anomaly.

There are a number of comorbidities associated with Down syndrome that increase the difficulty in managing these patients at the time of cardiac surgery. Upper-airway crowding often results in difficulty with both in- and extubation. Atlanto-occipital cervical spine instability can further complicate anesthesia maneuvers. Tracheal stenosis and increased airway secretions often lead to lobar- or whole-lung atelectasis. There is a higher risk of early labile and fixed pulmonary hypertension. Although many studies have documented that Down syndrome is a risk factor for early mortality after cardiac surgery [2], this has not been a universal finding [1]. However, it is important to recognize that Down syndrome has been identified as a significant risk factor for many perioperative events in the setting of cardiac (heart) surgery (CHS), in particular the development of AV block specifically following closure of a perimembranous VSD, although this block is likely due to the anatomy of the defect rather than the genetic syndrome alone [1]. In addition, clinicians must remain mindful in the perioperative period of other medical concerns that occur with higher frequency in patients with trisomy 21, including respiratory disease, infections, and immune disorders [1].

From a surgical perspective, it has been reported that patients with Down syndrome who undergo repair of a complete AV canal have higher perioperative and late cardiac mortality compared to nonsyndromic patients [3, 4]. However, some reports have suggested that outcomes may be similar for Down syndrome and nonsyndromic patients with other forms of CHD [3, 4]. Nevertheless, there are some situations where the pulmonary hypertension associated with Down syndrome can be a contraindication for a specific cardiac surgical procedure, such as the Fontan operation, although this potential contraindication has not yet been well elucidated [5, 6]. Given that patients with Down syndrome are at risk for complete AV canal defects, the cardiologist and surgeon must appreciate that a Rastelli type C valve is often present. The Rastelli classification separates AV canal defects into three subtypes that are useful when describing surgical approaches. The type C valve is described as 'free floating' due to its superior bridging leaflet that is not attached to the ventricular septum at its midpoint; appreciation of this anatomy is crucial in planning optimal correction [7].

Various technical approaches have been described for the surgical management of complete AV canal defects (also known as AV septal defects). In the classic single-patch approach, the superior and inferior common valve leaflets are incised over the crest of the septum if they are Rastelli type C. If Rastelli type A is present, the superior common leaflet is naturally divided allowing a patch to be attached to the crest of the ventricular septum (fig. 1). The AV valve tissue is resuspended on the pericardial patch to develop separate right- and left-sided valves analogous to a tricuspid and mitral valve. The primum ASD is closed with the same pericardial patch. Great care must be taken in suturing the lower edge of the patch in the region of the AV node and bundle of His, which are displaced in this anomaly.

Alternative approaches to the traditional single-patch technique include the two-patch technique, in which separate patches are used to close the ASD and VSD components of the complete AV canal. In the 'Australian technique' or 'modified single patch' described by Nunn, the AV valve tissue is brought down to the crest of the ventricular septum, thereby obliterating the VSD component (fig. 2). Operative streaming videos depicting these procedures are available in the second edition of *Comprehensive*

Fig. 1. Traditional single-patch repair of complete AV canal. This anomaly is very common in patients with Down syndrome. Repair involves closure of VSD, ASD, and creation of two separate AV valves from the original single common AV valve. TV = Tricuspid valve; MV = mitral valve; RBB = right bundle branch; LBB = left bundle branch; RV = right ventricle; LV = left ventricle. **a** Apposition of the superior and inferior common leaflets is determined. Single suture placed through these leaflets to maintain accurate leaflet coaptation. **b** Superior and inferior common leaflets are incised. **c** Autologous pericardial patch sutured to the middle of the ventricular septum. **d** Bundle of His enters the ventricular septum close to the AV node, making it vulnerable to injury. **e, f** Superior and inferior leaflets are resuspended on the pericardial patch. **g** Closure of the cleft of the new mitral valve. **h** Closure of the primum ASD component of the complete AV canal.

(*For figure see next page.*)

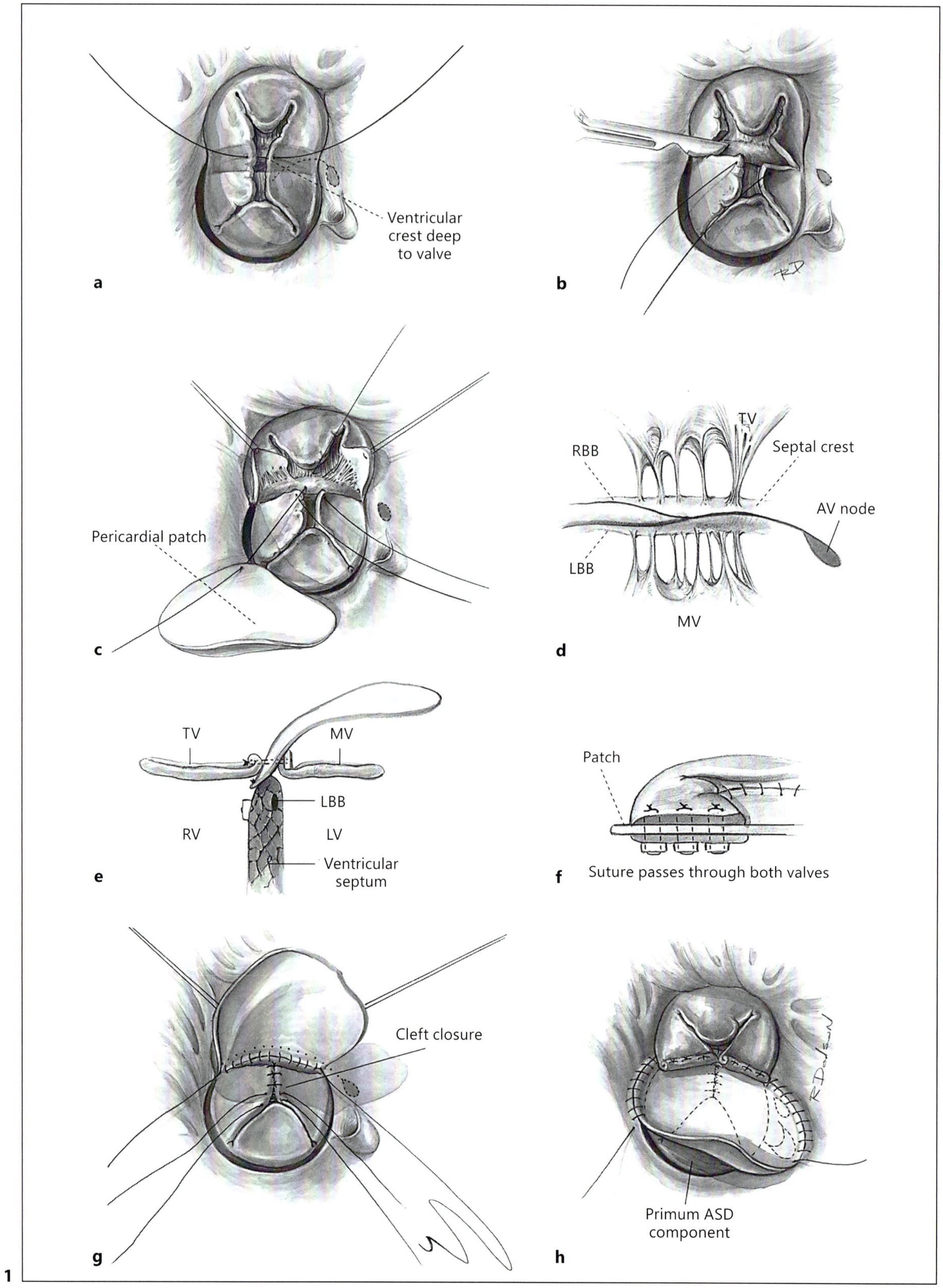

Ventricular crest deep to valve
a
b
Pericardial patch
c
TV
RBB
Septal crest
AV node
LBB
MV
d
TV
MV
LBB
RV
LV
Ventricular septum
e
Patch
Suture passes through both valves
f
Cleft closure
g
Primum ASD component
h

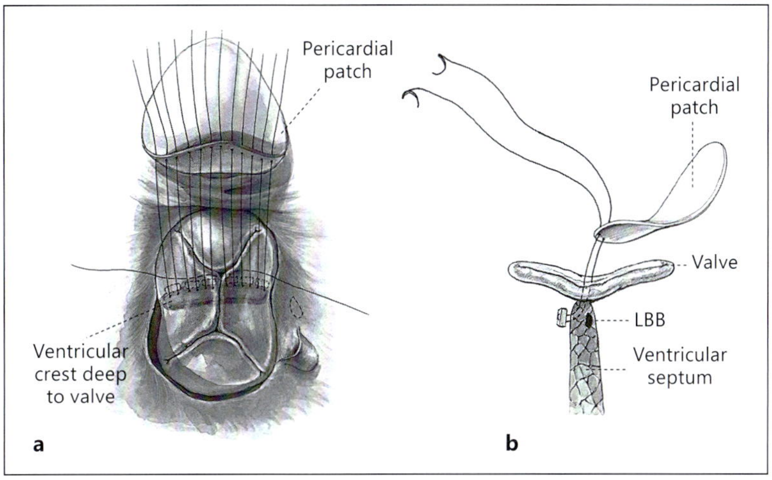

Fig. 2. The modified single-patch technique ('Australian technique') involves bringing the common AV valve down to the crest of the septum, thereby obliterating the VSD component. The pericardial patch reinforces the valve repair and is also used to close the ASD component of the complete AV canal defect. **a** Multiple sutures passed through the superior and inferior common leaflets and then through the pericardial patch. **b** Tying these sutures brings the common AV valve leaflets down to the crest of the septum. LBB = Left bundle branch.

Surgical Management of Congenital Heart Disease [8].

One additional consideration that medical professionals must be mindful of is the cost of hospitalization and surgical care for any patient, especially when evaluating the goals of care and treatment. When looking at the cost of cardiac care, at least one study has suggested that the hospital costs for providing cardiac surgery to Down syndrome patients with CHD are no different than the cost of care for CHS patients without diagnosed genetic syndromes [1].

The 22q11.2 Deletion – DiGeorge Syndrome

The most common congenital heart abnormalities seen in patients with the 22q11.2 deletion are conotruncal heart defects, including tetralogy of Fallot, pulmonary atresia with VSD, truncus arteriosus, interrupted aortic arch, isolated anomalies of the aortic arch, and VSD (see Goldmuntz chapter on 22q11.2 deletion syndrome on p. 100) [9]. As for Down syndrome, there is a high incidence of significant developmental delay. The risk of surgical management for DiGeorge syndrome patients varies depending on the nature of the underlying congenital heart lesion. In patients with tetralogy of Fallot, the presence of the 22q11.2 deletion does not worsen the surgical prognosis [9]. However, in patients with pulmonary atresia and VSD as well as interrupted aortic arch, the 22q11.2 deletion is a risk factor for surgical management [9].

Corrective cardiac surgery is commonly performed in the neonatal period or during the 1st year of life in the majority of DiGeorge syndrome infants with large VSD or conotruncal defects [10]. Lability of serum calcium can present a major challenge both intraoperatively as well as in the early postoperative period. Even without the parathyroid dysfunction that can characterize the DiGeorge syndrome, calcium management can be challenging in the neonate undergoing cardiopulmonary bypass. This is mainly a consequence of the large load of citrated blood and blood products that chelate free calcium. However, the inflammatory effects of bypass probably also play a role in calcium instability. Generally, calcium management is not a problem in the postoperative management of the patient with DiGeorge syndrome.

Following successful repair, it is important to recognize the occurrence of complications at later follow-up. Interestingly, late problems consequent to the immune deficiency that is a component of DiGeorge syndrome are not often seen by the cardiac team and are rarely an indication for readmission. However, after surgical repair of a interrupted aortic arch type B, aortic recoarctation and recurrence of left-ventricular outflow tract obstruction may be encountered [10]. Patients with truncus arteriosus who have undergone complete surgical repair may experience truncal valve stenosis or regurgitation, which may necessitate surgical reintervention [10]. In addition, the surgical burden that these patients experience is often increased due to the frequent need for surgical revision of the conduit connecting the branch pulmonary arteries to the right ventricle [10]. These potential surgical complications are seen not only following truncus arteriosus repair but can also occur in patients with tetralogy of Fallot as a result of recurrent right-sided obstruction [10]. When a transannular patch has been utilized in the original tetralogy of Fallot repair, pulmonary insufficiency and subsequent right-ventricular dilation and dysfunction can develop, which may necessitate replacement of the pulmonary valve [11]. All of these procedures, including primary repair and any subsequent cardiac operations, are notably more challenging in patients with the 22q11.2 deletion, as these patients are more likely than their nonsyndromic counterparts to have critically small pulmonary arteries and pulmonary blood supply predominantly from aortopulmonary collateral vessels [12].

Apart from specific operative considerations, there are other differences in surgical outcomes between DiGeorge syndrome and nonsyndromic patients. In particular, it has been demonstrated that patients with DiGeorge syndrome and either tetralogy of Fallot/pulmonary atresia or interrupted aortic arch type B have a greater risk of surgical mortality [13], and the 5-year survival rate in patients with tetralogy of Fallot/pulmonary atresia is lower [14]. In addition, it is important for the congenital cardiac surgeon and anesthesiology team to recognize that pediatric DiGeorge syndrome patients undergoing CHS have been found to have a greater incidence of poor direct laryngoscopic views at the time of intubation compared to nonsyndromic patients [15]. Of note, patients less than 1 year of age were significantly more likely to have poor direct laryngoscopic views compared to older patients [15]. In this same study, Down syndrome was not found to be associated with poor direct laryngoscopic views [15]. On the whole, pediatric cardiac surgery has an incidence of difficult laryngoscopy that is twice as high as in other fields of pediatric surgery [15].

Trisomy 13 (Patau Syndrome) and Trisomy 18 (Edwards Syndrome)

Patients with trisomies 13 and 18 are known to have significantly shortened lifespans in the setting of multiple congenital abnormalities. Until recently, patients with the Patau and Edwards syndrome and concomitant CHD were not routinely offered surgical repair due to their short expected lifespans and poor prognoses (see Boss and Shapiro chapter on Ethical Considerations in Congenital Heart Disease p. 301). However, recent reports have demonstrated encouraging outcomes following surgical repair of CHD in these patients and have put the focus on how surgical repair can help maximize the overall quality of life that these patients experience [16].

The most common forms of CHD that are seen in patients with trisomies 13 and 18 include VSD, ASD, and patent ductus arteriosus (PDA), although other critical cardiac anomalies are also seen. A recent retrospective study utilizing the Pediatric Cardiac Care Consortium registry provided great insight into the outcomes of these patient populations [16]. Upon review of this database, 35 patients with trisomy 13 (n = 11) or trisomy 18 (n = 24) who underwent CHS over an 18-year period were identified. The majority of these patients had VSD, but multiple cardiac lesions were also present in most patients. The surgical repair techniques utilized ranged from palliative approaches to complete repair, and resulted in a 91% hospital survival rate. These data demonstrate that the preponderance of patients with the Patau and Edwards syndromes can in fact survive palliative and corrective heart surgeries.

As studies have now shown that central apnea is the primary cause of death in these patients, this particular study also evaluated the occurrence of and need for preoperative mechanical ventilation. This analysis revealed that trisomy 13 and 18 patients who required less than or equal to 2 days or no mechanical ventilation preoperatively were unlikely to require prolonged ventilation following surgery, with 100% of these patients achieving successful extubation prior to hospital discharge [16].

Overall, the question still remains regarding what type of surgery should be offered to these patients, namely palliative procedures or complete surgical repair? Given these recent study findings, at present we advocate for and offer complete surgical repair of CHD to nearly all patients with the Patau or Edwards syndrome for whom operative intervention is indicated from the cardiovascular perspective.

Marfan Syndrome

Cardiovascular abnormalities are present in a majority of patients with Marfan syndrome (see Bondy chapter on Turner syndrome on p. 91). Although most of the morbidity from Marfan syndrome is manifested from the adolescent years to adults, clinically apparent morbidity can also affect young children. In pediatric Marfan syndrome, clinical cardiac abnormalities of syndromic etiology are most commonly the result of severe mitral valve prolapse and regurgitation [17]. This mitral regurgitation can be so severe that it leads to congestive heart failure, even in infants [10]. As a result, children with Marfan syndrome and clinically symptomatic mitral regurgitation may require operative mitral valve repair early in life [10]. In addition, these children are at risk for dilation of the root of the aorta, although vascular dissection remains an infrequent occurrence before the adolescent years [10]. If aortic dissection occurs prior to adolescence, it is of utmost importance to verify the Marfan syndrome diagnosis as the Loeys-Dietz syndrome could also be a possible causative etiology [18].

Prior to the availability of modern surgical therapeutic approaches, cardiovascular complications were the major contributor to mortality in patients with the Marfan syndrome [10]. As the surgical management of the Marfan syndrome has improved dramatically in recent years, this has enabled Marfan patients to achieve long-term survival [10]. Regardless of the course of care a particular Marfan patient has received, it is imperative that the adult with Marfan syndrome is actively managed by a cardiovascular disease specialist with frequent clinical and imaging follow-up [10, 19]. Criteria for replacement of the aortic root in Marfan syndrome patients are clearly established, and operative aortic intervention is well tolerated [19]. However, practitioners must be aware that the risk of recurrent aneurysm and redissection of the aorta in Marfan syndrome patients is much higher than that seen in patients with other aortic diseases [19].

Turner Syndrome

Turner syndrome is classically associated with coarctation of the aorta, but recent imaging studies have shown that elongation of the transverse aortic arch (and the potential for pseudocoarctation) and other vascular abnormalities also occur in these patients (see Bondy chapter on Turner syndrome on p. 91) [20, 21]. From a surgical perspective, it has been reported that the aortic wall in pediatric Turner syndrome patients with coarctation is friable, leading to a higher risk of hemorrhage after stent implantation and at the time of surgery [22–24]. Specifically in hypoplastic left-heart syndrome, although there are conflicting reports regarding whether or not the presence of Turner syndrome is a risk factor for operative mortality, Turner syndrome has been shown to be a predictor of inferior outcomes mid-term [25].

Although aortic dissection and rupture can occur in Turner syndrome patients with aortic dilation (even early in life), it is crucial to appreciate that Turner syndrome is an independent risk factor for aortic dissection itself, as dissection can occur in the absence of systemic hypertension and CHD in Turner syndrome patients [26]. In addition, these patients frequently have prominent lymph nodes within the chest that surgeons must be careful to avoid. Due to these lymphatic structures, Turner syndrome patients are at risk for the development of chylothoraces following cardiac or thoracic surgery.

Noonan Syndrome

As the great majority of Noonan syndrome patients have comorbid cardiac anomalies [10], it is common for this patient population to require expert medical and surgical cardiac evaluation. Pediatric patients with Noonan syndrome frequently have pulmonary valve stenosis, and, in certain children, this stenosis can be associated with dysplastic valve leaflets that result in severe obstruction of the right-ventricular outflow tract [10] (see Gelb et al. chapter on Noonan syndrome on p. 122). Nonsurgical, percutaneous balloon valvuloplasty of these dysplastic valve leaflets can be of great benefit in reducing this obstruction; however, surgical intervention is often required. The specific surgical approach utilized in these patients is usually excision of the dysplastic valve leaflets [10]. Valvotomy alone is rarely adequate because of the bulky, thickened nature of the valve leaflets. Placement of a transannular patch may be needed if there is concomitant annular hypoplasia.

It is important to recognize that 20–30% of pediatric patients with Noonan syndrome have comorbid hypertrophic cardiomyopathy [10]. The hypertrophic cardiomyopathy seen in Noonan syndrome is recognized as an entity that is clinically and macroscopically distinct from familial hypertrophic cardiomyopathy, even though tissue analysis of both entities reveals similar histologic findings, namely myocyte fiber disarray; oftentimes the right ventricle is affected, and pulmonary stenosis and other cardiac abnormalities may occur [10]. As these patients may require surgery to relieve ventricular outflow tract obstruction, this macroscopic difference has direct and important surgical implications as a different surgical approach needs to be undertaken in patients with Noonan syndrome to address the right-sided abnormalities. Branch pulmonary stenosis can also occur in Noonan syndrome. As the constraints of the mediastinum limit what can be accessed during cardiac surgery in these patients, it may not be possible to address the stenotic branch pulmonary arteries while in the operating room. This may result in the need for a combined sequential open surgical and percutaneous catheterization approach to correct this stenosis in these patients.

Other Syndromes

There are many other genetic syndromes in which congenital heart anomalies often coexist. Although CHD is rarely seen in patients with isolated Klinefelter syndrome, a variety of lesions can still be encountered [27, 28]. A notable case of double aortic arch in a patient with the combined Down-Klinefelter syndrome has even been reported [29]. When looking at conotruncal cardiac defects outside of the Down syndrome and 22q11.2 deletion populations, syndromes such as the Cantrell and Alagille syndromes, and the VACTERL association are considered to increase the risk of surgical intervention [1]. Given the overall clinical variety among these relatively uncommon syndromes, surgical management of CHD in these patients may need to be handled on a more individual basis.

Special Considerations

Despite clear differences in outcomes among these genetic syndromes in relation to CHD, it is important to recognize that survival also varies when considering specific cardiac lesions, tetralogy of Fallot in particular. In a study of 306 consecutive pediatric patients who underwent primary or staged tetralogy of Fallot repair, it was demonstrated that patients with comorbid genetic syndromes had decreased long-term (10-year) survival compared to nonsyndromic patients. In addition, genetic syndromes other than the 22q11.2 deletion and Down syndrome were found to have negative impacts on tetralogy of Fallot surgical outcomes [30]. Overall, patients with any genetic abnormality in the setting of tetralogy of Fallot were found to have less freedom from reintervention following operative repair compared to nonsyndromic patients [30]. Most important, given that the probability of survival 10 years after primary tetralogy of Fallot repair is 90% in patients with genetic syndromes with normal anatomy of the pulmonary arteries, these findings support the notion that a genetic syndrome alone should not be preclusive for primary surgical repair in these patients [30]. The authors concluded that performing primary tetralogy of Fallot repair in patients with genetic syndromes in the setting of normal pulmonary arterial anatomy is a valid surgical approach that does not increase the risk of mortality and results in a higher freedom from procedural reintervention compared to nonsyndromic patients [30].

A controversial topic in the surgical management of patients with CHD in the setting of genetic syndromes is the use of heart transplantation and mechanical circulatory support (MCS), particularly in syndromes with associated cognitive impairment. In the most recent summary statement from the American Heart Association (AHA) regarding the indications for heart transplantation in pediatric patients, the presence of a genetic syndrome is not considered an outright contraindication to transplantation [31]. Likewise, the 2013 International Society for Heart and Lung Transplantation guidelines for MCS do not directly limit its use in patients with genetic syndromes [32]; however, a recent AHA scientific statement on the use of MCS does include impaired cognitive function as a relative contraindication to durable MCS [33]. However, when considering trisomy 21, for example, where there is a wide range of cognitive and functional capacities, there is documented evidence of the successful use of heart transplantation and MCS (specifically, the use of ventricular assist devices) in both pediatric and adult Down syndrome patients for heart failure treatment [34, 35]. However, as overall evidence-based data are lacking and as the diversity that exists among these genetic syndromes is substantial, the current consensus remains that these therapies should be considered on a case-by-case basis following comprehensive evaluation of each individual patient.

References

1 Formigari R, Michielon G, Digilio MC, et al: Genetic syndromes and congenital heart defects: how is surgical management affected? Eur J Cardiothorac Surg 2009;35:606–614.
2 Patel SS, Burns TL, Kochilas L: Early outcomes and prognostic factors for left atrioventricular valve reoperation after primary atrioventricular septal defect repair. Pediatr Cardiol 2012;33:129–140.
3 Marino B, Diociaiuti L, Calcagni G, Mastroiacovo P: Outcome in Down syndrome fetuses with cardiac anomalies. Am J Med Genet 2004;128A:101–102.
4 Reller MD, Morris CD: Is Down syndrome a risk factor for poor outcome after repair of congenital heart defects? J Pediatr 1998;132:738–741.
5 Fiore AC, Turrentine M, Rodefeld M, et al: Fontan operation: a comparison of lateral tunnel with extracardiac conduit. Ann Thorac Surg 2007;83:622–629.
6 Jacobs ML, Pelletier GJ, Pourmoghadam KK, et al: Protocols associated with no mortality in 100 consecutive Fontan procedures. Eur J Cardiothorac Surg 2008;33:626–632.
7 Shiokawa Y, Becker AE: The left ventricular outflow tract in atrioventricular septal defect revisited: surgical considerations regarding preservation of aortic valve integrity in the perspective of anatomic observations. J Thorac Cardiovasc Surg 1997;114:586–593.
8 Jonas RA: Comprehensive Surgical Management of Congenital Heart Disease, ed 2. Boca Raton, CRC Press, 2014.
9 Carotti A, Digilio MC, Piacentini G, Saffirio C, Di Donato RM, Marino B: Cardiac defects and results of cardiac surgery in 22q11.2 deletion syndrome. Dev Disabil Res Rev 2008;14:35–42.
10 Lin AE, Basson CT, Goldmuntz E, et al: Adults with genetic syndromes and cardiovascular abnormalities: clinical history and management. Gen Med 2008;10:469–494.
11 McElhinney DB, Clark BJ 3rd, Weinberg PM, et al: Association of chromosome 22q11 deletion with isolated anomalies of aortic arch laterality and branching. J Am Coll Cardiol 2001;37:2114–2119.
12 Carotti A, Marino B, Di Donato RM: Influence of chromosome 22q11.2 microdeletion on surgical outcome after treatment of tetralogy of Fallot with pulmonary atresia. J Thorac Cardiovasc Surg 2003;126:1666–1667.
13 Anaclerio S, Di Ciommo V, Michielon G, et al: Conotruncal heart defects: impact of genetic syndromes on immediate operative mortality. Ital Heart J 2004;5:624–628.
14 Mahle WT, Crisalli J, Coleman K, et al: Deletion of chromosome 22q11.2 and outcome in patients with pulmonary atresia and ventricular septal defect. Ann Thorac Surg 2003;76:567–571.
15 Heinrich S, Birkholz T, Ihmsen H, et al: Incidence and predictors of poor laryngoscopic view in children undergoing pediatric cardiac surgery. J Cardiothorac Vasc Anesth 2013;27:516–521.
16 Graham EM, Bradley SM, Shirali GS, Hills CB, Atz AM, Pediatric Cardiac Care Consortium: Effectiveness of cardiac surgery in trisomies 13 and 18 (from the Pediatric Cardiac Care Consortium). Am J Cardiol 2004;93:801–803.
17 Morse RP, Rockenmacher S, Pyeritz RE, et al: Diagnosis and management of infantile Marfan syndrome. Pediatrics 1990;86:888–895.
18 Loeys BL, Chen J, Neptune ER, et al: A syndrome of altered cardiovascular, craniofacial, neurocognitive and skeletal development caused by mutations in TGF-BR1 or TGFBR2. Nat Genet 2005;37:275–281.
19 Baumgartner H, Bonhoeffer P, De Groot NM, et al: ESC Guidelines for the management of grown-up congenital heart disease (new version 2010). Eur Heart J 2010;31:2915–2957.
20 Bechtold SM, Dalla Pozza R, Becker A, Meidert A, Dohlemann C, Schwarz HP: Partial anomalous pulmonary vein connection: an underestimated cardiovascular defect in Ullrich-Turner syndrome. Eur J Pediatr 2004;163:158–162.
21 Ho VB, Bakalov VK, Cooley M, et al: Major vascular anomalies in Turner syndrome: prevalence and magnetic resonance angiographic features. Circulation 2004;110:1694–1700.
22 Brandt B 3rd, Heintz SE, Rose EF, Ehrenhaft JL, Clark EB: Repair of coarctation of the aorta in children with Turner syndrome. Pediatr Cardiol 1984;5:175–177.
23 Fejzic Z, van Oort A: Fatal dissection of the descending aorta after implantation of a stent in a 19-year-old female with Turner's syndrome. Cardiol Young 2005;15:529–531.
24 Ravelo HR, Stephenson LW, Friedman S, et al: Coarctation resection in children with Turner's syndrome: a note of caution. J Thorac Cardiovasc Surg 1980;80:427–430.
25 Gaynor JW, Mahle WT, Cohen MI, et al: Risk factors for mortality after the Norwood procedure. Eur J Cardiothorac Surg 2002;22:82–89.
26 Carlson M, Silberbach M: Dissection of the aorta in Turner syndrome: two cases and review of 85 cases in the literature. J Med Genet 2007;44:745–749.

27 Adatia I, Coe JY, Harder J: Transposition of the great arteries in a neonate with Klinefelter's syndrome. Pediatr Cardiol 1987;8: 285–286.

28 Rosenthal A: Cardiovascular malformations in Klinefelter's syndrome: report of three cases. J Pediatr 1972;80:471–473.

29 Gerretsen MF, Peelen W, Rammeloo LA, Koolbergen DR, Hruda J: Double aortic arch with double aneuploidy – rare anomaly in combined Down and Klinefelter syndrome. Eur J Pediatr 2009;168:1479–1481.

30 Michielon G, Marino B, Formigari R, et al: Genetic syndromes and outcome after surgical correction of tetralogy of Fallot. Ann Thorac Surg 2006;81:968–975.

31 Canter CE, Shaddy RE, Bernstein D, et al: Indications for heart transplantation in pediatric heart disease: a scientific statement from the American Heart Association Council on Cardiovascular Disease in the Young; the Councils on Clinical Cardiology, Cardiovascular Nursing, and Cardiovascular Surgery and Anesthesia; and the Quality of Care and Outcomes Research Interdisciplinary Working Group. Circulation 2007; 115:658–676.

32 Feldman D, Pamboukian SV, Teuteberg JJ, et al: The 2013 International Society for Heart and Lung Transplantation Guidelines for mechanical circulatory support: executive summary. J Heart Lung Trans 2013;32:157–187.

33 Peura JL, Colvin-Adams M, Francis GS, et al: Recommendations for the use of mechanical circulatory support: device strategies and patient selection: a scientific statement from the American Heart Association. Circulation 2012;126:2648–2667.

34 Irving CA, Chaudhari MP: Cardiovascular abnormalities in Down's syndrome: spectrum, management and survival over 22 years. Arch Dis Child 2012;97:326–330.

35 Nunes AJ, Buchholz H, Sinnadurai S, MacArthur RG: Long-term mechanical circulatory support of an adult patient with Down syndrome. Ann Thorac Surg 2012; 93:1305–1307.

Dr. Richard A. Jonas
Division of Cardiac Surgery, Children's National Medical Center
111 Michigan Avenue NW
Washington, DC 20010 (USA)
E-Mail rjonas@childrensnational.org

Muenke M, Kruszka PS, Sable CA, Belmont JW (eds): Congenital Heart Disease: Molecular Genetics, Principles of Diagnosis and Treatment. Basel, Karger, 2015, pp 289–297
DOI: 10.1159/000375225

Interventional Cardiology

Gareth J. Morgan · Shakeel A. Qureshi

Evelina London Children's Hospital, Guy's and St. Thomas' NHS Foundation Trust, London, UK

Abstract

The development of interventional techniques and practice in congenital cardiology has progressed significantly over the last 20 years. Various elements have contributed to the growth in this new field, including antenatal diagnosis, surgical and interventional techniques, intensive care medicine and tertiary-care collaborative research networks. These factors have created a huge pool of patients with residual structural defects and chronic pathophysiological morbidity, which has demanded the development of interventional cardiology. Paediatric interventional catheterisation is a rapidly developing subspecialty with new techniques and technologies coming through at a steady pace. This chapter describes exciting developments in interventional cardiac catheterisation in paediatric cardiology, neonatal intervention, infant and paediatric procedures, stent technology, fetal intervention and hybrid techniques.

Interventional Cardiac Catheterisation in Paediatric Cardiology

The development of interventional techniques and practice in congenital cardiology can be attributed to many factors over the last 20 years. Congenital heart disease in infants and children in the developed world has changed from a high-mortality condition to a low-mortality, high-morbidity condition; as such, survival into adulthood has become the expected norm even in patients with the most severe malformations. Various elements have contributed to this shift in demographics, including antenatal diagnosis, surgical and interventional techniques, intensive care medicine and tertiary-care collaborative research networks.

These factors have created a huge pool of patients with residual structural defects and chronic pathophysiological morbidity, which has demanded the development of our subspecialty. As we react and respond to these demands, we have also continued to be proactive, developing alternate techniques to cardiopulmonary bypass surgery using interventional as well as hybrid techniques and combining surgical and interventional skills at the same operating table.

We will discuss a number of standard interventional procedures in the context of age ranges and then look at some of the more cutting-edge technologies in interventional congenital catheterisation.

Neonatal Intervention

The application of interventional techniques in the neonatal period (<4 weeks old) is limited due to the size mismatch between interventional equipment and the babies who require treatment. Despite this, huge steps forward in intensive care for sick neonates have allowed percutaneous intervention to be the primary intervention in many pathologies [1]. A few examples are given below.

Atrial Septostomy

Although it may seem counter-intuitive to intentionally create or enlarge a defect in a child's heart, there is a diverse range of cardiac conditions in which allowing free flow of blood between the left and right atria is beneficial. The most common indication for atrial septostomy is in transposition of the great arteries. In this condition, the pulmonary and systemic circulations run in parallel to each other disallowing oxygenated blood returning from the lungs to find its way into the systemic circulation. An unrestrictive septal communication is vital to allow stability for the baby prior to surgical correction [2].

The most common technique for achieving a septostomy involves the passage of a catheter via femoral venous access. Patience and technique then allow manipulation of a balloon-tipped catheter up the inferior vena cava, into the right atrium then across the septum into the left atrium. Here, the balloon is inflated, before briskly withdrawing it across the septum, tearing the septum to allow free communication of the blood from one side to the other. Access can also be achieved via the umbilical vein in the cord stump in babies where the umbilical vessels can still be instrumented. This allows a relatively easy approach angle towards the atrial septum. Unlike most other interventional procedures, septostomies are often performed in the intensive care unit, under echo guidance only, without the need for transfer to the catheterisation laboratory and without the need for radiation exposure (fig. 1).

Aortic Valvoplasty

In neonatal critical aortic stenosis, the systemic circulation cannot be maintained by the flow through the stenotic aortic valve; adequate cardiac output is maintained via right-to-left shunting at the ductus arteriosus (fig. 2). This ductal dependence necessitates maintenance of ductal patency

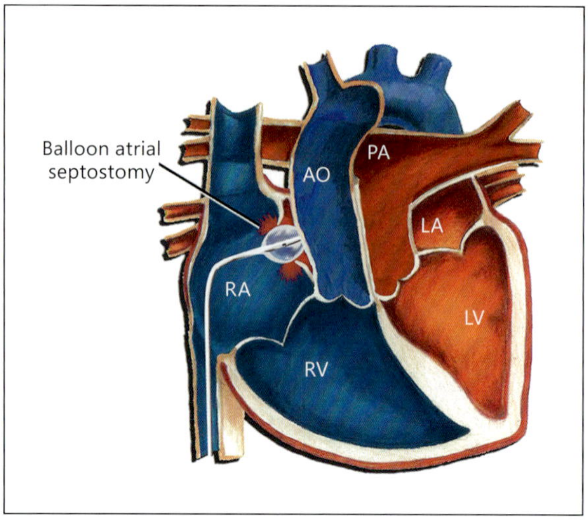

Fig. 1. Septostomy form transposition of the great arteries. The inflated balloon is rapidly withdrawn across the atrial septum enlarging the septal communication and allowing unrestricted flow between the left atrium (LA) and right atrium (RA). LV = Left ventricle; PA = pulmonary artery; RV = right ventricle.

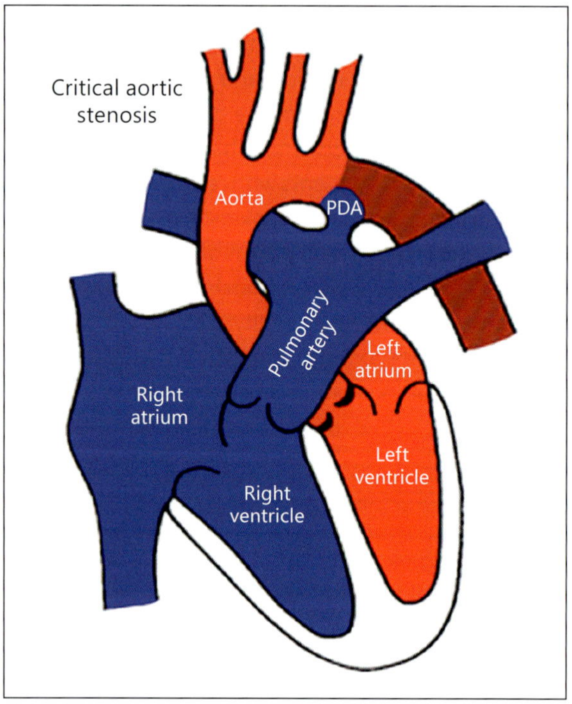

Fig. 2. Cardiac output which would normally steam through the stenosed aortic valve instead has to be diverted into the systemic circulation (aorta) via the ductus arteriosus away from the lung arteries. The oxygen content and saturation of this blood depends on the amount of intracardiac mixing, but it will usually be significantly desaturated compared to normal. PDA = Patent ductus arteriosus.

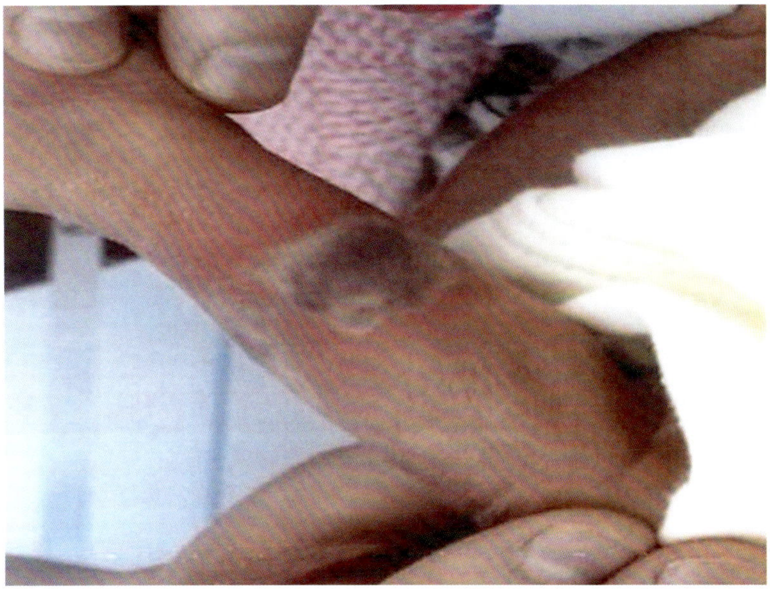

Fig. 3. Evidence of arterial thrombo-embolism following arterial cannulation in a 1.4-kg neonate. The demarcated ulcerated area relates to partial occlusion of the femoral artery with related distal embolism.

(usually with a prostaglandin infusion) until the time the valve stenosis can be relieved. Balloon valvoplasty to the aortic valve in the neonatal period can be a delicate procedure. The choice of the vascular access site and technique is critical to optimise the angulation towards the aortic valve and also to decrease the risk of permanent loss of the arterial pulse with its associated perfusion risks (fig. 3). Even the lowest-profile, 3- or 4-Fr access sheath will present a significant mismatch to the femoral artery in a neonate <4 kg. Some interventionists have moved towards carotid or axillary cut-down techniques, which allow straightforward repair of the access vessel and an excellent angle of approach to allow crossing of the stenotic aortic valve. Once the valve has been crossed with a wire, a low-profile angioplasty balloon measuring usually between 80 and 90% of the diameter of the valve is positioned across it and inflated (fig. 4). Low pressures of only 2–3 Pa are required to significantly relieve stenoses in neonates [3].

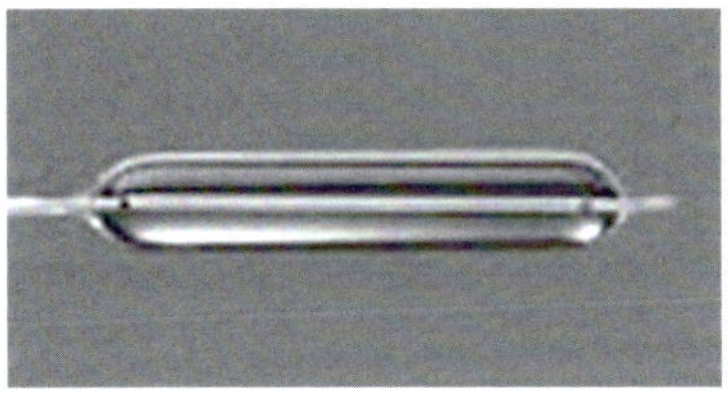

Fig. 4. Tyshak® percutaneous angioplasty balloon (low profile with a low inflation and burst pressure) suited for valvoplasty in neonates and small children.

Pulmonary Valvoplasty

As with the aortic valve, dependency of the pulmonary circulation on the ductus arteriosus due to pulmonary valvar stenosis may necessitate urgent neonatal intervention. As the pulmonary valve is approached via the transvenous route, vascular access is rarely a major issue. Successfully crossing a critically stenosed or atretic valve can be challenging in either the pulmonary or aortic position and might necessitate the use of various wires and catheter curves. Perforation of atretic valves can be achieved using radiofrequency energy delivered through the tip of a fine wire; once perforated, the valve can be balloon dilated to relieve outflow obstruction. In patients with critical tetralogy of Fallot, stent implantation in the right-ventricular outflow tract may also be required [4] (fig. 5).

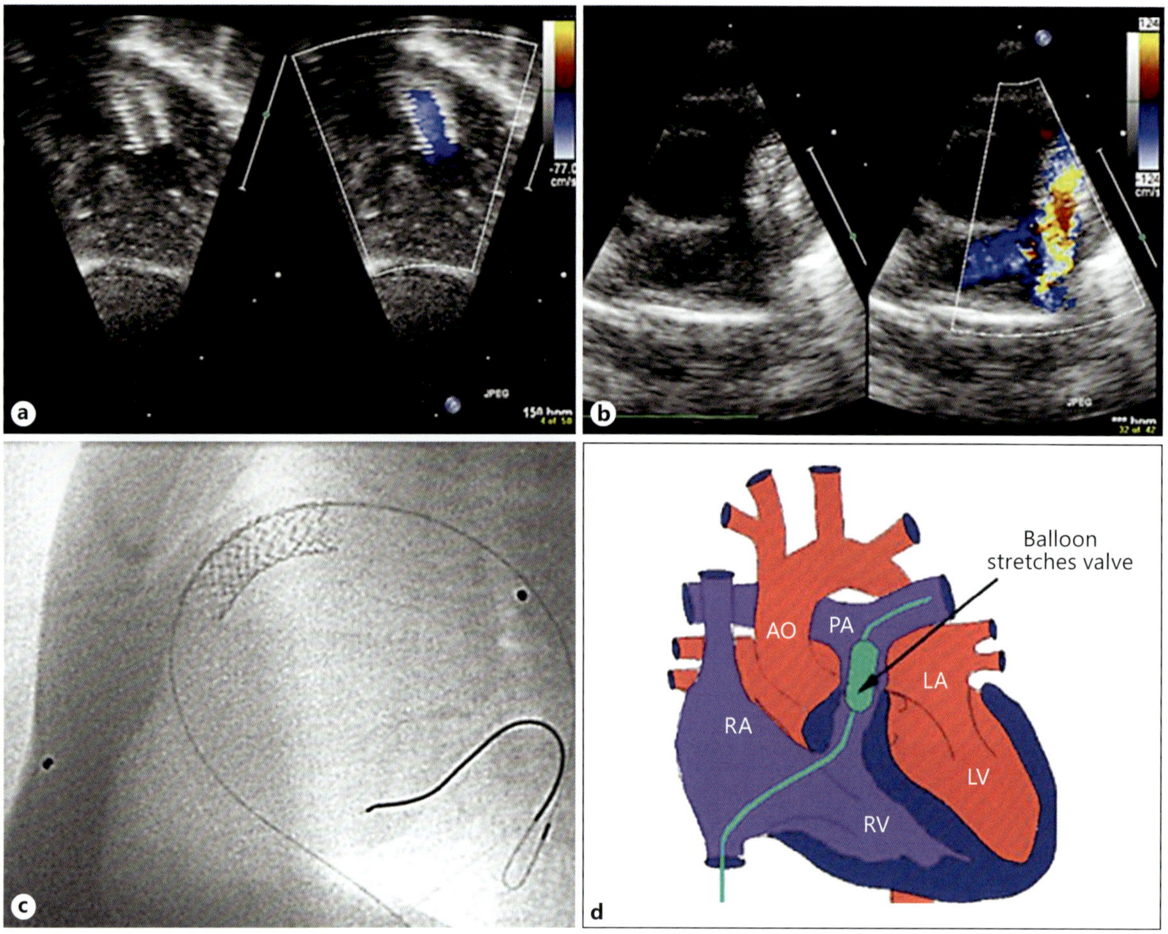

Fig. 5. a Right-ventricular outflow tract stent in situ by echocardiography. **b** The same patient showing the bifurcation of the branch pulmonary arteries. **c** The stent after insertion on fluoroscopy (the guide wire is still in position across the stent). **d** The anatomical position of the balloon or stent for pulmonary valvoplasty or stent implantation in the right-ventricular outflow tract. Ao = Aorta; LA = left atrium; LV = left ventricle; PA = pulmonary artery; RA = right atrium; RV = right ventricle;

Infant and Paediatric Procedures

Outside of the neonatal period, most interventions in everyday practice are performed on a more elective basis. There are always particular circumstances which require emergency work, such as percutaneous drainage of effusions causing cardiac tamponade; atrial septostomy in patients requiring mechanical circulatory support (extracorporeal membrane oxygenation) and procedures to relieve residual lesions in postsurgical patients.

Elective indications for catheterisation outside the neonatal period include pulmonary and aortic valvoplasty, a variation of the technique described in the Neonatal Intervention section.

Atrial Septal Defect Occlusion

Closure of atrial septal defects (ASDs) is also increasingly common in older paediatric patients in an effort to reduce the long-term detrimental effects of right-atrial and -ventricular volume loading associated with ASDs and to prevent arrhythmia. There is a growing number of devices on the market which purport to be ideal platforms for ASD closure; however, in truth, the availability of multiple platforms, all of which have specific limitations and

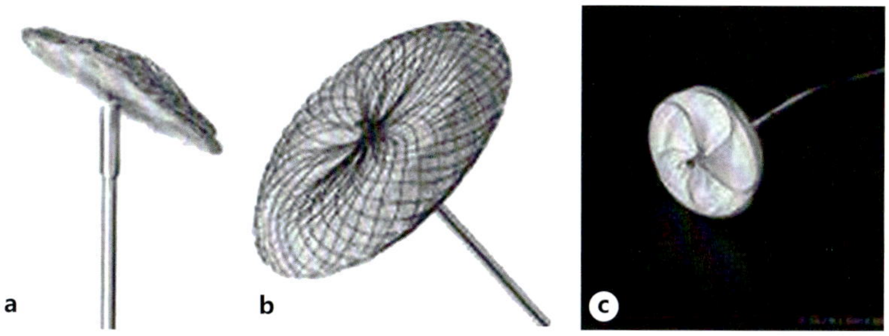

Fig. 6. Three of the current most commonly used devices for ASD closure. **a** St Jude Amplatzer atrial septal occluder. **b** Occlutech Figula Flex II. **c** Gore septal occluder.

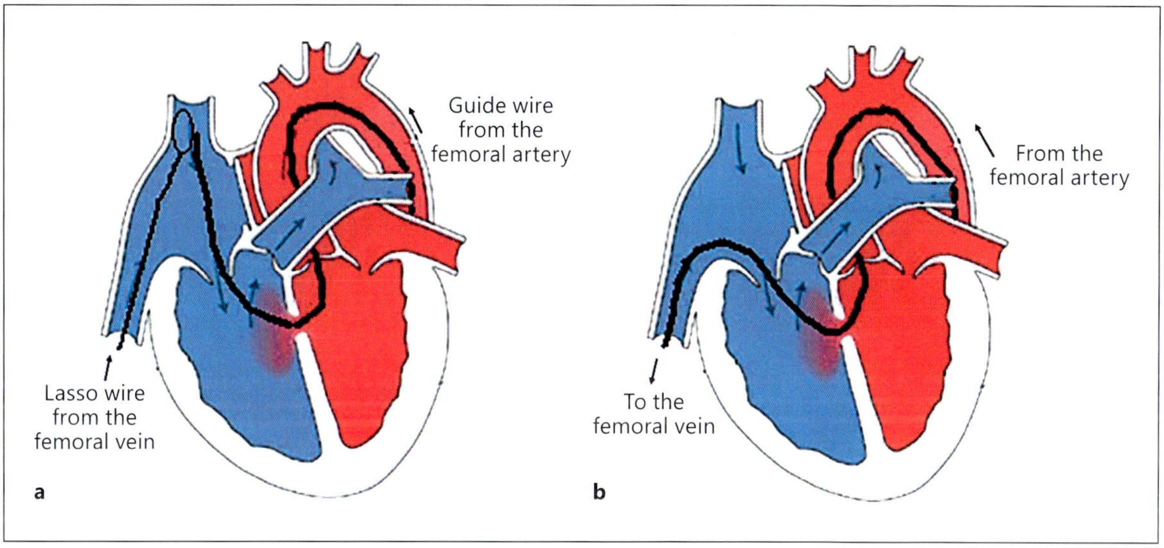

Fig. 7. Arteriovenous loop for stabilisation of wire position during device closure of a VSD. The thick black line represents a guide wire which has been passed from the femoral artery across the aortic valve and through the VSD before being manipulated backwards across the tricuspid valve. Once the tip of this wire is in either the superior vena cava or one of the pulmonary arteries, it can be snared using a lasso wire guided from the femoral vein or the internal jugular vein (**a**). Pulling the lassoed wire out of the delivery sheath, and hence the body, creates a continuous arteriovenous rail or loop over which sheaths and devices can be delivered (**b**).

indications, ensures that the widest variety of defects can be closed in the widest range of patients. There is rarely a strong indication to close an ASD before the child reaches 3 years or 20 kg; thereafter, the defect is likely to be more easily and safely corrected (fig. 6) [5].

Ventricular Septal Defect Occlusion

Closure of ventricular septal defects (VSDs) by cardiac catheterisation is also feasible, usually in patients weighing more than 10 kg. A pathophysiological understanding of the anatomy of the ventricular septum and the position of the defect to be closed is crucial to understand the associated risks and complications. Heart block, device embolism, haemolysis, and aortic and tricuspid valve damage are all possibilities when closing VSDs in the catheterisation laboratory. The technique itself requires placing a large-calibre, long sheath across the septal defect in order to deploy the septal closure device. Positioning of the sheath usually requires approaching and crossing the VSD from the left-ventricular side of the septum and then forming a VA circuit (fig. 7) before drawing the delivery sheath through the right side of the heart coaxially over the wire. Recognition of the excellent results achievable by

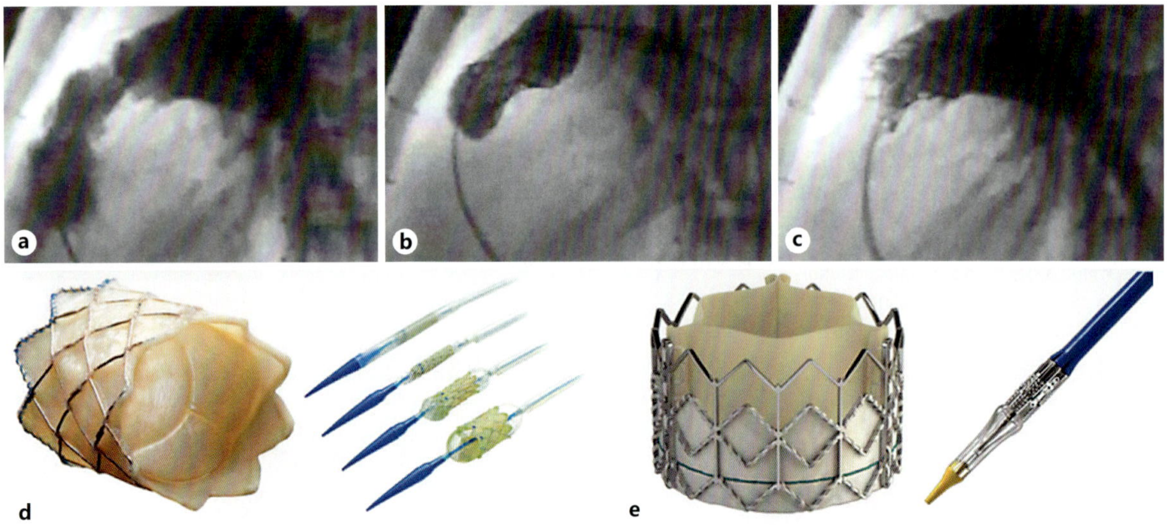

Fig. 8. Adapted from Singh et al. [15]. **a–c** Delivery of a transcatheter valve in the pulmonary position. **d, e** The two most commonly used transcatheter pulmonary valves. **d** Medtronic Melody® transcatheter pulmonary valve device (left) and its delivery system (right) showing several stages of device expansion (d). **e** Edwards SAPIEN® transcatheter heart valve (Edwards Lifesciences, Irvine, Calif., USA) valve (left) and its delivery system (right).

cardiac surgery for most morphologies of VSD is important; therefore, VSD closure in the catheterisation laboratory will likely remain a technique with limited indications for the foreseeable future [6].

Transcatheter Pulmonary Valve Implantation

Surgical pulmonary valve replacement is usually associated with low mortality and morbidity and a good outcome; however, many patients, such as those with tetralogy of Fallot or pulmonary atresia, require pulmonary valve surgery from infancy, meaning that they may require multiple follow-up operations as they grow. This is due to a combination of mismatch of the original valve size to the requirements of the growing patient and deterioration in valve function, which occurs more aggressively in young patients compared to adults. We now have the ability to implant valves in the pulmonary position in the catheterisation laboratory via sheaths placed through femoral or internal jugular access. This may avoid higher mortality and the morbidity of 'multiple redo' sternotomy operations. Although many of the patients currently having transcatheter pulmonary valve implants are adults, improvement in valve technology and design are widening the age range and anatomical range at which transcatheter replacement can be performed (fig. 8) [7].

Coarctation Stent Implantation

Stent implantation for treatment of coarctation of the aorta has become the procedure of choice in most institutions for patients presenting with native or postsurgical stenosis in the descending thoracic aorta. Again, this is not a blanket indication and an intimate knowledge of the anatomy of the patient's specific aortic arch, branching pattern and the area surrounding the coarctation is key. Associated connective tissue and genetic disorders also have important implications regarding the indication, conduct and equipment choice for this procedure.

The key practical points relate to procedure planning. Cross-sectional imaging is almost always advisable to delineate the exact anatomy and preselect equipment to have available. One of the key limitations on this therapy relates to the size of the sheath required to deliver a stent into a coarctation. Large-diameter stents require large-diameter sheaths and this needs to be taken into account when making treatment decisions and planning the intervention [8].

Stent Technology

Stents allow us to more definitively enlarge the size of stenosed vessels with more permanency than simple balloon angioplasty, and their use has revolutionised the treatment of coarctation of the aorta and pulmonary artery stenosis. They can also be used to hold ASDs open when a shunt across the atria needs to be maintained and to hold the ductus arteriosus open in some patients with so-called *'duct-dependant'* congenital heart disease.

Safe delivery of stents within the paediatric population is often difficult due to the requirement to implant them via large-calibre long sheaths. Achieving stable appropriate stent positioning is challenging and may involve multiple imaging modalities, including 3D echo, rotational angiography and fusion imaging with cardiac MRI and CT.

The implications of stent implantation in paediatric patients for any indication require careful consideration. The vessel in which the stent is implanted will usually have a requirement to grow as the patient grows, therefore implanting a fixed-size stent, which may not allow the vessel to reach adult size, may have significant consequences [9, 10].

Fetal Interventions

Disease-modifying interventions in critical congenital heart disease often happen in the presymptomatic patient to decrease the duration of negative remodelling, which occurs in chronic pathophysiological haemodynamic states. As an extension of this, an intervention performed in the fetal period has the possibility of improving the haemodynamic situation prior to birth, with the attendant hope that this may lessen the degree of neonatal pathology.

The overall approach is variable. Access to the fetus may be through the maternal abdominal wall using ultrasound guidance or directly through the uterus with a laparotomy. Maternal general anaesthesia or sedation and delivery of appropriate sedation to the fetus are important considerations. The focus so far has been on two procedures; the first is fetal aortic valvoplasty. Poor flow through an abnormal aortic valve has been linked to the progressive development of hypoplastic left-heart syndrome (HLHS). To try and interrupt this natural history, relieving aortic valve stenosis in fetal life and hence promoting forward flow may halt or even reverse the development of HLHS, leading to improved postnatal haemodynamics and a lesser form of the disease. Case selection, timing of the intervention as well as the complication rate and lack of definitive proof of concept have limited this procedure to only a few centres around the world.

The other procedure is atrial septal decompression in HLHS. Atrial septal restriction in HLHS is associated with poor outcomes, and early decompression of the atrial septum may stop the progressive pulmonary congestion, which is thought to irreversibly damage the pulmonary vasculature. This can be achieved with needle or radiofrequency perforation, followed by dilation and stent implantation. Again, there are no hard data to suggest that these interventions are beneficial. Fetal cardiac interventions remain a small field with ongoing problems with the production of appropriately sized equipment and the risk to fetal and maternal well-being [11].

Hybrid Techniques

Although the concept of joint working between surgeons and interventional cardiologists is not a new concept, the specific development of techniques requiring both skill sets has only become commonplace in the last 10–15 years. Recognition of the potential in hybrid working has led to growing numbers of conditions which can be treated more safely and efficiently by this route. Although most hybrid techniques are performed through a median sternotomy incision, thoracotomy access to the cardiac apex and vascular cut-down access also exemplify when the two subspecialties combine. Some applications of hybrid approaches are detailed below.

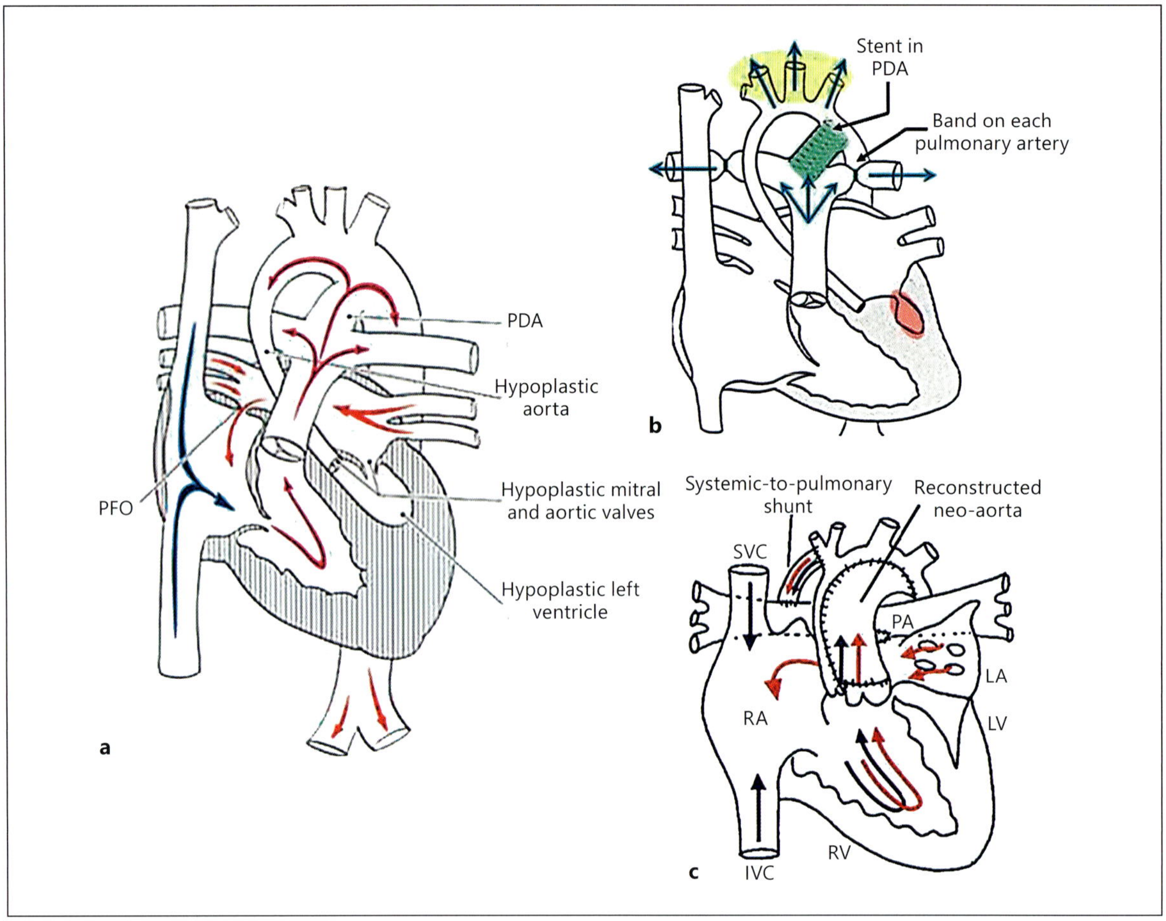

Fig. 9. These schematic drawings demonstrate the anatomy and physiology of HLHS in its unoperated form (**a**), following the recently developed hybrid palliation strategy (**b**) and following a traditional Norwood operation (**c**). IVC = Inferior vena cava; LA = left atrium; LV = left ventricle; PA = pulmonary artery; PDA = patent ductus arteriosus; PFO = patent foramen ovale; RA = right atrium; RV = right ventricle; SVC = superior vena cava.

Hybrid Palliation of Hypoplastic Left Heart Disease

First described back in the mid-1990s, hybrid palliation of HLHS has made a comeback with several large institutions introducing the procedure to offset the high mortality and morbidity of the traditional Norwood procedure, which requires neonatal cardiopulmonary bypass for the highest-risk neonates with this condition. The key principles of the hybrid palliation relate to the avoidance of neonatal cardiopulmonary bypass and the delay of major reconstruction of the aortic arch until later in infancy [12]. Figure 9 demonstrates the anatomy of the patient with unoperated HLHS (fig. 9a), following hybrid palliation of HLHS (fig. 9b) and following a traditional Norwood operation (fig. 9c).

Muscular Ventricular Septal Defect Closure

Closure of some muscular VSDs can be challenging due to a combination of the size of the patient and the position of the VSD in the ventricular septum. These features can combine to make surgical closure of muscular VSDs very challenging from either the traditional surgical or the percutaneous route. In order to overcome this, the VSD can be approached via a sternotomy and a direct insertion through the right-ventricular free wall of a delivery sheath [13].

Paravalvar Leak Occlusion

The position of some paravalvar aortic and mitral valve leaks can make percutaneous closure very challenging. These defects can sometimes be effectively crossed and occluded by using a transapical approach, with access to the left-ventricular apex gained by a limited left thoracotomy. This allows placement of an occlusion device in the paravalvar leak via a much physically straighter and easier approach [14].

Conclusion

Paediatric interventional catheterisation is a rapidly developing subspecialty with new techniques and technologies coming through at a steady pace. Confidence in hybrid techniques and neonatal interventions is making major differences to patients in whom early mortality would previously have been an expectation.

References

1 Lee JY: Clinical presentations of critical cardiac defects in the newborn: decision making and initial management. Korean J Pediatr 2010;53:669–679.
2 Cinteza E, Carminati M: Balloon atrial septostomy – almost half a century after (review). Maedica (Buchar) 2013;8:280–284.
3 McElhinney DB, Lock JE, Keane JF, Moran AM, Colan SD: Left heart growth, function, and reintervention after balloon aortic valvuloplasty for neonatal aortic stenosis (review). Circulation 2005;111:451–458.
4 Tulzer G, Arzt W, Franklin RC, Loughna PV, Mair R, Gardiner HM: Fetal pulmonary valvuloplasty for critical pulmonary stenosis or atresia with intact septum. Lancet 2002;360:1567–1568.
5 Huang TC, Hsieh KS, Lin CC, Lee CL: Clinical results of percutaneous closure of large secundum atrial septal defects in children using the Amplatzer septal occluder. Heart Vessels 2008;23:187–192.
6 Kenny D, Morgan G, Bajwa A, Farrow C, Parry A, Caputo M, Tometzki A, Martin R: Evolution of transcatheter closure of perimembranous ventricular septal defects in a single centre. Catheter Cardiovasc Interv 2009;73:568–575.
7 Ringewald JM, Suh EJ: Transcatheter pulmonary valve insertion, expanded use and future directions. Cardiol Young 2013;23:910–914.
8 Bozzani A, Odero A: Stent implantation in the native and recurrent aortic coarctation in children. Am J Cardiol 2012;109:1822.
9 Veeram Reddy SR, Welch TR, Wang J, Richardson JA, Forbess JM, Riegel M, Nugent AW: A novel design biodegradable stent for use in congenital heart disease: mid-term results in rabbit descending aorta. Catheter Cardiovasc Interv 2014, Epub ahead of print.
10 Hascoët S, Baruteau A, Jalal Z, Mauri L, Acar P, Elbaz M, Boudjemline Y, Fraisse A: Stents in paediatric and adult congenital interventional cardiac catheterization. Arch Cardiovasc Dis 2014;107:462–475.
11 Mellander M, Gardiner H: Foetal therapy, what works? An overview. Cardiol Young 2014:1–5.
12 Honjo O, Caldarone CA: Hybrid palliation for neonates with hypoplastic left heart syndrome: current strategies and outcomes. Korean Circ J 2010;40:103–111.
13 Michel-Behnke I, Ewert P, Koch A, Bertram H, Emmel M, Fischer G, Gitter R, Kozlik-Feldman R, Motz R, Kitzmüller E, Kretschmar O; Investigators of the Working Group Interventional Cardiology of the German Association of Pediatric Cardiology: Device closure of ventricular septal defects by hybrid procedures: a multicenter retrospective study. Catheter Cardiovasc Interv 2011;77:242–251.
14 Davidavicius G, Rucinskas K, Drasutiene A, Samalavicius R, Bilkis V, Zakarkaite D, Aidietis A: Hybrid approach for transcatheter paravalvular leak closure of mitral prosthesis in high-risk patients through transapical access. J Thorac Cardiovasc Surg 2014;148:1965–1969.
15 Singh HS, Horlick E, Osten M, Benson LN: Interventional cardiology in adults with congenital heart disease. Nat Rev Cardiol 2013;10:662–678.

Dr. Shakeel A. Qureshi
Evelina Children's Hospital, Guy's and St. Thomas NHS Foundation Trust
London SE1 7EH (UK)
E-Mail adam.philpott@gstt.nhs.uk

Muenke M, Kruszka PS, Sable CA, Belmont JW (eds): Congenital Heart Disease: Molecular Genetics, Principles of Diagnosis and Treatment. Basel, Karger, 2015, pp 298–305
DOI: 10.1159/000375226

Ethical Considerations in Congenital Heart Disease

Renee D. Boss · Miriam C. Shapiro

Berman Institute of Bioethics, Johns Hopkins University School of Medicine, Baltimore, Md., USA

Abstract

This chapter reviews important ethical issues related to the diagnosis, evaluation, and management of congenital heart disease (CHD). We highlight the social injustices and political forces which may impact pregnancy risk, prenatal diagnosis, and perinatal interventions for CHD. We explore complex decision points that juxtapose competing interests of the patient, family, clinician, and society. We review the conflicts that can arise when these ethically complex decisions are navigated by diverse medical teams, and consider ways in which individual clinician's treatment recommendations for patients differ from what they would choose for their own child. We examine the implications that novel therapies have on our understanding of 'lethal' anomalies and on the role of palliative care in the treatment of these patients. We debate the thorny issues raised in talking with families about what is a life worth living. Many of the ethical complexities raised in this chapter center around this pivotal issue: *Just because we could provide an intervention, should we?*

This chapter will review important ethical issues related to the diagnosis, evaluation and management of congenital heart disease (CHD). We will highlight the social injustices and political forces which may impact pregnancy risk, prenatal diagnosis, and perinatal interventions for CHD. We will explore complex decision points that juxtapose competing interests of the patient, family, clinician, and society. We will review the conflicts that can arise when these ethically complex decisions are navigated by diverse medical teams, and will consider ways in which individual clinician's treatment recommendations for patients differ from what they would choose for their own child. We will examine the implications that novel therapies have on our understanding of 'lethal' anomalies and on the role of palliative care in the treatment of these patients. We will debate the thorny issues raised in talking with families about what is a life worth living. Many of the ethical complexities raised in this chapter center around this pivotal issue: *Just because we could provide an intervention, should we?*

Social Justice and Congenital Heart Disease Risk

Preconceptional and pregnancy risk factors for abnormal fetal cardiac formation are not randomly distributed among women of child-bearing age. Maternal-child race, ethnicity, and socioeconomic status impact CHD incidence and outcomes. Infants of Hispanic and non-Hispanic black women are less likely to have had prenatal detection of their CHD than are infants born to white women, likely reflecting barriers in access to adequate prenatal care [1]. Prenatal CHD detection is lower among pregnant women of lower socioeconomic status, those with public insurance, and those in more rural locales [2, 3]. Incidence of CHD is related to environmental risks, such as exposure to organic solvents or cigarette smoke, which also tend to disproportionately impact socioeconomically vulnerable populations [4, 5]. Specific types of CHD seem to vary by race [6]. Mortality related to several CHD phenotypes, such as tetralogy of Fallot, varies by maternal race and ethnicity, with non-Hispanic black race conferring the highest risk [7]. The likelihood that a fetus with CHD will be born prematurely, or of low birth weight, also varies by maternal race [8], which parallels variability in overall rates of prematurity and low birth weight by maternal race [9].

These prenatal disparities, some immutable and some reflecting social inequalities, can only partially account for the excess CHD mortality rates among patients in the neonatal and early childhood periods [10]. Pediatric disparities in access to and outcomes from CHD interventions also occur, and are closely linked to socioeconomic inequalities. Children with CHD who are covered by managed care plans, versus indemnity insurance, are more likely to receive care in hospitals with higher mortality rates [11]. Infants born with CHD in areas of high poverty may experience delay in referral to a cardiac center [12]. Nearly 25 years ago, Allen et al. [13] writing for the American Heart Association described challenges in the diagnosis and long-term management of children with CHD born into poverty. Health literacy, reliable transportation, good nutrition, medication adherence, stable housing, and safe childcare are all important to successful CHD outcomes. These critical elements are unequally distributed and play important, if underappreciated, roles in the medical care of pediatric CHD.

Such disparities have clear implications for medical decision making. Early fetal diagnosis of CHD is essential to perinatal options, including pregnancy termination, fetal therapy, local delivery for palliative care only, delivery at a regional hospital for lifesaving prostaglandin, and planning for postnatal management [14]. When CHD is diagnosed as part of an overall syndrome, early fetal detection permits time for further testing and discussion of whether CHD interventions can enhance quality of life and survival. Early diagnosis facilitates relationships between parents and clinicians, establishing the trust and communication that enables high-stake medical decision making. Because of disparities in fetal diagnosis, those women with the fewest social supports are least likely to have these discussions or establish these relationships. Their newborn's clinical status may be compromised, physical separation of the mother and neonate may be necessary postpartum, and the experience of diagnosis and decision making becomes shocking and urgent.

Just and fair medical care demands that we consider how health inequities impact disease management and family counseling. Exploration of family resources, relationships, and values can tailor the decision-making process to address their needs more closely. Early identification of family vulnerabilities permits integration of community resources and enhances discharge planning. Assistance in planning for acute and lifetime costs of care associated with pediatric CHD should be offered. Without frank and compassionate discussions about these very real issues, clinicians cannot adequately foster informed consent. Given their own social advantages, physicians can also advocate for the broader economic and legislative efforts that can improve access to coordinated, high-quality maternal-child health care.

Prenatal Diagnosis: Promises and Harms

The realm of what is possible to diagnose prenatally has evolved quickly over the last 50 years. Once over-the-counter pregnancy tests became available in the 1970s, women could present for prenatal care early enough that elective termination or fetal therapies were feasible. Because fetal testing until recently entailed risks of infection, premature labor, and fetal loss, clinicians and parents had to balance their desire for information to permit pregnancy termination or fetal interventions for an affected fetus against the possibility that a healthy fetus could be endangered by that prenatal testing. This risk/benefit ratio often led parents to forgo invasive prenatal testing, such as amniocentesis. As a result, prenatal decision making about conditions such as CHD were often made without genetic information.

The last decade has brought important refinements in prenatal testing. Importantly, a much broader range of fetal diagnoses may be confirmed with little, even no, increased risk to the fetus from that testing. Analysis of fetal DNA fragments in the maternal circulation and whole fetal genome sequencing promise greater certainty about potentially life-limiting conditions, such as trisomy 13 and 18, and may permit earlier pregnancy termination. At the same time, emerging forms of prenatal testing have the potential to uncover many abnormalities which may be of uncertain clinical significance. The potential harms of prenatal testing are shifting towards a greater burden of information for families and clinicians [15]. Due to the broad range of potential diagnoses, genetic counselors cannot practically inform parents about the potential pros and cons of uncovering particular fetal diagnoses until the results are in hand. The growth of private industries advertising genetic testing may encourage prenatal diagnosis without any prenatal counseling. Parents may learn of fetal predilections, traits, or minor conditions; this could lead to requests for pregnancy termination on bases untenable to the medical profession or to society at large.

Earlier, broader, and more certain prenatal diagnoses will impact prenatal counseling for and management of CHD. Currently, in the United States, >90% of pregnancy terminations occur in the first trimester [16]. Historically, fetal CHD and associated conditions have been diagnosed after the first trimester; earlier detection may lead to more requests for therapeutic terminations. Alternatively, knowing that a fetus does not have the genetic abnormality known to worsen outcomes from a particular CHD phenotype may lead a family to reject termination. Enhanced prenatal diagnosis could also shift the balance of maternal-fetal risks and benefits related to fetal therapies for progressive CHD, such as aortic valve obstruction [17, 18]. Perhaps confirmation that a fetus does not have a genetic syndrome will endorse fetal listing for heart transplant [19].

Greater certainty about prenatal diagnoses is also likely to draw interest from stakeholders outside of the patient-clinician relationship. A wide range of proposed restrictions on physician counseling of pregnant patients have gotten traction in several locales. Some US states bar malpractice claims against clinicians who choose to withhold information from women about fetal health problems, such as CHD, to prevent pregnancy termination. Legislation to restrict access to abortion in general, and second-trimester abortion in particular, will reduce the choice about therapeutic terminations. As options for prenatal testing are expanded, it will be important to consider the utility of this information in light of evolving pregnancy options.

A Life Worth Living – Can We Agree?

Management of serious medical conditions should result from reflections about what we can do, and what we ought to do, for the patient. These reflections inherently involve judgments about benefits and burdens, oftentimes subjective assessments that differ among family members and among clinicians. In situations where there exist robust outcome data to guide deliberations, as for isolated CHD, counseling of families may be fairly straightforward. But when CHD is only one part of an underlying genetic syndrome, outcome data may not exist. As genetic testing evolves, we are likely to see less 'isolated CHD', and more patients who also have genetic abnormalities of uncertain significance. How can we know what ought to be done for such patients?

Whether low-risk surgeries ought to be performed to extend life in patients with underlying syndromes, especially syndromes involving neurodevelopmental disabilities, became a topic for social consideration with the Baby Doe cases that inspired the film *Who Should Survive?* At that time, the prevailing professional ethic was that clinicians should not compel life-prolonging therapies for a child who would have cognitive disabilities. Today, while many consider that life-prolonging therapies should not be forgone solely based on underlying cognitive disabilities, there is not clear consensus about the boundaries around quality-of-life concerns. Increasingly, we face decisions not about low-risk surgeries for patients with syndromes compatible with a lifespan of decades, but of high-risk surgeries for patients with syndromes likely to result in death in the first months or years of life. One example is the consideration of parental requests for surgical management of hypoplastic left heart syndrome (HLHS) in a neonate with trisomy 18 [20]. Some argue that historical morbidity and mortality estimates for such patients are self-fulfilling prophecies – if medical interventions are withheld from patients with trisomy 18, these patients will die quickly (see Costello et al. chapter on Surgical Management on p. 284 for further discussion of surgical therapy in Trisomy 18). Others assert that patients with serious genetic syndromes may be considered surgical candidates, based on their individual clinical condition [21].

Similar complexities characterize decisions about CHD management for the emerging group of premature and low-birth-weight patients. Even without CHD, premature and low-birth-weight infants are often chronically and critically ill with pulmonary, nutritional, and neurologic complications, require prolonged ICU care and surgical feeding tubes or mechanical ventilation, and are at significant risk of early death and disability. How then, should we assess the risk/benefit ratio when such patients also have CHD which may require cardiopulmonary bypass or staged procedures [22]? When surgical intervention is elected, how should we balance the technical complications related to infant size against the potential advantages of early surgical correction [23]? And to what extent should these decisions be shared with the family?

As standards of care about these patients continue to evolve, the interventions offered to some patients are inherently of uncertain outcome. While staged reconstruction may have favorable results in otherwise healthy patients, we do not know how the underlying nutritional or immunologic complications of trisomy 18 may impact those results. It is not surprising that there is disagreement among clinicians about which as-yet-unproven therapies should be offered or recommended to families [24]. It remains difficult to navigate this calculus of uncertainty, the promise of beating the odds versus the possibility of survival with intolerable deficits. Transparency about these complex judgments can enhance trust and communication with families, and improves decision making [25].

Survivors of Congenital Heart Disease and Demand for Destination Therapies

As more and more children with CHD survive after surgical palliation, salvage options such as a ventricular assist device (VAD) and transplant will be increasingly sought. These therapies raise unique ethical concerns in the pediatric population. Foremost issues include the scarcity of organs for transplantation, particularly for the smallest patients, and the limited viability of a transplanted heart. Though survival data for pediatric heart transplant show continued improvement, with median survival of 19.7 years for infants and 12.4 years for adolescents, heart transplantation does not provide permanent cure [26]. We must assume the potential need for cardiac retransplantation throughout a lifetime, with outcomes generally poorer than for initial transplants [27, 28]. Should a second- or third-time candidate get less consideration for repeat transplant of a limited organ be cause of expectation of poorer outcome? Justice in pediatric organ allocation must also address the disparities in pre- and post-transplant outcomes for patients based on race and socioeconomic status [29–31]. How should we consider the fact that, among children with HLHS, those of black race or lower socioeconomic status are more likely to experience graft failure after cardiac transplant [30, 32]?

The limited availability of organs via brain death led to the development of a pediatric protocol for heart transplantation following donation after cardiac death [33]. In this pathway, life-sustaining care is withdrawn, resulting in cardiorespiratory arrest, and is followed by organ procurement. Donation after cardiac death has sparked much debate [34, 35]. Opponents argue that the ability to resuscitate the heart following transplantation into the recipient is inconsistent with having declared the donor dead by virtue of cardiac arrest, violating the dead donor rule [34, 36]. Though beyond the scope of this review, there remains active discussion in the medical, bioethical, and lay press about the definitions of death that allow for organ transplantation in adults and children.

The long-term medication adherence essential for successful cardiac transplant also raises unique concerns among the pediatric population. Long-term medication adherence is continually challenged by a child's evolving autonomy, reason, and ability to understand consequences, as well as by family context. Pediatric medication adherence for serious medical conditions, including transplant, is often suboptimal [37, 38]; determining which children are likely to be nonadherent after transplant has proved elusive [39]. Yet immunosuppressive regimens must be followed strictly, and have side effects and toxicities including life-threatening infection, malignancy, and renal failure, which could necessitate pediatric kidney transplantation [40]. How should pediatric nonadherence affect considerations of organ allocation? Should a child be penalized for the failings of their guardians to follow up with medical requirements? Should a child be placed in medical foster care to improve adherence? These questions are routinely faced in the clinical setting, though consensus is elusive [41].

Scarcity of pediatric organs has also driven the development of other methods for expanding survival in children with CHD. Extracorporeal membrane oxygenation (also referred to as extracorporeal life support) has historically been a bridge to transplant for children with significant hemodynamic compromise, though extracorporeal membrane oxygenation/extracorporeal life support has significant risk of morbidity and mortality itself [26]. The VAD was initially designed for, tested in, and used with an adult population with the goal of improving outcomes after transplantation for patients suffering from end-stage heart failure associated with cardiomyopathy. Pediatric use in the US became possible via compassionate exception by the Food and Drug Administration, not through traditional methods of device study and approval [42]. While initial data suggest that VAD may function as a bridge to transplant for children [42–45], the associated ethical issues are myriad. They include the need to rigorously monitor and report all outcomes associated with VAD use, given the lack of rigorous pediatric device approval methods. The VAD may result in long-term ICU stays with high costs [46]. If smaller implantable devices were available, VAD could become a destination therapy and would reduce the demand for transplant, ease the burden on the inpatient health care system, and potentially improve quality of life for children with CHD.

Palliative Care – Clinicians' Personal Choices versus Professional Recommendations

Pediatric palliative care has traditionally been associated with end of life care, considered only after curative therapies had failed, were not available, or were intentionally forgone in the face of impending death. The Institute of Medicine [47] and the American Academy of Pediatrics [48] advocate for much earlier integration of palliative care, beginning at the time of diagnosis of a potentially life-limiting disease. Interdisciplinary palliative care can be delivered alongside curative care, with the goal of enhancing pain and symptom management and quality of life for patients, as well as assisting families in understanding prognosis and making decisions that reflect their goals and values. Pediatric hospice, one aspect of pediatric palliative care, can be offered to families whose child is likely to die. In the context of CHD, palliative care has most often been considered for children with HLHS or with multiple serious congenital anomalies [49, 50]. Though HLHS was considered 'lethal' 30 years ago, improvements in staged palliation techniques raise the question of whether it is reasonable to withhold these interventions from HLHS patients.

Evolving standards of care have led to significant variability in counseling about treatment options for HLHS. While physicians consistently offer the Norwood-staged palliation pathway to parents, there is less consensus about offering other treatment options, including the option to pursue palliative or comfort care only [50–55]. One interesting area of inquiry has highlighted the differences between what physicians recommend to patients and what they would choose themselves. A not insignificant proportion of physicians who regularly counsel families about HLHS would personally consider or choose palliative care only if their child were diagnosed with HLHS [52, 56]. That physicians who may choose palliative care for their own child do not offer that option to parents raises concerns about informed consent and justice. Kon [57] and Feudtner [58] argue that, according to the principal of reasonableness, if reasonable people would and do choose palliative care for HLHS, then it should always be discussed as a treatment option. Others hold that it is no longer acceptable to offer palliative care alone because surgical outcomes are 'too good' [54]. This argument is similar to that regarding extremely premature infants: technological successes have defined a new threshold beyond which parents may not opt out of attempted neonatal resuscitation and intensive care [59].

Yet for many, survivability should not be used exclusively to compel surgical interventions for high-risk lesions. In Kon's repeat 2007 survey asking physicians what they would choose if their own child were diagnosed with HLHS, physicians were just as likely, and in some cases more likely than those surveyed in 1999, to forgo surgery for their child [56]. Improvements in survival alone from surgical interventions was not enough to change the risk-benefit calculus for physicians. Ross and Frader [25] argue that reasonableness ought to take into account not just the likelihood for survival with a good outcome, but also the chance of survival with intolerable deficit. If this chance is 'not miniscule', they argue that treatment should be optional, and further that, because of comorbidities associated with HLHS and with surgical palliation, this standard is met and palliative care remains reasonable.

It is also important to note that there is clear variability in HLHS outcomes, including survival, depending on the site of intervention. Infants treated at high-volume centers have better outcomes compared to those treated elsewhere [57, 59]. This raises concerns about equity, and about justifications for palliative care. Should parents be offered the option to transfer their child's care to a high volume center? Is that feasible in our medical system? Should certain high volume centers be allowed to assert that, since their outcomes are sufficiently good, offering palliative care alone is unacceptable, while lower volume centers should continue to offer that option?

Conclusions

As the management of CHD evolves, so do the boundaries around what is considered fair, just, reasonable, compulsory, and optimal in the care of these patients and their families. These ethical complexities are best navigated via professional consensus, transparent decision making, and excellent communication.

References

1 Waller DK, Pujazon MA, Canfield MA, Scheuerle AE, Byrne JL: Frequency of prenatal diagnosis of birth defects in Houston, Galveston and the Lower Rio Grande Valley, Texas 1995. Fetal Diagn Ther 2000;15:348–354.

2 Sekar P, Heydarian HC, Cnota JF, Hornberger LK, Michelfelder EC: Diagnosis of congenital heart disease in an era of universal prenatal ultrasound screening in southwest Ohio. Cardiol Young 2015;25:35–41.

3 Peiris V, Singh TP, Tworetzky W, Chong EC, Gauvreau K, Brown DW: Association of socioeconomic position and medical insurance with fetal diagnosis of critical congenital heart disease. Circ Cardiovasc Qual Outcomes 2009;2:354–360.

4 Patel SS, Burns TL, Botto LD, et al: Analysis of selected maternal exposures and non-syndromic atrioventricular septal defects in the National Birth Defects Prevention Study, 1997–2005. Am J Med Genet A 2012; 158A:2447–2455.

5 Jenkins KJ, Correa A, Feinstein JA, et al: Noninherited risk factors and congenital cardiovascular defects: current knowledge: a scientific statement from the American Heart Association Council on Cardiovascular Disease in the Young: endorsed by the American Academy of Pediatrics. Circulation 2007;115:2995–3014.

6 Nembhard WN, Salemi JL, Wang T, Loscalzo ML, Hauser KW: Is the prevalence of specific types of congenital heart defects different for non-Hispanic white, non-Hispanic black and Hispanic infants? Matern Child Health J 2010;14:184–193.

7 Wang Y, Liu G, Druschel CM, Kirby RS: Maternal race/ethnicity and survival experience of children with congenital heart disease. J Pediatr 2013;163:1437–1442.e2.

8 Nembhard WN, Salemi JL, Loscalzo ML, Wang T, Hauser KW: Are black and Hispanic infants with specific congenital heart defects at increased risk of preterm birth? Pediatr Cardiol 2009;30:800–809.
9 MacDorman MF: Race and ethnic disparities in fetal mortality, preterm birth, and infant mortality in the United States: an overview. Semin Perinatol 2011;35:200–208.
10 Nembhard WN, Xu P, Ethen MK, Fixler DE, Salemi JL, Canfield MA: Racial/ethnic disparities in timing of death during childhood among children with congenital heart defects. Birth Defects Res A Clin Mol Teratol 2013;97:628–640.
11 Erickson LC, Wise PH, Cook EF, Beiser A, Newburger JW: The impact of managed care insurance on use of lower-mortality hospitals by children undergoing cardiac surgery in California. Pediatrics 2000;105: 1271–1278.
12 Fixler DE, Nembhard WN, Xu P, Ethen MK, Canfield MA: Effect of acculturation and distance from cardiac center on congenital heart disease mortality. Pediatrics 2012; 129:1118–1124.
13 Allen HD, Taubert KA, Deckelbaum RJ, et al: Poverty and cardiac disease in children. Am J Dis Child 1991;145:550–553.
14 Tibballs J, Cantwell-Bartl A: Outcomes of management decisions by parents for their infants with hypoplastic left heart syndrome born with and without a prenatal diagnosis. J Paediatr Child Health 2008;44: 321–324.
15 Benn PA, Chapman AR: Ethical challenges in providing noninvasive prenatal diagnosis. Curr Opin Obstet Gynecol 2010;22:128–134.
16 Pazol K, Creanga AA, Burley KD, Hayes B, Jamieson DJ: Abortion surveillance – United States, 2010. MMWR Surveill Summ 2013;62:1–44.
17 Mavroudis CD: Foetal cardiac intervention: an ethical perspective. Cardiol Young 2011; 21(suppl 2):141–147.
18 Nelle M, Raio L, Pavlovic M, Carrel T, Surbek D, Meyer-Wittkopf M: Prenatal diagnosis and treatment planning of congenital heart defects – possibilities and limits. World J Pediatr 2009;5:18–22.
19 Russell BJ: Fetal listing for organ transplantation in Canada. Transplant Proc 2006;38: 2737–2741.
20 Boss RD, Holmes KW, Althaus J, Rushton CH, McNee H, McNee T: Trisomy 18 and complex congenital heart disease: seeking the threshold benefit. Pediatrics 2013;132: 161–165.
21 Robinson WM, Newburger JW: Ethical issues concerning cardiac surgery in patients with syndromic abnormalities. Semin Thorac Cardiovasc Surg Pediatr Card Surg Annu 2003;6:147–151.
22 Borowski A, Schickendantz S, Mennicken U, Korb H: Open heart interventions in premature low- and very-low-birth-weight neonates: risk profile and ethical considerations. Thorac Cardiovasc Surg 1997;45: 238–241.
23 Reddy VM, Hanley FL: Cardiac surgery in infants with very low birth weight. Semin Pediatr Surg 2000;9:91–95.
24 Cooper TR, Garcia-Prats JA, Brody BA: Managing disagreements in the management of short bowel and hypoplastic left heart syndrome. Pediatrics 1999;104:e48.
25 Ross LF, Frader J: Hypoplastic left heart syndrome: a paradigm case for examining conscientious objection in pediatric practice. J Pediatr 2009;155:12–15.
26 Dipchand AI, Kirk R, Edwards LB, et al: The Registry of the International Society for Heart and Lung Transplantation: sixteenth official pediatric heart transplantation report – 2013; focus theme: age. J Heart Lung Transplant 2013;32:979–988.
27 Kaufman BD, Jessup M: Adult and pediatric perspectives on heart retransplant. World J Pediatr Congenit Heart Surg 2013;4:75–79.
28 Mahle WT: Cardiac retransplantation in children. Pediatr Transplant 2008;12:274–280.
29 Mahle WT, Kanter KR, Vincent RN: Disparities in outcome for black patients after pediatric heart transplantation. J Pediatr 2005;147:739–743.
30 Singh TP, Naftel DC, Addonizio L, et al: Association of race and socioeconomic position with outcomes in pediatric heart transplant recipients. Am J Transplant 2010;10: 2116–2123.
31 Davies RR, Russo MJ, Reinhartz O, et al: Lower socioeconomic status is associated with worse outcomes after both listing and transplanting children with heart failure. Pediatr Transplant 2013;17:573–581.
32 Singh TP, Gauvreau K, Bastardi HJ, Blume ED, Mayer JE: Socioeconomic position and graft failure in pediatric heart transplant recipients. Circ Heart Fail 2009;2:160–165.
33 Boucek MM, Mashburn C, Dunn SM, et al: Pediatric heart transplantation after declaration of cardiocirculatory death. N Engl J Med 2008;359:709–714.
34 Potts M, Byrne PA, Evans DW: Infant heart transplantation after cardiac death: ethical and legal problems. J Clin Ethics 2010;21: 224–228.
35 Antommaria AH: Dying but not killing: donation after cardiac death donors and the recovery of vital organs. J Clin Ethics 2010; 21:229–231.
36 Joffe AR, Carcillo J, Anton N, et al: Donation after cardiocirculatory death: a call for a moratorium pending full public disclosure and fully informed consent. Philos Ethics Humanit Med 2011;6:17.
37 McGrady ME, Williams SN, Davies SM, Pai AL: Adherence to outpatient oral medication regimens in adolescent hematopoietic stem cell transplant recipients. Eur J Oncol Nurs 2014;18:140–144.
38 Berquist RK, Berquist WE, Esquivel CO, Cox KL, Wayman KI, Litt IF: Non-adherence to post-transplant care: prevalence, risk factors and outcomes in adolescent liver transplant recipients. Pediatr Transplant 2008;12:194–200.
39 Fisher M, Storfer-Isser A, Shaw RJ, et al: Inter-rater reliability of the Pediatric Transplant Rating Instrument (P-TRI): challenges to reliably identifying adherence risk factors during pediatric pre-transplant evaluations. Pediatr Transplant 2011;15: 142–147.
40 Sweet SC, Wong HH, Webber SA, et al: Pediatric transplantation in the United States, 1995–2004. Am J Transplant 2006;6:1132–1152.
41 Suddaby EC: No simple answers: ethical conflicts in pediatric heart transplantation. J Transpl Coord 1999;9:266–270.
42 Eghtesady P, Almond CS, Tjossem C, et al: Post-transplant outcomes of children bridged to transplant with the Berlin Heart EXCOR Pediatric ventricular assist device. Circulation 2013;128(11 suppl 1): S24–S31.
43 Ezon DS, Khan MS, Adachi I, et al: Pediatric ventricular assist device use as a bridge to transplantation does not affect long-term quality of life. J Thorac Cardiovasc Surg 2014;147:1334–1343.
44 Moreno GE, Charroqui A, Pilan ML, et al: Clinical experience with Berlin Heart Excor in pediatric patients in Argentina: 1373 days of cardiac support. Pediatr Cardiol 2011;32:652–658.
45 Brancaccio G, Filippelli S, Michielon G, et al: Ventricular assist devices as a bridge to heart transplantation or as destination therapy in pediatric patients. Transplant Proc 2012;44:2007–2012.
46 Rossano JW, Kaufman BD, Rame JE: Ethical considerations related to the use of mechanical support in congenital heart disease. World J Pediatr Congenit Heart Surg 2013;4:70–74.
47 Institute of Medicine of the National Academies: When Children Die: Improving Palliative and End-of-Life Care for Children and Their Families. Washington, National Acedemies, 2003.
48 American Academy of Pediatrics. Committee on Bioethics and Committee on Hospital Care. Palliative care for children. Pediatrics 2000;106:351–357.
49 Rychik J: What does palliative care mean in prenatal diagnosis of congenital heart disease? World J Pediatr Congenit Heart Surg 2013;4:80–84.

50 Yates AR, Hoffman TM, Boettner B, Feltes TF, Cua CL: Initial counseling prior to palliation for hypoplastic left heart syndrome. Congenit Heart Dis 2011;6:347–358.
51 Paris JJ, Moore MP, Schreiber MD: Physician counseling, informed consent and parental decision making for infants with hypoplastic left-heart syndrome. J Perinatol 2012;32:748–751.
52 Prsa M, Holly CD, Carnevale FA, Justino H, Rohlicek CV: Attitudes and practices of cardiologists and surgeons who manage HLHS. Pediatrics 2010;125:e625–e630.
53 Kon AA, Ackerson L, Lo B: How pediatricians counsel parents when no 'best-choice' management exists: lessons to be learned from hypoplastic left heart syndrome. Arch Pediatr Adolesc Med 2004; 158:436–441.
54 Wernovsky G: The paradigm shift toward surgical intervention for neonates with hypoplastic left heart syndrome. Arch Pediatr Adolesc Med 2008;162:849–854.
55 Wernovsky G, Ghanayem N, Ohye RG, et al: Hypoplastic left heart syndrome: consensus and controversies in 2007. Cardiol Young 2007;17(suppl 2):75–86.
56 Kon AA, Prsa M, Rohlicek CV: Choices doctors would make if their infant had hypoplastic left heart syndrome: comparison of survey data from 1999 and 2007. Pediatr Cardiol 2013;34:348–353.
57 Kon AA: Healthcare providers must offer palliative treatment to parents of neonates with hypoplastic left heart syndrome. Arch Pediatr Adolesc Med 2008;162:844–848.
58 Feudtner C: Ethics in the midst of therapeutic evolution. Arch Pediatr Adolesc Med 2008;162:854–857.
59 Mercurio MR, Peterec SM, Weeks B: Hypoplastic left heart syndrome, extreme prematurity, comfort care only, and the principle of justice. Pediatrics 2008;122:186–189.

Dr. Renee D. Boss
Berman Institute of Bioethics, Johns Hopkins School of Medicine
1809 Ashland Avenue 212
Baltimore, MD 21287 (USA)
E-Mail rboss1@jhmi.edu

Muenke M, Kruszka PS, Sable CA, Belmont JW (eds): Congenital Heart Disease: Molecular Genetics, Principles of Diagnosis and Treatment. Basel, Karger, 2015, pp 306–316
DOI: 10.1159/000375227

The Future of Therapeutics: Stem Cells, Tissue Plasticity, and Tissue Engineering

Ge Tao[a] · James F. Martin[a, b]

[a]Department of Molecular Physiology and Biophysics, Baylor College of Medicine, and [b]Cardiomyocyte Renewal Laboratory, Texas Heart Institute, Houston, Tex., USA

Abstract

Effective therapies for congenital heart disease (CHD) are an urgent clinical need. Insights gained from fundamental scientific research, together with the results of clinical trials, are beginning to yield potential new strategies for treating CHD. Novel discoveries in tissue engineering, intrinsic cardiac stem cells, regeneration-triggering factors, and gene-editing technologies are beginning to change the appearance of cardiovascular therapies. Investigators worldwide are intensively studying ways to harness, modify, and combine these interdisciplinary techniques in order to develop the most effective therapeutic strategies.

Congenital heart disease (CHD) is characterized by a combination of structural and functional defects arising from abnormal development of the heart or major blood vessels [1, 2]. Most CHD have specific anatomic or hemodynamic lesions; the severity of lesions ranges from small pinholes in the chamber septum that may spontaneously resolve to major life-threatening malformations that require serial surgeries during early life. Current surgical and pharmacological-based therapies for CHD may improve, but often cannot eliminate clinical symptoms, which may lead to severe sequelae later in life [3]. Presently, the only available cure for CHD is heart transplantation, which is hampered by the limited number of donor hearts. This lack of a cure has made CHD a global medical problem. Thus, reconstitution of a healthy heart in vivo, or even de novo, has become a major goal of modern bioengineering and cardiovascular science. Here, we will discuss recent advances in stem cell biology, bioengineering, and prototypical gene therapies that have provided important strides toward achieving this goal.

Cardiac Tissue Engineering

Early intervention of CHD usually involves a surgical procedure for reconstructing the gross structure of the heart, such as filling defective or missing tissue with artificial patches [4]. Ideally, bioengineered patches should mimic and be biocompatible with human tissue, and have the ability to grow with surrounding tissue. However, commonly used materials lack dynamic growth potential, and their use may result in stenosis, thromboembolization, calcium deposition, and infection in the long term [5].

The challenges in this field are substantial because of the highly intricate and exquisitely organized cardiac anatomy. Mature cardiomyocytes are coupled end to end in myofibers that are further integrated into diversely oriented sheets [6]. These highly energetic sheets are stacked and bound by extracellular matrix (ECM) and synchronized by highly specialized myocardial conduction cells, which initiate and coordinate cardiac contraction [3]. To maintain cardiac structure, meshworks of supportive cardiac ECM intertwine within the cardiac myofibers, along with essential blood vessels, fibroblasts, and conduction system cells [3]. Modern biological tissue engineering includes not only the manipulation of live cells, but also the development of favorable microenvironments, for the cells to thrive and function [5].

Several critical factors are required for in vitro development of cardiac tissue. First, a suitable biological matrix that contains one or several different substances is necessary. Second, a mix of healthy cardiomyocytes and supporting cells must be seeded into a preformed matrix, and, lastly, application of a proper mechanical load with electrical stimulation is necessary during the construction of the tissue (fig. 1) [5].

Supportive Matrix in Favor of Tissue Formation

The concept of engineered heart tissue (EHT) started from a simple culture of suspended chicken heart cells that aggregate into 'cardiac spheres' under frequent disturbance [7]. It was soon discovered that gels made of collagen provided a favorable three-dimensional (3D) environment that promoted cell aggregation and differentiation [8, 9]. Interestingly, supplementing the collagen with Engelbreth-Swarm tumors (Matrigel) promotes EHT maturation [10], indicating that extra ECM components or growth factors may facilitate tissue formation. Artificial ECM composed primarily of collagen and laminin (present in high concentration in Matrigel) is presently believed to be the optimal scaffold material in cardiac tissue engineering because collagen I, collagen III, and laminin are the most abundant ECM components in endogenous myocardium [3]. Addition of growth factors to biopolymer patches has stimulated vascularization and angiogenesis, and reduced scar size when patches were implanted on the epicardial surface of an infarcted myocardium [11, 12].

Tissue-Forming Cell Population

Spatial organization of myocardium during embryogenesis requires signaling interactions between cardiomyocytes and the ECM [13]. The local microenvironment appears to be crucial for the function of mature cardiomyocytes. Embryonic stem (ES) cell-derived cardiomyocytes engraft more efficiently into intact myocardium than into infarcted zone, in which the balance among ECM components has been disturbed [14]. Although an artificial gel structure could potentially involve all essential components, current gaps in our knowledge about ECM prevent the assembly of all potentially crucial factors. To address this shortcoming, a mixture of cardiomyocytes and supporting cells, including cardiac fibroblasts, endothelial cells, and smooth muscle cells, are seeded into the in vitro matrix scaffold [15]. This complex mixture prepared from whole-heart tissue enhanced the cellularization of scaffolds [15]. Because these supporting cells are involved in myocardial development, it is reasonable to anticipate that they will also be required during the construction of an artificial ECM.

Pioneer EHT studies showed that immature cardiomyocytes had greater potential to form tissue-like structures than did mature cardiomyocytes [5]. Thus, researchers assumed that cardiac progenitors were a better cell source for EHT. Hypothetically, when placed in an environment with essential sig-

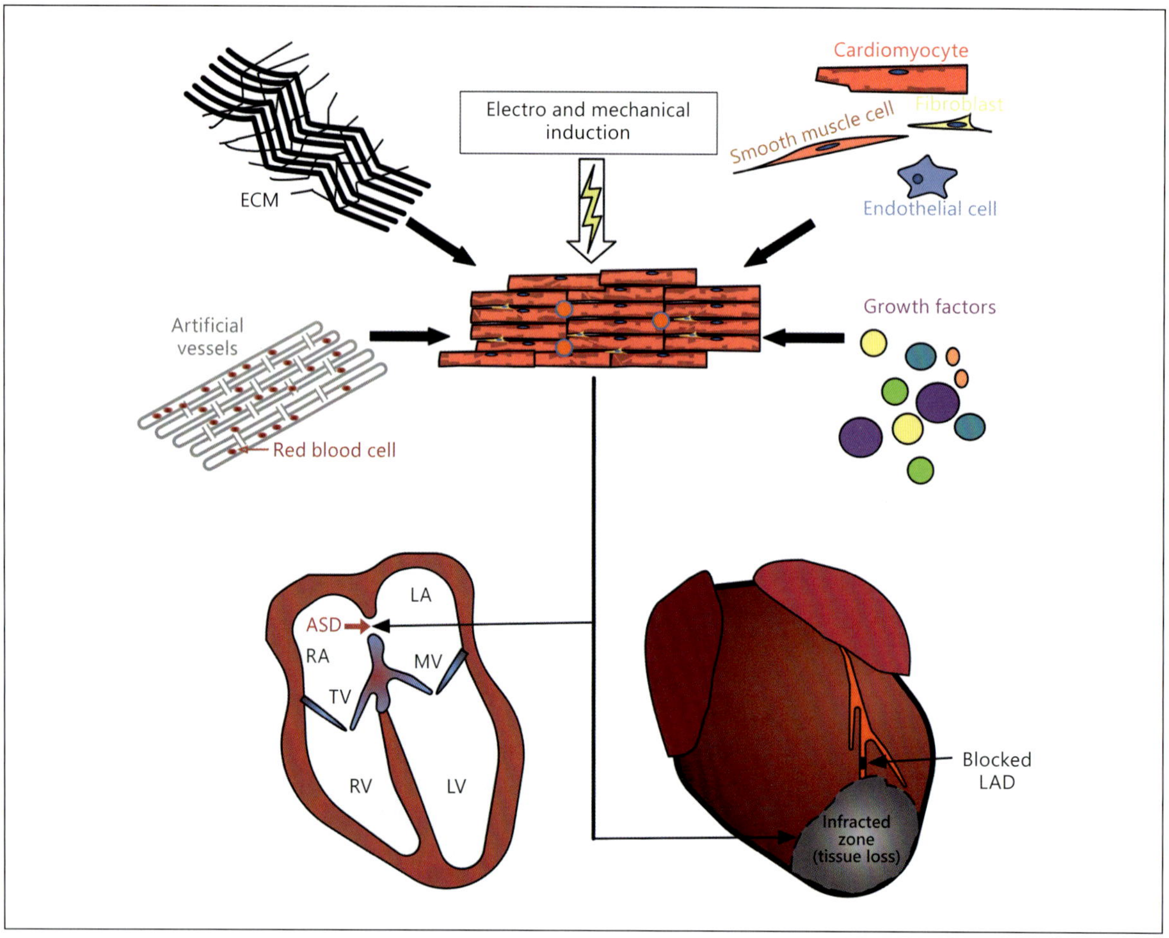

Fig. 1. The construction and application of EHT. Effective EHT includes structurally and physiologically coupled cardiomyocytes, supported by vessels, fibroblasts and proper ECM. After mechanical force and electronic stimulation, the matured EHT can be transplanted into a patient's heart for repairing defects and damage, including atrial septal defect (ASD) and infracted zone. LA = Left atrium; RA = right atrium; LV = left ventricle; RV = right ventricle; MV = mitral valve; TV = tricuspid valve; LAD = left anterior descending artery.

naling factors, cardiac progenitors should be able to differentiate into a population of multiple cell types that mimic the in vivo myocardial composition. Many studies were dedicated to the identification of cardiac progenitors, and the progress made so far is discussed below.

Mechanical Load and Electrical Stimulation

The embryonic mouse heart starts to beat on embryonic day 8; thus, the native myocardium is electronically synchronized and eventually matured during repetitive cycles of contraction and relaxation [13]. To imitate this activity in vitro, mechanical strain or electrical stimulation must be applied to the EHT. Vandenburgh et al. [16] and Terracio et al. [17] employed cybernated devices to stretch cultured skeletal myocytes and cardiomyocytes. Other investigators electrically stimulated collagen sponges seeded with neonatal rat heart cells and improved EHT morphology, contractility, and molecular marker profiles [18]. Together, these reports unveiled the favorable roles of mechanical and electrical stimulation during the maturation of cardiomyocytes in vitro.

Bioreactors – A Breeding Ground for Engineered Heart Tissue

The proper bioreactor combines all features required for the construction of EHT. After the discovery that cell growth was affected by the underlying matrix, various approaches for generating the optimal EHT have been studied, with the use of modern technologies of material and computer science, tissue engineering, and matrix biology [5].

The earliest bioreactor, comprising a culture medium-containing receptacle under constant gyration [7], has evolved over the decades into a more sophisticated modern bioreactor [19, 20]. Most bioreactors now include supplemented collagen matrix, cardiomyocytes, supporting cells, and mechanical-electric stimulation-generating systems [15]. There are also distinctive systems such as the matrix-free bioreactor, in which the EHT comprises multiple cultured cardiomyocyte monolayers [21]. The beating monolayers can be stacked and grown together to form integrated 3D tissue sheets up to 50–75 μm thick [21]. Beating aggregates of neonatal rat heart cells have also been generated in bioreactors by exposing cell-matrix mixture to microgravity [22]. Further improvement in the standard system includes the invention of molds [11], reusable devices that allow large-scale production of high-quality EHT with minimal handling [11].

In 2007, the generation of human induced pluripotent stem cells (hiPSCs) provided an exceptional opportunity to create patient-specific cardiac tissue in vitro [23, 24]. In addition, early findings showed that the cardiomyocytes need to be oriented by underlying substrates or an auxiliary device in order to couple better with adjacent cardiomyocytes [25]. Recently, Nunes et al. [19] described a novel system designated 'biowire', which better incorporates cardiomyocytes prepared from hiPSCs and human ES cells (hESCs) into an EHT bioreactor. Usually, hiPSC-derived cardiomyocytes are proliferative and less differentiated [26, 27]; besides, they show immature action potentials and Ca^{2+} profiles [28, 29]. hESC-based EHT share the same immature characteristics [30]. The biowire is a micro-environmental platform that combines architectural and functional cues favorable to maturation of hESC- and hiPSC-derived 3D EHTs [19]. The investigators seeded cells in collagen gel around a template suture (the 'wire') in a microfabricated well and subjected them to electrical stimulation with a progressive increase in frequency [19]. The cardiomyocytes in the matured biowires showed improved ultrastructures and conduction velocity, better-defined sarcomere and desmosome structures, and enhanced Ca^{2+} handling [19]. These findings suggest that a simple template can significantly enhance EHT quality. Although effective, the biowire is a microtemplate that will need to be streamlined before large-scale clinical application is practical.

Current Challenges for Engineered Heart Tissue Production

Cardiomyocyte Maturation

Engineered tissues with sufficient quality have been tested in clinical trials such as the 'chain mail' device (ACORN; CorCap Cardiac Support Device), a therapeutic device expected to support both diastolic and systolic functions of a failing heart (NCT00630266) [31]. The physiological traits of the myocardium include high mechanical stability, pliability, and resilience. Moreover, muscle fibers and bundles within the heart form layers with different orientations to provide optimal pump function [32]. Despite the advances of current technologies, there are no fabricated materials that mimic such a sophisticated structure. Furthermore, the purified or stem cell-derived cardiac cells have to survive and physiologically integrate into a cell-free space. There are still differences in the quantity and quality of contractility between EHT and native myocardium due to a lower cellular occupancy of the EHT by cardiomyocytes and less well-developed sarcomeres [33]. Future studies should include characterizing the native cardiomyocyte microenvironment, filling the gaps of our knowledge about ECM, thus informing the future EHT technology.

Host Immune Response

An important drawback of biopolymer-based technology is the potential for adverse host reactions to biomaterials. This issue led to the development of scaffold-free cardiac tissue grafts [34]. These second-generation patches comprise only cells and the ECM that these cells produce [34]. In a rat model of this type of patch graft, vessels from patches integrated into the native circulation, and cardiomyocytes from the patches were electromechanically coupled into host myocardium [34]. However, the native cardiac ECM established during development requires signaling far more sophisticated than the artificial environment can provide, making it difficult for cells in EHT to excrete the correct quantity and quality of ECM components.

Ischemia within Engineered Heart Tissue

Tissue constructs harboring physiologic cell densities have been generated; however, optimal methods for sustaining the construct with a functional vascular system have not been identified. Without vascular networks, 3D engineered tissues quickly develop a necrotic core [35]. To create perfusable channels in engineered tissues, investigators have studied the use of layer-by-layer assembly [5, 36]. In this approach, a trench is molded into a basal layer of EHT, so a second layer can be aligned on top, to form channels. However, this method is time consuming and limited by the availability of bio-materials. A potential way to overcome this problem is bioprinting, in which the cells and matrix are deposited drop-wise [37]. This 3D printing approach is a cutting-edge technology for artificial human tissue manufacture and provides a broad stage for testing ideas. The value of 3D printing is tremendous, particularly in cardiology, and could have a significant impact on future patient therapies [38]. Currently, 3D printing is being developed as a potential approach to repair or replace defective organs, including the heart. Theoretically, the computer-controlled printing process could incorporate a vascular system into the EHT, using endothelial and smooth muscle cells, to achieve artificial angiogenesis. However, the inability to rapidly construct such networks is still a major challenge for 3D printing and culture [39]. The extremely long printing process results in the loss of living cells, and the lack of oxygen and nutrients limits tissue thickness to microns. Current research to solve this issue includes optimizing the microenvironment in which the tissue is printed and identifying more perfusable artificial materials that can substitute for living cells [40]. Such strategies include the application of printed rigid filament networks of carbohydrate glass that function as a cell-compatible sacrificial template in engineered tissues [41]. This system is able to generate conduit networks that could be lined with endothelial cells and perfused with blood [41]. These vascular channels are compatible with a wide variety of cell types [41]. This modified 3D sacrificial molding is a promising alternative for native vasculature.

Decellularized Heart as an Artificial Scaffold for Engineered Heart Tissue

In the challenge to generate a scaffold that mimics the endogenous cardiac ECM, Taylor and colleagues took direct advantage of in vivo cardiac matrices by decellularizing a whole rat heart and repopulating it with neonatal cardiomyocytes [42]. This innovative study addressed several critical issues involved in all tissue engineering approaches [5]. Existing scaffold technologies are limited by unfavorable matrix properties including low mechanical compliance, material toxicity, cellular incompatibility, and limited size caused by low diffusion capacity [43]. Contracting cardiomyocytes have a very high metabolic activity that requires an extensive capillary density, making the development of a thick tissue patch difficult [21]. These issues could be solved by the presence of a preexisting blood vessel mold that preserves the complex coronary vascular system. Using perfusion-based decellularization methods, Taylor's group produced a mostly intact, biocompatible cardiac matrix template with a perfusable vascular system, which could be reseeded either by intramural injection of cardiac-derived cells or by perfusion of endothelial cells through the remaining outflow tract [42]. The recellularized construct was able to contract and was drug responsive after 8 days of culture in a bioreactor [42]. Further effort is required to improve the maturation and integrity of the reconstructed heart and to develop an optimized cell perfusion protocol for better dispersion of cells throughout the construct. This promising strategy could eventually provide transplantable heart tissue or an entire heart for treating heart disease.

Stem Cells in Engineered Heart Tissue

A bioartificial heart requires an architectural construct and an appropriate cell composition and maturation environment (fig. 1). Successful reconstitution of defective cardiac tissue cannot rely solely on recreation of the natural geometry, and the greatest challenge of EHT relates to a suitable cell source. An unpurified heart cell preparation generates EHT with better function than does a pure cardiomyocyte fraction [15]. Moreover, to avoid lifelong immunosuppression regimens, the use of patient-derived cells is desirable. There are about 40 million cardiomyocytes per gram of tissue in the native myocardium [44]. Thus, creating even a small tissue patch would require significantly more cells than that could be currently obtained from a patient heart biopsy. Therefore, the primary EHT cell source used at present serves only as a proof of principle.

Early in mouse embryogenesis, mesodermal cells that are destined to form the heart gather into two anatomically distinct groups: the primary and secondary heart fields [13]. The identification of the homeobox gene *NKX2.5* and the LIM domain transcription factor *Isl-1* led to the identification of two cardiac progenitor populations that reside in the primary and secondary heart fields, which form the primary heart tube early in embryogenesis [45, 46]. Knowledge of these cell populations helps identifying molecular cues that establish cell fate of early progenitors. After reaching adulthood, a small group of cells marked by Wt1 and Tbx18 persist within the epicardium, a source of progenitors during embryogenesis that give rise to fibroblasts, smooth muscle cells, and perhaps cardiomyocytes [47]. Although largely quiescent, adult epicardial cells respond to myocardial injury by secreting a mixture of growth factors into the underlying myocardium [32, 48]. This cell population can also be activated by paracrine factors such as thymosin β_4 [49]. In addition, there is evidence that cardiac progenitors found in the mature human heart retain pluripotency and are able to differentiate into cardiomyocytes, smooth muscle cells, and endothelial cells after being sorted and cultured [50].

Adult stem cells have been found in bone marrow [51], peripheral blood [52], and adipose tissue [53]. Some of them have also been identified as cardiac progenitors [51]. Beltrami et al. [54] described small, round c-Kit+ cells in the adult rat heart that could be clonally expanded and that generated new viable myocardium when injected into infarcted hearts. Since then, several groups confirmed that c-Kit+CD45–tryptase– cardiac progenitors participate in the adaptation to myocardial stress [55, 56]. In another study, Sca-1+ cells isolated from an adult mouse heart were able to acquire a cardiac phenotype when induced [57]. Genetic labeling studies show that Sca-1+CD31–Isl1– cells home to the injured myocardium when injected intravenously and have the capacity to differentiate into cardiomyocytes and fuse with host cells in the presence of fibroblast growth factor-2 [57–59]. Although the role of c-Kit+ cardiac cells in response to injury was questioned and will require more precise phenotype definition [32, 60], these findings suggest the possibility of using EHT derived from autologous cells, which would avoid immune rejection concerns. However, the rarity of these cell populations would make it difficult to generate enough cells for clinical application [5]. An alternative to adult cardiac progenitors is ES cells, which are self-renewing pluripotent cells capable of forming any cell type under appropriate in vitro conditions [61]. The potential of a cardiac fate varies significantly between ES cell lines, and pharmacological strategies could be employed to promote a heart lineage from certain ES cell lines [62]. However, therapeutic injection of ES-cell-derived cardiomyocytes is unlikely to be used clinically because of ethical issues and requirement of immunosuppression therapy.

New tactics have been inspired by the findings of Takahashi and Yamanaka who designed an in vitro reprogramming protocol to transform terminally differentiated skin fibroblasts into pluripotent cells

7

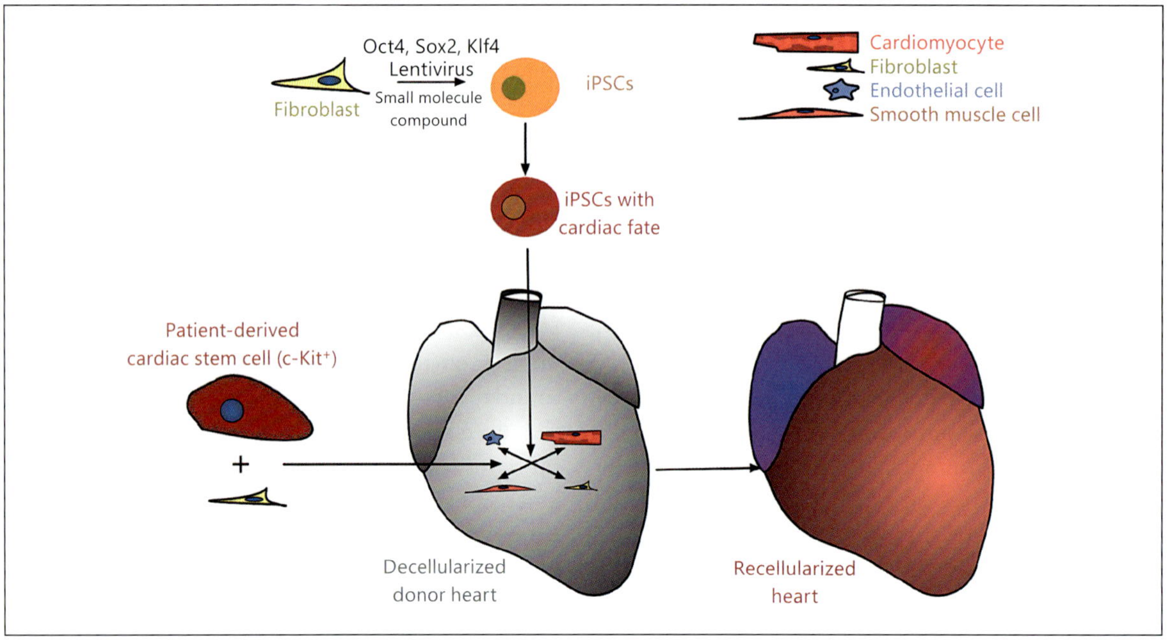

Fig. 2. Repopulation of a decellularized donor heart with patient-derived cardiac stem cells. A donor cadaveric heart wil be decellularized by antegrade coronary perfusion and then seeded with live cells by intramural injection or coronary perfusion. The cell source for recellularization could be either in vitro expanded cardiac stem cells, such as c-Kit$^+$ cells, obtained from patient biopsy, or cardiac progenitors derived from iPSCs, generated with patient-specific fibroblasts.

that closely resemble ES cells [23]. These reprogrammed cells (iPSCs) can be derived from an individual patient without the need for ES cells and can be used to generate cardiac cells in vitro [23, 63]. Autologous cell transplantation may be possible using this technique, with a theoretical reduction in the risk of immune rejection. The virus-based 4-factor-combination method used in the original study has been associated with an increased risk of malignant carcinogenesis [23], but has been optimized by leaving out unnecessary tumorigenic factors, which have been substituted with safer factors [24, 64], or even using chemical compounds only [65]. Moreover, iPSCs retain the epigenetic pattern of the cell type from which they were derived, therefore making left-ventricular cells a better cell source than skin fibroblasts when considering treating heart disease with iPSC-derived tissue [66]. Taken together, it is reasonable to believe that iPSC-derived cardiac cells are suitable to be incorporated into EHT or serve as a reliable cell source to repopulate a decellularized donor heart (fig. 2).

A majority of stem cell studies are still focusing on developing therapies for treating heart failure caused by myocardial infarction [4, 32]. A key question is whether engrafted cells survive, differentiate, and integrate after being injected into the infarcted myocardium. Importantly, the insight gained from these studies could guide us in the treatment of other heart diseases, including CHD. The major barrier scientists encountered during many clinical trials is the low efficiency of cell delivery by intramural or intracoronary injection [67–69]. Improper delivery methods could stress the introduced cells, preventing them from differentiating and integrating. Thus, the development of a minimally invasive, highly efficient cell delivery procedure is required.

Reentry of Mature Cardiomyocytes into the Cell Cycle

Besides introducing extraneous cells, novel methods of cardiac repair include augmenting endogenous regenerative activity. It is believed that adult mammalian myocardium cannot regenerate as observed in lower vertebrates [70, 71]. In a mature heart, the progressive scarring and dilation of left ventricles after myocardial infarction led to the belief that mature cardiomyocytes are not responsive to injury; however, high-definition labeling and imaging techniques have recently shown a notable population of proliferative cardiomyocytes in the area adjacent to the infarct (up to 3.2%) [72], which suggests that mature cardiomyocytes possess regenerative potential. Moreover, neonatal mouse myocardium has shown robust regeneration after trauma but only during a limited time window (before postnatal day 7) [73]. In two recent studies, postmitotic cardiomyocytes were reintroduced into the cell cycle, forcing the elongation of the regenerative window, by genetically inactivating Hippo signaling [74, 75]. By regulating Yes-associated protein (Yap) and PDZ-binding motif (TAZ), the Hippo kinase cascade serves as a mechanical sensor that relays signals from the cell membrane into the nucleus where it controls the expression of a series of target genes that control cell proliferation, survival, and differentiation [76]. Our group showed that Hippo signaling restricts heart size and cardiomyocyte hyperplasia during mouse embryonic development, and genetic disruption of Hippo signaling reintroduces cardiomyocytes into the cell cycle, thus promoting myocardial regeneration after apex resection and myocardial infarction [74, 77]. These findings suggest a novel way for potentially expanding mature cardiomyocytes both in vitro and in vivo and for producing a large cell population sufficient for EHT preparation. Also, the effect of Yap on survival signaling may promote the survivability of cardiomyocytes during construction for artificial tissue.

Novel Possibilities for Treating Hypertrophic Cardiomyopathy

Hypertrophic cardiomyopathy can result in arrhythmias, sudden collapse, and possible death [78]. Although some symptoms are treatable, the heart enlargement associated with cardiomyopathies is not reversible [78]. In a recent report, Lee and Wager's groups surgically connected two mice to create a shared blood circulation [79]. This so-called parabiosis technique is a powerful model for determining whether circulating factors can alter tissue function. By coupling aged and young mice, Lee and Wager's groups were able to reverse hypertrophy in the aged heart by exposing it to a young circulatory environment [79]. Furthermore, they identified a growth differentiation factor (GDF 11) as the responsible factor for reversing age-related cardiac hypertrophy [79, 80]. This finding emphasized the effect of a single factor in reversing hypertrophy, especially considering that these factors can be easily manipulated and administered [80]. Although the mechanisms that cause age-related hypertrophy may not be identical to those that cause hypertrophic cardiomyopathy [81], it is worthwhile to examine if GDF 11 can reverse hypertrophy caused by genetic mutation and to identify novel factors that may reverse the hypertrophic cardiomyopathy phenotype.

Gene Therapy as Early Intervening Strategies

Although the top priority is to eliminate the symptoms and phenotypes of CHD, editing the genome to repair the disease-causing mutations may have long-term benefits. In genetic diseases, genes that play critical roles during development are often mutated, such as *TBX5* in the Holt-Oram syndrome or *FBN1* in the Marfan syndrome [82]. Scientists have been manipulating the genome for decades, and modern advances in gene-editing techniques have evolved from a random to a more targeted application that can break DNA at specific spots by using synthetic zinc finger nucleases or transcription activator-like effectors nucleases [83, 84]. Recently, the development of a more efficient strategy, named CRISPR (clustered regularly interspaced short palindromic repeats), further simplified the gene manipulation [85].

CRISPR, a faster and more versatile technique, was developed from the immune system of bacteria [85]. Using a guide RNA to locate the target gene and Cas9 nuclease, researchers showed that the CRISPR system could target and cut specific DNA, knocking out a gene or enabling a partial replacement by substitute DNA [85]. Further modification of Cas9 allows delivery of a repressor or activator to the adjacent region of a target gene, thus regulating its expression [86, 87]. CRISPR has been shown to be more efficient than transcription activator-like effector nucleases [88], and convenient guide RNA libraries are being completed to target every affected gene in human CHD. Although off-targeting is still a concern, with better understanding of the functional mechanisms and proper modifications, CRISPR technology may eventually be useful for gene therapies targeting human disease.

Perspectives

The heart is a complex organ that possesses distinct anatomical elements, which may be disrupted in CHD. This complexity makes restoration of the cardiac function extremely challenging. Ideally, the native architecture of a defective heart should be rebuilt with proper EHTs, comprised of sustainable, cell-friendly matrices and a mixture of healthy, functional donor cells that will cause minimal immune activity. Ideally, this type of EHT will mature and become viable cardiac tissue with all functional features. The in vitro development of a contracting tissue patch that can correct heart defects requires a profound knowledge of both tissue engineering and stem cells. Therefore, to achieve a clinically meaningful therapy, combined efforts from the areas of stem cell biology, tissue engineering, transplantation biology, cardiovascular medicine, and material science will be required.

References

1 Yuan S, Zaidi S, Brueckner M: Congenital heart disease: emerging themes linking genetics and development. Curr Opin Genet Dev 2013;23:352–359.
2 Preuss C, Andelfinger G: Genetics of heart failure in congenital heart disease. Can J Cardiol 2013;29:803–810.
3 Mishra PK, Givvimani S, Chavali V, et al: Cardiac matrix: a clue for future therapy. Biochim Biophys Acta 2013;1832:2271–2276.
4 Roger VL, Go AS, Lloyd-Jones DM, et al: Heart disease and stroke statistics – 2012 update: a report from the American Heart Association. Circulation 2012;125:e2–e220.
5 Eschenhagen T, Zimmermann WH: Engineering myocardial tissue. Circ Res 2005; 97:1220–1231.
6 Bers DM: Cardiac excitation-contraction coupling. Nature 2002;415:198–205.
7 Moscona AA: Tissues from dissociated cells. Sci Am 1959;200:132–134 passim.
8 Chambard M, Gabrion J, Mauchamp J: Influence of collagen gel on the orientation of epithelial cell polarity: follicle formation from isolated thyroid cells and from preformed monolayers. J Cell Biol 1981;91:157–166.
9 Hall HG, Farson DA, Bissell MJ: Lumen formation by epithelial cell lines in response to collagen overlay: a morphogenetic model in culture. Proc Natl Acad Sci USA 1982;79: 4672–4676.
10 Zimmermann WH, Fink C, Kralisch D, et al: Three-dimensional engineered heart tissue from neonatal rat cardiac myocytes. Biotechnol Bioeng 2000;68:106–114.
11 Zimmermann WH, Schneiderbanger K, Schubert P, et al: Tissue engineering of a differentiated cardiac muscle construct. Circ Res 2002;90:223–230.
12 Ahmed TA, Dare EV, Hincke M: Fibrin: a versatile scaffold for tissue engineering applications. Tissue Eng Part B Rev 2008;14: 199–215.
13 Srivastava D, Olson EN: A genetic blueprint for cardiac development. Nature 2000;407: 221–226.
14 Laflamme MA, Chen KY, Naumova AV, et al: Cardiomyocytes derived from human embryonic stem cells in pro-survival factors enhance function of infarcted rat hearts. Nat Biotechnol 2007;25:1015–1024.
15 Zimmermann WH, Eschenhagen T: Cardiac tissue engineering for replacement therapy. Heart Fail Rev 2003;8:259–269.
16 Vandenburgh H, Karlisch H, Farr L: Maintenance of highly contractile tissue-cultured avian skeletal myotubes in collagen gel. In Vitro Cell Dev Biol 1988;24:166–174.
17 Terracio L, Miller B, Borg TK: Effects of cyclic mechanical stimulation of the cellular components of the heart: in vitro. In Vitro Cell Dev Biol 1988;24:53–58.
18 Radisic M, Park H, Shing H, et al: Functional assembly of engineered myocardium by electrical stimulation of cardiac myocytes cultured on scaffolds. Proc Natl Acad Sci USA 2004;101:18129–18134.
19 Nunes SS, Miklas JW, Liu J, et al: Biowire: a platform for maturation of human pluripotent stem cell-derived cardiomyocytes. Nat Methods 2013;10:781–187.
20 Thavandiran N, Dubois N, Mikryukov A, et al: Design and formulation of functional pluripotent stem cell-derived cardiac microtissues. Proc Natl Acad Sci USA 2013; 110:E4698–E4707.
21 Shimizu T, Yamato M, Isoi Y, et al: Fabrication of pulsatile cardiac tissue grafts using a novel 3-dimensional cell sheet manipulation technique and temperature-responsive cell culture surfaces. Circ Res 2002;90:e40.
22 Akins RE, Boyce RA, Madonna ML, et al: Cardiac organogenesis in vitro: reestablishment of three-dimensional tissue architecture by dissociated neonatal rat ventricular cells. Tissue Eng 1999;5:103–118.
23 Takahashi K, Tanabe K, Ohnuki M, et al: Induction of pluripotent stem cells from adult human fibroblasts by defined factors. Cell 2007;131:861–872.
24 Nakagawa M, Koyanagi M, Tanabe K, et al: Generation of induced pluripotent stem cells without Myc from mouse and human fibroblasts. Nat Biotechnol 2008;26:101–106.
25 Simpson DG, Terracio L, Terracio M, et al: Modulation of cardiac myocyte phenotype in vitro by the composition and orientation of the extracellular matrix. J Cell Physiol 1994;161:89–105.
26 Snir M, Kehat I, Gepstein A, et al: Assessment of the ultrastructural and proliferative properties of human embryonic stem cell-derived cardiomyocytes. Am J Physiol Heart Circ Physiol 2003;285:H2355–H2363.
27 McDevitt TC, Laflamme MA, Murry CE: Proliferation of cardiomyocytes derived from human embryonic stem cells is mediated via the IGF/PI 3-kinase/Akt signaling pathway. J Mol Cell Cardiol 2005;39:865–873.

28 Mummery C, Ward-van Oostwaard D, Doevendans P, et al: Differentiation of human embryonic stem cells to cardiomyocytes: role of coculture with visceral endoderm-like cells. Circulation 2003;107:2733–2740.
29 Dolnikov K, Shilkrut M, Zeevi-Levin N, et al: Functional properties of human embryonic stem cell-derived cardiomyocytes: intracellular Ca2+ handling and the role of sarcoplasmic reticulum in the contraction. Stem Cells 2006;24:236–245.
30 Frank D, Kuhn C, Brors B, et al: Gene expression pattern in biomechanically stretched cardiomyocytes: evidence for a stretch-specific gene program. Hypertension 2008;51:309–318.
31 Starling RC, Jessup M: Worldwide clinical experience with the CorCap Cardiac Support Device. J Card Fail 2004;10(6 suppl):S225–S233.
32 Ptaszek LM, Mansour M, Ruskin JN, Chien KR: Towards regenerative therapy for cardiac disease. Lancet 2012;379:933–942.
33 Zimmermann WH, Didié M, Wasmeier GH, et al: Cardiac grafting of engineered heart tissue in syngenic rats. Circulation 2002;106(12 suppl 1):I151–I157.
34 Stevens KR, Kreutziger KL, Dupras SK , et al: Physiological function and transplantation of scaffold-free and vascularized human cardiac muscle tissue. Proc Natl Acad Sci U S A 2009;106:16568–16573.
35 Radisic M, Yang L, Boublik J, et al: Medium perfusion enables engineering of compact and contractile cardiac tissue. Am J Physiol Heart Circ Physiol 2004;286:H507–H516.
36 Cuchiara MP, Allen AC, Chen TM, et al: Multilayer microfluidic PEGDA hydrogels. Biomaterials 2010;31:5491–5497.
37 Visconti RP, Kasyanov V, Gentile C, et al: Towards organ printing: engineering an intra-organ branched vascular tree. Expert Opin Biol Ther 2010;10.409–420.
38 Schubert C, van Langeveld MC, Donoso LA: Innovations in 3D printing: a 3D overview from optics to organs. Br J Ophthalmol 2014;98:159–161.
39 Vunjak-Novakovic G, Scadden DT: Biomimetic platforms for human stem cell research. Cell Stem Cell 2011;8:252–261.
40 Villar G, Graham AD, Bayley H: A tissue-like printed material. Science 2013;340:48–52.
41 Miller JS, Stevens KR, Yang MT, et al: Rapid casting of patterned vascular networks for perfusable engineered three-dimensional tissues. Nat Mater 2012;11:768–774.
42 Ott HC, Matthiesen TS, Goh SK, et al: Perfusion-decellularized matrix: using nature's platform to engineer a bioartificial heart. Nat Med 2008;14:213–221.
43 Badylak SF, Taylor D, Uygun K: Whole-organ tissue engineering: decellularization and recellularization of three-dimensional matrix scaffolds. Annu Rev Biomed Eng 2011;13:27–53.
44 Beltrami CA, Finato N, Rocco M, et al: Structural basis of end-stage failure in ischemic cardiomyopathy in humans. Circulation 1994;89:151–163.
45 Harvey RP: NK-2 homeobox genes and heart development. Dev Biol 1996;178:203–216.
46 Cai CL, Liang X, Shi Y, et al: Isl1 identifies a cardiac progenitor population that proliferates prior to differentiation and contributes a majority of cells to the heart. Dev Cell 2003;5:877–889.
47 Zhou B, Ma Q, Rajagopal S, et al: Epicardial progenitors contribute to the cardiomyocyte lineage in the developing heart. Nature 2008;454:109–113.
48 Zhou B, Honor LB, He H, et al: Adult mouse epicardium modulates myocardial injury by secreting paracrine factors. J Clin Invest 2011;121:1894–1904.
49 Smart N, Bollini S, Dubé KN, et al: De novo cardiomyocytes from within the activated adult heart after injury. Nature 2011;474:640–644.
50 Bu L, Jiang X, Martin-Puig S, et al: Human ISL1 heart progenitors generate diverse multipotent cardiovascular cell lineages. Nature 2009;460:113–117.
51 Orlic D, Kajstura J, Chimenti S, et al: Bone marrow cells regenerate infarcted myocardium. Nature 2001;410:701–705.
52 Asahara T, Murohara T, Sullivan A, et al: Isolation of putative progenitor endothelial cells for angiogenesis. Science 1997;275:964–796.
53 Zuk PA, Zhu M, Mizuno H, et al: Multilineage cells from human adipose tissue: implications for cell-based therapies. Tissue Eng 2001;7:211–228.
54 Beltrami AP, Barlucchi L, Torella D, et al: Adult cardiac stem cells are multipotent and support myocardial regeneration. Cell 2003;114:763–776.
55 Ellison GM, Torella D, Karakikes I, et al: Myocyte death and renewal: modern concepts of cardiac cellular homeostasis. Nat Clin Pract Cardiovasc Med 2007;4(suppl 1):S52–S59.
56 Waring CD, Vicinanza C, Papalamprou A, et al: The adult heart responds to increased workload with physiologic hypertrophy, cardiac stem cell activation, and new myocyte formation. Eur Heart J 2014;35:2722–2731.
57 Rosenblatt-Velin N, Lepore MG, Cartoni C, et al: FGF-2 controls the differentiation of resident cardiac precursors into functional cardiomyocytes. J Clin Invest 2005;115:1724–1733.
58 Matsuura K, Nagai T, Nishigaki N, et al: Adult cardiac Sca-1-positive cells differentiate into beating cardiomyocytes. J Biol Chem 2004;279:11384–11391.
59 Pfister O, Mouquet F, Jain M, et al: CD31- but not CD31+ cardiac side population cells exhibit functional cardiomyogenic differentiation. Circ Res 2005;97:52–61.
60 Andersen DC, Andersen P, Schneider M, et al: Murine 'cardiospheres' are not a source of stem cells with cardiomyogenic potential. Stem Cells 2009;27:1571–1581.
61 Wobus AM, Wallukat G, Hescheler J: Pluripotent mouse embryonic stem cells are able to differentiate into cardiomyocytes expressing chronotropic responses to adrenergic and cholinergic agents and Ca^{2+} channel blockers. Differentiation 1991;48:173–182.
62 Yang L, Soonpaa MH, Adler ED, et al: Human cardiovascular progenitor cells develop from a KDR+ embryonic-stem-cell-derived population. Nature 2008;453:524–528.
63 Zhang J, Wilson GF, Soerens AG, et al: Functional cardiomyocytes derived from human induced pluripotent stem cells. Circ Res 2009;104:e30–e41.
64 Maekawa M, Yamaguchi K, Nakamura T, et al: Direct reprogramming of somatic cells is promoted by maternal transcription factor Glis1. Nature 2011;474:225–229.
65 Hou P, Li Y, Zhang X, et al: Pluripotent stem cells induced from mouse somatic cells by small-molecule compounds. Science 2015;341:651–654.
66 Xu H, Yi BA, Wu H, et al: Highly efficient derivation of ventricular cardiomyocytes from induced pluripotent stem cells with a distinct epigenetic signature. Cell Res 2012;22:142–154.
67 Menasche P, Alfieri O, Janssens S, et al: The Myoblast Autologous Grafting in Ischemic Cardiomyopathy (MAGIC) trial: first randomized placebo-controlled study of myoblast transplantation. Circulation 2008;117:1189–1200.
68 Bolli R, Chugh AR, D'Amario D, et al: Cardiac stem cells in patients with ischaemic cardiomyopathy (SCIPIO): initial results of a randomised phase 1 trial. Lancet 2011;378:1847–1857.
69 Makkar RR, Smith RR, Cheng K, et al: Intracoronary cardiosphere-derived cells for heart regeneration after myocardial infarction (CADUCEUS): a prospective, randomised phase 1 trial. Lancet 2012;379:895–904.
70 Addis RC, Epstein JA: Induced regeneration – the progress and promise of direct reprogramming for heart repair. Nat Med 2013;19:829–836.
71 Poss KD, Wilson LG, Keating MT: Heart regeneration in zebrafish. Science 2002;298:2188–2190.
72 Senyo SE, Steinhauser ML, Pizzimenti CL, et al: Mammalian heart renewal by pre-existing cardiomyocytes. Nature 2013;493:433–436.

73 Porrello ER, Mahmoud AI, Simpson E, et al: Transient regenerative potential of the neonatal mouse heart. Science 2011;331:1078–1080.
74 Heallen T, Morikawa Y, Leach J, et al: Hippo signaling impedes adult heart regeneration. Development 2013;140:4683–4690.
75 Xin M, Kim Y, Sutherland LB, et al: Hippo pathway effector Yap promotes cardiac regeneration. Proc Natl Acad Sci USA 2013;110:13839–13844.
76 Johnson R, Halder G: The two faces of Hippo: targeting the Hippo pathway for regenerative medicine and cancer treatment. Nat Rev Drug Discov 2014;13:63–79.
77 Heallen T, Zhang M, Wang J, et al: Hippo pathway inhibits Wnt signaling to restrain cardiomyocyte proliferation and heart size. Science 2011;332:458–461.
78 Maron BJ, McKenna WJ, Danielson GK, et al: American College of Cardiology/European Society of Cardiology clinical expert consensus document on hypertrophic cardiomyopathy. A report of the American College of Cardiology Foundation Task Force on Clinical Expert Consensus Documents and the European Society of Cardiology Committee for Practice Guidelines. J Am Coll Cardiol 2003;42:1687–1713.
79 Loffredo FS, Steinhauser ML, Jay SM, et al: Growth differentiation factor 11 is a circulating factor that reverses age-related cardiac hypertrophy. Cell 2013;153:828–839.
80 McPherron AC, Lawler AM, Lee SJ: Regulation of anterior/posterior patterning of the axial skeleton by growth/differentiation factor 11. Nat Genet 1999;22:260–264.
81 Cirino AL, Ho C: Hypertrophic cardiomyopathy overview (2008, updated 2014); in Pagon RA, Adam MP, Ardinger HH, et al (eds): GeneReviews [Internet]. Seattle, University of Washington, 1993–2015.
82 Dietz HC: New therapeutic approaches to mendelian disorders. N Engl J Med 2010;363:852–863.
83 Handel EM, Cathomen T: Zinc-finger nuclease based genome surgery: it's all about specificity. Curr Gene Ther 2011;11:28–37.
84 Mussolino C, Cathomen T: TALE nucleases: tailored genome engineering made easy. Curr Opin Biotechnol 2012;23:644–650.
85 Mali P, Esvelt KM, Church GM: Cas9 as a versatile tool for engineering biology. Nat Methods 2013;10:957–963.
86 Qi LS, Larson MH, Gilbert LA, et al: Repurposing CRISPR as an RNA-guided platform for sequence-specific control of gene expression. Cell 2013;152:1173–1183.
87 Larson MH, Gilbert LA, Wang X, et al: CRISPR interference (CRISPRi) for sequence-specific control of gene expression. Nat Protoc 2013;8:2180–2196.
88 Mali P, Yang L, Esvelt KM, et al: RNA-guided human genome engineering via Cas9. Science 2013;339:823–826.

Prof. James F. Martin
Department of Molecular Physiology and Biophysics
Baylor College of Medicine
One Baylor Plaza 512E, Houston, TX 77030 (USA)
E-Mail jfmartin@bcm.edu

Author Index

Subject Index